Workbook and Competency Evaluation Review

MOSBY'S® TEXTBOOK FOR NURSING ASSISTANTS

T0294902

Eleventh Edition

Candice K. Kumagai, RN, MSN
Formerly, Instructor in Clinical Nursing
School of Nursing
University of Texas at Austin
Austin, Texas

ELSEVIER

Elsevier
3251 Riverport Lane
St. Louis, Missouri 63043

WORKBOOK AND COMPETENCY EVALUATION REVIEW
MOSBY'S® TEXTBOOK FOR NURSING ASSISTANTS, ELEVENTH EDITION ISBN: 978-0-443-12133-3

Previous editions copyrighted 2021, 2017, 2012, 2008 and 2004.

Content Strategist: Sonya Seigafuse
Content Development Specialist: Brooke R. Kannady
Publishing Services Manager: Deepthi Unni
Senior Project Manager: Beula Christopher

Printed in India

Last digit is the print number: 9 8 7 6 5 4 3 2 1

PREFACE

This workbook is written to be used with Remmert's *Mosby's Textbook for Nursing Assistants*, Eleventh Edition. You will not need other resources to complete the exercises in this workbook.

This workbook is designed to help you apply what you have learned in each chapter of this textbook. You are encouraged to use this book as a study guide. Each chapter is thoroughly covered in the multiple-choice questions, which will help prepare you to take the Nurse Aide Training and Competency Evaluation Program (NATCEP) test. In addition, other exercises such as fill in the blanks, matching, labeling, and crossword puzzles are used in many chapters. The section titled Optional Learning Activities may be used as an alternative exercise to give you more practice in studying the materials. The FOCUS ON PRIDE critical thinking and discussion questions offer opportunities to reflect on and improve clinical practice. The answer key for each chapter can be viewed on Evolve within TEACH. The Evolve Student Learning Resources also include Independent Learning Activities for each chapter that can be used to apply the information you will learn in a practical setting.

In addition, Procedure Checklists that correspond with the procedures in the textbook are provided. These checklists are designed to help you become skilled at performing procedures that affect quality of care. In addition to NATCEP skills being identified for you, icons indicate skills that are (1) in Mosby's Nursing Assistant Video Skills 4.0 and (2) on the Evolve Student Learning Resources website (video clips).

The Competency Evaluation Review includes a general review section and two practice exams with answers to help you prepare for the written certification exam. It also features a skills evaluation review to help you practice the procedures required for certification.

Assistive personnel are important members of the health team. Completing the exercises in this workbook will increase your knowledge and skills. The goal is to prepare you to provide the best possible care and to encourage pride in a job well done.

Candice K. Kumagai

CONTENTS

1 Health Care Agencies

Fill in the Blanks: Key Terms

Chain of command
Licensed practical nurse (LPN)
Licensed vocational nurse (LVN)
Health care system
Regulations
Registered nurse (RN)
Survey

1. A nurse who has completed a practical nursing program and has passed a licensing test is a ________________.
2. A ________________ has training and licensing that is similar to the LPN.
3. A ________________ is a nurse who has completed a 2-, 3-, or 4-year nursing program and has passed a licensing test.
4. ________________ is the order of authority in an agency.
5. A ________________ is a coordinated network of health care agencies and services.
6. It is important to know the ____________ or rules made by government agencies that affect nursing care.
7. A ________________ is the formal review of an agency through the collection of facts and observations.

Circle the Best Answer

8. Which team member is responsible for the person's total care when primary care nursing is the care pattern?
   A. Nursing assistant
   B. Physician
   C. Functional nurse
   D. Registered nurse
9. Which patient condition is an example where care could be coordinated using the case management nursing care pattern?
   A. Throat infection
   B. Influenza
   C. Diabetes
   D. Sprained ankle
10. Which person would be included in the nursing team?
    A. Nursing assistant
    B. Physician assistant
    C. Surveyor
    D. Phlebotomist
11. What would the nursing assistant expect when the facility uses the nursing care pattern known as functional nursing?
    A. To be assigned certain tasks
    B. To care for a large number of patients
    C. To make independent decisions
    D. To be responsible for total patient care
12. Which team member performs delegated nursing tasks under the supervision of an RN or LPN/LVN?
    A. Case manager
    B. Nursing assistant
    C. Surveyor
    D. Task nurse
13. Which health care agency or program promotes comfort and quality of life for the dying person and the family?
    A. Case management
    B. Assisted living residence
    C. Hospice
    D. Patient-focused care
14. Which member of the health care team is responsible for deciding the amount and kind of care each person needs?
    A. Licensed practical nurse
    B. Registered nurse
    C. Licensed vocational nurse
    D. Nursing assistant
15. Which person has an acute illness?
    A. Person A has pancreatic cancer.
    B. Person B has an ear infection.
    C. Person C has arthritis.
    D. Person D has high blood pressure.
16. Which setting would be best for a person who needs help with daily activities and desires access to support services, health care, and social activities?
    A. Hospice
    B. Home health care
    C. Acute care hospital
    D. Assisted living residence
17. Which condition does a person have when they are not likely to recover?
    A. Acute injury
    B. Terminal illness
    C. Chronic illness
    D. Functional injury
18. Which person is most likely to need the type of care that is provided in a memory care unit?
    A. Has chronic cardiac and respiratory problems
    B. Has Alzheimer disease with wandering behaviors
    C. Needs some assistance with activities of daily living
    D. Has cancer and death is expected within 6 months
19. Which nursing assistant action contributes to health promotion?
    A. Assists doctor with the person's physical examination
    B. Obtains stool and urine specimens as ordered
    C. Encourages person to do daily recommended exercises
    D. Holds infant while RN administers an immunization

20. Which nursing assistant action contributes to detection and medical diagnosis of disease?
    A. Transports person to the radiology department
    B. Assists elderly person to a standing position
    C. Shows respect and maintains person's privacy
    D. Assists vision-impaired person to read a lunch menu
21. Which nursing assistant action helps the person to meet the goal of rehabilitation and restorative care?
    A. Reassures person that all needs will be met in a timely manner
    B. Encourages person to independently do as much self-care as possible
    C. Takes and reports vital signs according to facility protocol
    D. Helps to organize and pack person's belongings for discharge
22. Which health care agency offers care and treatment for an acute illness?
    A. A hospital
    B. A long-term care center
    C. An assisted living facility
    D. A rehabilitation agency
23. Which person needs subacute care?
    A. Had minor surgery for a skin condition
    B. Discharged from hospital but needs complex wound care
    C. Needs help with toileting, bathing, and meal preparation
    D. Has terminal illness and death is imminent
24. Which elderly person needs the care that is provided in a long-term care center?
    A. Developed pneumonia and now has trouble breathing
    B. Sustained a hip fracture and needs surgery
    C. Has chronic heart and respiratory problems
    D. Has depression and thoughts about suicide
25. What is the primary difference between long-term care centers and skilled nursing facilities?
    A. Length of stay
    B. Complexity of care
    C. Funding sources
    D. Certification of staff
26. Which care situation is suitable for a person who wants apartment-style living but also needs help with personal care?
    A. A long-term care center
    B. An assisted living facility
    C. A rehabilitation care agency
    D. A skilled nursing facility
27. Which health care facility is appropriate for a person who has thoughts of harm to self or others?
    A. Mental health center
    B. Long-term care center
    C. Skilled care facility
    D. Hospice
28. What is expected of nursing assistants who work for home care agencies?
    A. Ability to perform more complex nursing care
    B. Willingness to call the doctor if the person is very ill
    C. Competent to provide care with offsite supervision
    D. Skilled at helping families resolve interpersonal problems
29. Which action would the nursing assistant perform to fulfill the role in hospice care?
    A. Do everything for person until they recover
    B. Ensure that person is clean and comfortable
    C. Encourage person to eat and exercise to regain strength
    D. Provide care only to meet person's physical needs
30. What is the primary goal of a health care system that includes several clinics, a hospital, a pharmacy, a skilled nursing facility, and a home health agency?
    A. Decrease the overall cost of comprehensive health care
    B. Share resources and cross-train members of the health team
    C. Make medical records readily accessible across the system
    D. Meet all health care needs for persons and their families
31. Which member of the health care team can recommend treatments for a person who is having trouble swallowing?
    A. Speech therapist
    B. Podiatrist
    C. Occupational therapist
    D. Physician
32. Who would the nursing assistant notify if a family member has a complaint about the nursing care?
    A. Person's primary care doctor
    B. RN team leader
    C. Director of nursing
    D. All health care team members
33. In which circumstance would the nursing assistant seek help from the nursing education staff?
    A. Needs tutoring to pass the NATCEP competency evaluation
    B. Is unsure how to use a new automatic blood pressure machine
    C. Knows that an elderly person has questions about his medications
    D. Suspects that an LPN is doing tasks that should be done by an RN
34. Which health care team member would the nursing assistant notify if a resident says he has pain in his foot?
    A. Podiatrist
    B. Physician's assistant
    C. Physical therapist
    D. Supervising RN

35. What is included in the role and responsibilities of the RN?
    A. Has liability for the nursing assistant's actions and performance
    B. Is expected to give the nursing assistant clear and specific instructions
    C. Will complete the nursing assistant's tasks if they are unfinished
    D. Has authority to fire the nursing assistant for using assertive communication
36. Which action is the LPN/LVN most likely to perform?
    A. Assists the nursing assistants to complete tasks
    B. Assists the RN in caring for an acutely ill person
    C. Assumes RN responsibilities if no RN is available
    D. Claims limited authority in supervising nursing assistants
37. What is the best description of the nursing assistant's role in the nursing care pattern of team nursing?
    A. Team leader assigns several patients and nursing assistant performs all of the care.
    B. Team leader creates teams by pairing nursing assistants for tasks.
    C. Nursing assistant describes skills and abilities to the team leader.
    D. Nursing assistant reports observations and the care given to the team leader.
38. Which action would the nursing assistant perform in the nursing care pattern of functional nursing?
    A. Help patients with bathing and hygiene and assist with meals
    B. Talk to the other nursing assistants and decide how to divide duties
    C. Assist the RNs and LPNs after receiving specific instructions
    D. Perform total care for all patients who are assigned
39. What would you expect to observe in patient-focused care?
    A. You would transport the patient to diagnostic testing center.
    B. The patient directs the focus and type of care and treatment.
    C. The RN would draw blood sample at the patient's bedside.
    D. The patient is invited to actively participate in care conferences.
40. Which action would the nursing assistant perform to contain health care costs for a person who has Medicare coverage?
    A. Complete care and duties as quickly and efficiently as possible
    B. Assist the person to be discharged to home as soon as possible
    C. Limit the amount and use of supplies that are charged to the person
    D. Follow the RN's instructions for the prevention of pressure injuries
41. Which action should the nursing assistant perform to help the health care agency to meet the standards of licensure, certification, or accreditation?
    A. Maintain safety when assisting a patient or resident to bathe
    B. Describe the NATCEP testing process to the surveyor
    C. Memorize all policies and procedures related to the job
    D. Do whatever the patients or residents want or need
42. What should the nursing assistant do when a confused elderly resident says he does not have any money to pay for help or to pay the bill for the long-term care center?
    A. Reassure him that care will continue no matter how much money he has
    B. Tell him not to worry about it and change the subject
    C. Find out who is paying the bills for the resident
    D. Tell the charge nurse about the resident's concerns
43. Which rationale would support the nursing assistant's choice to work for an accredited health care agency?
    A. All health care team members are licensed and experienced.
    B. Any person needing care is accepted regardless of income level.
    C. Voluntary review shows that a high quality of care is provided.
    D. Facility is likely to offer promotions, a good salary, and benefits.
44. Which action should you take if a deficiency is found during a survey of a health care agency where you work?
    A. Seek a new job with a different agency within 60 days
    B. Ask if your responses to surveyor's questions created a problem
    C. Give honest information about the deficiency to patients/residents
    D. Follow instructions from the team leader to correct the deficiency
45. If you do not understand a question that is posed by a surveyor, what should you do?
    A. Explain that you are not allowed to answer any questions
    B. Answer the question to the best of your ability
    C. Tell the surveyor that you do not know the answer
    D. Ask the surveyor to restate or rephrase the question

Matching

Match the Type of Health Care Agency With the Service Provided

A. Hospital
B. Rehabilitation agency
C. Long-term care center
D. Mental health center
E. Home care agency
F. Hospice
G. Skilled nursing facility
H. Assisted living residence

46. ________ promotes comfort and quality of life for dying persons and the families.
47. ________ provides complex care for persons with health problems that require skilled care.
48. ________ provides services to persons who do not need hospital care but cannot care for themselves at home.
49. ________ serves people of all ages for acute, chronic, or terminal illnesses.
50. ________ treats people who may have difficulty dealing with social or personal events in life.
51. ________ provides housing, personal care, and other services in a home-like setting.
52. ________ serves people who do not need hospital care but require complex care and equipment to recover function.
53. ________ provides care to persons at home.

Fill in the Blanks

54. Write out the abbreviations.
    A. ALR ________________________________
    B. OSHA ________________________________
    C. APRN ________________________________
    D. HHS ________________________________
    E. SNF ________________________________
    F. PPS ________________________________

Write the Name of the Health Team Member Described

55. ______________________ supervises LPNs/LVNs and assistive personnel.
56. ______________________ diagnoses and prescribes treatment for diseases and injuries.
57. ______________________ collects samples and performs tests on blood, urine, and other body fluids.
58. ______________________ takes x-rays and processes film for viewing.
59. ______________________ gives respiratory treatments and therapies.
60. ______________________ assesses and plans for nutritional needs.
61. ______________________ assists persons with movement, prevention of disability, and rehabilitation.
62. ______________________ assists persons to learn or retain skills needed for activities of daily living.
63. ______________________ treats persons with communication and swallowing disorders.
64. ______________________ assists persons with their spiritual needs.
65. ______________________ helps patients and families with social, emotional, and environmental issues affecting illness and recovery.
66. ______________________ treats hearing, balance, and ear problems.
67. ________________ gives drugs as allowed by state law under the supervision of a licensed nurse.
68. ________________ performs exams and provides diagnoses and treatments under a doctor's direction.

Optional Learning Exercises

Name the Member of the Health Team Who Provides the Service Described

69. Mr. Williams needs assistance to regain skills to dress, shave, and feed himself (ADLs). He is assisted by the ________________________________.
70. Mrs. Young needs the corns on her feet treated. The nurse notifies the ______________________.
71. Ms. Stewart has the responsibility of doing physical examinations, health assessments, and health education in the center where she works. She is a ________________________________.
72. Mr. Gomez keeps turning up the volume of his TV. His hearing is tested by the ______________________.
73. The ________________ meets with a new resident and his family to discuss his nutritional needs.
74. Mr. Fox had a stroke and has weakness on his left side. The ________________ assists him by developing a plan that focuses on restoring function and preventing disability from his illness.
75. The doctor orders x-rays after Mr. Jackson falls. The x-rays are done by the ______________________.
76. Mr. Ling has chronic lung disease and needs respiratory treatments. These are given by the ________________________________.
77. Ms. Walker plans the recreational needs of a nursing center. She is an ______________________.
78. After a stroke, Mr. Stubbs has difficulty swallowing. He is evaluated by the ______________________.
79. When the doctor orders blood tests, the samples are collected by the ______________________.
80. Mr. Suny needs to see a ____________ so that he can get his teeth cleaned and learn about preventive care.
81. A ________________ can help Mrs. Jansten who lives at home but needs help with daily activities, such as laundry, bedmaking, grocery shopping, meals, hygiene, dressing, and grooming.
82. The ______________ fills drug orders and advises about safe prescription use.
83. When Ms. Kia returns home after surgery, the ____________ can help to coordinate community agencies to assist Ms. Kia and the family.

Name the Nursing Care Pattern Described in the Following Examples

84. Ms. Hines works with Dr. Hogan. When patient, Harry Forbes, is admitted to the hospital, Ms. Hines coordinates the care from admission to discharge. She also communicates with the insurance company and community agencies involved in Mr. Forbes' care. This is an example of ______________________________.

85. When Mr. Holcomb reports for work as a nursing assistant, he is assigned to make all beds on the unit. The RN gives all intravenous medications and the LPN gives all oral medications. This nursing care pattern is ______________________________.

86. Ms. Conroy works on the same nursing unit each day. She has a group of patients, and she gives total care to each of them. She teaches and counsels the person and family and plans for home care or long-term care when needed. This is an example of ______________.

87. Ms. Ryan is a nursing assistant. She gives care that is delegated by an RN. The RN leads a team of nursing staff members, and she decides the amount and kind of care each person needs. This is called ______________________________.

88. Mrs. Young receives her care and physical therapy on the nursing unit. She does not have to go to different departments to receive treatments and care. This care is provided by the nursing team instead of by other health team members. This is called ______________________________.

Use the FOCUS ON PRIDE Section to Complete These Statements and Then Use the Critical Thinking and Discussion Questions to Develop Your Ideas

89. The word PRIDE used in the chapter stands for:
P______________________________
R______________________________
I______________________________
D______________________________
E______________________________

Critical Thinking and Discussion Questions

90. List three or four personal behaviors that will help you achieve your goals in the nursing assistant program; then share, compare, and discuss your list with your classmates.
91. Identify three or four professional behaviors that you believe are necessary to be an excellent nursing assistant. Discuss your rationale for identifying those professional behaviors with your classmates.

2 The Person's Rights

Fill in the Blanks: Key Terms

Involuntary seclusion | Ombudsman | Representative | Treatment

1. A ______________________________ is any person who has the legal right to act on the resident's behalf when they cannot do so for themselves.
2. Separating a person from others against their will, keeping the person in a certain area, or keeping the person away from their room without consent is ______________________________.
3. The care provided to maintain or restore health, improve function, or relieve symptoms is ______________________________.
4. An ______________________ is someone who supports or promotes the needs and interests of another person.

Circle the Best Answer

5. Which factor is a part of the patient care partnership?
   A. The person must follow all recommended treatments or plans of care.
   B. The doctor makes the treatment decisions if the person is unable to do so.
   C. The person should know when students or other trainees are involved in their care.
   D. Hospital charges are not given to the person, only to the insurance companies.
6. Which action violates a resident's rights?
   A. The resident is asked to share a room with another resident.
   B. You help the resident to arrange personal items and clothing.
   C. You decline to discuss a resident's care with another resident.
   D. The resident is not told that their health status has changed.
7. For which circumstance must the resident's representative be consulted?
   A. The resident refuses to brush their teeth or comb their hair.
   B. A resident with dementia needs a medical procedure.
   C. The resident has out-of-town visitors including children.
   D. A resident would like to see a physical therapist.
8. If a resident refuses treatment, what should the nursing assistant do?
   A. Avoid giving care and move on to other duties
   B. Report the refusal to the nurse
   C. Tell the resident the treatment is necessary
   D. Tell the resident's family
9. Which action is correct if a student wants to observe a treatment, but the resident does not want any observers?
   A. Student cannot watch as this violates the resident's right to privacy.
   B. Student may observe from the doorway out of sight of the resident.
   C. Staff nurse tells the resident that the student must be allowed to watch.
   D. Nurse calls the resident's spouse to get permission.
10. Which consideration is the most important when a resident is making a personal choice?
    A. Safety
    B. Personal rights
    C. Doctor's orders
    D. Personal pride
11. Which resident is exercising their right to voice a dispute or grievance?
    A. Resident A tells Resident B that he talks too much.
    B. Resident C tells the doctor that he is not getting his pain medication.
    C. Resident D requests extra sugar packets for his coffee.
    D. Resident E refuses to allow anyone to take his blood pressure.
12. When a resident volunteers to take care of houseplants at the center, which action violates residents' rights?
    A. The resident's desire to work is reflected in the care plan.
    B. The resident tends the plants in exchange for care items.
    C. The resident incorporates the plant care into his schedule.
    D. The resident's rehabilitation goals include volunteering.
13. Which action violates residents' right to participate in resident and family groups?
    A. Residents are encouraged to meet and discuss concerns about the care center.
    B. Several families gather to celebrate birthdays and holidays.
    C. Resident is invited to attend a church service, but invitation is declined.
    D. Residents with dementia are not invited to attend a musical performance.

14. Which action denies the resident their rights to keep and use personal items?
    A. Storing the resident's belongings when they leave for emergency surgery
    B. Taking soiled items to the laundry and hanging clean clothes in the closet
    C. Throwing away old holiday decorations without direct permission
    D. Wiping off the surface of the nightstand and dusting picture frames
15. Which action infringes on residents' right to freedom from abuse, mistreatment, and neglect?
    A. A staff member tells a resident that he cannot leave his room because he talks too much.
    B. A nurse explains the problems that can result when a resident refuses a medication.
    C. A nursing assistant coaches a resident to do portions of self-care as identified by the RN.
    D. A nurse accompanies a resident to a private room to discuss an upsetting incident.
16. Which right is denied to a resident when they are given a drug that affects mood and restricts body movement or mental function?
    A. Right to information
    B. Freedom to express personal choice
    C. Right to have privacy
    D. Freedom from restraint
17. Which of these actions will promote courteous and dignified care?
    A. Using terms of endearment such as "Honey" or "Sweetheart" to address the residents
    B. Assisting with dressing the resident in clothing appropriate to the time of day
    C. Using frequent touch, hugs, and handshakes with all residents and staff
    D. Leaving the bathroom door open so that the resident can be observed
18. Which question is a surveyor most likely to ask to determine if you are promoting residents' rights?
    A. What can the resident expect from the treatment plans?
    B. How much time does it take you to help a resident to bathe?
    C. What tasks must you complete when a resident is discharged?
    D. How do you prevent unnecessary exposure of the resident's body?
19. Which information is the most important for the nursing assistant to give to a coworker who will help assist residents to and from activities?
    A. Which residents require a wheelchair, cane, or walker
    B. How to politely address the residents using proper name and title
    C. Which residents take offense to scolding or hurried actions
    D. How to provide privacy and draping during transport
20. Which nursing assistant action provides privacy and self-determination for a resident?
    A. Knocking on the door before entering and waiting to be asked in
    B. Allowing the resident to smoke in designated areas
    C. Listening with interest to what the person is saying
    D. Grooming hair and beard as requested by the resident
21. Which nursing assistant action allows the resident to maintain personal choice and independence?
    A. Obtaining resident's attention before interacting
    B. Providing extra clothing for warmth such as a sweater or lap robe
    C. Assisting resident to take part in activities according to their interests
    D. Using curtains or screens during personal care and procedures
22. What is the best action to encourage social interaction among residents?
    A. Tell residents about activities and offer help to and from activities
    B. Place wheelchair residents in a close circle after mealtimes
    C. Talk to individual residents whenever there is extra time
    D. Encourage residents to sit by different people during meals
23. Which people should be present when the nursing assistant is giving a report about a resident's care to the oncoming staff?
    A. All oncoming staff including nursing students
    B. Resident's family and legal representative
    C. Any licensed health care professional
    D. Any staff directly involved in the resident's care
24. Which response is best to give a family member who asks about a resident's weight?
    A. "I weigh him every morning and his weight is about the same as it has been."
    B. "I told the nurse about your question and she will speak to you soon."
    C. "It will take me a couple of minutes, but I can go and look at the records."
    D. "I am sorry, but I am not allowed to give you any information."
25. Which of these activities would be carried out by an ombudsman?
    A. Organize activities for a group of residents
    B. Accompany residents to a religious service at a house of worship
    C. Investigate and resolve complaints made by a resident
    D. Assist the resident to choose friends
26. What is the purpose of the Omnibus Budget Reconciliation Act of 1987 (OBRA)?
    A. Protects the rights of health care staff who work in nursing centers
    B. Sets minimum standards for quality of care in nursing centers
    C. Ensures equal access to care in a nursing center for those under Medicare
    D. Creates a partnership between staff, residents, and families in nursing centers

27. Which action would the nursing assistant take when a resident says, "I don't like the food on this lunch tray."?
   A. Give the lunch tray to another resident
   B. Ask dietary to make a different lunch tray
   C. Report the comment to the charge nurse
   D. Encourage the resident to try eating some of it
28. According to the patient care partnership, what does the patient need to understand to make informed decisions about treatment choices?
   A. Benefits and risks of the treatment
   B. Other patients' experience with the treatment
   C. Doctor's personal feelings about the treatment
   D. Time frame for expected cure after treatment is completed
29. What would the nursing assistant do if a person refuses cancer treatment?
   A. Suggest other treatment options
   B. Explain what will happen if treatment does not occur
   C. Find out why the person is refusing the treatment
   D. Continue to assist with activities of daily living
30. Which nursing assistant action is an example of involuntary seclusion?
   A. Nursing assistant A blocks doorway when resident tries to enter another person's room.
   B. Nursing assistant B confines resident in bedroom because she is argumentative.
   C. Nursing assistant C encourages a reluctant resident to go to an activity.
   D. Nursing assistant D is disrespectful toward resident when he is forgetful.

Optional Learning Activities

OBRA-Required Actions to Promote Dignity and Privacy (see Box 2.3, p. 17)

Match the Action to Promote Dignity and Privacy With the Example

A. Courteous and dignified interaction
B. Courteous and dignified care
C. Privacy and self-determination
D. Maintain personal choice and independence

31. ________ use good eye contact.
32. ________ cover the resident with a blanket during a bath.
33. ________ gain the person's attention before giving care.
34. ________ show interest when a resident tells stories about his past.
35. ________ move person's items only with the person's consent.
36. ________ close the door when the person asks for privacy.
37. ________ allow a resident to smoke in a designated area.
38. ________ make sure the resident is wearing his dentures when he goes to the dining room.
39. ________ take the resident to her weekly card game.

Use the FOCUS ON PRIDE section and the critical thinking and discussion questions to develop your ideas

Critical Thinking and Discussion Questions

40. Discuss how leaving the familiar setting of home and community to move into a nursing care facility would influence a person's independence.
41. Identify ways to help residents maintain their independence.

3 The Nursing Assistant

Fill in the Blanks: Key Terms

Certification | Endorsement | Job description | Preceptor

1. A ____________________ is an experienced staff member who mentors a new employee at the start of a job.
2. ____ means that a state recognizes the certificate, license, or registration issued by another state.
3. A ____________________________ is a document that describes what the agency expects you to do.
4. Official recognition by a state that standards or requirements have been met is ____________________.

Circle the Best Answer

5. What do OBRA and other federal and state laws require for nursing assistants who apply to work in long-term care agencies?
   A. Background check
   B. High school diploma
   C. Two forms of identification
   D. Bank account information
6. A nursing assistant who works in Texas is told that some states have reciprocity. Which documentation would be included in the application to another state?
   A. Birth certificate
   B. Passport
   C. Proof of citizenship
   D. Fingerprint cards
7. Which state registration policy would benefit nursing assistants who complete NATCEP in their home state and later desire to work in a different state?
   A. Acceptance
   B. Impartiality
   C. Equivalency
   D. Acknowledgment
8. Based on background check findings and self-report on applications, which nursing assistant would be eligible to be employed in a long-term care agency?
   A. Nursing assistant A has a history of misappropriation at a previous job.
   B. Nursing assistant B recently divorced and has relocated to another state.
   C. Nursing assistant C has a history of exploitation before becoming a nursing assistant.
   D. Nursing assistant D was convicted of neglect of an older family member.
9. What would the nursing assistant do if a nurse is performing an action that violates the state's nurse practice act?
   A. Do nothing because the nurse has more authority
   B. Watch to see if the nurse's actions are causing harm to anyone
   C. Call the Board of Nursing and make an anonymous report
   D. Go up the chain of command and give the facts to the nurse's supervisor
10. Which nurse is performing an action that violates the nurse practice act?
    A. Nurse A recently graduated and seems unsure about the facility policies.
    B. Nurse B makes many unreasonable demands on the nursing assistants.
    C. Nurse C comes to work and is under the influence of alcohol and drugs.
    D. Nurse D is tired after working day shift but agrees to stay and cover night shift.
11. How are the state's nurse practice acts relevant to nursing assistants?
    A. RNs and LPNs/LVNs are affected; nursing assistants are not affected.
    B. Nurse practice acts bestow protection from liability for nursing assistants.
    C. Roles, tasks, actions, and education of nursing assistants can be affected.
    D. Nurse practice acts are less relevant for nursing assistants than facility policies.
12. Which outcome is likely if a nursing assistant does something beyond the legal limits of the role?
    A. The nursing assistant is protected by the nurse practice act.
    B. The nursing assistant's actions will be investigated.
    C. The nursing assistant is protected by the supervising nurse.
    D. The nursing assistant will be accused of a criminal act.
13. Which nursing assistant is likely to face disciplinary charges and possible loss of certification?
    A. Nursing assistant A is frequently absent from work.
    B. Nursing assistant B releases confidential information.
    C. Nursing assistant C refuses to care for a certain patient.
    D. Nursing assistant D has frequent arguments with coworkers.
14. How many hours of instruction are required by OBRA for nursing assistant training and competency evaluation programs?
    A. 16 hours
    B. 75 hours
    C. 120 hours
    D. 200 hours
15. Which skill would nursing assistants be expected to master in a training program?
    A. Interpreting vital signs
    B. Positioning people in bed
    C. Transcribing the doctor's orders
    D. Drawing blood for laboratory testing

16. What should you say first when you meet a patient in your student clinical experience?
    A. "Hello. Please state your name and may I see your identification band."
    B. "Hello. Are you Mr. Smith? I will be caring for you today."
    C. "Hello. My name is Ms. Jones. I am a student nursing assistant."
    D. "Hello. Would you like me to call you Mr. Smith or use your first name?"
17. According to the nursing assistant registry, if there is an incident of misappropriation, what rights would the nursing assistant have?
    A. Right to include a statement disputing the findings
    B. Right to have record expunged for good behavior
    C. Right to sue the nursing assistant registry
    D. Right to have incident withheld from employers
18. How does the nursing assistant registry benefit the nursing assistant as an individual?
    A. Records dates and times of excellent work ethic
    B. Is a permanent record of interactions with patients
    C. Allows freedom to move from state to state for work
    D. Shows successful completion of the state's approved NATCEP
19. OBRA requires that retraining and a new competency evaluation test must be taken if you have not worked as a certified nursing assistant for
    A. 24 months
    B. 5 years
    C. 1 year
    D. 6 months
20. Which action is best if a mandatory in-service training is scheduled during the middle of the shift?
    A. Tell the nurse that patient care duties have priority over in-service training
    B. Ask the in-service trainer to provide you with copies of the handouts
    C. Explain to the patients that you must go and to call the nurse as needed
    D. Plan with coworkers; some do patient care while others attend the training
21. Which nursing assistant action could result in a discipline with a possible loss of certification?
    A. Goes to a patient's home after discharge and provides care without the supervision of a nurse
    B. Informs the nurse that vital signs were recorded on the wrong person's medical records
    C. Informs the nurse about leaving because there is family emergency in the middle of the shift
    D. Reports that a confused resident made rude and offensive remarks during morning hygiene
22. Which circumstance is most important for the nursing assistant to report to the supervising nurse?
    A. A new nursing assistant is unable to complete her duties and is frequently asking for help.
    B. The offgoing nursing assistant frequently fails to tidy up work areas and expects others to do the cleaning.
    C. Another nursing assistant is overheard asking a resident to lend her money for a child's school fees.
    D. An experienced nursing assistant gives tips about how to interact with confused residents.
23. In which circumstance would the nursing assistant give medications?
    A. The nurse is busy and asks the nursing assistant to give the medications.
    B. The person is in the shower and the nurse leaves the medications at the bedside.
    C. The nursing assistant has completed a state-approved medication assistant training program.
    D. The nursing assistant is feeding the person and the nurse suggests mixing the medications with the food.
24. Which action would you take upon answering the phone and the doctor begins to give verbal orders?
    A. Tell the doctor that you are not allowed to take phone orders
    B. Politely give your name and title and then promptly get the nurse
    C. Quickly write down the orders and promptly give them to the nurse
    D. Politely tell the doctor to call back later when the nurse is there
25. Which action would the nursing assistant take when the nurse asks for assistance with a sterile dressing change?
    A. Assist the nurse as needed
    B. Explain nursing assistant role limitations
    C. Offer to change the dressings
    D. Report the nurse to the director of nursing.
26. Which member of the health care staff can tell the person or family a diagnosis or prescribe treatments?
    A. Director of nursing
    B. RN
    C. Physician
    D. Experienced nursing assistant
27. Which action would the nursing assistant take when a nurse assigns a task that is unfamiliar?
    A. Ignore the assignment because it would not be safe to carry out the task
    B. Promptly explain to the nurse why the task cannot be carried out
    C. Look up information about the task and then do the task
    D. Ask another nursing assistant to demonstrate how to carry out the task
28. Which action would the nursing assistant take when the nurse delegates the task of starting an IV on a patient because the nursing assistant is also an emergency medical technician (EMT)?
    A. Tell the nurse that starting an IV is outside the role of a nursing assistant
    B. Start the IV since starting IVs is a routine task of an EMT
    C. Ask the nurse to spend a few minutes supervising the task of IV insertion
    D. Report the nurse to the director of nursing services.

29. In a home care setting, which action would the nursing assistant be expected to do?
    A. Give medications and physical therapy treatments
    B. Provide personal care and prepare meals
    C. Do any household chores that the person is unable to do
    D. Drive the person's car so the person can shop or run errands
30. Which action would the nursing assistant take if an elderly home care patient offers extra money for helping the spouse to paint the house?
    A. Make private arrangements to do the work on days off
    B. Consult the supervising nurse about what to do and say
    C. Help the family locate a reliable handyman to help
    D. Explain that it would be illegal to accept any money
31. Which information must be immediately reported to the nurse?
    A. Resident is upset because he did not get any coffee with breakfast.
    B. Resident wants to take a tub bath, but his doctor has ordered showering.
    C. Resident's blood pressure and pulse are higher than usual.
    D. Resident's daily weight was recorded on the flow sheet.
32. Which job description would cause the nursing assistant to decline a job offer?
    A. Requires doing duties that are unpleasant
    B. Demands function that exceeds training limits
    C. Involves maintaining required certification
    D. Mandates attendance to in-service training

Fill in the Blanks

33. Write out the abbreviations
    A. CNA ______________________________
    B. LNA ______________________________
    C. NATCEP ___________________________
    D. BON ______________________________
    E. RNA ______________________________
    F. SRNA _____________________________
    G. STNA _____________________________
    H. NCSBN ____________________________
34. Which task would be taught in a nursing assistant training program so that nursing assistants can perform basic nursing skills and personal care?
    A. Measuring vital signs
    B. Identifying a mental health problem
    C. Teaching how to perform hand hygiene
    D. Selecting and suggesting personal care products
35. Which task is an example of basic restorative care that would be included in a nursing assistant training program?
    A. Interacting with confused patients
    B. Performing range-of-motion exercises
    C. Assisting with bathing and hygiene
    D. Using respectful and courteous language
36. What information does the nursing assistant registry have about each nursing assistant?
    A. Full name, including maiden name and any married names
    B. Gender, pronoun, and sexual preference
    C. Health status and chronic illness that impacts the job
    D. Salary range and benefits expectations
37. In compliance with OBRA, how many hours of educational programs and performance reviews each year are required for every nursing assistant?
    A. 10 hours
    B. 12 hours
    C. 20 hours
    D. 40 hours
38. Which reason would justify a nursing assistant's decision to decline a job offer based on a written job description?
    A. Salary increases are not given during the probation period.
    B. Actions and duties are beyond the legal limits of the nursing assistants' role.
    C. Attendance to educational and training opportunities is mandatory.
    D. Errors in patient care must be reported to the charge nurse.
39. Which task is included in the responsibilities for nursing assistants who provide home care?
    A. Carrying firewood or coal and stoking fireplace, and cleaning ash containers
    B. Washing windows, and cleaning rugs, drapes, or furniture that is soiled
    C. Waxing floors and shampooing carpets or upholstery as needed
    D. Washing and drying clothing and linens; this may include family laundry
40. Which nursing assistant is performing duties within the role limits?
    A. Nursing assistant A takes a doctor's phone order because the nurse is busy.
    B. Nursing assistant B supervises a new assistant to ensure a task is correctly done.
    C. Nursing assistant C ignores a request from the LPN to give a medication.
    D. Nursing assistant D declines to give information about a patient's medical diagnosis.
41. List at least four observations that a surveyor could make to assess your competence to perform your job.
    A. ______________________________
    B. ______________________________
    C. ______________________________
    D. ______________________________
42. If you wanted to work in another state, what would you do first? ______________________________
    ____

43. Identify at least seven of the Nursing Assistant Standards in Box 3.3 (p. 27) that are particularly meaningful to you.
    A. ______________________________
    B. ______________________________
    C. ______________________________
    D. ______________________________
    E. ______________________________
    F. ______________________________
    G. ______________________________

Optional Learning Exercises

OBRA Requirements Related to the Nursing Assistant

44. OBRA requires many areas of study. Write the area of study where you learn the skill used in each example.
    A. ______________________ You assist an unsteady resident to stand up.
    B. ______________________ You close Mr. Smith's door to give him privacy.
    C. ______________________ You tell Mrs. Forbes the time of day and the day of the week frequently because she is mildly confused.
    D. ______________________ You apply lotion to a resident's skin.
    E. ______________________ You assist a person to put on his shirt.
    F. ________________ When assigned to a new unit, you check the location of the fire alarm.
    G. ______________________ You practice hand hygiene before and after giving care.
    H. ____________________ You get help to move a person from his bed to the chair.
    I. ______________________ When speaking to Mr. Jackson, you maintain good eye contact.
    J. ______________________ The nurse tells you to exercise a person's extremities (limbs).
    K. ____________________ You position a urinal for a resident in bed.
    L. ______________________ You provide privacy when Mr. Jones is talking on the phone.
    M. ________________ You gently redirect a confused resident who is trying to leave the nursing center.
    N. ____________________ You cut up the meat on Mr. Sanyo's plate before helping him to eat.

Use the FOCUS ON PRIDE Section to Complete These Statements and Then Use the Critical Thinking and Discussion Questions to Develop Your Ideas

45. If a patient refuses to have a student care for him, you should respectfully ____________ the person's rights to choose who is involved in his care.
46. Practicing skills in the classroom or laboratory will make you feel more ______________________.
47. When the nurse asks you to do a task, the nurse is ______________________ the task to you.

Critical Thinking and Discussion Questions

Recall the areas of knowledge and skills that will be included in your training program: (1) communication, (2) infection control, (3) safety and emergency procedures, (4) resident's rights, (5) basic nursing skills, (6) personal care skills, (7) feeding methods, (8) elimination methods, (9) skin care, (10) transferring, positioning and turning methods, (11) dressing, (12) helping the person to walk, (13) range-of-motion exercises, and (14) care for cognitively impaired persons.

48. After considering the list, identify three or four areas that seem the most difficult or challenging for you. Discuss your selections and your concerns with your classmates or instructors.
49. Discuss how you plan to take personal and professional responsibility for achieving excellence and mastery in the areas that seem to be the most difficult for you.

4 Delegation

Fill in the Blanks: Key Terms

Accountable | Delegate | Routine nursing task

1. Being ______________________ is to answer to one's self and others about one's choices, decisions, and actions.
2. To ________________ means to authorize or direct a nursing assistant to perform a nursing task.
3. A ________________ is a nursing task that is part of a nursing assistant's routine job description; a nursing task that was learned in a Nursing Assistant Training and Competency Evaluation Program (NATCEP).

Circle the Best Answer

4. Which task is an example of a delegated nursing task that a nursing assistant could be asked to perform with appropriate training and supervision?
   A. Changing the linen on a resident's bed
   B. Helping a resident to comb her hair
   C. Assisting a patient with morning hygiene
   D. Measuring a patient's blood glucose
5. Which task would the nursing assistant decline to perform because it requires a nurse's professional knowledge and judgment?
   A. Taking and reporting vital signs
   B. Supervising a newly hired nursing assistant
   C. Walking with a confused resident in the garden area
   D. Transporting a patient who is in a wheelchair
6. Which circumstance is an example of correct delegation?
   A. APRN tells the nursing assistant to answer all phone queries while the nurse is at lunch.
   B. Charge nurse instructs the nursing assistant to report all abnormal vital signs.
   C. RN tells the nursing assistant to assess a resident who fell in the bathroom.
   D. LPN/LVN asks the nursing assistant to help residents to go to the dining hall.
7. Which health care team member is exceeding their authority to delegate?
   A. An APRN delegates a task to a nursing assistant.
   B. An RN delegates a task to a nursing assistant.
   C. An LPN/LVN delegates a task to a nursing assistant.
   D. A nursing assistant delegates a task to another nursing assistant.
8. Which factor is the most important when a nurse is delegating care for patients on the unit?
   A. What is the best care for the patient at the time
   B. How many staff members are available to assist
   C. Personal requests from patients needing care
   D. Whether the patient likes the nursing assistant
9. Which factor affects the nurse's decision to take over the care of a patient who has been assigned to the same nursing assistant for the past several weeks?
   A. How well the nursing assistant gave care in the past
   B. Changes in the patient's current condition
   C. Assistant's need to spend time caring for other patients
   D. How much supervision the nursing assistant needs
10. At which step of the delegation process would the nursing assistant tell the nurse that the assigned task is unfamiliar?
    A. Assess and plan
    B. Communication
    C. Supervision
    D. Evaluation and feedback
11. Which nurse is performing the supervision step of the delegation process?
    A. Nurse A tells the nursing assistant how to perform and complete the task.
    B. Nurse B determines the skills that are needed to safely perform the nursing task.
    C. Nurse C observes as the nursing assistant performs the nursing task.
    D. Nurse D gives the nursing assistant feedback about task performance.
12. Which nursing assistant has the greatest need for a good communication plan with the supervising nurse?
    A. Nursing assistant A has been asked to do a task that she has never done before.
    B. Nursing assistant B does home care for an elderly person with many health problems.
    C. Nursing assistant C is assisting in the orientation of a newly hired assistant.
    D. Nursing assistant D is assigned extra patients because someone called in sick.
13. Which of these tasks cannot be delegated to a nursing assistant?
    A. Give perineal care
    B. Supervise others
    C. Assist with range-of-motion exercises
    D. Collect specimens
14. In which situation would the nursing assistant have the right to refuse a task?
    A. The nursing assistant has never cared for the person before.
    B. The task is too time-consuming for the nursing assistant.
    C. The task is not in the nursing assistant job description.
    D. It is the end of the nursing assistant's shift.

15. Which task would generally be considered a routine nursing task for a nursing assistant?
    A. Measuring the height and weight
    B. Inserting a urinary catheter
    C. Administering an enema
    D. Helping a person to swallow medication
16. Which action would the nursing assistant take when a newly graduated nurse says to check on a patient and see if his breathing is okay and start oxygen if needed?
    A. Tell the charge nurse about the new nurse's inappropriate delegation
    B. Count the respiratory rate, put the oxygen on, and report back to the nurse
    C. Check on the patient and ask if he is okay and if he needs oxygen
    D. Explain that nursing assistants are not trained to assess breathing or need for oxygen
17. Which direction given by the nurse is unethical and would therefore justify the nurse assistant's refusal to participate?
    A. Report immediately if the patient is having chest pain or seems short of breath
    B. Help the new nursing assistant to complete care if she seems to be having difficulties
    C. Take incontinence supplies from a resident who has more money and family support
    D. First perform morning hygiene for other residents then help a confused resident
18. Which nursing assistant has the right to refuse to perform the nurse's request?
    A. Nursing assistant A is asked to feed a resident who cannot hold a spoon.
    B. Nursing assistant B is asked to complete assigned tasks before leaving.
    C. Nursing assistant C is expected recognize when a patient's condition has changed.
    D. Nursing assistant D is told to show a new nursing assistant where the linens are stored.
19. Which directions must be given when the nurse communicates with the nursing assistant about a delegated task?
    A. How much time is allotted to complete a task
    B. Mistakes that other nursing assistants have made
    C. Consequences for failure to perform the task correctly
    D. What observations to report and record

Fill in the Blanks

20. What are the five rights of delegation?
    A. ______________________________
    B. ______________________________
    C. ______________________________
    D. ______________________________
    E. ______________________________

Optional Learning Experiences

21. What are the four steps in the delegation process in the correct order? (See Fig. 4.2, p. 35, in the textbook)
    A. Step 1 ______________________________
    B. Step 2 ______________________________
    C. Step 3 ______________________________
    D. Step 4 ______________________________
22. Read the following statements and indicate which of the four steps of the delegation process it describes.
    A. The nurse makes sure that you complete the task correctly. ______________________________
    B. How will delegating the task help the person? What are the risks to the person?
    ____
    C. The nurse tells you when to report observations.
    ____
    D. Was the desired result achieved?
    ____
23. Look at the Five Rights of Delegation for Nursing Assistants in Box 4.1 (p. 37). For each question, list the Right that is fulfilled.
    A. Did you review the task with the nurse?
    ____
    B. Were you trained to do the task? ______________________________
    C. Do you have concerns about performing the task?
    ____
    D. Is the nurse available if the person's condition changes or if problems occur?
    ____
    E. Do you have the equipment and supplies to safely complete the task? ______________________________

Use the FOCUS ON PRIDE Section to Complete These Statements and Then Use the Critical Thinking And Discussion Questions to Develop Your Ideas

24. If uncertain about your ability to safely perform a task, tell the nurse. Take pride in protecting the person from ______________________________.
25. List five behaviors that indicate that you are respectful and willing to receive corrective feedback from the supervising nurse who will help to improve your performance.
    A. ______________________________
    B. ______________________________
    C. ______________________________
    D. ______________________________
    E. ______________________________
26. List four things that the staff can do to facilitate positive interactions during delegation experiences.
    A. ______________________________
    B. ______________________________
    C. ______________________________
    D. ______________________________

Critical Thinking and Discussion Questions

27. You are providing care for an elderly resident who lives in a long-term care center. What should you do if the nurse delegates the nursing task (measuring blood glucose) that is beyond your routine nursing assistant role?

28. You are caring for a resident who falls in the bathroom. You tell the nurse at once. The nurse says: "Take him to the dining room. I'll check him after lunch." You are aware that the agency policy states that a nurse must immediately assess the resident after a fall. What should you do?

5 Ethics and Laws

Fill in the Blanks: Key Terms

Abuse	Defamation	Malpractice	Slander
Assault	Elder abuse	Misappropriation	Standard of care
Battery	Ethics	Neglect	Tort
Boundary crossing	False imprisonment	Negligence	Vulnerable adult
Boundary sign	Fraud	Professional sexual misconduct	
Boundary violation	Informed consent	Protected health information	
Code of ethics	Intimate partner violence	Self-neglect	
Criminal law	Invasion of privacy		

1. Abuse or aggression that occurs in a romantic relationship is ________________.
2. Any intentional act, or failure to act, by a caregiver or other trusted person that causes harm or risk of harm to an older adult is ________________.
3. The dishonest use of property is ________________.
4. ________________ is injuring a person's name and reputation by making false statements to a third person.
5. A violation of professional interactions with an act, behavior, or comment that is sexual in nature is ________________.
6. Touching a person's body without their consent is ________________.
7. ________________ are laws concerned with offenses against the public and society in general.
8. ________________ is the failure by caregiver or other person to protect a vulnerable person or failure to provide food, water, clothing shelter, health care, or other basic activities of daily living.
9. ________________ are rules, or standards of conduct, for group members to follow.
10. An act, behavior, or thought that warns of a boundary crossing or violation is a ________________.
11. ________________ is the skills, care, and judgments required by a health team member under similar conditions.
12. ________________ is the process by which a person receives and understands information about a treatment or procedure and is able to decide to receive or refuse the treatment or procedure.
13. ________________ is saying or doing something to trick, fool, or deceive a person.
14. The willful infliction of injury, unreasonable confinement, intimidation, or punishment that results in physical harm, pain, or mental anguish is ________________.
15. An unintentional wrong in which a person did not act in a reasonable and careful manner and causes harm to a person or to the person's property is ________________.
16. ________________ is a person's behaviors and way of living that threaten their health, safety, and well-being.
17. A wrong committed against a person or the person's property is a ________________.
18. ________________ is a brief act or behavior of being overinvolved with the person.
19. ________________ is intentionally attempting or threatening to touch a person's body without the person's consent.
20. Unlawful restraint or restriction of a person's freedom of movement is ________________.
21. ________________ is knowledge of what is right and wrong conduct.
22. Violating a person's right not to have his or her name, photo, or private affairs exposed or made public without giving consent is an ________________.
23. Identifying information and information about the person's health care that is maintained or sent in any form (paper, electronic, oral) is ________________.
24. A ________________ is a person 18 years old or older who has a disability or condition that makes them at risk for harm.
25. A ________________ is an act or behavior that meets your needs, not the person's.
26. Negligence by a professional person is ________________.
27. Making false statements orally or by using sign language ________________.

Circle the Best Answer

28. Which nursing assistant is exploiting the person?
    - A. Nursing assistant A spends extra time with a person because she is helpless and needy.
    - B. Nursing assistant B scolds a person who keeps falling because they will not ask for help.
    - C. Nursing assistant C spreads rumors about a person who is difficult to satisfy.
    - D. Nursing assistant D accepts money from a person who appreciates the care that is given.

29. Which health care staff's action would be considered drug diversion?
    A. There is a delay for the LPN/LVN to administer the patients' medications because of an emergency situation.
    B. RN takes opioid medication from one patient and gives it to another patient who is having pain.
    C. The home health nursing assistant reaches a medication bottle from the top shelf of a cabinet for a person.
    D. The doctor tells the nursing assistant to give the medication after the patient finishes eating lunch.
30. In which circumstance would the health care staff suspect child abuse?
    A. Nursing assistant observes that a 6-year-old child has an abrasion on the knee.
    B. Doctor observes that a 4-month-old infant has burns on both feet and ankles.
    C. RN notices that an 8-month-old infant cries when approached by strangers.
    D. LPN/LVN takes vital signs on a 5-year-old child who is crying and has a fever.
31. Which penalty is likely if a nursing assistant is guilty of breaking a civil law?
    A. Will be put on probation and performance review
    B. Must pay a sum of money to injured person
    C. Must serve time in jail or do community service
    D. Will be removed from the nursing assistant registry
32. In which case should the nursing assistant decline to witness a will?
    A. The person had a sound mind when will was prepared and is now 99 years old.
    B. The will was prepared by a lawyer who is related to the nursing assistant.
    C. RN says that nursing assistants do not have the legal right to witness.
    D. Nursing assistant is named in the will to receive some property.
33. Which action would the nursing assistant take when a doctor keeps making unwelcome sexual advances?
    A. Call the police and make a report
    B. Ask another nursing assistant to stay close by
    C. Report the doctor's behavior to the charge nurse
    D. Refuse to assist the doctor with procedures
34. Which situation is unethical behavior for a nursing assistant?
    A. Nursing assistant believes that children should care for their elderly parents.
    B. Nursing assistant asks to be assigned to care for people of the same race.
    C. Nursing assistant reports that an elderly patient's son is hitting the patient.
    D. Nursing assistant disagrees with a man's decision to refuse lifesaving measures.
35. Which action would the nursing assistant take upon observing a coworker drinking alcohol at work?
    A. Report the facts and details of the event to the nurse
    B. Tell the coworker this behavior is endangering the patients
    C. Give the coworker information about a program for alcoholics
    D. Ignore the behavior to be loyal to the coworker
36. According to the code of conduct for nursing assistants, which principle is the nursing assistant following when taking the lunch break after finishing personal care for a person?
    A. Perform no act that will cause the person harm
    B. Know the limits of the role and knowledge
    C. Consider the person's needs to be more important
    D. Respect each person as an individual
37. Which action constitutes boundary crossing?
    A. Telling the patient the steps of a procedure
    B. Inviting the patient to your house for Thanksgiving dinner
    C. Avoiding a patient because they have made sexual advances
    D. Showing interest when the patient is talking
38. In which circumstance may the nursing assistant be accused of negligence while giving care?
    A. Tells the nurse that the assigned person is a friend of the family
    B. Assists a person to the bathroom and the toilet paper dispenser is empty
    C. Gives the wrong care to the wrong person because of similar names
    D. Reports to the nurse that the person is complaining of chest pain
39. The nursing assistant tells a coworker that the housekeeper is stealing money from the staff. This is an example of
    A. Defamation
    B. Boundary crossing
    C. Invasion of privacy
    D. Libel
40. In the cafeteria, the nursing assistant overhears two nursing assistants talking about a person they are caring for. This is an example of
    A. Defamation
    B. Libel
    C. Boundary crossing
    D. Invasion of privacy
41. If care is given to a person without asking, the nursing assistant may be guilty of
    A. Battery
    B. Assault
    C. Invasion of privacy
    D. Slander
42. Which person can give informed consent for treatment?
    A. They are under the legal age (usually 18 years).
    B. They are the responsible party.
    C. They are sedated.
    D. They have dementia.
43. Which action applies if the nursing assistant is asked to witness the signing of a consent?
    A. Must know the agency policy related to this task
    B. Should always refuse as it is not legal to do this
    C. Cannot ethically or legally witness a will
    D. Cannot refuse as it is part of the role.
44. What happens to the incident-specific information if a nursing assistant is convicted of abuse, neglect, or mistreatment?
    A. Will be in the nursing assistant registry data
    B. Should not be disclosed during a job application or interview
    C. Is available only in the court records and attorney's notes
    D. Is deleted if you make amends to the abused person.

45. What does the nursing assistant suspect upon noticing that a home care patient has no food in the house and the water has been turned off?
A. Self-neglect
B. Physical abuse
C. Involuntary seclusion
D. Emotional abuse

46. Which action would the nursing assistant take for suspicion that an elderly person is being abused?
A. Ask the person who is doing the abusing
B. Discuss suspicions with the caregiver
C. Call the police or social services
D. Discuss observations with the nurse

47. What does the nursing assistant suspect when a child asks for food or money for food because "Mom's not home and there's nothing to eat."?
A. Physical abuse
B. Neglect
C. Sexual abuse
D. Emotional abuse

48. Which action would the nursing assistant take for suspicion that a child is being abused?
A. Exam the child for bruises or laceration
B. Share concerns with the nurse
C. Call the local child welfare agency
D. Observe parents' interaction with the child

49. Which health care team member is committing wrongful use of electronic communications?
A. Physical therapist uses a cell phone to make an appointment for a home visit.
B. Nurse uses a computer to enter assessment data and treatment outcomes.
C. Physician obtains informed consent to photograph a wound on a patient's foot.
D. Nursing assistant student takes photos of residents and posts them on social media.

50. Which action would the nursing assistant take to avoid being accused of assault and battery when assisting a person to take a shower?
A. Ask the nurse to give specific instructions related to the procedure
B. Keep the person covered and warm before and after showering
C. Explain actions and get verbal or implied consent
D. Validate with the nurse that general consent was obtained which covers duties

51. Which nursing assistant could be accused of abandonment?
A. Nursing assistant is doing home care an elderly person but leaves before giving report to a nurse who will assume responsibility.
B. Nursing assistant spends extra time with the resident and often trades assignments to care for that resident.
C. Nursing assistant does not like to answer questions about the care given or the relationship with the resident.
D. Nursing assistant sends text messages about patient's health condition to family members and the patient's friends.

52. What does the nursing assistant suspect upon observing that the person who has home care is not taking the prescribed medications?
A. Substance abuse
B. Self-neglect
C. Physical abuse
D. Financial misappropriation

53. Which action would the nursing assistant take upon noticing that another nursing assistant is forcing food into a 90-year-old person's mouth because "They need to eat and this is the only way I can get done with my assignments."?
A. Offer to feed the person, so that the other assistant can finish assignments
B. Remind that force feeding is considered a form of physical abuse
C. Demonstrate how to feed the person and share tips for time management
D. Discuss the observations and the assistant's remarks with the nurse

54. Which rationale defines negligence when a person sustains a hot water burn while showering because the water temperature was not tested?
A. Nursing assistant did not act in a reasonable and careful manner.
B. Nursing assistant was acting outside scope of practice.
C. Nursing assistant did not ask for clarification and supervision.
D. Nursing assistant was focusing on the task, not the person.

55. In which circumstance would the nursing assistant be liable?
A. Nurse tells the nursing assistant to see if a pain pill relieved the patient's pain.
B. Nurse tells the nursing assistant that hygiene is deferred because of patient's condition.
C. Nursing assistant is correctly assisting a resident to eat, but he chokes and coughs.
D. Nursing assistant records the vital signs and weight on the wrong chart.

56. Which nursing assistant could be accused of committing slander?
A. Nursing assistant A puts a humiliating picture on the RN's locker.
B. Nursing assistant B spreads false rumors about a coworker.
C. Nursing assistant C expresses disgust when a person soils his pants.
D. Nursing assistant D tells a doctor to stop being so rude to everyone.

57. Which person would be considered a vulnerable adult?
A. A 60-year-old male who has a hard labor construction job
B. A 71-year-old female who lives alone in her own home
C. A 15-year-old girl who is living on the streets
D. A 35-year-old man who had a serious brain injury

58. Which nursing assistant has violated the Health Insurance Portability and Accountability Act of 1996 (HIPAA)?
    A. Nursing assistant A posts pictures of patients on social media.
    B. Nursing assistant B hands a doctor the patient's medical records.
    C. Nursing assistant C tells the nurse that the spouse has a question.
    D. Nursing assistant D logs off computer screen after entering vital signs.
59. What does the nursing assistant suspect upon overhearing a husband telling the wife that she is stupid and worthless?
    A. Stalking
    B. Psychological aggression
    C. Physical violence
    D. Sexual abuse
60. Which action by a member of the health care team is most likely to be investigated for false imprisonment?
    A. RN will not allow a confused resident to go outside by himself.
    B. Nursing assistant ties resident in a chair to prevent falls.
    C. Doctor closes door when doing a physical assessment of a resident.
    D. LPN/LVN asks residents to sit in the dayroom for an activity.

Match the Statements to the Correct Term

A. Rules for maintaining professional boundaries
B. Boundary signs
C. Boundary crossing
D. Boundary violation

61. ________ You keep the person's information confidential.
62. ________ You borrow money from a patient's family.
63. ________ You do not go out on a date with a current patient or resident or family members of a current patient or resident.
64. ________ You believe you are the only person who understands the person and their needs.
65. ________ You hug a person because they are crying.
66. ________ You tell a person about your personal relationships or problems.
67. ________ You select what you report and record. You do not give complete information.
68. ________ You trade assignments with other nursing assistants so you can provide the person's care.

Fill in the Blanks

69. Write out the meaning of the abbreviations
    A. CDC ____________________
    B. HIPAA ____________________
    C. IPV ____________________
70. If a nursing assistant causes unintentional harm to a person, it is called ____________________. If a nurse or other professional person causes unintentional harm, it is called ____________________.
71. Name the type of child abuse described in these examples.
    A. The child is injured mentally.
    ____
    B. The child was left in circumstances where the child suffered serious harm.
    ____
    C. The child has been kicked, burned, or bitten.
    ____
    D. The child has engaged in sexual activity with a family member.
    ____
    E. Drug activity has taken place when the child is present.
    ____
    F. Parents withhold praise and affection.
    ____

Optional Learning Exercises

Which Principle in the Code of Conduct for Nursing Assistants Applies to the Situations?

72. A nursing assistant has back pain and takes her mother's medication to treat it.
    ____
73. A nursing assistant is caring for a person her sister knows. The sister asks for information about the person. ____________________
74. A nursing assistant changes her lunchtime because her assigned patient needs unexpected care.
    ____
75. The nursing assistant tells the nurse that he recorded information on the wrong patient. ____________________
    ____
76. The nursing assistant knows that she is not allowed to care for very ill patients by herself.
    ____
77. The nursing assistant declines to start an IV when the nurse delegates that task.
    ____
    ____
78. The nursing assistant carefully cleans and stores the resident's dentures. ____________________
    ____

Use the FOCUS ON PRIDE Section to Complete These Statements and Then Use the Critical Thinking and Discussion Questions to Develop Your Ideas

79. Persons who must report abuse and neglect are called ____________________.
80. If you suspect a person is being abused, tell ____________________.
81. Accepting a task beyond the legal limits of your role can lead to ____________________.

Critical Thinking and Discussion Questions

You notice that the door to a resident's room is shut, when you enter the room, you see that the call bell has been removed. This resident frequently calls out, demands help, and never seems to be satisfied with the care that any of the staff provides. The resident has been rude toward staff.

82. Discuss the ethical and legal implications of the staff's reaction and behaviors toward this resident.
83. What can the staff do to improve the situation?

6 Student and Work Ethics

Fill in the Blanks: Key Terms

Burnout	Courtesy	Priority	Teamwork
Confidentiality	Gossip	Professionalism	Work ethics
Conflict	Harassment	Stress	

1. A clash between opposing interests or ideas is ________________________________.
2. ____________________ is job stress resulting in being physically or mentally exhausted.
3. Following laws, being ethical, having good work ethics, and having the skills to do your work is ________________________________.
4. The most important thing at the time is the ________________________________.
5. Trusting others with personal and private information is ________________________________.
6. ____________________ is behavior in the workplace.
7. ____________________ is to spread rumors or talk about the private matters of others.
8. The response or change in the body caused by any emotional, physical, social, or economic factor is ________________________________.
9. ____________________ is a polite, considerate, or helpful comment or act.
10. ____________________ means to trouble, torment, offend, or worry a person by one's behavior or comments.
11. When staff members work together as a group, it is called ________________________________.

Circle the Best Answer

12. Which situation would be a stressor for a new nursing assistant?
    A. Charge nurse assigns patients who have less complex needs.
    B. Experienced nursing assistant offers tips for time management.
    C. New nursing assistant is paired with a coworker during orientation.
    D. RN gives insufficient instructions to safely complete the task.
13. Which nursing assistant demonstrates good work ethics?
    A. Nursing assistant A does duties quickly and avoids interaction.
    B. Nursing assistant B shares personal religious beliefs at work.
    C. Nursing assistant C respects others and works well with others.
    D. Nursing assistant D has similar cultural beliefs as the residents.
14. Which nursing assistant action involves the use of good body mechanics?
    A. Turning a patient during a bed bath
    B. Opening a milk carton for a patient
    C. Recording a patient's vital signs
    D. Buttoning a patient's shirt
15. Which action will best help the nursing assistant to maintain a healthy weight?
    A. Limits intake of salty and sweet foods
    B. Eats fewer sweets during vacations and holidays
    C. Avoids consumption of fat and oils
    D. Balances calorie intake and energy needs
16. Adults need about ____________ hours of sleep daily.
    A. 7 to 8
    B. 10 to 11
    C. Less than 6
    D. 12
17. Which form of exercise is the best to start with when the student nursing assistant has spent the past several months sitting and studying?
    A. Hiking
    B. Running
    C. Cycling
    D. Walking
18. Which information about smoking odors applies to the use of cigarettes?
    A. The odors disappear quickly when the person finishes smoking.
    B. Smoke odors can be covered up by using mouthwash or gum.
    C. The smoker is the only one who can actually smell residual odor.
    D. Odors stay on a person's breath, hands, clothing, and hair.
19. Which rationale is the best explanation for healthcare workers to avoid using drugs or alcohol while on the job?
    A. Usage affects the safety of self and others.
    B. Intoxication creates personal disorganization.
    C. Drug usage is an unlawful criminal offense.
    D. Alcohol or drug use can result in termination.
20. Which rationale best supports the nursing assistant's decision to cover tattoos at work?
    A. May offend persons who are cared for, their families, or coworkers.
    B. Can become infected while caring for persons who have infections.
    C. May cause persons with dementia to hallucinate or become fearful.
    D. May increase risk of injuries because the skin has been pierced.

21. When working, the nursing assistant may wear
    A. Any type of clothing if it is clean and neat
    B. Wristwatch with a second hand
    C. Decorative pins that relate to healthcare
    D. Professionally applied nail polish
22. Which nursing assistant needs to be counseled to change and correct professional presentation?
    A. Nursing assistant A has a beard and mustache that is clean and trimmed.
    B. Nursing assistant B has long hair that is pulled back in a ponytail.
    C. Nursing assistant C uses fragrant smelling cologne and aftershave.
    D. Nursing assistant D wears a large black wristwatch with a second hand.
23. Which reason is the most important for a student or an experienced nursing assistant to plan good childcare and transportation in advance?
    A. Makes the instructor or employer like the nursing assistant
    B. Shows that nursing assistant is a responsible student or employee
    C. Prevents undue stress for nursing assistant and children
    D. Shows that nursing assistant is a conscientious parent
24. What is a common reason for losing a job?
    A. Lacking knowledge about a task
    B. Being absent or tardy
    C. Being disorganized or slow
    D. Lacking self-confidence
25. Which plan is best for a nursing assistant who is scheduled to begin work at 3:00 p.m.?
    A. To arrive by 2:30 p.m. and clock in just before 3:00 p.m.
    B. To arrive at exactly 3:00 p.m. and ready to work at 3:05 p.m.
    C. To arrive a few minutes early and be ready to work at 3:00 p.m.
    D. To arrive within a few minutes before or after 3:00 p.m.
26. Which of these statements would signal that the nursing assistant has a good attitude?
    A. "I will do that right away."
    B. "My turn is tomorrow."
    C. "That's not my patient."
    D. "It's not my fault."
27. Which action would the nursing assistant take to avoid being part of gossip?
    A. Remain quiet when people in the group are gossiping
    B. Talk about patients and their family only to coworkers
    C. Advise others that gossiping is unethical and grounds for dismissal
    D. Remove self from a situation where gossip is occurring
28. Which person or persons should be allowed to share the patient's information?
    A. Patient's immediate family
    B. Staff members involved in the care
    C. Coworkers who know the patient
    D. Healthcare facility administrators
29. Which rationale supports avoiding slang or swearing at work?
    A. This language can be offensive to others.
    B. Older people may not understand.
    C. Communication should be clear and precise.
    D. Usage violates the professional code of ethics.
30. Which nursing assistant is displaying a courtesy act?
    A. Nursing assistant A completes their work in a timely manner.
    B. Nursing assistant B arrives for work at the scheduled time.
    C. Nursing assistant C understands their job description.
    D. Nursing assistant D greets a family member who is visiting.
31. Which nursing assistant is demonstrating a behavior that is acceptable at work?
    A. Borrows a pen from the nurses' station to use at home
    B. Sells cookies for own child's school project
    C. Uses a cell phone during break to make a personal call
    D. Uses the copier to copy several textbook pages
32. What is the best rationale for the nursing assistant to tell the nurse when leaving and returning for breaks or lunch?
    A. Nurse expects you to behave professionally.
    B. Nurse will do your tasks while you are gone.
    C. Nurse knows when you are available.
    D. Nurse knows why your tasks are not done.
33. Which action will help the nursing assistant to maintain safety practices?
    A. Allow family members to enter the elevator first
    B. Follow the agency's rules, policies, and procedures
    C. Be mindful of the cost and usage of supplies
    D. Be cheerful, friendly, and have a good attitude
34. Which nursing assistant's action is contributing to unsafe practice?
    A. Nursing assistant A checks the stability of the person's walker.
    B. Nursing assistant B asks the nurse to clarify instructions for a task.
    C. Nursing assistant C forgets to take vital signs and no one notices.
    D. Nursing assistant D requests training to use a new piece of equipment.
35. Which factor is most important when planning and setting priorities for care?
    A. The nursing assistant's break times
    B. The person's needs
    C. The time of day
    D. The time scheduled by the nurse

36. Which circumstance would be considered a pleasant stressor?
    A. You and a coworker are competing for the same promotion.
    B. You plan a celebration for your grandmother's 85th birthday.
    C. You feel like you need to lose weight; so, you go on a diet.
    D. You experience stress every day because of work.
37. Which physical effects of stress are the most dangerous and life-threatening?
    A. High blood pressure, heart attack, strokes, ulcers
    B. Increased heart rate, faster and deeper breathing
    C. Anxiety, fear, anger, depression
    D. Headaches, insomnia, muscle tension
38. Which step is first when dealing with a conflict and trying to resolve the problem?
    A. Talk to the supervisor
    B. Collect the information
    C. Define the problem
    D. Identify possible solutions
39. Which outcome is most likely for a nursing assistant who is experiencing burnout?
    A. Caring for people becomes stressful and unsafe
    B. Can lead to quitting the job or changing occupations
    C. Can cause physical and mental health problems
    D. Will improve if the symptoms and discomfort are ignored
40. Which of these actions is harassment?
    A. Offending others with gestures or remarks
    B. Gossiping about a patient or his family
    C. Voicing doubts about the nurse's instructions
    D. Ignoring a conflict among staff members
41. What is best practice when you resign from a job?
    A. To give 1 week's notice
    B. To provide 2 weeks' notice
    C. To go part-time for 4 weeks
    D. To offer to stay 3 months
42. Which nursing assistant is displaying a courtesy?
    A. While working with Mr. Smith, nursing assistant A tries to understand and feel what it must be like to be paralyzed on one side.
    B. Nursing assistant B realizes that her basic care skills are good but recognizes the need to improve communication skills.
    C. Nursing assistant C works with attention to detail and performs delegated tasks quickly and efficiently.
    D. Nursing assistant D thanks coworkers when they help and remembers to wish residents happy birthday as appropriate.
43. Which nursing assistant is performing an action that contributes to patient safety?
    A. When Mrs. Gibson is upset and angry, nursing assistant A remembers to respect her feelings and to be kind.
    B. Nursing assistant B reports the blood pressure and temperature readings promptly and accurately to the nurse.
    C. Nursing assistant C realizes that giving care to residents is important and is excited about the work.
    D. Even though Mr. Acevado has different cultural and religious views, nursing assistant D values his feelings and beliefs.
44. Which nursing assistant is managing their personal matters in a professional way?
    A. Nursing assistant A had a terrible argument with family but makes an effort to be pleasant and cheerful at work.
    B. The nurse discusses a resident problem, and nursing assistant B knows to keep the information confidential.
    C. Nursing assistant C is assigned to give care to a resident and made sure that the care is done thoroughly and exactly as instructed.
    D. Nursing assistant D adjusts the schedule when the patient has a visitor and care cannot be given when planned.
45. Which nursing assistant is demonstrating the best example of good teamwork?
    A. Nursing assistant A knows that patients, residents, families, visitors, and coworkers depend on assistants to give safe and effective care.
    B. Nursing assistant B cheerfully offers to help when a coworker needs help to turn and bathe a resident.
    C. Nursing assistant C tries to do small things to make elderly residents happy or to find ways to ease their pain.
    D. Nursing assistant D plans for childcare in advance and makes sure that the car has enough gas.
46. Which situation would be considered a legitimate reason to be absent from class or clinical?
    A. You are unable to get a babysitter.
    B. You cannot afford to get your car fixed.
    C. You have a high fever and a cough.
    D. You have not finished your assignment.
47. What is the ethical or legal outcome if a nursing assistant leaves before the care of a home health patient is completed?
    A. Conflict that can be fixed with the problem-solving process
    B. Abandonment if no other healthcare staff arrives to assume care
    C. Discourteous to the patient, but not a serious legal error
    D. Acceptable if the patient can independently finish the care

48. Which type of bullying is occurring when other nursing assistants will not talk to or welcome a newly hired nursing assistant?
   A. Verbal bullying
   B. Cyberbullying
   C. Emotional bullying
   D. Prejudicial bullying
49. Which action would the nursing assistant take first when experiencing burnout because the schedule, assignments, or workloads are difficult?
   A. Report to the director of nursing because staffing is unsafe
   B. Seek a job at a facility that has better patient-to-caregiver ratio
   C. Ask other nursing assistants for support in protesting assignments
   D. Talk to the supervisor about the stress related to the workload
50. Which action would the nursing assistant take first if fever, muscle aches, and sore throat are noted upon waking up in the morning?
   A. Take an antipyretic and pain reliever and wear a mask at work
   B. Complete a written form and request an excused absence for illness
   C. Call supervisor as soon as possible before shift begins and explain illness
   D. Call primary care provider and obtain a note to be excused for illness
51. To promote teamwork and time management, which action would the nursing assistant take when another staff member is late or does not show up for work?
   A. Ask the nurse to call another nursing assistant and to come to work
   B. Care for assigned patients first and then help others if there is time
   C. Ask the nurse to list the most important tasks and care measures
   D. Contact administration because staffing shortages cause patient dissatisfaction
52. How does the nursing assistant interpret this coworker's comment, "It's not my turn. I did it yesterday."?
   A. Coworker does not like to do the required task.
   B. Coworker has burnout and is preparing to quit.
   C. Coworker should be advised to seek a new job.
   D. Coworker has a bad attitude and poor work ethic.
53. Which violation of ethical behavior has the nursing assistant made by repeating a comment that is untrue, or a comment that can hurt a person or family member?
   A. Harassment
   B. Gossiping
   C. Bullying
   D. Discourtesy
54. Which violation of the person's legal rights has the nursing assistant made when giving information about the person's illness to a family friend?
   A. Right to be free of harassment
   B. Right to be treated in a respectful way
   C. Right to feel safe and not threatened
   D. Right to privacy and confidentiality

Matching

Match the Related Health, Hygiene, or Appearance Factor With the Examples

A. Smoking	E. Exercise
B. Alcohol	F. Eyes
C. Diet	G. Body mechanics
D. Drugs	H. Sleep and rest

55. ________ Handwashing and good personal hygiene are needed to remove odors on your breath, hands, clothing, and hair.
56. ________ If you have fatigue, lack of energy, and irritability, it may mean you need more of this.
57. ________ You will feel better physically and mentally if you walk, run, swim, or bike regularly.
58. ________ Some of these affect thinking, feeling, behavior, and function. This may affect the person's safety.
59. ________ Avoid foods from the fats, oils, and sweets group. Also avoid salty foods and crash diets.
60. ________ You may not be able to read instructions and take measurements accurately if you do not have these checked.
61. ________ Practice this when you bend, carry heavy objects, and lift, move, and turn persons.
62. ________ This substance depresses the brain and affects thinking, balance, coordination, and mental alertness.

Fill in the Blanks

63. List factors to consider when setting priorities
   A. ____________________
   B. ____________________
   C. ____________________
   D. ____________________
   E. ____________________
   F. ____________________
   G. ____________________
64. What physical symptoms may occur when a person has stress?
   A. ____________________
   B. ____________________
   C. ____________________
   D. ____________________
   E. ____________________
65. When you have a conflict with another person, what are steps (in correct order) to take when resolving the conflict?
   A. Step 1 ____________________
   B. Step 2 ____________________
   C. Step 3 ____________________
   D. Step 4 ____________________
   E. Step 5 ____________________
   F. Step 6 ____________________

Optional Learning Exercises

66. Use Box 6.1 (p. 58), Professional Appearance, in the text to answer these questions.
    A. It is best to wear your name badge ______________________________
    B. Why should undergarments be the correct color for your skin tone? ______________________________
    C. You should follow the dress code for jewelry and not wear necklaces or dangling earrings because ______________________________.
    D. Chipped nail polish may provide a ______________________________.
    E. Perfume, cologne, or aftershave lotion scents may ______________________________.

Use the FOCUS ON PRIDE section to complete these statements and then use the critical thinking and discussion question to develop your ideas

67. When you greet patients and residents and politely introduce yourself, you are displaying good social ______________________________.
68. When you offer to help others, ask the nurse if you can help others, and return from breaks on time, you are displaying actions that help build a strong ______________________________.

Critical Thinking and Discussion Questions

69. Think back to the first time you entered the nursing school or the first time you walked into a new clinical unit. Discuss: How were you greeted? Who made you feel welcome? Were people friendly? How did they act toward you and each other? Did anyone offer to help? Why is it important to smile and greet people as they enter a new environment?
70. Two nursing assistants are having a conflict. Nursing assistant A who works the day shift says that nursing assistant B who works the night shift leaves patient care tasks undone. Nursing assistant B says that the comments are unfounded and unsubstantiated. Discuss how this conflict can be resolved.

7 The Person and Family

Fill in the Blanks: Key Terms

Bariatrics	Esteem	Obstetrics	Religion
Body language	Geriatrics	Optimal level of functioning	Self-actualization
Comatose	Holism	Paraphrasing	Self-esteem
Communication	Need	Pediatrics	Sexuality
Culture	Nonverbal communication	Psychiatry	Verbal communication
Disability	Obesity		

1. ____________________ is a weight that is higher than what is healthy for a given height.
2. __________________ is the characteristics of a group of people—language, values, beliefs, habits, likes, dislikes, customs—passed from one generation to the next.
3. Communication that uses spoken words is ______________________________________.
4. ______________________ is restating the person's message in your own words.
5. The branch of medicine concerned with the problems and diseases of old age and older persons is ________ ______________________________.
6. Messages sent through facial expressions, gestures, posture, hand and body movements, gait, eye contact, and appearance is ____________________________.
7. The field of medicine focused on the treatment and control of obesity is __________________________.
8. The worth, value, or opinion one has of a person is ______________________________________.
9. ______________________________________ is communication that does not use words.
10. The branch of medicine concerned with mental health disorders is ________________________________.
11. Thinking well of oneself and seeing oneself as useful and having value is ________________________.
12. ____________ is a concept that considers the whole person; physical, social, psychological, and spiritual parts are woven together and cannot be separated.
13. A lost, absent, or impaired physical or mental function is a _______________________________.
14. The branch of medicine concerned with the care of women during pregnancy, labor, and childbirth and for 6 to 8 weeks after birth is___________________.
15. __________________________ is experiencing one's potential.
16. _______________________ is the branch of medicine concerned with the growth, development, and care of children who range in age from newborn to teenagers.
17. A ________________________ is something necessary or desired for maintaining life and well-being.
18. ____________________________________ is an organized system of spiritual beliefs and practices.
19. A person who is unable to respond to stimuli is ______________________________________.
20. __________________________ is a person's desired level of ability.
21. The physical, emotional, social, cultural, and spiritual factors that affect a person's feelings, attitudes, and behaviors about one's gender identity and sexual behavior is _____________________________.
22. ______________________________ is the exchange of information—a message sent is received and correctly interpreted by the intended person.

Circle the Best Answer

23. Who is the most important person in the health-care relationship?
    A. The patient or resident
    B. The doctor
    C. The director of nursing
    D. The administrator
24. Which action would the nursing assistant take to identify and respect a person's gender identity?
    A. Focus on the person's priority physical problems or needs
    B. Address older persons by using Mr., Mrs., Ms., or Miss
    C. Ask what name and pronouns the person prefers
    D. Consider the whole person—physical, social, psychological, and spiritual
25. Which of these statements shows that the nursing assistant respects the person as a whole person?
    A. "I need to give a bath to the gallbladder."
    B. "The gentleman in 220 needs pain medication."
    C. "Mrs. Jones reports having pain in the right leg."
    D. "Room 235 needs to speak to the charge nurse."
26. Which basic needs have the highest priority?
    A. Physical needs
    B. Safety and security needs
    C. Love and belonging needs
    D. Self-esteem needs

27. Oxygen, food, water, elimination, rest, and shelter needs
    A. Relate to feeling safe from harm and danger
    B. Relate to the needs to live and survive
    C. Relate to love, closeness, and affection
    D. Relate to feelings of self-worth and value
28. Which rationale supports explaining routines to a resident who was recently admitted to a long-term care center?
    A. Helps the resident feel more secure
    B. Makes the resident feel important
    C. Fulfills the resident's legal rights
    D. Helps the resident to self-actualize
29. Why would the nursing assistant need to repeat information many times to a resident who is newly admitted to a long-term care nursing center?
    A. May have hearing or visual loss
    B. Is elderly and cannot remember details
    C. Is in a strange place with strange routines
    D. Is not able to understand what is being said
30. Who can meet love and belonging needs?
    A. The spouse or relationship partner
    B. Family, friends, and the health-care team
    C. The mother and the father
    D. Best friends if family is unavailable
31. Which need is rarely, if ever, totally met?
    A. Safety and security
    B. Love and belonging
    C. Self-actualization
    D. Self-esteem
32. Which action would the nursing assistant take when caring for a person from a different culture or religion?
    A. Judge the person's behavior according to the community norms
    B. Assume that standard health practices override cultural beliefs
    C. Give needed care and not worry about culture or religious beliefs
    D. Respect and accept the person's culture and religion
33. Which culture has a traditional belief that hot and cold imbalances cause disease?
    A. Mexican
    B. African
    C. American
    D. Russian
34. Which action would the nursing assistant take when a person does not follow all beliefs and practices of their religion?
    A. Assume that the person is not religious or that their beliefs are not important
    B. Should know and accept that each person is unique in beliefs and practices
    C. Call a spiritual leader to help the person follow the religious beliefs
    D. Should not be concerned about the person's religious beliefs when giving care
35. What is a common response that the nursing assistant may observe when a person becomes ill or disabled?
    A. They may be angry and say hurtful things
    B. They may ruminate about death and dying
    C. They want to be left alone with their thoughts
    D. They want someone to do everything for them
36. Which phrase would the nursing assistant use when preparing to help a new patient whose gender identity is unknown and could be male, female, a combination of male and female, or neither male nor female?
    A. "May I help you, sir to put on your shirt?"
    B. "May I help you, miss to get dressed?
    C. "May I help you, mam to adjust your clothes?"
    D. "May I help you with donning your clothes?"
37. Which of these persons would need to see a pediatrician?
    A. A woman who has breast cancer
    B. An older person with disorders of old age
    C. A 7-year-old child with pneumonia
    D. A person receiving kidney dialysis
38. Which type of care would be appropriate for a person who weighs 600 pounds?
    A. Subacute care
    B. Bariatric care
    C. Psychiatric care
    D. Geriatric care
39. Which of these persons is not a candidate for a long-term care center?
    A. A man who is recovering from minor surgery and needs antibiotics
    B. An alert person with a chronic illness who needs help with personal care
    C. A 63-year-old who is unable to care for himself due to dementia
    D. A person with a terminal illness who needs assistance with care
40. Which nursing assistant is not using effective communication?
    A. Nursing assistant A uses words that the person understands.
    B. Nursing assistant B communicates in a logical and orderly manner.
    C. Nursing assistant C gives specific facts and information to the person.
    D. Nursing assistant D uses medical terminology when talking to the person.
41. Which rule applies when using verbal communication?
    A. Ask one question at a time, then wait for an answer
    B. Speak in a loud voice so the person can hear you
    C. Ask several questions at a time, then wait for answers
    D. Use slang words to make the person comfortable

42. What is the best way to replace verbal communication when a person cannot speak?
 A. Use touch, as a nonverbal method
 B. Use body language to send messages
 C. Use gestures to communicate
 D. Use written messages on a pad of paper
43. Which action would the nursing assistant take when using touch to communicate?
 A. Be aware of the person's culture and practices about touch
 B. Write a note to the person to ask if touch is permitted
 C. Check the doctor's order to see if touch is ordered
 D. Touch the person before speaking or beginning care
44. Which of these would be a sign that Mrs. Green is not happy or is not feeling well?
 A. Her hair is well groomed.
 B. She has a slumped posture.
 C. She smiles when she is greeted.
 D. She has applied her makeup.
45. Which action shows that the nursing assistant is effectively listening?
 A. Focuses on what is said and observes nonverbals
 B. Leans back, relaxes, smiles, and crosses arms
 C. Frequently interrupts to offer suggestions
 D. Changes the subject to a more interesting topic
46. Mrs. Smith says, "I am used to farm life. I am not sure what I am supposed to do here at the nursing center." Which of these is paraphrasing?
 A. "The routine is different than what you are used to."
 B. "That's okay. We are here to help you with things."
 C. "Tell me about living on a farm and your daily life."
 D. "Can you explain what you mean? I don't understand."
47. Which communication technique is the nursing assistant using when saying "Mr. Davis, have you taken a shower this morning?"
 A. Paraphrasing his thoughts
 B. Asking a direct question
 C. Focusing his thoughts
 D. Asking an open-ended question
48. What is the purpose of asking an open-ended question?
 A. Invites the sharing of thoughts, feelings, or ideas
 B. Requests "yes" or "no" answer
 C. Ensures that the message is understood
 D. Response focuses conversation on a certain topic
49. Which communication technique would the nursing assistant use if trying to understand the person's message?
 A. Ask an open-ended question
 B. Clarify what was said
 C. Use nonverbal communication
 D. Use silence and wait
50. Mr. Parker often rambles and his thoughts wander while he tells long stories. Which communication technique would the nursing assistant use to find out if he had a bowel movement today?
 A. Make a clarifying statement
 B. Ask an open-ended question
 C. Ask a direct question
 D. Paraphrase his thoughts
51. What is the best action to use if the person takes long pauses between statements?
 A. Be present to demonstrate caring
 B. Try to cheer the person up by talking
 C. Leave the room and come back later
 D. Find another resident to talk with him
52. Which nursing assistant is using a barrier to communication?
 A. Nursing assistant A asks, "Are you saying that you want to go home?"
 B. Nursing assistant B says, "I think you should follow your doctor's advice."
 C. Nursing assistant C asks, "Would you like me to help you take a shower?"
 D. Nursing assistant D says, "I understand that this is upsetting for you."
53. Which action would the nursing assistant take when caring for a patient who is comatose?
 A. Explain purpose and steps of procedure
 B. Remain silent to avoid disturbing the patient
 C. Enter the room quietly to avoid startling the patient
 D. Speak in a loud voice so the patient can hear
54. Which action would the nursing assistant take when Mrs. Duke has visitors and it is time to give care?
 A. Tell the nurse that visitors are present and so care was deferred
 B. Politely ask the visitors to leave the room until care is finished
 C. Ask the visitors if they would like to participate in the care
 D. Tell the visitors that they must leave the nursing center
55. Which action would the nursing assistant take when a patient becomes very angry?
 A. Avoid the patient until they calm down
 B. Stay calm. Listen to their concerns
 C. Explain to the patient why being angry is hurtful
 D. Tell the patient that nursing assistants have rights too
56. If a person hits, pinches, or bites during care, what is the first action that a nursing assistant should take?
 A. Protect the person, others, and self from harm
 B. Write a report and explain the incident to the nurse
 C. Firmly tell the person to stop being so aggressive
 D. Ask for help when assigned to care for the person

57. What is the meaning of touching the head for people from China?
    A. Some would feel embarrassed.
    B. Some would feel comforted.
    C. Some would consider it a friendly gesture.
    D. Some would think it is rude behavior.
58. What would a male family member who is East India Hindu do to greet people?
    A. He will lightly touch hands.
    B. He will clasp his hands together and bow.
    C. He will hug or handhold.
    D. He will give a long, firm handshake.
59. What should the nursing assistant do first when caring for a person who cannot speak or hear?
    A. Find someone on the staff who knows sign language to help
    B. Ask the nurse or check the care plan for the communication method
    C. Get a pad of paper and a felt pen and write messages in large block letters
    D. Get a picture board and point at the figures that convey the message
60. Which outcome is the most serious when a nursing assistant is not listening to the person as care is provided?
    A. Person feels unnoticed and disrespected, and this decreases their self-esteem.
    B. Person feels that the nursing assistant does not like them, so they stop talking.
    C. Person's requests are ignored, and they make an official complaint.
    D. Person has pain and other symptoms that do not get reported to the nurse.
61. Which nursing assistant is performing an action that supports the social part of the whole person?
    A. Nursing assistant A assists the person with grooming and hygiene.
    B. Nursing assistant B tells the nurse that the person seems upset.
    C. Nursing assistant C provides privacy when person wants to meditate.
    D. Nursing assistant D invites the person to join in a group game.
62. Which person is demonstrating the need for love and belonging according to Maslow's theory?
    A. Elderly person is confused and expresses feelings of fear and persecution.
    B. Teenage chooses to go out with friends despite having a fever and cough.
    C. Student nursing assistant feels successful upon passing a skills test.
    D. Nurse decides to get extra sleep and rest because work has been very hectic.
63. Which communication technique would the nursing assistant use if a person can hear but cannot speak or read?
    A. Use sign language
    B. Use brief messages
    C. Use a language translator
    D. Use "yes or no" questions
64. Which nursing assistant is using the guidelines for good communication?
    A. Nursing assistant A smiles a lot and chats about self.
    B. Nursing assistant B frequently offers own opinions.
    C. Nursing assistant C faces the person during the conversation.
    D. Nursing assistant D makes the bed and cleans up while talking.

Fill in the Blanks

65. Name the culture that may follow the listed belief or custom.
    A. ________________ or ________________ Food and medicine is given to restore the hot-cold balance.
    B. ______________________ Folk healers called *yerbero* may use herbs and spices to prevent or cure disease.
    C. ________________________ and __________ Eye contact is impolite and an invasion of privacy.
    D. ______________________ Eyes are rolled upward to express disapproval.
    E. ________________________ Facial expressions may mean the opposite of what the person is feeling. Negative emotions may be concealed with a smile.
66. Nonverbal communication messages reflect a person's ________________ more accurately than words do.
67. Body language is nonverbal communication that is shown with
    A. ______________________________
    B. ______________________________
    C. ______________________________
    D. ______________________________
    E. ______________________________
    F. ______________________________
    G. ______________________________
68. List nine communication barriers
    A. ______________________________
    B. ______________________________
    C. ______________________________
    D. ______________________________
    E. ______________________________
    F. ______________________________
    G. ______________________________
    H. ______________________________
    I. ______________________________

Crossword

Fill in the crossword by answering the clues below with the words from this list

Clarifying	Esteem	Nonverbal	Touch
Comatose	Focusing	Paraphrasing	Verbal
Culture	Holism	Silence	
Direct	Need		

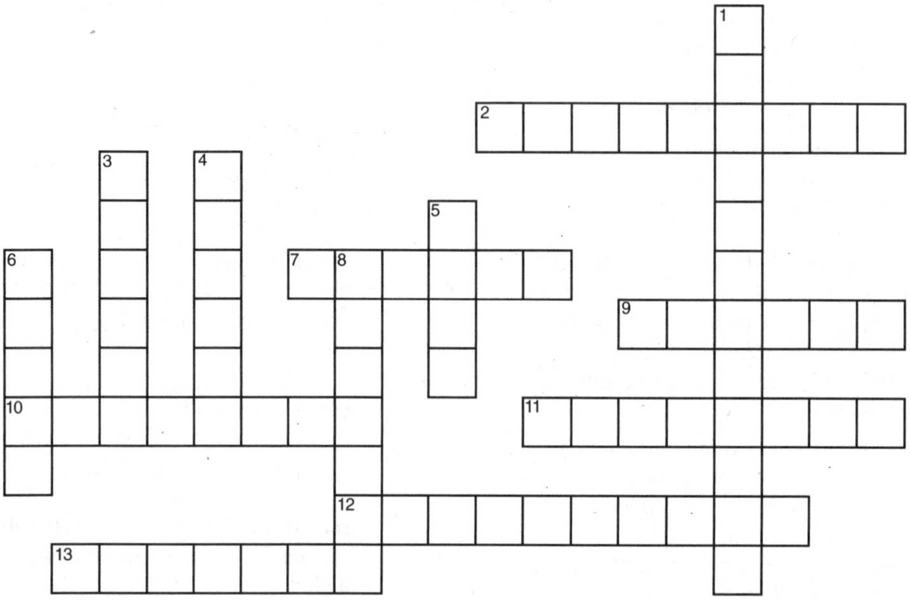

Across

2. Communication expressed with gestures, facial expressions, posture, body movements, touch, and smell
7. The worth, value, or opinion one has of a person
9. Communication in which the words are spoken
10. An unconscious person who cannot respond to others
11. A communication method that is useful when a person rambles or wanders in thought
12. A communication method in which you can ask the person to repeat the message, say you do not understand, or restate the message
13. The characteristics of a group of people—language, values, beliefs, habits, likes, dislikes, customs—passed from one generation to another

Down

1. Restating the person's message in your own words
3. A concept that considers the whole person—physical, social, psychological, and spiritual parts
4. A question that focuses on certain information and may require a "yes" or "no" answer or more information
5. Something necessary or desired for maintaining life and mental well-being
6. Nonverbal communication that conveys comfort, caring, loving, affection, interest, concern, and reassurance
8. Communicating by not saying anything

Optional Learning Exercises

Basic Needs

Physical Needs

69. What are the six physical needs required for survival?
    A. ___
    B. ___
    C. ___
    D. ___
    E. ___
    F. ___
70. Give one example of how a serious problem with urinary elimination could cause death.
    ___

Safety and Security

71. Safety and security needs relate to protection from
    A. ___
    B. ___
    C. ___
72. You can help meet safety and security needs when you explain the following for every task.
    A. ___
    B. ___
    C. ___
    D. ___

Love and Belonging

73. The need for love and belonging relates to
    A. ___
    B. ___
    C. ___

Self-Esteem

74. Self-esteem means to
    A. Think ___
    B. See ___
    C. See oneself as having ___
75. Why is it important to encourage residents to do as much as possible for themselves? ___
    ___

Self-Actualization

76. What does self-actualization involve?
    A. ___
    B. ___
    C. ___

Culture and Religion Practices

Religion

77. How can you help a resident observe religious practices if services are held in the nursing center?
    ___
78. If the resident wants a spiritual leader or advisor to visit in the room, you should tell the nurse and
    A. ___
    B. ___
    C. ___

Cultural Health-Care Beliefs

79. List three examples of "hot" conditions according health beliefs for people from Mexico.
    A. ___
    B. ___
    C. ___

Cultural Sick Practices

80. How are Vietnamese folk practices used to treat these illnesses?
    A. Common cold ___
    B. Headache and sore throat ___
81. An elderly person from ___ may believe that an infection (caused by yang forces) can be treated with green vegetables and fruits (foods with yin qualities).

Cultural Touch Practices

82. People from ___
    ___ do not usually touch each other while speaking.
83. A hug or handholding while walking is common among close friends may be observed in ___culture.

Eye Contact Practices

84. ___ eye contact may be avoided in African American cultures.
85. Eye contact in American culture signals ___
    ___.

Using Communication Methods

You have completed your duties for the morning and have some free time. Mr. Harry Donal is a resident of the nursing center. He rarely has visitors and you try to spend time with him when you can. Answer the following questions about communication techniques you use when you visit with Mr. Donal.

86. You ___ Mr. Donal. Smile and show that you are happy to see him.
87. You sit in a chair next to Mr. Donal so you can see each other. This position will help you to have better
    ___.
88. You should lean ___ Mr. Donal to show interest.
89. Mr. Donal says, "I know this is the best place for me but I miss my flower garden at home." You respond, "You miss your home." This is an example of ___
    ___.
90. You ask Mr. Donal, "You told me you did not sleep well last night. Can you tell me what was happening?" He replies, "There was a lot of noise in the hall." This is an example of a ___
    ___ question.
91. You say to Mr. Donal, "Tell me about your flower garden at home." This is an ___ question.
92. When you say, "Can you explain what that means?" you are asking a person to ___.

93. Mr. Donal says he "hurts all over" and then begins to talk about the weather. You say, "Tell me more about where you hurt. You said you hurt all over." This statement helps in ______________________ the topic.
94. Mr. Donal begins to cry when he talks about his flower garden. How can you show caring and respect for his situation and feelings? ______________________ ______________________.
95. When Mr. Donal begins to cry, you quickly begin to talk about the activities planned this morning. Changing the subject is a ______________________ ______________________.

Use the FOCUS ON PRIDE section to complete these statements and then use the critical thinking and discussion questions to develop your ideas

96. To promote a sense of identity, worth, and belonging when communicating, you should
    A. ______________________
    B. ______________________
    C. ______________________
    D. ______________________
    E. ______________________
    F. ______________________

Critical Thinking and Discussion Questions

Think back to a conversation that you recently had with someone who needed you to listen, for example, your child was trying to explain a school project, or a friend just ended a serious romantic relationship. Cite examples of good (attentive listening, making good eye contact, asking questions, using open-ended questions, or paraphrasing) and poor (changing the subject, giving opinions, talking too much, failure to listen, or pat answers) communication that you used during the conversation with your child or friend.

97. What can you do to improve?

You are assigned to take care of a resident who has recently moved into the long-term care facility. During the shift, the resident calls you repeatedly and orders you around using a commanding tone. Whatever you do, does not seem to please the resident and she asks you to do things over and over. At the end of the day, you feel exhausted and frustrated. The next day you are assigned to the same resident and her behavior is the same.

98. A. Discuss some of the reasons that may be causing the resident to be so demanding.
    B. What can you do to improve the care experience for the resident and yourself?

8 Health Team Communications

Fill in the Blanks: Key Terms

Analysis	Evaluation	Nursing intervention	Progress note
Assessment	Implementation	Nursing process	Recording
Electronic health record	Medical record	Observation	Reporting
End-of-shift report	Nursing care plan (care plan)	Planning	Subjective data

1. An electronic version of a person's medical record is the ____________________, also called electronic medical record.
2. Interpreting data and identifying problems is ____.
3. ________________________________ describes the care given and the person's response and progress.
4. The legal account of a person's condition and response to treatment and care is the ______________ ______________________, also referred to as the chart.
5. ________________________ are things a person tells you about that you cannot observe through your senses, symptoms.
6. The method RNs use to plan and deliver nursing care is the ____________________________________.
7. ________________________________ is to perform or carry out measures in the care plan, a step in the nursing process.
8. ____ is the written account of care and observations.
9. A written guide about the person's nursing care is the ____.
10. ___________________________ is collecting information about the person, a step in the nursing process.
11. A report that the nurse gives at the end of the shift to the oncoming staff is ____________________________.
12. Using the senses of sight, hearing, touch, and smell to collect information is ___________________________.
13. The verbal account of care and observations is ____.
14. A step in the nursing process that is used to measure if goals in the planning step were met is called ____.
15. __________________________ is setting priorities and goals, a step in the nursing process.
16. A ______________________________ is an action or measure taken by the nursing team to help the person reach a goal.

Circle the Best Answer

17. Which question would the nursing assistant ask for the basic observation of ability to respond?
    A. What is your name?
    B. What would you like for breakfast?
    C. Where is your cane?
    D. What would you like to do today?
18. Which observation is a sign that the nursing assistant would report to the nurse?
    A. Patient reports painful urination.
    B. Patient has a feeling of urgency.
    C. Urine has a foul smell and a dark color.
    D. Patient wants assistance to go to the bathroom.
19. Which subjective data are the most important for the nursing assistant to report to the nurse?
    A. Patient reports severe left-sided chest pain.
    B. Patient reports dizziness when standing up.
    C. Patient says arm feels numb after lying on it.
    D. Patient says he can't hear very well this morning.
20. Which finding is a symptom that the nursing assistant would report to the nurse?
    A. Patient's skin is cool to the touch.
    B. Patient reports feeling very nauseated.
    C. Patient's blood pressure is higher than usual.
    D. Patient vomits a large amount of green liquid.
21. Which objective data are the most important for the nursing assistant to report to the nurse?
    A. Respiratory rate is 50 breaths per minute.
    B. Patient is sleeping longer than usual.
    C. Pulse rate is 80 beats per minute.
    D. Skin feels hot to the touch.
22. In which section of the medical record will the nursing assistants do most of the recording for their assigned tasks?
    A. Admission records
    B. Therapy records
    C. Flow sheets and graphic sheets
    D. Progress notes
23. Which member of the healthcare team needs a reminder about inappropriate sharing of patient information?
    A. Nurse relates a personal story about the patient and his family.
    B. Nursing assistant reports that the patient's vital signs are recorded.
    C. Nursing assistant informs the nurse that patient is reporting pain.
    D. Doctor informs the team that the patient is not responding to therapy.
24. What would the nurse think when a nursing assistant says, "Mr. Jones ate a small amount of his lunch?"
    A. Mr. Jones ate one-half of his meal.
    B. Mr. Jones ate two or three bites of food.
    C. Mr. Jones ate between 0% and 25% of his meal.
    D. Mr. Jones ate but exact amount is unknown.

25. Which action would the nursing assistant take when giving information to another health team member?
    A. Be brief and concise and include important details.
    B. Be professional and use new or unfamiliar medical terminology.
    C. Give many details, so that nothing is overlooked.
    D. Use general phases, such as "He's doing great."
26. The medical record or chart is
    A. A temporary tool for staff
    B. Discarded when the person dies
    C. A permanent legal document
    D. Given to the person upon discharge
27. Which information can be found in the person's chart?
    A. Person's selections from the daily menu
    B. Person's current and previous X-ray reports
    C. Outstanding debt that the person owes the agency
    D. History of person bring lawsuits against staff
28. Which responsibility, related to the medical records, applies to the nursing assistant?
    A. May read the medical records in all healthcare agencies
    B. Is never allowed to read the person's medical records
    C. Must know the agency policy before reading the medical records
    D. Can tell the person and family what is in the medical records
29. Which action would the nursing assistant take if a person asks to see their record?
    A. Advise that the nurse will be notified about the request
    B. Check agency policy about letting a person see the chart
    C. Give the chart to the person's legal representative
    D. Make a photocopy of the chart for the person
30. Which information is contained in the admission record?
    A. Doctor's orders for medications and treatments
    B. Name, birth date, age, and biological sex of the person
    C. Test results, such as laboratory and radiology
    D. Special diet information related to religion or culture
31. When is the health history completed?
    A. When the person is discharged.
    B. When the person is admitted.
    C. When the doctor has time.
    D. When the person has time.
32. In which section of the chart would the nursing assistant find the patient's reason for seeking health care?
    A. Health history
    B. Graphic sheet
    C. Progress notes
    D. Kardex
33. In which area of the chart, would the nursing assistant record the vital signs taken during the shift?
    A. Health history
    B. Nurses notes
    C. Flow sheet
    D. Progress notes
34. In long-term care, what is the nursing assistant's role in making sure that the medical record reflects the requirements of the Centers for Medicare and Medicaid?
    A. On the monthly summary, the nursing assistant records actions for each shift.
    B. Nursing assistant summarizes actions for the nurse every 3 months.
    C. Nursing assistant contributes to the written summary every 3 months.
    D. On the weekly record, the nursing assistant records on the day care is given.
35. In which setting, is the nursing assistant more likely to document on a weekly care record on the day care was given?
    A. Home care
    B. Hospital
    C. Long-term care
    D. Special care unit
36. What is the purpose of the Kardex?
    A. Used to record visits by health team members
    B. A sheet used to record vital signs taken every 15 minutes
    C. A record of the person's family history
    D. A quick, concise source of information about the person
37. What is the primary purpose of the nursing process?
    A. The doctor communicates orders for diagnosis and treatment.
    B. Care is planned and delivered according to the person's needs.
    C. Care tasks are described in detail with step-by-step instructions.
    D. Process describes tasks that can delegated to nursing assistants.
38. Which member of the health-care team is correctly using and safeguarding electronic communications?
    A. Nursing assistant changes password at recommended intervals.
    B. Doctor leaves the computer unattended while talking to the patient.
    C. Student nursing assistant takes a printout to complete homework assignments.
    D. Nurse uses the unit computer to send personal email messages.
39. What is the nursing assistant's role in nursing process?
    A. Nursing assistant reports observations to the nurse.
    B. Nursing assistant plans care and develops the care plan.
    C. Nursing assistant assesses symptoms as instructed by the nurse.
    D. Nursing assistant chooses tasks according to the care plan.
40. Which observation displays the sense of hearing?
    A. Nursing assistant notices that the person's ankle is swollen.
    B. Nursing assistant uses a stethoscope to take blood pressure.
    C. Nursing assistant smells a strong odor on the person's breath.
    D. Nursing assistant touches a person's wrist to take a pulse.

41. In which step of the nursing process is the nursing assistant contributing when noticing and reporting to the nurse that the person feels hot to the touch?
    A. Assessment of the person
    B. Planning how to reduce fever
    C. Ensuring that the person is comfortable
    D. Evaluating the person's response to touch
42. Which of these is an example of objective data that the nursing assistant can collect?
    A. Mrs. Hewitt complains of pain and nausea.
    B. Mr. Stewart says he has a dull ache in his stomach.
    C. While taking Mrs. Jensen's pulse, it is noted that she is very pale.
    D. Mrs. Murano says she is tired because she could not sleep last night.
43. Which action would the nursing assistant take upon noticing that Mr. Young's blood pressure is 50 points higher than it was in the morning?
    A. Chart the results on the flow sheet
    B. Report the difference at the end of the shift
    C. Tell the nurse immediately
    D. Ask Mr. Young if he feels okay
44. In which circumstance is a Minimum Data Set (MDS) required by Centers for Medicare and Medicaid Services (CMS)?
    A. In long-term nursing centers
    B. In all health-care settings
    C. In acute care settings
    D. In home care settings
45. What is an important role for the nursing assistants related to the MDS?
    A. Be courtesy and polite and respond to the nurses' requests
    B. Report changes in the level of assistance required for ADLs
    C. Attend and actively contribute at the care conferences
    D. Record and report vital signs promptly and accurately
46. To clarify duties, which question would the nursing assistant ask the nurse after reading in the care plan that the person needs help with hygiene and bathing?
    A. "When should I help the person with hygiene?"
    B. "Which part of the hygiene can the person do independently?"
    C. "Are the supplies in the person's room?"
    D. "Should I explain my actions to the person?"
47. What does the nursing assistant say first to a caller when assigned to answer the unit phone while the nurse is taking care of a critically ill patient?
    A. "Let me give you a phone number to call back in case we are disconnected."
    B. "What is your name and phone number? The nurse will your return call."
    C. "I'm sorry we are having an emergency, could you call back later?"
    D. "Hello, 5th floor nurse's station, this is Ms. Jones, nursing assistant."
48. Which nursing assistant is contributing to the planning step of the nursing process?
    A. Nursing assistant A tells the nurse that the person prefers to shower in the evening.
    B. Nursing assistant B assists the person to ambulate in the hallway after lunch.
    C. Nursing assistant C tells the nurse that the person ate 75% of her breakfast.
    D. Nursing assistant D reports that the person is following the toilet schedule.
49. What is the most important reason for nursing assistants to attend care conferences?
    A. Conferences are educational because the nurses teach new skills.
    B. Attendance demonstrates interest and commitment to the job and agency.
    C. Nursing assistants spend time caring for people and make many observations.
    D. Conferences are required for funding from Medicare and Medicaid.
50. What is the purpose of the comprehensive care plan, which is required by the CMS?
    A. Conference held to update the care plan
    B. Written guide about the person's care
    C. Discussion about problems that affect the care
    D. Conference held regularly to review care plans
51. What part of the nursing process is being carried out when you give personal care to a person?
    A. Assessing
    B. Planning
    C. Implementation
    D. Evaluation
52. Which step of the nursing process is the nursing assistant contributing to by reporting to the nurse that the person continues to need help with brushing his teeth, when the patient's goal is to achieve independence with morning hygiene?
    A. Assessing
    B. Planning
    C. Implementation
    D. Evaluation
53. When is the nursing assistant expected to report information about the person?
    A. Only at the end of the shift
    B. When a change in condition occurs
    C. Each time care is given
    D. Only if the nurse asks for a report
54. The oncoming staff is listening to the end-of-shift report, who should answer the call lights?
    A. The oncoming staff will answer when the report is finished.
    B. The staff going off duty will answer so the report can continue.
    C. The lights are answered by the first person who is available.
    D. The nurse will assign one nursing assistant to answer all lights.

55. Below is a section of the assignment sheet. When would the nursing assistant obtain Ms. Jones' weight?

Room # 202 Name: Mary Jones ID Number: S1514491530
Date of birth: 11/04/1934 VS: Daily at 0700 T ______
P ______ R ______ BP ______
Wt: Weekly (Monday at 0700) Intake ______________
Output ______________ BM ____________ Bath________
or Shower____

A. Every day at 0700
B. Every Monday at 0700
C. After the shower
D. At Ms. Jones' request

56. If the nursing assistant is recording using the 24-hour clock, which of these is correct?
A. 1 AM
B. 0100 PM
C. 1300
D. 2500

57. Which action would the nursing assistant take when given a computer password?
A. Must never change or alter it in anyway
B. Can share it with the nursing supervisor
C. Should never tell anyone the password
D. Can use a friend's password with their permission

58. Which staff member has made an error in using the agency computer?
A. Laboratory technician sends the blood work results to the nursing unit.
B. Physician prints outs an X-ray report, reads it, and then shreds it.
C. Nurse updates the family on the patient's condition via email.
D. Nursing assistant enters vital sign data for assigned patients.

59. Which staff member has created a potential lack of privacy?
A. Nurse A responds to a call light and leaves the computer screen on.
B. Social worker changes their password every 3 to 4 months.
C. Nursing assistant puts their assignment worksheets through the shredder.
D. Nursing assistant logs off as soon as they are done using the computer.

60. In which circumstance when answering the telephone, would the nursing assistant avoid putting the caller on hold?
A. Person has an emergency
B. Caller is a physician
C. Call needs to be transferred
D. Everyone is too busy

61. Which action would the nursing assistant take when answering the patient's phone during a home care visit?
A. Give name, title, and location.
B. Simply answer with "Hello"
C. Explain role as the home care assistant
D. Hand the receiver to whoever lives in the home

62. Which action would the nursing assistant take when the care plan indicates that the person is unable to independently complete hygiene because he is having trouble remembering how to do it?
A. Do everything for him
B. Teach him how to perform hygiene
C. Coach him through steps as needed
D. Tell the nurse that the patient is having trouble

Fill in the Blanks

63. Write out the meaning of the abbreviations
A. ADL ______________________________
B. BMs ______________________________
C. CAA ______________________________
D. CMS ______________________________
E. EHR ______________________________
F. EMR ______________________________
G. EPHI; ePHI ______________________________
H. PHI ______________________________
I. MDS ______________________________
J. OASIS ______________________________

64. When the nursing assistant makes observations while giving care, what senses are used?
A. ______________________________
B. ______________________________
C. ______________________________
D. ______________________________

65. Name the body system or other area that the nursing assistant is observing in each of these examples (from Box 8.3, p. 90, Basic Observations).
A. Is the abdomen firm or soft?
____
B. Is the person sensitive to bright lights?
____
C. Are sores or reddened areas present?
____
D. What is the frequency of the person's breathing?
____
E. Can the person bathe without help?
____
F. Is the person eating and drinking?
____
G. What is the position of comfort?
____
H. Does the person answer questions correctly?
____
I. Does the person report stiff or painful joints?
____

66. When planning care, needs that are required for life and survival must be met before ______________________________.

67. List at least six observations that the nursing assistant needs to immediately report to the nurse.
    A. ____________________
    B. ____________________
    C. ____________________
    D. ____________________
    E. ____________________
    F. ____________________
68. What information can be found on the assignment sheet?
    A. ____________________
    B. ____________________
    C. ____________________
69. How does the nursing assistant's actions assist the nurse in the nursing process?
    A. The nurse uses the nursing assistant's observations for ____________________, planning, and evaluation.
    B. In the ____________________ step, the nursing assistant performs nursing actions and measures.
70. Next to each time, write the military time using the 24-hour clock. Use the figure as a guide.

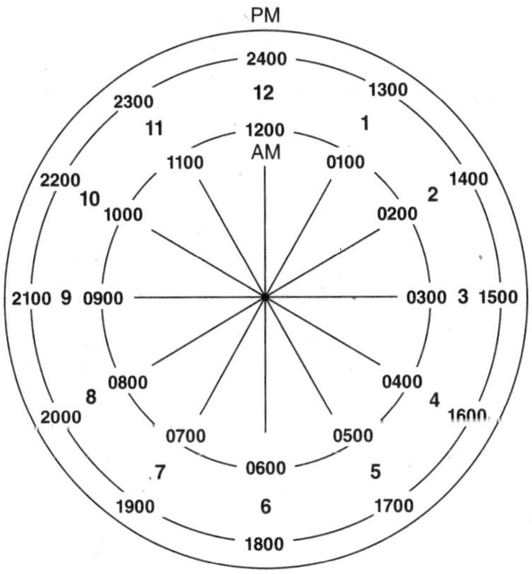

A.	_______	11:00 AM	G.	_______	3:00 AM
B.	_______	8:00 AM	H.	_______	4:50 AM
C.	_______	4:00 PM	I.	_______	5:30 PM
D.	_______	7:30 AM	J.	_______	10:45 PM
E.	_______	6:45 PM	K.	_______	11:55 PM
F.	_______	12 Noon	L.	_______	9:15 PM

71. Convert the times from military time to standard time
    A. 0200 = ____________________ AM/PM
    B. 2030 = ____________________ AM/PM
    C. 0500 = ____________________ AM/PM
    D. 0930 = ____________________ AM/PM
    E. 1545 = ____________________ AM/PM
    F. 2345 = ____________________ AM/PM
    G. 0600 = ____________________ AM/PM
    H. 1145 = ____________________ AM/PM
    I. 1800 = ____________________ AM/PM
    J. 2200 = ____________________ AM/PM
72. Mr. Duke is having trouble feeding himself because of weakness in the right arm and he is right-hand dominant. Briefly describe how you might help Mr. Duke. ____________________

Optional Learning Exercises

Case Study

Mr. Larsen was admitted to a subacute care center after his abdominal surgery 1 week ago. This morning, the nursing assistant gave Mr. Larsen a shower and assisted him to sit in a comfortable chair. The nursing assistant noticed that he sat there very still and held his arms across his abdomen. He asked for a pillow and held it tightly against his abdomen.

73. Imagine how Mr. Larsen would answer these questions.
    A. What would Mr. Larsen like the nursing assistant to ask?
    ____
    B. How would Mr. Larsen communicate his feelings to the nursing assistant?
    ____
    C. How could Mr. Larsen let the nursing assistant know that he was having pain without directly saying anything?
    ____
74. Imagine how the nursing assistant would answer these questions.
    A. As the nursing assistant, what observations would be important to make about Mr. Larsen?
    ____
    B. What questions would the nursing assistant ask Mr. Larsen?
    ____
    C. What nonverbal communication would give the nursing assistant information about Mr. Larsen?
    ____

Case Study
Mrs. Miller was just admitted to the health-care center and the nursing assistant last worked 3 days ago. The nursing assistant has just started the shift and has been assigned to Mrs. Miller.

75. What information would the nursing assistant need to know before giving care?
____
____
____

Use the FOCUS ON PRIDE Section to Complete the Statements

76. The person has the right to take part in the care ______________________________.

77. ______________________________ action can be taken against persons who record false information.

Review the Assignment Sheet and Use the Principles of Communication and Teamwork to Answer the Questions

Room # 501 A Name: Mrs. Ann Lopez
ID Number: S1514491530 Date of birth: 11/04/1934
VS: Daily at 0700 T ______ P ______ R ______ BP ______
Wt: Weekly (Monday at 0700) Intake __________
Output __________ BM _______ Bath: Portable tub
Functional status/care measures and procedures
- Total assist with ADL
- Stand-pivot transfers
- Uses w/c
- Incontinent of bowel and bladder – uses briefs
- Passive ROM exercises to extremities twice daily
- Turn and re-position q2h when in bed
- Wears eyeglasses and dentures
- Diet: High fiber (total assist)

78. It is 0650 on Tuesday morning. You are assigned to care for Ms. Lopez. Review the assignment sheet and answer the following questions:
A. What will you do first?
____
____
____
B. What (if anything) do you need to clarify with the nurse?
____
____
____
C. What do you need help with?
____
____
____

9 Medical Terminology

Fill in the Blanks: Key Terms

Anterior (ventral)
Deep
Distal
Lateral
Medial
Posterior (dorsal)
Prefix
Proximal
Suffix
Superficial

1. ______________________ is at or near the middle or midline of the body or body part.
2. ______________________ is at or toward the back of the body or body part.
3. At or toward the front of the body or body part is ______________________.
4. The part nearest to the center or the point of origin is ______________________.
5. At the side of the body or body part is ______________________.
6. ______________________ is the part farthest from the center or from the point of attachment.
7. A ______________ is at the beginning of a word; it changes the meaning of the word.
8. On the surface is ______________________.
9. Below the surface is ______________________.
10. A ___________ is at the end of a word; it changes the meaning of the word.

Circle the Best Answer

11. Which task has the priority?
    A. Patient needs to drink extra water after meals.
    B. Patient is assisted to the bathroom prn.
    C. Nurse says collect a specimen for an urinalysis.
    D. Doctor asks for a set of vital signs stat.
12. Which position is a side-lying position?
    A. Dorsal
    B. Lateral
    C. Anterior
    D. Posterior
13. Which term describes the position of the foot in relation to the knee?
    A. Inferior to
    B. Anterior to
    C. Posterior to
    D. Superior to
14. What will the nursing assistant tell the nurse if a person points to the left side of the body below the umbilicus and says that he has pain?
    A. Person has pain in the right upper quadrant.
    B. Person has pain in the left lower quadrant.
    C. Person has pain in the left upper quadrant.
    D. Person has pain in the right lower quadrant.
15. Which term describes the position of the fingers in relation to the hand?
    A. Medial
    B. Distal
    C. Proximal
    D. Posterior
16. Which type of assistance would the nursing assistant be prepared to offer for a person who has paraplegia?
    A. Opening a milk carton
    B. Reminding to use the hearing aid
    C. Assisting in moving the legs
    D. Fastening the shirt and pants
17. What does the nursing assistant watch for when the nurse says that the patient has occasional episodes of cyanosis that need to be reported?
    A. Bluish hue to the skin
    B. Tremors in the hands
    C. Difficulty swallowing
    D. Blood in the urine
18. Which equipment will the nursing assistant obtain when caring for a person who has fecal incontinence?
    A. Disposable pads for the bed
    B. Blood pressure cuff
    C. Measurement cylinder
    D. Thermometer
19. Which type of pain and discomfort is the person likely to report if they have a gastrointestinal disorder?
    A. Headache
    B. Joint stiffness
    C. Abdominal pain
    D. Backache
20. Which vital sign data indicate that the person is having tachycardia?
    A. 130/80 mm Hg
    B. 103 °F (39.4°C)
    C. 40 breaths/min
    D. 130 beats/min
21. What does the nursing assistant watch for when the nurse says to immediately report hematemesis?
    A. Blood in the person's vomit
    B. Redness and warmth of the skin
    C. Bleeding at a wound site
    D. Red or pinkish urine
22. Which patient is most likely to need a glucometer measurement?
    A. Patient has a tracheostomy.
    B. Patient has a urinary tract infection.
    C. Patient had a stroke last year.
    D. Patient has diabetes mellitus.
23. Which type of equipment will the nursing assistant use to protect self in caring for a person who has dermatitis?
    A. Radiation badge
    B. Eyeshield
    C. Gloves
    D. Mask
24. Which type of equipment will the nursing assistant obtain for a person who has rhinorrhea?
    A. Stethoscope
    B. Box of tissues
    C. Extra laundry bags
    D. Otoscope

25. Which question would the nursing assistant ask to clarify duties when the nurse says that the person has risk for polyuria?
    A. Should I apply the gait belt for ambulation?
    B. How often should I measure the urine output?
    C. How often should I perform range-of-motion?
    D. Should I cut up the food in smaller bites?
26. Which action would the nursing assistant take when caring for a person who has dysphagia?
    A. Allow extra time for communication
    B. Ask the nurse for feeding instructions
    C. Assist the person to the bathroom
    D. Watch for vaginal bleeding
27. Which condition is the most serious and needs to be immediately reported?
    A. Dyspnea
    B. Polyphagia
    C. Dermatitis
    D. Otitis
28. Which person is most likely to have dysmenorrhea?
    A. A 3-year-old female
    B. A 23-year-old female
    C. An 84-year-old male
    D. A 55-year-old male
29. Anemia is a condition of the
    A. Heart
    B. Lungs
    C. Blood
    D. Bones
30. Which question would the nursing assistant ask to clarify duties when caring for a person who has pharyngitis?
    A. What types of food and fluids should I offer?
    B. How often should I offer to help with toileting?
    C. How often should I take the vital signs?
    D. Is the person on fall precautions?

In questions 31 to 38, choose the correct spelling of the medical term

31. Slow heart rate
    A. Bradecardia
    B. Bradycardia
    C. Bradacordia
    D. Bradicardia
32. Difficulty urinating
    A. Dysuria
    B. Dysurya
    C. Dysuira
    D. Disuria
33. Blue color or condition
    A. Cyonosis
    B. Cyinosis
    C. Cyanosis
    D. Cianosys
34. Rapid breathing
    A. Tachepnea
    B. Tachypinea
    C. Tachypnea
    D. Tachypnia
35. Opening into the trachea
    A. Tracheastomy
    B. Trachiostomy
    C. Tracheostome
    D. Tracheostomy
36. Inflammation of the kidneys
    A. Nephytisis
    B. Nephretis
    C. Nefritis
    D. Nephritis
37. Removal of the breast
    A. Mastectomy
    B. Massectomy
    C. Masectomy
    D. Mastecomy
38. Record of the electrical activity in the heart
    A. Electrocartiogram
    B. Electrocardiogram
    C. Eletrocardeogram
    D. Elegtocardeeogram

Matching

Match the word with the correct definition

A. Arthroscopy
B. Bronchoscope
C. Cholecystectomy
D. Colostomy
E. Cyanotic
F. Dermatology
G. Dysuria
H. Enteritis
I. Gastrostomy
J. Gastritis
K. Glossitis
L. Nephritis
M. Neuralgia
N. Oophorectomy
O. Proctoscopy

39. ________ Difficulty urinating
40. ________ Inflammation of kidneys
41. ________ Pertaining to blue coloration
42. ________ Joint examination with a scope
43. ________ Study of the skin
44. ________ Creating an opening into the large intestine
45. ________ Instrument used to examine bronchi
46. ________ Inflammation of the tongue
47. ________ Nerve pain
48. ________ Examination of rectum with instrument
49. ________ Excision of gallbladder
50. ________ Excision of ovary
51. ________ Creating an opening into stomach
52. ________ Inflammation of stomach
53. ________ Inflammation of intestine

Fill in the Blanks

54. Write out the meaning of these abbreviations
    A. ADL ________________
    B. BP ________________
    C. TPR ________________
    D. NPO ________________
    E. ROM ________________
    F. I&O ________________

Write the definition of each prefix

55. anti- ________________
56. auto- ________________
57. brady- ________________
58. dys- ________________
59. ecto- ________________
60. leuk- ________________
61. macro- ________________
62. neo- ________________
63. supra- ________________
64. uni- ________________

Write the definition of each root word

65. adeno ________________
66. angio ________________
67. broncho ________________

68. cranio ______
69. duodeno ______
70. entero ______
71. gyneco ______
72. masto ______
73. pyo ______

Write the definition of each suffix

74. -asis ______
75. -genic ______
76. -oma ______
77. -phasia ______
78. -ptosis ______
79. -plegia ______
80. -megaly ______
81. -scopy ______
82. -stasis ______

Write the correct abbreviations

83. Weight ______
84. Fahrenheit ______
85. Bowel movement ______
86. Intake and output ______
87. Lower left quadrant ______
88. Vital signs ______
89. Urinary tract infection ______
90. Milliliter ______
91. Centigrade; Celsius ______

Labeling

92. Label the four abdominal regions. Use RUQ, LUQ, RLQ, LLQ to label.

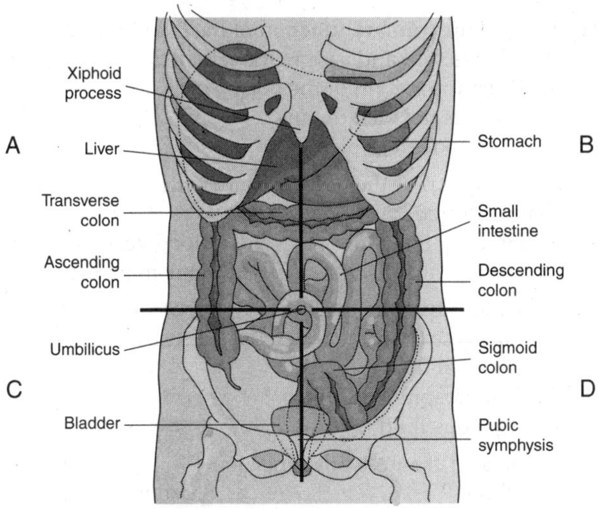

A. ______
B. ______
C. ______
D. ______

Optional Learning Exercises

Use the FOCUS ON PRIDE section to complete the statement and then take pride in learning and conduct the class experiment.

93. Only use abbreviations allowed by the ______.

Class Experiment

94. It is often difficult to describe fluids in a clear and precise manner. Set up the following examples that imitate situations where you need to describe intake, output, or drainage. Describe as accurately as possible what you see in terms of amounts, colors, and textures. Compare your notes with classmates to see if you are using words that all have the same meaning. What words were used that were easy to understand? What words were used that had more than one meaning?
    1. Bloody drainage: Mix a teaspoon of ketchup and a teaspoon of water. Pour onto the center of a paper napkin.
    2. Urine: Pour a tablespoon of tea into the center of a paper towel.
    3. Bleeding: Smear a teaspoon of red jelly in the center of a paper towel.
    4. Broth: Pour 4 ounces of tea into a bowl.

Class Experiment	
Substance	**Observations**
Bloody drainage	
Urine	
Bleeding	
Broth	

10 Body Structure and Function

Fill in the Blanks: Key Terms

Artery
Capillary
Cell
Digestion
Hemoglobin
Hormone
Immunity
Menstruation
Metabolism
Organ
Peristalsis
Respiration
System
Tissue
Vein

1. The substance in red blood cells that carries oxygen and gives blood its color is ____________________.
2. ____________________ is protection against a disease or condition.
3. The process of supplying the cells with oxygen and removing carbon dioxide from them is ____________________.
4. The process of physically and chemically breaking down food so that it can be absorbed for use by the cells is ____________________.
5. ____________________ is the burning of food for heat and energy by the cells.
6. A blood vessel that carries blood away from the heart is an ____________________.
7. ____________________ is the alternating contraction and relaxation of muscles that moves food through the digestive system.
8. Organs that work together to perform special functions form a ____________________.
9. The basic unit of body structure is a ____________________.
10. Groups of tissues with the same function form an ____________________.
11. A ____________________ is a tiny blood vessel.
12. A group of cells with similar function is ____________________.
13. ____________________ is the process in which the lining of the uterus breaks up and is discharged from the body through the vagina.
14. A chemical substance secreted by the glands into the bloodstream is a ____________________.
15. A ____________________ is a blood vessel that carries blood back to the heart.

Circle the Best Answer

16. During which task would the nursing assistant observe and care for the person's mucous membranes?
    A. Helping the person to stand up
    B. Assisting with oral hygiene
    C. Washing the lower back and buttocks
    D. Shampooing and combing the hair
17. Which action is an example of a reflex?
    A. You enjoy your day off with family and friends
    B. You immediately document assigned tasks after completion
    C. You take your lunch break after you have finished your duties
    D. You immediately pull your hand away when it touches a hot object
18. Genes control a person's
    A. Level of physical activity
    B. Dietary practices
    C. Skin and eye color
    D. Hygiene and odor
19. What is an example of connective tissue?
    A. Stomach
    B. Brain
    C. Pelvic bone
    D. Heart
20. How would the person be affected if the epidermis is damaged?
    A. There is a loss of sensation to touch and pain.
    B. Hair growth could cease because of root damage.
    C. There is an increased risk of infection.
    D. Sensitivity to temperature would decrease.
21. What is the function of sweat glands?
    A. Helps to regulate body temperature
    B. Keeps the nails healthy and shiny
    C. Protects the nose from dust
    D. Allows the skin to interpret sensations
22. What is the primary function of the long bones?
    A. Allows skill and ease in movement
    B. Bears the weight of the body
    C. Protects the vital organs
    D. Allows degrees of flexion
23. In which part of the body are blood cells manufactured?
    A. Heart
    B. Liver
    C. Blood vessels
    D. Bone marrow
24. Which fluid allows the joints to move smoothly?
    A. Cartilage fluid
    B. Synovial fluid
    C. Cerebrospinal fluid
    D. Aqueous fluid
25. What is an example of a hinge joint?
    A. Elbow
    B. Hip
    C. Shoulder
    D. Spine

26. Where are voluntary muscles located?
    A. Found in the stomach
    B. Attached to bones
    C. Found in the heart
    D. Attached to sphincters
27. What is the expected result when a person exercises and this causes the muscles to contract?
    A. Heat production
    B. Shivering
    C. Cooling down
    D. Involuntary movement
28. Which problem would the nursing assistant expect to observe for a patient who has damage to the right hemisphere of the cerebrum?
    A. Difficulty moving the upper body
    B. Difficulty moving the lower body
    C. Difficulty moving the left arm or leg
    D. Difficulty moving the right arm or leg
29. How would the person be affected if the medulla was damaged?
    A. Muscle control would stop.
    B. Breathing could cease.
    C. Memory loss would occur.
    D. Vision would be blurry.
30. Which safety precaution would the nursing assistant use if a person has a disorder that affects the cerebellum?
    A. Watch for and immediately report problems with swallowing
    B. Remind to test water temperature before getting in the shower
    C. Use a gait belt when assisting person to stand or ambulate
    D. Help the person to clean and don corrective eyewear
31. Which behavior would the nursing assistant observe if the person has a disorder that affects the cerebral cortex?
    A. Can't recall the name of eldest grandchild.
    B. Movements are jerky and has muscle weakness.
    C. Has a hard time coughing up secretions.
    D. Seems a little unsteady when first getting up.
32. What is the purpose of cerebrospinal fluid?
    A. Cushions the brain and spinal cord
    B. Controls voluntary muscles
    C. Lubricates movement
    D. Controls involuntary muscles
33. Which problem is a person likely to experience if there is damage to the optic nerve?
    A. Visual disturbance
    B. Difficulty walking
    C. Memory loss
    D. Irregular pulse
34. Which part of the nervous system is stimulated when a person gets frightened?
    A. Sympathetic
    B. Parasympathetic
    C. Central
    D. Cranial
35. Which instruction is the nurse likely to give to the nursing assistant who is caring for a person who has a corneal abrasion?
    A. Remind the person to use the hearing aid
    B. Watch for and report bleeding or pus
    C. Watch and report if the person has eye pain
    D. Be gentle when cleaning and drying the affected area
36. What happens to a person if the semicircular canals of the ear are not functioning properly?
    A. Ability to interpret sounds is lost
    B. Person will have inner ear pain
    C. Ability to hear low tones will occur
    D. Person will have trouble with balance
37. Which important function does hemoglobin perform?
    A. Carries oxygen
    B. Helps blood to clot
    C. Fights infection
    D. Contains water
38. Which component of the blood is likely to be contributing to the problem for a person who must be gently handled because of bruising and bleeding?
    A. There are too few red blood cells.
    B. There are too few white blood cells.
    C. The number of platelets is insufficient.
    D. The amount of plasma is decreased.
39. Which problem would the person experience if there is a disturbance or disorder of the white blood cells (leukocytes)?
    A. Decreased ability to protect against infection
    B. Increased bruising because blood cannot clot
    C. Retention of waste products and toxins
    D. Shortness of breath because oxygen in blood is decreased
40. Which observation needs to be immediately reported because it suggests that the left atrium of the heart is failing to perform its important function?
    A. Pulse is irregular and weak.
    B. Hiccupping will not stop.
    C. Knee joints appear red and swollen.
    D. Urine is pink-tinged with small clots.
41. Which blood vessels carry oxygenated blood to the body?
    A. Venules
    B. Capillaries
    C. Veins
    D. Arteries
42. Which problem would occur first if a person's spleen is seriously damaged in an accident?
    A. Old red blood cells would remain in the bloodstream.
    B. Bacteria and other substances would not be filtered.
    C. There would be significant blood loss, at least 500 milliliters.
    D. The recovered and stored iron would not be available for use.

43. Which action could the person take to get more oxygen into the lungs?
    A. Deep exhalation
    B. Rapid expiration
    C. Shallow inhalation
    D. Deep inspiration
44. Which organ could potentially be damaged if a person sustains a sternum fracture in a car accident?
    A. Kidney
    B. Ovary
    C. Lung
    D. Urinary bladder
45. In which location would the patient most likely experience discomfort and pain if peristalsis stops?
    A. Neck
    B. Abdomen
    C. Head
    D. Legs
46. In which circumstance would the nursing assistant be most likely to observe bile?
    A. Patient has dental pain and spits out unchewed food.
    B. Patient has an unusually heavy menstrual period.
    C. Patient frequently urinates because of infection.
    D. Patient has vomiting related to gallbladder disorder.
47. Which equipment would the nursing assistant need to provide care for a patient who is having an increase in fecal elimination because of a gastrointestinal disorder?
    A. Blood pressure cuff
    B. Wheelchair
    C. Gloves
    D. Stethoscope
48. What is a function of the urinary system?
    A. Removes waste products from the blood
    B. Rids the body of solid waste
    C. Removes oxygen from the blood
    D. Burns food for energy
49. Which amount in the urinary bladder will trigger the urge to urinate?
    A. 1000 mL of urine
    B. 500 mL of urine
    C. 250 mL of urine
    D. 125 mL of urine
50. Which observation would the nursing assistant report to the nurse because sodium (one type of electrolyte) and water loss are being lost?
    A. Headache
    B. Vomiting
    C. Nausea
    D. Constipation
51. Which secondary sexual characteristics would the nursing assistant expect to see in a young male patient with adequate testosterone production?
    A. Facial hair; pubic and axillary hair
    B. Widening and rounding of the hips
    C. Urethra within the penis
    D. Vas deferens in the scrotum
52. Which question would the nursing assistant ask about the care and cleaning of a male patient's genital area?
    A. "Can the patient clean the labia by himself?"
    B. "What type of soap should I use on the prostate gland?"
    C. "Does the foreskin need special care?"
    D. "Is the patient able to clean his own urethra?"
53. Which secondary female sexual characteristics could be affected for a young female patient who lacks estrogen and progesterone because the ovaries were surgically removed?
    A. Development of breasts
    B. Strength of long bones
    C. Coloration of the skin
    D. Maintenance of muscle tone
54. Where does the ovum travel through first when it is released from an ovary?
    A. Uterus
    B. Fallopian tubes
    C. Endometrium
    D. Vagina
55. Which time frame for menstrual flow is expected to appear in the care plan, for a newly admitted female patient who is unable to perform the self-care related to menstruation?
    A. 1 to 3 days
    B. 3 to 7 days
    C. 5 to 10 days
    D. 7 to 14 days
56. What would the nursing assistant expect to observe when the adrenal medulla excretes epinephrine?
    A. Slow respiratory rate
    B. Subnormal temperature
    C. Increased pulse
    D. Decreased blood pressure
57. What would the nursing assistant expect to observe if a person has excessive thyroid hormone?
    A. Short stature
    B. Lethargy
    C. Weight loss
    D. Increased facial hair
58. What would the nursing assistant expect to observe if a person has insufficient thyroid hormone?
    A. Nervous behavior
    B. Slowed movements
    C. Muscle spasms
    D. Delayed secondary sexual characteristics
59. If too little insulin is produced by the pancreas, the person has
    A. Decrease urine output
    B. Irregular menstruation
    C. Diabetes mellitus
    D. High blood pressure
60. When abnormal or unwanted substances enter the body, they are attacked and destroyed by
    A. Antibodies
    B. Red blood cells
    C. Antigens
    D. Platelets

Fill in the Blanks

61. Write out these abbreviations
    A. CNS ________________
    B. CO_2 ________________
    C. GI ________________
    D. mL ________________
    E. O_2 ________________
    F. RBC ________________
    G. WBC ________________
    H. PNS ________________

Matching

Match the Terms With the Descriptions

Musculoskeletal System

A. Periosteum
B. Joint
C. Cartilage
D. Synovial fluid
E. Striated muscle
F. Smooth muscle
G. Voluntary muscle
H. Tendons

62. ________ Connective tissue at the end of long bones
63. ________ Skeletal muscle
64. ________ Membrane that covers bone
65. ________ Connects muscle to bone
66. ________ Point at which two or more bones meet
67. ________ Consciously controlled
68. ________ Involuntary muscle
69. ________ Acts as a lubricant so the joint can move smoothly

Sensory System

A. Sclera
B. Cornea
C. Retina
D. Cerumen
E. Middle ear
F. Inner ear

70. ________ Contains Eustachian tubes and ossicles
71. ________ White of the eye
72. ________ Inner layer of the eye; receptors for vision are contained here
73. ________ Light enters the eye through this structure
74. ________ Waxy substance secreted in the auditory canal
75. ________ Contains the semicircular canal and cochlea

Nervous System

A. Autonomic nervous system
B. Cerebral cortex
C. Brainstem
D. Peripheral nervous system

76. ________ Has 12 pairs of cranial nerves and 31 pairs of spinal nerves
77. ________ Outside of the cerebrum; controls highest function of the brain
78. ________ Contain the midbrain, pons, and medulla
79. ________ Controls involuntary muscles, heartbeat, blood pressure, and other functions

Circulatory System

A. Plasma
B. Erythrocytes
C. Hemoglobin
D. Leukocytes
E. Thrombocytes
F. Pericardium
G. Myocardium
H. Endocardium
I. Arteries
J. Veins
K. Capillaries

80. ________ Liquid part of blood
81. ________ Thin sac covering the heart
82. ________ Very tiny blood vessels
83. ________ Substance in blood that picks up oxygen
84. ________ Carry blood away from the heart
85. ________ White blood cells
86. ________ Carry blood toward the heart
87. ________ Red blood cells
88. ________ Thick muscular portion of the heart
89. ________ Platelets; necessary for clotting
90. ________ Membrane lining inner surface of the heart

Lymphatic System

A. Lymph nodes
B. Tonsils
C. Spleen

91. ________ Stores blood and saves iron
92. ________ Bean shaped and found in the neck, underarm, groin, chest, abdomen, and pelvis
93. ________ Traps microorganisms in the mouth to prevent infection

Respiratory System

A. Epiglottis
B. Larynx
C. Bronchiole
D. Trachea
E. Aveoli
F. Diaphragm
G. Pleura

94. ________ Air passes from the larynx into this structure
95. ________ A two-layered sac that covers the lungs
96. ________ Piece of cartilage that acts like a lid over the larynx
97. ________ Separates the lungs from the abdominal cavity
98. ________ The voice box
99. ________ Several small branches that divide from the bronchus
100. ________ Tiny one-celled air sacs

Digestive System

A. Liver
B. Chyme
C. Colon
D. Rectum
E. Anus
F. Saliva
G. Pancreas
H. Gallbladder

101. ________ Feces passes out of the body
102. ________ Semiliquid food mixture formed in the stomach
103. ________ Receives feces passed from the colon
104. ________ Stores bile
105. ________ Portion of GI tract that absorbs water
106. ________ Produces bile
107. ________ Moistens food particles in the mouth
108. ________ Produces digestive juices

Urinary System

A. Bladder
B. Urethra
C. Kidney
D. Meatus
E. Nephrons
F. Ureter
G. Tubule

109. ________ Basic working unit of the kidney
110. ________ Fluid and waste products form urine in this structure
111. ________ Bean-shaped structure that produces urine
112. ________ Opening at the end of the urethra
113. ________ Structure that allows urine to pass from the bladder
114. ________ A tube attached to the renal pelvis of the kidney
115. ________ Hollow muscular sac that stores urine

Reproductive System

A. Scrotum
B. Testes
C. Urethra
D. Gonads
E. Vagina
G. Labia
H. Vulva
F. Endometrium

116. ________ Male or female sex organs
117. ________ Two folds of tissue on each side of the vagina
118. ________ Sac between thighs that contains testes
119. ________ External genitalia of female
120. ________ Testicles; sperm produced here
121. ________ Muscular canal that receives the penis during intercourse
122. ________ Outlet for urine and semen
123. ________ Tissue lining the uterus

Endocrine System

A. Epinephrine
B. Estrogen
C. Insulin
D. Parathormone
E. Testosterone
F. Thyroxine

124. ________ Regulates sugar in blood; allows sugar to enter the cells
125. ________ Sex hormone secreted by testes
126. ________ Sex hormone secreted by ovaries
127. ________ Regulates metabolism
128. ________ Regulates calcium levels in the body
129. ________ Stimulates the body to produce energy during emergencies

Immune System

A. Antibodies
B. Antigens
C. Phagocytes
D. Lymphocytes
E. B cells
F. T cells

130. ________ Normal body substances that recognize abnormal or unwanted substances
131. ________ Type of cell that destroys invading cells
132. ________ Type of white blood cell that digests and destroys microorganisms
133. ________ Type of cell that causes production of antibodies
134. ________ Substances that cause an immune response
135. ________ Type of white blood cell that produces antibodies

Labeling

136. Identify the subcutaneous fatty tissue, dermis, and epidermis in the skin.

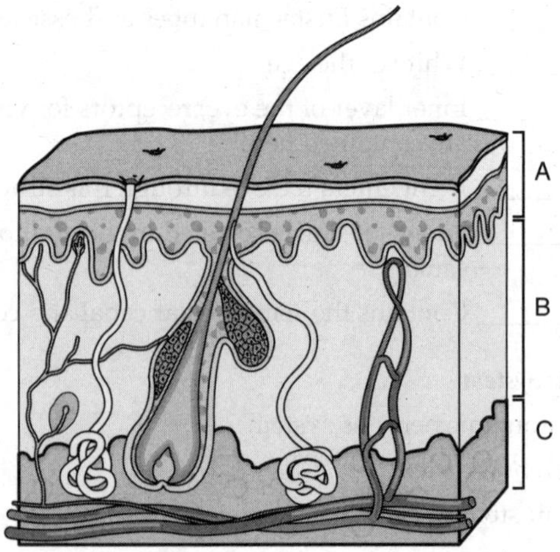

A. ______________________________
B. ______________________________
C. ______________________________

137. Name each type of joint in the figures.

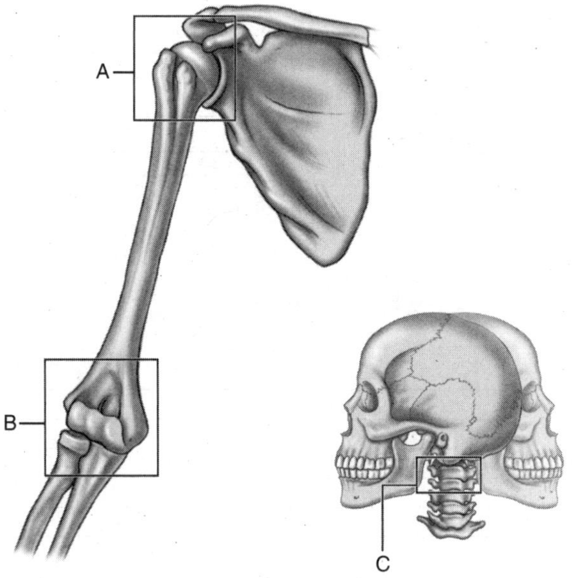

Modified from Herlihy B. The Human Body in Health and Illness. 6 ed. Elsevier; 2018.

A. ______________________
B. ______________________
C. ______________________

138. Identify the structures in the chest cavity.

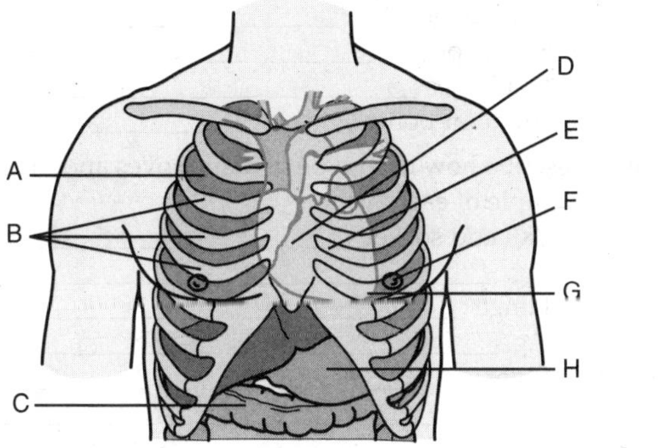

A. ______________________
B. ______________________
C. ______________________
D. ______________________
E. ______________________
F. ______________________
G. ______________________
H. ______________________

139. Name the structures of the respiratory system in the figure.

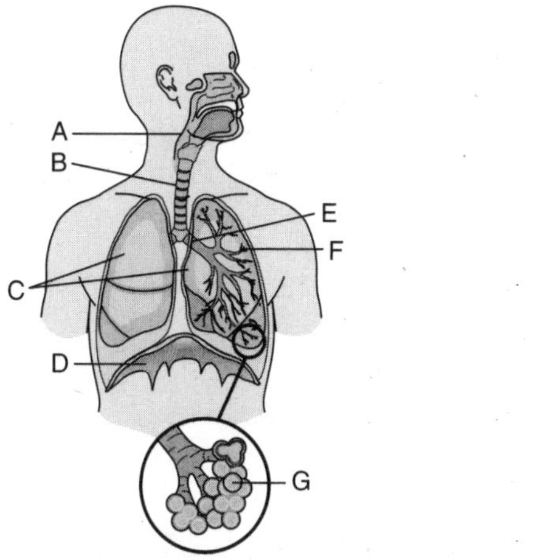

A. ______________________
B. ______________________
C. ______________________
D. ______________________
E. ______________________
F. ______________________
G. ______________________

140. Name the structures of the digestive system in the figure.

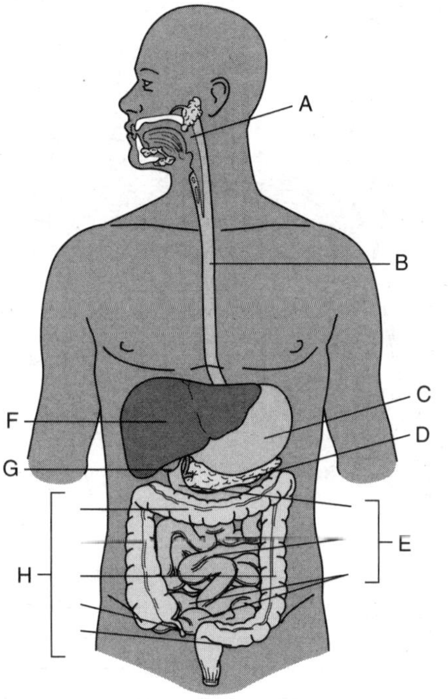

A. ______________________
B. ______________________
C. ______________________
D. ______________________
E. ______________________
F. ______________________
G. ______________________
H. ______________________

141. Name the structures of the urinary system in the figure.

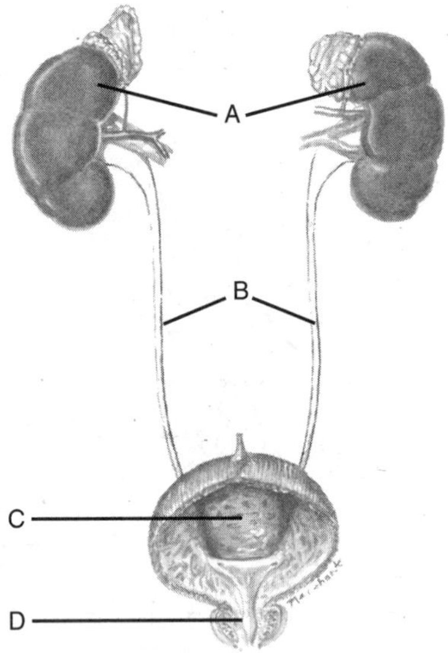

A. ______________________
B. ______________________
C. ______________________
D. ______________________

142. Name the structures of the male reproductive system in the figure.

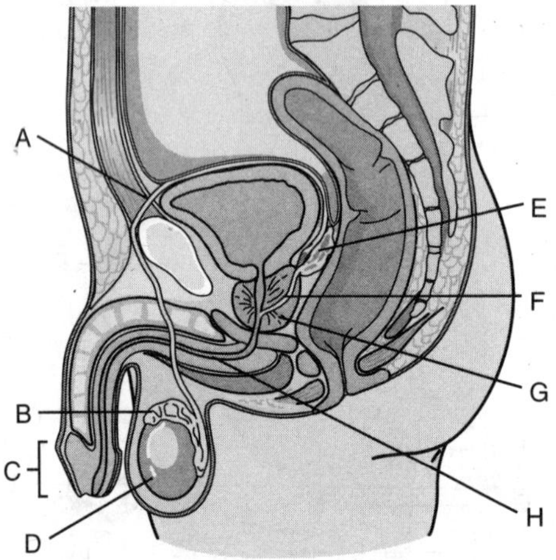

A. ______________________
B. ______________________
C. ______________________
D. ______________________
E. ______________________
F. ______________________
G. ______________________
H. ______________________

143. Name the external female genitalia in the figure.

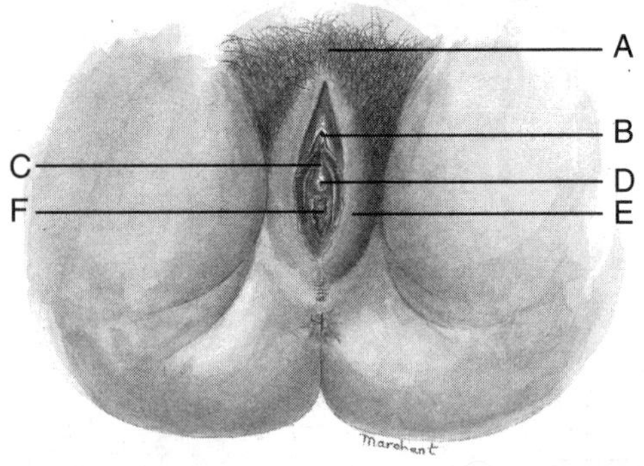

A. ______________________
B. ______________________
C. ______________________
D. ______________________
E. ______________________
F. ______________________

Optional Learning Exercises

144. List what structures are contained in the two skin layers.
    A. Epidermis ______________________
    B. Dermis ______________________

145. Explain the function of the types of bone.
    A. Long bones ______________________
    B. Short bones ______________________
    C. Flat bones ______________________
    D. Irregular bones ______________________

146. Describe how each type of joint moves and give an example of each type.
    A. Ball and socket ______________________
    E.g. ______________________
    B. Hinge ______________________
    E.g. ______________________
    C. Pivot ______________________
    E.g. ______________________

147. Explain what happens when muscles contract.
    ____

148. Explain how the sympathetic and parasympathetic nervous systems balance each other.
    ____

149. What happens to the pupil of the eye in bright light?
    ____

150. What is the function of the acoustic nerve?
    ____

151. When an infection occurs, what do white blood cells do?
____
____
____

152. Explain the function of the four atria of the heart.
A. Right atrium ______________________________
B. Left atrium ______________________________
C. Right ventricle ______________________________
D. Left ventricle ______________________________

153. Explain what happens in the aveoli.
____
____

154. After food is swallowed, explain what happens in each of these parts of the digestive tract.
A. Stomach ______________________________
B. Duodenum ______________________________
C. Jejunum and ileum ______________________________
D. Colon ______________________________
E. Rectum ______________________________
F. Anus ______________________________

155. What is the function of the endometrium?
____
____

156. Menstruation occurs about every ____________ days. Ovulation usually occurs on or about day __________ of the cycle.

157. What is the function of each of these pituitary hormones?
A. Growth hormone ______________________________
B. Antidiuretic hormone ______________________________
C. Oxytocin ______________________________

158. What is the function of insulin? ________________
____

159. What happens if too little insulin is produced?
____

160. What happens when the body senses an antigen?
____
____

161. What is a reflex? ______________________________
____

Optional Learning Exercises

Use the FOCUS ON PRIDE Section to Complete the Statement and Then Use the Critical Thinking and Discussion Question to Develop Your Ideas

162. If the person's decision about his own body may cause __________, tell the nurse at once.

Critical Thinking and Discussion Question

163. You are caring for a person who can walk independently, but he moves very slowly. He also has pain in his finger joints, and this causes problems with tasks, such as buttoning his shirt. He is otherwise healthy and other body systems function properly.
A. Discuss how these changes in the musculoskeletal system could affect his toileting abilities.
B. What could you do to help this person?

164. You are caring for a person with a low red blood cell count.
A. Based on your knowledge of the function of red blood cells, what would you expect to observe?
B. What could you do to assist him?

11 Growth and Development

Fill in the Blanks: Key Terms

Adolescence	Growth	Peer	Sexuality
Development	Menarche	Primary caregiver	Sexual orientation
Developmental task	Menopause	Puberty	Stage
Ejaculation	Milestone	Sex	Teen dating violence

1. The first menstruation and the start of menstrual cycles is ______________________.
2. ______________________ is the time between puberty and adulthood, a time of rapid growth and physical and social maturity.
3. The release of semen is ______________________.
4. The period when reproductive organs begin to function and secondary sex characteristics appear is ______________________.
5. ______________________ is the physical interaction between people involving the body and reproductive organs.
6. Changes in mental, emotional, and social function is ______________________.
7. ______________________ is the physical, emotional, social, cultural, and spiritual factors that affect a person's feelings, attitudes, and behaviors about one's gender identity and sexual behavior.
8. ______________________ is the physical changes that can be measured and that occur in a steady, orderly manner.
9. The person mainly responsible for providing or assisting with the child's basic needs is the ______________________.
10. A skill that must be completed during a stage of development is a ______________________.
11. ______________________ is the time when menstruation stops and menstrual cycles end; there has been at least 1 year without a menstrual period.
12. A person of the same age-group and background is a ______________________.
13. ______________________ refers to a person's emotional, romantic, or physical attraction to males, females, both, or neither.
14. ______________________ is the physical, sexual, psychological, or emotional violence within a dating relationship as well as stalking.
15. ______________________ is a behavior or skill that occurs in a stage of development.
16. ______________________ is a period of time (age range) in which a person learns certain skills.

Circle the Best Answer

17. When do growth and development begin?
    A. At fertilization
    B. At birth
    C. When the baby sits up
    D. When children have growth spurts
18. Based on the principle that growth and development occur from the center of the body outward, what would the nursing assistant expect to observe about a baby's movements?
    A. Baby would move legs and arms, but movements would be uncontrolled.
    B. Baby would control shoulder movements before controlling hand movements.
    C. Baby would control the hand movements before controlling the legs.
    D. Baby would move the legs before moving the arms or hands.
19. What would the nursing assistant do upon observing that a neonate is not cooing or babbling?
    A. Immediately report the observation to the nurse
    B. Ask the mother if she has heard the baby making any sounds
    C. Verify with nurse that this is normal behavior for the neonate
    D. Talk to and play with the neonate to stimulate a social response
20. Which newborn is within the range of average birth weight?
    A. Newborn A weighs 12 pounds.
    B. Newborn B weighs 10 pounds.
    C. Newborn C weighs 8 pounds.
    D. Newborn D weighs 5 pounds.
21. Which reflex would be useful for a newborn and a mother who are attempting to master breastfeeding?
    A. Moro reflex
    B. Rooting reflex
    C. Palmar grasp reflex
    D. Step reflex
22. Which result would the nursing assistant expect to observe when the nurse is teaching the mother of a newborn to gently touch the cheek near the mouth?
    A. Newborn opens mouth and turns head toward the nipple.
    B. Newborn opens eyes and looks at the mother's face.
    C. Newborn begins to coo and socialize with the mother.
    D. Newborn closes his fingers around the mother's finger.

23. When can infants start playing peekaboo?
    A. 2 to 3 months
    B. 4 to 5 months
    C. 8 to 9 months
    D. The first birthday
24. Which child is most likely to have a temper tantrum and say "no"?
    A. You are changing the diaper of a 9-month-old child.
    B. You are helping an 18-month-old child to get undressed.
    C. You are bathing and dressing a 4-month-old child.
    D. You are reading a bedtime story to a 4-year-old child.
25. Which task will begin in toddlerhood?
    A. Learning to stand and walk
    B. Learning to feed themselves
    C. Learning to share toys with others
    D. Learning to control bowel and bladder function
26. Which circumstance helps toddlers learn to feel secure?
    A. Primary caregivers are consistently present when needed.
    B. Long periods of separation from primary caregivers are planned.
    C. Primary caregivers teach that needs cannot be met quickly.
    D. They are alone for long periods of time with primary caregivers.
27. Which activity would the nursing assistant use to engage a 3-year-old child whose mother is undergoing a laboratory test?
    A. Have the child name and number objects in the waiting room
    B. Ask the child to draw mommy and self going to the hospital
    C. Ask the child to start counting numbers until mommy is done
    D. Have the child play make believe hospital with dolls and animals
28. Which growth pattern occurs during the preschool years?
    A. Growth is much more rapid than during infancy
    B. 2 to 3 inches per year and gain about 5 pounds per year
    C. Very slowly, if at all, especially if parents are short
    D. 6 to 7 inches per year and gain about 10 pounds per year
29. At which age baby teeth are lost and permanent teeth erupt?
    A. 2 years of age
    B. 12 months of age
    C. 6 years of age
    D. 9 or 10 years of age
30. When do reading, writing, grammar, and math skills develop?
    A. Toddlerhood
    B. Preschool years
    C. School-age years
    D. Late childhood
31. At which age is a girl most likely to be taller and heavier than the boys in her age-group?
    A. 3-year old
    B. 8-year old
    C. 12-year old
    D. 17-year old
32. Which child is most likely to be interested in "helping" to take the vital signs to get praise and a token reward?
    A. 7-year old
    B. 2-year old
    C. 18-year old
    D. 12-year old
33. When do girls reach puberty?
    A. When menarche occurs
    B. When they demonstrate gender identity
    C. When they stop growing in height
    D. When they begin to show interest in sex
34. You are volunteering at your child's school. Which behavior would you report to the school nurse who has asked you to watch for signs of bullying on the playground?
    A. Children are running, and one child cannot keep up.
    B. Children are playing, and one child falls on the grass.
    C. Children are teasing and pointing at one child.
    D. Children are sitting together and trading snack items.
35. Which adolescent behavior indicates that there is a need for guidance and discipline?
    A. Adolescent asks their parents for spending money.
    B. Adolescent drinks some beer because a friend does.
    C. Adolescent thinks they should be allowed to date.
    D. Adolescent asks a teacher for clarification of homework.
36. Which rationale explains why teens usually do not understand when parents worry about sexual activities, pregnancy, and sexually transmitted diseases?
    A. They are emotionally unstable and mood swings take over.
    B. Independence from adults is the overriding task for this age-group.
    C. They do not always consider the consequences of sexual activity.
    D. They do not have a sense of right and wrong, or good and bad.
37. Which teenager is experiencing teen dating violence?
    A. 15-year old female consents to kissing another female teenage.
    B. 16-year old frequently disagrees with parents about dating.
    C. 13-year old female gets unwelcome sexting from a 17-year old male.
    D. 16-year old male has occasional sex with a 17-year old male partner.
38. When does development end?
    A. When puberty occurs
    B. When physical growth is complete
    C. At young adulthood
    D. At death
39. Which behavior is expected for a young adult?
    A. Adjusting to physical changes
    B. Adjusting to aging parents
    C. Developing a satisfactory sex life
    D. Accepting changes in appearance

40. Which information is a 45-year-old adult likely to share with the nursing assistant?
    A. Plans for traveling during retirement
    B. Embarking on a chosen career path
    C. Death of a partner or spouse
    D. A daughter's upcoming wedding
41. Which observations would the home health nursing assistant report to the nurse as a possible sign that a child in the household is being bullied?
    A. Child likes to help his grandfather build and repair things.
    B. Child is very competitive and blames others for his failures at school sports.
    C. Child likes to do chores around the house in exchange for a small allowance.
    D. Child has unexplained minor injuries and does not want to go to school.
42. Which action would trigger the Moro reflex in an infant?
    A. Baby is startled by a loud noise.
    B. Mother touches the baby's cheek near the mouth.
    C. Mother strokes the baby's palm.
    D. Baby is held upright and the feet touch a surface.
43. Which behavior would an adolescent use to express gender identity?
    A. Improves school performance and grades
    B. Adopts selected styles of clothing
    C. Displays a birth certificate on social media
    D. Changes to healthier eating habits
44. Which physical changes would be observed around the same time that menopause occurs?
    A. Hips widen and breasts develop.
    B. Change of gender occurs.
    C. Facial wrinkles and gray hair appear.
    D. Growth happens in a steady and orderly manner.
45. Which adolescent comment is the most serious and needs to be immediately reported to the nurse?
    A. "My parents are so stupid."
    B. "I often fantasize about suicide."
    C. "I tried smoking a cigarette today."
    D. "My boyfriend told me that I look fat."
46. Which teenager is experiencing teen dating violence?
    A. A 17-year-old female pairs off with an 18-year-old male.
    B. A 15-year-old female participates in group dating.
    C. A 16-year-old male pairs off with another 16-year-old male.
    D. A 16-year-old female gets repeated attention that causes fear.

Match the Milestone/Task With the Correct Age-Group

A. Infancy (birth–1 year)
B. Toddler (1–3 years)
C. Preschooler (3–6 years)
D. School age (6–9 or 10 years)
E. Late childhood (9 or 10–12 years)
F. Adolescence (12–18 years)
G. Young adulthood (18–40 years)
H. Middle adulthood (40–65 years)
I. Late adulthood (65 years and older)

47. ________ Accepting changes in body and appearance
48. ________ Developing leisure-time activities
49. ________ Gaining control of bowel and bladder functions
50. ________ Becoming independent from parents and adults
51. ________ Learning to eat solid foods
52. ________ Adjusting to decreased strength and loss of health
53. ________ Learning how to study
54. ________ Learning how to get along with persons of the same age-group and background
55. ________ Increasing ability to communicate and understand others
56. ________ Tolerating separation from primary caregiver
57. ________ Learning to live with a partner
58. ________ Developing moral or ethical behavior
59. ________ Learning basic reading, writing, and arithmetic skills
60. ________ Developing stable sleep and feeding patterns
61. ________ Performing self-care
62. ________ Using words to communicate with others
63. ________ Adjusting to aging parents
64. ________ Develop appropriate relationships with others and begin to attract partners
65. ________ Cope with a partner's death
66. ________ Choosing education and a career

Optional Learning Exercises

Infancy

67. List six tasks of growth and development that occur during the stage of infancy.
    A. ________________________________
    B. ________________________________
    C. ________________________________
    D. ________________________________
    E. ________________________________
    F. ________________________________
68. What are the three language and communication behaviors that a 2-month old should display?
    A. ________________________________
    B. ________________________________
    C. ________________________________

Toddlerhood

69. What are the four developmental tasks of toddlerhood?
    A. ______________________
    B. ______________________
    C. ______________________
    D. ______________________

Preschool

70. What personal self-care skills can be performed by 3-year olds?
    A. Put on ______________________
71. What are the five communication skills that 5-year olds should be using?
    A. ______________________.
    B. ______________________.
    C. ______________________.
    D. ______________________.
    E. ______________________.

School-Age

72. Play activities in school-age children have a purpose and involve ______________.
    A. They like household tasks such as ______________________.
    B. Rewards are important, such as ______________________.

Late Childhood

73. What are the six developmental tasks of late childhood?
    A. ______________________
    B. ______________________
    C. ______________________
    D. ______________________
    E. ______________________
    F. ______________________

Adolescence

74. What are the six developmental tasks of adolescence?
    A. ______________________
    B. ______________________
    C. ______________________
    D. ______________________
    E. ______________________
    F. ______________________
75. During adolescence, girls and boys need about ______________________ hours of sleep at night because of ______________________.
76. Girls usually complete development by age ________. Boys usually stop growing between __________ years.
77. What is the definition of teen dating violence? ______________________

Young Adulthood

78. What are five developmental tasks of young adulthood
    A. ______________________
    B. ______________________
    C. ______________________
    D. ______________________
    E. ______________________

Middle Adulthood

79. During middle adulthood, weight control becomes a problem because ______________________.
80. What are the four developmental tasks of middle adulthood?
    A. ______________________
    B. ______________________
    C. ______________________
    D. ______________________

Late Adulthood

81. What are the five developmental tasks of late adulthood?
    A. ______________________
    B. ______________________
    C. ______________________
    D. ______________________
    E. ______________________

Use the FOCUS ON PRIDE Section to Complete the Statements and then Use the Critical Thinking and Discussion Questions to Develop Your Ideas

82. For children, the ______________________ is an important part of the health team.
83. When interacting with parents or the child's primary caregivers you should
    A. ______________________
    B. ______________________
    C. ______________________
    D. ______________________
    E. ______________________

Critical Thinking and Discussion Questions

84. You are making a home visit to assist an adult who had surgery and who needs some temporary assistance to bath and ambulate. During the visit, you notice that there is a 4-month-old infant who has been crying continuously for the past hour.
    A. What could be causing the infant to cry?
    B. If the crying continues and you and the caregiver cannot calm and comfort the infant, what would you do?
    C. Discuss how you feel about advocating or intervening for someone (such as this infant) who is not your responsibility or the person who is assigned to your care.

Crossword

Fill in the crossword by answering the clues below with the words from this list

Development	Menopause	Preadolescence	Step
Grasp	Moro	Puberty	Sucking
Growth	Neonatal	Rooting	

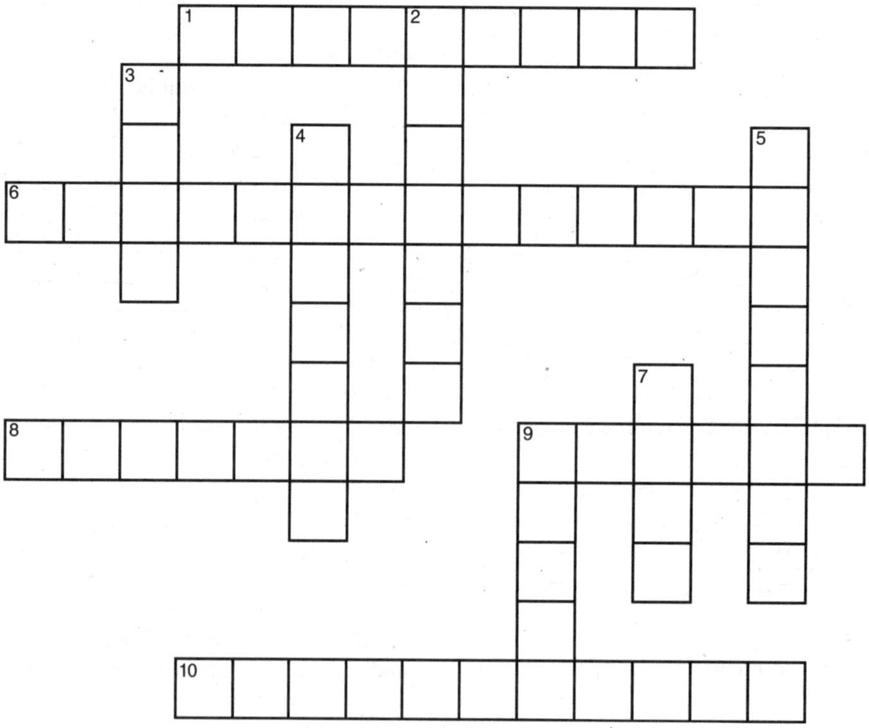

Across

1. Event that occurs to women between ages of 45 and 55 years
6. Time between childhood and adolescence (late childhood)
8. Reflex that occurs when the lips are touched
9. Physical changes that can be measured and that occur in a steady, orderly manner
10. Changes in mental, emotional, and social function

Down

2. Period between ages of 9 and 16 years that girls reach; period between ages of 13 and 15 years that boys reach
3. Reflex in which the feet move up and down as in stepping motions
4. Reflex that occurs when the cheek is touched near the mouth
5. Period of infancy from birth to 1 month of age
7. Reflex that occurs when a loud noise, a sudden movement, or the head falling back startles the baby
9. Reflex that occurs when the palm is stroked

12 The Older Person

Fill in the Blanks: Key Terms

Erectile dysfunction (ED) Gerontology
Geriatrics

1. ______________________ is the care of aging people.
2. ___________ is the inability of the male to have or maintain an erection.
3. The study of the aging process is _______________.

Circle the Best Answer

4. Which everyday activity is most likely to be included in the nursing assistant's assigned tasks in the care of an elderly person who had hip surgery?
   A. Helping them to visit with family
   B. Feeding them the prescribed diet
   C. Assisting them with toileting and hygiene
   D. Doing their shopping and housework
5. Which action is the nursing assistant most likely to use when caring for an 86-year-old man who retains physical mobility but needs help with everyday activities because of dementia?
   A. Supervise him while he prepares meals
   B. Coach him step-by-step to put on his shirt
   C. Spoon feed him and hold his drink cup
   D. Escort him around the shopping center
6. Which nursing assistant has provided a care measure that is insufficient to meet the needs of an elderly person who has limited mobility?
   A. Nursing assistant A assists the person in a wheelchair and to the dining area.
   B. Nursing assistant B helps the person to sit up and to wash their hands before eating.
   C. Nursing assistant C places the unwrapped food tray on a table in the person's room.
   D. Nursing assistant D cuts up the meat and puts the food within the person's reach.
7. Which belief is a myth about aging?
   A. Many older people enjoy a fulfilling sex life.
   B. Most older people have memory loss and dementia.
   C. Many older persons have jobs or do volunteer work.
   D. Most older persons frequently interact with family.
8. Which topic is the oldest of the old most likely to talk about based on the social changes that occur with aging?
   A. Changes in physical appearance
   B. Attending a family reunion in the summer
   C. Death of a friend or family member
   D. Investments and savings for retirement
9. Which basic need, as described by Maslow, is met when a retired older person decides to do volunteer work?
   A. Self-actualization
   B. Physical
   C. Love and belonging
   D. Safety and security
10. Which observation would the home health nursing assistant report to the supervising nurse because the elderly person is probably experiencing a reduced income?
    A. Elderly person is living with an adult child.
    B. Elderly person rarely goes out to eat dinner.
    C. Elderly person often talks about trips he used to take.
    D. Elderly person has stopped taking prescribed medication.
11. Which goal would the health-care team try to meet for a person with no family in the area who speaks a foreign language and rarely interacts with the other residents in the nursing center?
    A. Hire more interpreters to join the staff
    B. Have everyone accept persons from different cultures
    C. Promote a sense of belonging and self-worth
    D. Be pleasant but recognize nothing can be done
12. Which older person may be having trouble adjusting to changes in social relationships?
    A. Person stays at home alone to save money.
    B. Person attends church and community activities.
    C. Person takes up a new hobby to meet new people.
    D. Person maintains regular contact with family.
13. What is a source of disagreement when an older person moves in with an adult child?
    A. Older person tries to maintain dignity.
    B. Older person expresses a feeling of security.
    C. Family members need time alone.
    D. Grandchildren spend time with the older person.
14. Which observation would the home health nursing assistant, who is assigned to care for an older married couple, report to the nurse when the wife dies after a long illness?
    A. Husband seems to accept his wife's death as a part of life.
    B. Husband develops headaches, and insomnia and seems sad.
    C. Husband starts socializing and forming new friendships.
    D. Husband has prepared for this change and he seems at peace.

15. What changes in the integumentary system would the nursing assistant expect to observe in an older person?
   A. Skin is fragile and is easily bruised.
   B. Skin is moist and the fatty layer increases.
   C. Skin appears pale or a may be slightly bluish.
   D. Skin appears puffy and indents with pressure.
16. Which observation needs to be immediately reported to the nurse?
   A. Person gets up slowly from bed or chair.
   B. There is a small skin tear on the buttocks.
   C. Person refuses to wear his hearing aid.
   D. There is a thin layer of earwax in the ear.
17. What is the best rationale for avoiding the use of hot water bottles and heating pads on the feet for older persons?
   A. Older people do not understand how to adjust the temperature for safety.
   B. Nursing assistant is liable if the equipment fails and the person is injured.
   C. Fragile skin and changes in sensation create an increased risk for burns.
   D. Heat causes the blood vessels to dilate, and this causes changes in circulation.
18. Which self-care measure can older persons do to prevent bone loss and loss of muscle strength?
   A. Exercise and balanced nutrition
   B. Take hormones
   C. Rest with feet elevated
   D. Take vitamins
19. Which care measure would the nursing assistant use when assisting an elderly person who has risk for fractures of the bones?
   A. Ask the nurse for permission to leave the person in bed
   B. Put the person into a wheelchair; never let him walk
   C. Remind the person that the bones are weak
   D. Turn and move the person gently and carefully
20. Which care measure would the nursing assistant use for an older person who is experiencing dizziness?
   A. Encourage the person to take naps in the daytime
   B. Remind the person to get up slowly from bed or chair
   C. Have the person eat a snack before exercise or activity
   D. Use memory aids and prompts according to the care plan
21. Which older person is displaying expected behavior related to aging of the nervous system?
   A. Person A talks happily and continuously but most of it is nonsense.
   B. Person B talks about events that happened when they were a teenager.
   C. Person C is usually calm and cooperative, but today is angry and hostile.
   D. Person D has periods of confusion that seem to be related to medication.
22. Which patient comment will the nursing assistant immediately report to the nurse when caring for an older person has a reduced sensitivity to touch, pressure, or pain?
   A. Person asks for an icepack because the ankle is swollen and deformed.
   B. Person asks the nursing assistant to give a soothing back rub with warmed lotion.
   C. Person wants the air-conditioning turned down, even though it is hot weather.
   D. Person wants to take a deep warm bath to relieve muscle aches and stiffness.
23. Which care measure would the nursing assistant use when an older person says that the taste of the food is unpleasant?
   A. Provide or encourage oral hygiene
   B. Offer the person salt and pepper
   C. Tell the person to drink extra fluids
   D. Suggest raw fruits and vegetables
24. Which care measure would the nursing assistant use for an older person who reports decreased vision in dark rooms and at night?
   A. Tell the person to wear his glasses all the time
   B. Open curtains in the day and turn on a night light
   C. Ask the nurse if the person needs eye drops
   D. Advise the person not to walk around at night
25. Which sound is an older person most likely to have difficulty in hearing?
   A. Loud music on television
   B. High-pitched alarm on cell phone
   C. Pastor giving a sermon in church
   D. German shepherd dog barking outside
26. Which action would the nursing assistant reinforce, as instructed by the nurse, for a person who has severe circulatory changes?
   A. Encourage to walk long distances
   B. Rest during the day, as needed
   C. Avoid doing any kind of exercise
   D. Exercise only once a week
27. Which position facilitates breathing when a person has difficulty breathing?
   A. Lying flat in bed
   B. Lying prone with light bed linens
   C. Bed rest in side-lying position
   D. Resting in a semi-Fowler's position
28. Which types of food should generally be avoided by most older people?
   A. Fried food
   B. Whole grain food
   C. Puddings
   D. Fruit juices
29. Which types of foods would be included in the care plan to prevent constipation?
   A. Foods with fewer calories
   B. High-fiber foods
   C. Foods that supply calcium
   D. Low-protein foods

30. The nursing assistant is assigned to care for four people. Which person is likely to need the most assistance throughout the day?
    A. Person has flatulence.
    B. Person has genitalia atrophy.
    C. Person has urinary incontinence.
    D. Person has earwax impaction.
31. Which physical change would make intercourse uncomfortable or painful for an older woman?
    A. Partner has a delayed erection.
    B. There is vaginal dryness.
    C. Arousal takes longer.
    D. Orgasm is less intense.
32. Which care measure would the nursing assistant use upon noticing that an older person living in a nursing center seems lonely?
    A. Visit with the person a few times during the shift
    B. Take the person to own home during the holidays
    C. Call the family and tell them that the person is lonely
    D. Tell the person that he must attend social activities
33. What is the purpose of adult day-care centers?
    A. To provide meals, supervision, and activities for older persons
    B. To cater to self-care persons and those who can walk without help
    C. To provide complete care for physical, social, and emotional needs
    D. To offer sleeping facilities for older persons who have no family
34. What is the advantage of an older person renting an apartment?
    A. Allows person to remain independent and keep personal items
    B. Provides sharing common meals with other older persons
    C. Permits enjoyment of gardening and yard work
    D. Allows access to medical services and dental care
35. What is the advantage of the Elder Cottage Housing Opportunity or accessory dwelling units?
    A. Have meals with other people
    B. Have supervision and activities
    C. Live independently but near family
    D. Receive medical care in the home
36. Which care measure would the nursing assistant use for a female patient who has a weakened urinary bladder related to aging?
    A. Provide lap blankets and sweaters
    B. Assist with range-of-motion exercises
    C. Answer call lights promptly
    D. Turn and position according to care plan
37. Which care measure would the nursing assistant use for a person who has dizziness related to age-related changes in the nervous system?
    A. Remind person to get up slowly from the bed or a chair
    B. Encourage diet and fluid intake as ordered
    C. Discourage overexertion and encourage rest as needed
    D. Give good skin care and report skin breakdown
38. Which person would be best suited for an assisted living facility?
    A. Person A needs daily nursing care.
    B. Person B needs help getting in and out of bed.
    C. Person C needs help with daily living.
    D. Person D is dependent on others for all care.
39. What is the main advantage of a continuing care retirement community?
    A. Provides less costly independent living units
    B. Offers around the clock personal live-in assistant
    C. Delivers added services as care needs change
    D. Is fully funded for anyone who has Medicare
40. Which person is most likely to need a nursing center?
    A. Person A needs companionship only.
    B. Person B cannot care for themselves.
    C. Person C needs care during the daytime.
    D. Person D is developmentally disabled.
41. Which member of the health-care team is demonstrating a myth about aging?
    A. Nurse says that older people are irritable, lonely, and depressed.
    B. Social worker observes that most older people live in a family setting.
    C. Nursing assistant observes that as people mature, they are generally positive.
    D. Doctor assumes that older people want information about sexual health.
42. Which environmental observation needs to be reported because it reflects poorly on the quality of the nursing center?
    A. Ventilation is adequate to control odors.
    B. Temperature levels are comfortable and safe.
    C. Bed and bath linens are clean and in good condition.
    D. Rear exit hallway is being used as a storage space
43. What is a feature of a quality nursing center?
    A. Handrails are provided in hallways.
    B. Each resident has a private bathroom.
    C. Residents provide furniture for their rooms.
    D. Tablecloths and cloth napkins are used for dining.

Matching

Match Physical Changes During the Aging Process With the Body System Affected

A. Integumentary
B. Musculoskeletal
C. Nervous
D. Cardiovascular
E. Respiratory
F. Digestive
G. Urinary

44. ________ Reduced blood flow to the kidneys
45. ________ Arteries narrow and become stiffer
46. ________ Forgetfulness
47. ________ Gradual loss of height
48. ________ Decreased strength for coughing
49. ________ Decreased secretion of oil and sweat glands
50. ________ Difficulty digesting fried and fatty foods
51. ________ Heart pumps with less force
52. ________ Bladder muscles weaken
53. ________ Difficulty seeing green and blue colors
54. ________ Difficulty swallowing
55. ________ Lung tissue less elastic
56. ________ Bone mass decreases
57. ________ Facial hair in some women

Fill in the Blanks

58. A quality nursing center must meet Omnibus Budget Reconciliation Act of 1987 (OBRA) and Centers for Medicare and Medicaid Services (CMS) requirements to ________________.
59. List 11 everyday activities that can be affected by disabilities, illness, or changes related to aging.
    A. ________________
    B. ________________
    C. ________________
    D. ________________
    E. ________________
    F. ________________
    G. ________________
    H. ________________
    I. ________________
    J. ________________
    K. ________________
60. What changes can be made in the bathroom to make it safer for a person with poor eyesight?
    A. ________________ flooring
    B. Grab bars by ________________
    C. ________________ surfaces in showers and tubs
    D. Rugs with ________________
    E. ________________ devices on faucets and showerheads
    F. Toilet with raised ________________ or toilet ________________
    G. ________________ lighting
61. Name the housing options described in each of the following:
    A. A small portable home that can be placed in the yard of a single-family home ________________.
    B. Provides meals, supervision, activities, and sometimes rehabilitation to the elderly during daytime ________________.
    C. The elderly person lives with older brothers, sisters, or cousins for companionship or to share living expenses ________________.
    D. The elderly person pays rent and utility bills but does not need to do maintenance, yard work, or snow removal ________________.
    E. The elderly person who needs help with activities of daily living but does not need nursing care may live in a ________________.
    F. A ________________ meets the changing needs of older persons. Services change as the person's needs change.

Optional Learning Exercises

62. An older person may experience cognitive changes. The nursing assistant would follow the care plan to assist with ________________ or ________________ changes.
63. When bathing an older person, what kind of soap should be used? ________________ Often, no soap is used on the ________________.
64. Because bone mass decreases, why is it important to turn an older person carefully?
    ____
65. Why does an older person often have a gradual loss of height?
    ____
66. What types of exercise help prevent bone loss and loss of muscle strength?
    ____
67. What problems can occur because of the physiologic changes related to aging?
    A. Nerve conduction and reflexes are slower.
    ____
    ____
    B. Blood flow to the brain is reduced.
    ____
    C. Touch and sensitivity to pain and pressure are reduced. ________________
    ____
68. The nursing assistant notices that an older person puts salt on vegetables that are well seasoned by the dietary staff. What may be a reason for this?
    ____
69. What exercises will help a person with circulation changes who must stay in bed? ________________
    ____

70. What can the nursing assistant do to prevent respiratory complications from bed rest?

____

71. The stomach and colon empty slower and flatulence and constipation are common in the older person. What causes these problems? _______________

____

72. How will good oral hygiene and denture care improve food intake? _______________

____

73. How can a nursing assistant help prevent urinary tract infections in an older person? _______________

____

74. Why should the nursing assistant plan to give most fluids to the older person before 1700 (5:00 PM)?

____

Use the FOCUS ON PRIDE Section to Complete These Statements and Then Use the Critical Thinking and Discussion Question to Develop Your Ideas

75. List at least four ways that you can promote dignity and respect for the older person
    A. _______________
    B. _______________
    C. _______________
    D. _______________

Critical Thinking and Discussion Question

76. Discuss some beliefs or ideas that you have about older people. After studying and caring for older people in the clinical setting have your ideas changed? If so, give examples.

13 The Person's Unit

Fill in the Blanks: Key Terms

Entrapment | Full visual privacy | Hospital bed system | Person's unit

1. The space, furniture, and equipment used by the person in the agency is the ______________________________.
2. Getting caught, trapped, or entangled in spaces created by the bed rails, the mattress, the bed frame, the headboard, or the footboard is ______________________________.
3. ______________________________ is the bed frame and its parts: the mattress, bed rails, headboard and footboard, and bed attachments.
4. The person has the means to be completely free from public view while in bed when they have ______________________________.

Circle the Best Answer

5. Which nursing assistant has made an error in the daily maintenance of the person's unit?
   A. Nursing assistant A keeps call light within reach at all times.
   B. Nursing assistant B adjusts the temperature for the person's comfort.
   C. Nursing assistant C wipes the overbed table and moves it out of the way.
   D. Nursing assistant D empties the wastebaskets at least daily and when full.
6. What is the best rationale for leaving furniture or belongings in place for a person who has poor vision?
   A. Person may rely on memory or sense of touch to find items.
   B. It is disrespectful to the person to rearrange their personal items.
   C. Moving furniture causes too much noise and confusion.
   D. Moving belongings is not part of the nursing assistant's duties.
7. Which action would the nursing assistant take upon finding a resident with their head caught in the hospital bed entrapment zone 1?
   A. Lower the side rail
   B. Ask the resident how they got there
   C. Pull on the resident's head
   D. Call the nurse immediately for help
8. Which nursing assistant has made an error for completing the safety check before leaving the room?
   A. Nursing assistant A makes sure that the resident is wearing her eyeglasses.
   B. Nursing assistant B stores the resident's cane in the back corner of the closet.
   C. Nursing assistant C puts the bed in a low, safe, and comfortable position.
   D. Nursing assistant D checks to see that unused electrical equipment is turned off.
9. For which resident is the care plan likely to include keeping the head of the bed raised at least 30 degrees?
   A. Resident A is recovering from hip surgery.
   B. Resident B wants to listen to music while resting.
   C. Resident C is confused and has a tendency to wander.
   D. Resident D is currently having mild shortness of breath.
10. Which resident's behavior should be reported to the nurse?
    A. Resident A asks you to keep the door of her room closed.
    B. Resident B is using her roommate's shampoo and lotion.
    C. Resident C has placed family pictures on her bedside table.
    D. Resident D wants to borrow a novel from the community bookshelf.
11. Which temperature range is correct to meet the Centers for Medicare and Medicaid Services (CMS) requirement for nursing centers?
    A. 68°F to 74°F
    B. 61°F to 71°F
    C. 71°F to 81°F
    D. 78°F to 85°F
12. Which temperature adjustment may be necessary for older persons or those who are ill?
    A. Cooler room temperatures
    B. Higher room temperatures
    C. Decreased temperature in the night
    D. Warmer room in the morning
13. Which factor can the nursing staff control to enhance the residents' comfort?
    A. Illness
    B. Age
    C. Noise
    D. Facility design
14. Which nursing measure is the best way to protect a person who is sensitive to drafts?
    A. Putting the person to bed
    B. Giving the person a hot shower
    C. Offering a lap cover
    D. Turning off the air-conditioning
15. Which factor causes older persons to be more sensitive to the cold?
    A. Poor circulation and a loss of fatty tissue
    B. Confusion about the season and time of day
    C. Poor nutrition and low body weight
    D. Inability to select warm clothes and dress themselves

16. Which action would the nursing assistant use to reduce unpleasant odors?
    A. Use spray deodorizers before cleaning up feces or urine
    B. Report poor personal hygiene to the charge nurse
    C. Place soiled linens and clothing in the far corner of the room
    D. Empty and clean bedpans, commodes, and urinals promptly
17. Which circumstance is the surveyor most likely to query when observing for comfortable sound levels in a health-care agency?
    A. Noise levels in the evening are decreased as the residents get ready to retire to bed.
    B. During a social activity, the residents converse with each other in conversational tones.
    C. Nursing assistant calls across the dining room to ask about residents' drink preferences.
    D. Nurse answers the intercom at a low volume to prevent others from overhearing.
18. Which measure helps to reduce noises in a health-care agency?
    A. Control the volume and tone of your voice
    B. Use metal equipment, such as meal trays
    C. Step outside to answer your cell phone
    D. Move residents outside when housekeepers are cleaning
19. For which person and circumstance is bright lighting the best choice?
    A. A person with poor vision is trying to read a medication label.
    B. The nursing assistant is helping a person to put on a shirt.
    C. A person who is hard of hearing wants to watch television.
    D. The person had a busy day and wants to rest and relax.
20. What is the advantage of a low bed position?
    A. Is the safest position to give care, such as a bed bath
    B. Allows the person get out of bed with ease
    C. Facilitates the transfer of the person to a stretcher
    D. Helps the person to maintain good body alignment
21. What is the rationale for leaving the cranks on manual beds in a down position when not in use?
    A. Prevents persons from operating the bed
    B. Prevents anyone walking past the crank from bumping into it
    C. Keeps the bed in the correct position
    D. Ensures that bed crank is ready to use at all times
22. How can the staff prevent a person from adjusting an electric bed to unsafe positions?
    A. Lock the bed into a position
    B. Unplug the bed
    C. Put the person in a bed that cannot be repositioned
    D. Keep reminding the person not to change the position
23. Which action will the nursing assistant use when the nurse says to put the patient in a semi-Fowler's position?
    A. Lower the head of the bed until flat
    B. Raise the head of the bed to 30 degrees
    C. Raise the head of the bed to 45 to 60 degrees
    D. Raise the head of the bed to 60 to 90 degrees
24. When would the nursing assistant lock the bed wheels?
    A. Only when giving care
    B. When the person is not using bed rails
    C. At all times except when moving the bed
    D. When indicated in the care plan
25. Which person has the greatest risk for bed entrapment?
    A. Person A is alert and oriented.
    B. Person B moves easily and independently in bed.
    C. Person C is elderly, frail, and confused.
    D. Person D is morbidly obese.
26. Which bed is needed for a person who weighs 600 pounds?
    A. Electric bed
    B. Manual bed
    C. Bariatric bed
    D. Bed without rails
27. Which question will the nursing assistant ask the nurse because a confused bedridden resident has gotten his leg stuck in hospital bed entrapment zone 4 several times over the past few days?
    A. "How frequently should I check the resident for safe bed position?"
    B. "Should I raise all of the side rails or is it better if the rails are lowered?"
    C. "Can I restrain the resident's extremities, so he doesn't get injured?"
    D. "Could the resident be given a medication to decrease his restlessness?"
28. Which circumstance increases the risk for a child to become entrapped in a crib?
    A. Mattress is larger than the crib.
    B. Mattress is smaller than the crib.
    C. Mattress is too soft.
    D. Bumper pad does not fit correctly.
29. Which items are never placed on the overbed table?
    A. Meals, snacks, and drinks
    B. Personal care items
    C. Writing and reading materials
    D. Bedpans, urinals, and soiled linens
30. Where are the bedpan and urinal stored?
    A. Wherever the person wants them kept
    B. On the top shelf of the person's closet
    C. On the lower shelf or drawer of the bedside stand
    D. In the top drawer of the person's chest of drawers

31. Which nursing assistant is correctly using the privacy curtains?
    A. Nursing assistant A always closes curtains if there is more than one person in the room.
    B. Nursing assistant B always pulls curtains completely around the bed before giving care.
    C. Nursing assistant C closes the privacy curtains to block sounds and conversations.
    D. Nursing assistant D only closes the curtains if the person specifically requests privacy.
32. Which action achieves full visual privacy as required by the Centers for Medicare & Medicaid Services (CMS)?
    A. Covering the person with a bath blanket
    B. Placing a movable screen around the person
    C. Assisting the person to don a full-length robe
    D. Asking other persons in the room to look away
33. Which action would the nursing assistant take upon noticing that the person develops a light red rash after application of the lotion that is on the bedside table?
    A. Report the observation to the nurse
    B. Respect the person's choice of personal care product
    C. Ask the family if this has ever happened before
    D. Obtain a new bottle of lotion from the supply room
34. Where is the call light placed when the person is weak on the left side?
    A. On the left side
    B. On the headboard
    C. On the right side
    D. Attached to bed rail
35. Which nursing measure would the nursing assistant use if a confused person cannot use a call light?
    A. Use simple language to explain how to use the call light
    B. Instruct the person to call out loudly for assistance
    C. Ask the family to give suggestions for a solution
    D. Check the person often to make sure needs are met
36. When a person turns on a call light, who should answer it?
    A. Only the person assigned to give care to the person.
    B. Any available nursing team member should answer and assist the person.
    C. The charge nurse will decide and delegate the task to someone.
    D. Another team member may answer but is not expected to give any care.
37. Which person would benefit most from an elevated toilet seat?
    A. Person A has discomfort in hip and knee joints.
    B. Person B has a plaster cast because of a broken arm.
    C. Person C is transferred by using a mechanical lift.
    D. Person D is very short and overweight.
38. What would the nursing assistant watch and listen for in case a person uses a bathroom call light?
    A. Red flashing light above the room door and at the nurses' station
    B. Same sound as the room call lights
    C. Activation of the intercom, so the person can speak
    D. Yellow flashing light above the bathroom door
39. Which nursing assistant is compliant with the CMS requirements for the person's closet and drawer space?
    A. Nursing assistant A stores roommates' clothes and belonging in the same closet.
    B. Nursing assistant B cleans out the drawer whenever it is ajar and discards trash.
    C. Nursing assistant C ensures that person can reach the drawer to access belongings.
    D. Nursing assistant D suspects hoarding so closet is searched while person is asleep.
40. Which nursing assistant has exceeded their responsibilities in maintaining the person's unit?
    A. Nursing assistant A throws away papers and knickknacks that are cluttering the room.
    B. Nursing assistant B arranges personal items after discussing the person's preferences.
    C. Nursing assistant C empties the wastebasket and linen receptacle at least once a day.
    D. Nursing assistant D explains that the unusual noises are related to building repairs.
41. Which circumstance violates a "comfortable" sound level according to the Centers for Medicare & Medicaid Services (CMS) criteria?
    A. Singing songs in the activity center interferes with a resident's rest and sleep.
    B. Arrangement of the activity room allows everyone to take part in social activities.
    C. Distant between residents' rooms and dayroom promotes privacy when privacy is desired.
    D. Music from the chapel is at a level that allows conversation in residents' rooms.
42. Which action would the nursing assistant take before giving care to assigned patients after smoking a cigarette during lunch break?
    A. Perform dental hygiene with brushing, flossing, and mouthwash
    B. Ask the nurse what to do about patients who are sensitive to odors
    C. Change into a clean uniform and brush hair with a dry shampoo
    D. Perform handwashing and follow other agency procedures
43. What is an important function that is served by safe and comfortable lighting?
    A. Increases brightness, intensity, glare, and amount of available light.
    B. The nurse has central control over intensity, location, and direction of light.
    C. Visually impaired persons maintain or increase independent functioning.
    D. Older people feel safer and more relaxed when rooms are bright and well lit.
44. Which factor can the health-care staff control that would contribute to the residents' comfort?
    A. Gender preference
    B. Acute illness
    C. Ventilation
    D. Age-related disorders

45. Which staff member is performing an action that increases noise and decreases comfort for the residents in a nursing center?
    A. Doctor stands out in the hall and calls out for someone to bring the patient's lunch tray.
    B. Nursing assistant handles metal equipment carefully to decease banging and clanging.
    C. Nursing assistant immediately reports equipment that is not in good working order.
    D. Nurse answers the phones and intercoms promptly and quietly to maintain privacy.

Fill in the Blanks

46. Describe each hospital bed system entrapment zone
    A. Zone 1 ____________________
    B. Zone 2 ____________________
    C. Zone 3 ____________________
    D. Zone 4 ____________________
    E. Zone 5 ____________________
    F. Zone 6 ____________________
    G. Zone 7 ____________________

Labeling

47. In this figure

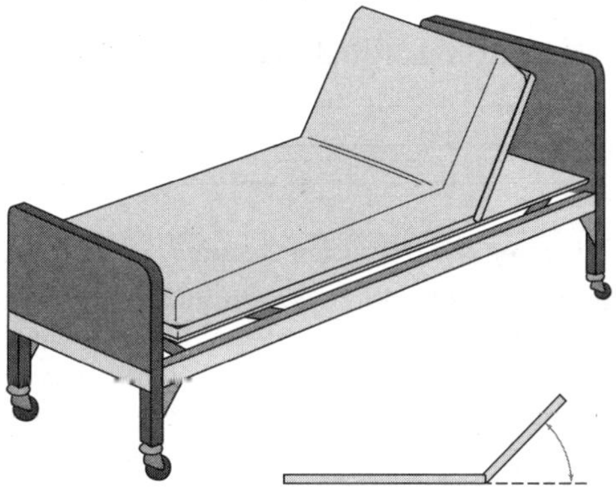

What is the bed position called?

____

48. In this figure

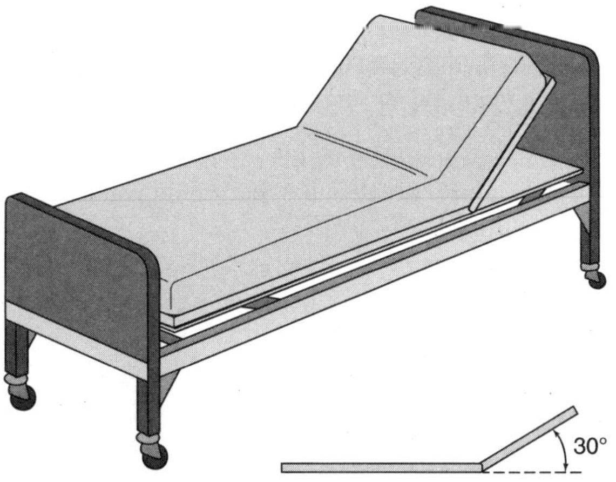

What is the bed position called?

____

49. In this figure

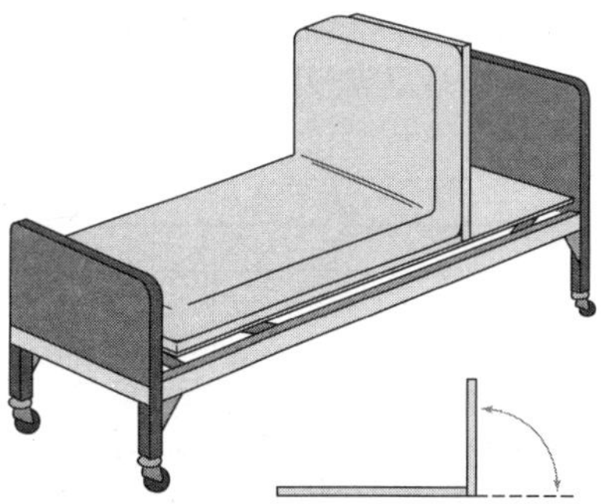

What is the bed position called?

____

50. In this figure

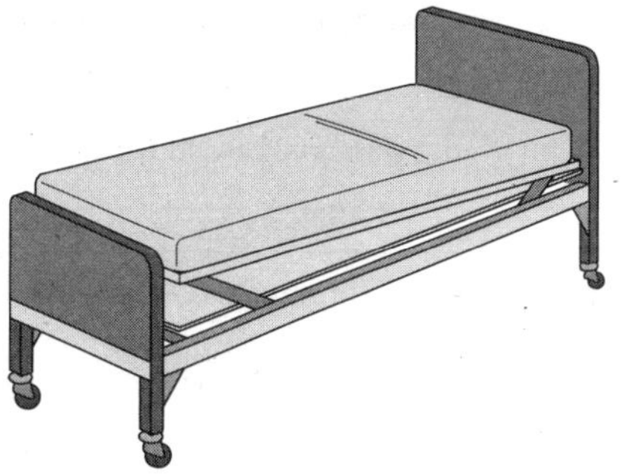

What is the bed position called?

____

51. In this figure

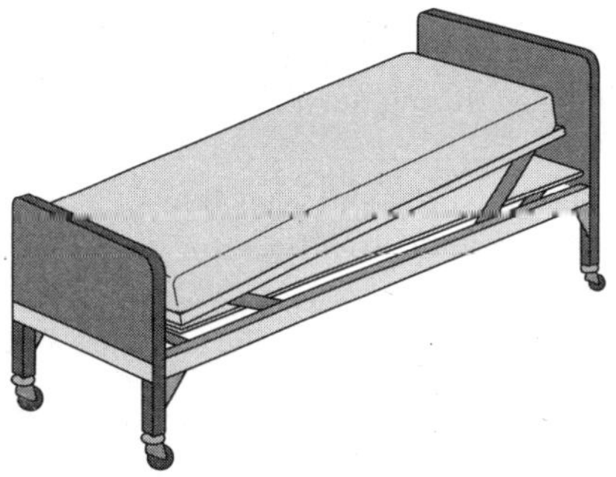

What is the bed position called?

____

Optional Learning Exercises

52. List five questions/statements that you could ask to determine if the person feels comfortable.
    A. ______
    B. ______
    C. ______
    D. ______
    E. ______
53. In these situations, how would you protect a person from drafts?
    A. The person is dressing for the day. ______
    B. The person is sitting in a wheelchair. ______
    C. You are assisting a person who is going to bed for the night. ______
    D. You are giving personal care to the person. ______
54. How can you help to eliminate odors in these situations?
    A. You are caring for a person who is frequently incontinent. ______
    B. The person is vomiting and has wound drainage. ______
    C. The person changes his own ostomy drainage bag in his bathroom. ______
    D. The person keeps a urinal at his bedside and uses it himself during the day. ______
55. For a person with poor vision, how does good lighting contribute to safety? ______
56. What does CMS require for the furniture and equipment listed?
    A. Closet space ______
    B. Bed and bath linens ______
    C. Chair ______
    D. Temperature ______
    E. Toilet seat ______
    F. Number of persons in a room ______
    G. Windows ______
    H. Call system ______
    I. Lighting ______
    J. Hand rails ______
57. When the nursing team uses the overbed table as a work area, which items can be placed on it? ______
58. What are your responsibilities in these situations regarding the call light?
    A. The person is sitting in a chair next to the bed. ______
    B. The person is weak on the right side. ______
    C. The person calls out instead of using the call light. ______
    D. The person is embarrassed because she soiled the bed after calling for assistance. ______
    E. The call light in a bathroom rings while you are busy in another room. ______

Use the FOCUS ON PRIDE section to complete these statements and then use the critical thinking and discussion question to develop your ideas

59. You will need to move items in the person's setting when giving care. What can you do to show respect?
    A. ______
    B. ______
    C. ______
60. You help to promote independence and safety by
    A. ______
    B. ______
    C. ______

Critical Thinking and Discussion Question

61. You know that Resident B's family brought a special box of candy for her yesterday. When you enter the room, Resident A says, "Look, my family brought this candy for me." Resident A proceeds to eat the candy and then stores the box with her personal items. Resident B looks tearful but says nothing and looks away. Later, you see Resident A walk up to Resident B and grab B's lap cover. Resident B says, nothing and acts like nothing has happened. The next day, you notice that Resident B's furniture and other personal items have been pushed into a far corner and Resident A has taken over much of the space in the room. When you ask Resident B about the furniture, she quietly says, "It's okay. I don't want any trouble." You suspect that Resident A is intimidating her roommate Resident B. What would you do?

14 Safety

Fill in the Blanks: Key Terms

Coma	Electrical shock	Hazard	Poison
Dementia	Elopement	Hazardous chemical	Suffocation
Disaster	Ground	Paralysis	Workplace violence

1. When a patient or resident leaves the agency without staff knowledge, it is ______________________.
2. The loss of cognitive function that interferes with daily life and activities is ______________________.
3. ______________________ are violent acts (including assault or threat of assault) directed toward persons at work or while on duty.
4. A ______________________ is anything in the person's setting that could cause injury or illness.
5. ______________________ is any chemical that is a physical hazard or a health hazard.
6. A ______________________ is harmful event that can affect the agency, patient or resident population, community, or larger geographic area.
7. ______________________ occurs when breathing stops from the lack of oxygen.
8. A ______________________ is any substance harmful to the body when ingested, inhaled, injected, or absorbed through the skin.
9. A ______________________ is prolonged state of unconsciousness.
10. That which carries leaking electricity to the earth and away from an electrical appliance is a ______________________.
11. ______________________ means loss of muscle function.
12. ______________________ occurs when electrical current passes through the body.

Circle the Best Answer

13. What will happen when the nursing assistant files an incident report about an equipment-related accident?
    A. Nurse will be responsible for any injuries that occurred.
    B. Nursing assistant must attend an equipment safety training.
    C. Report is reviewed by a risk management committee.
    D. Report will be used to justify buying new equipment.
14. Which action is the home care nursing assistant's responsibility in preventing accidental poisoning in the patient's home?
    A. Discard poisonous household plants and other poisonous substances.
    B. Ensure that the family buys products with child-resistant packaging.
    C. Administer drugs prescribed by a licensed health-care professional.
    D. Store personal care items, such as soap and shampoo, according to agency policy.
15. Which health disorder can be caused by hazardous chemicals?
    A. Viral infection
    B. Cancer
    C. Obesity
    D. Diabetes
16. Which action would you take when a person seems increasingly upset and may become aggressive?
    A. Take a strong stance and firmly tell the person to calm down
    B. Identify and remove any objects that can be used as weapons
    C. Point your finger to gain the person's attention
    D. Run from the room as quickly as possible
17. Which event is an example of an incident?
    A. Person always wants someone to hold her hand.
    B. Person tells the nursing assistant a joke.
    C. Person reports that someone took her necklace.
    D. Person asks the nursing assistant for an extra dessert.
18. Where would the nursing assistant look to find specific safety measures that are needed for resident in a long-term care center who is at risk for elopement?
    A. Doctor's orders
    B. Care plan
    C. Kardex
    D. Progress notes
19. Which action would the nursing assistant take upon finding the home health patient in a confused state and a strong odor of smoke throughout the house?
    A. Check the house to make sure that no one else is there
    B. Help the patient to immediately go outside and call 911
    C. Call the supervising nurse and report the patient's confusion
    D. Look for the source or location of the smoke or fire

20. Which safety issue is the biggest concern for a person who takes a drug that causes loss of balance as a side effect?
    A. Potential for suffocation
    B. Risk for injuries due to falls
    C. Burning self with hot water
    D. Unintentional poisoning
21. Which developmental factor places young children at risk for injury?
    A. They have not learned the difference between safety and danger.
    B. They have limited control over their environment.
    C. They have poor motor control and no self-discipline.
    D. They have not learned how to read and interpret information.
22. Which characteristic of dementia increases a person's risk for injury?
    A. There is an inability to smell and react to hazardous odors.
    B. Judgment and the ability to discriminate danger are lacking.
    C. Physical immobility prevents moving to a safe place.
    D. Dementia increases sensitive to hazardous materials.
23. What is the most important reason for the nursing assistant to correctly identify persons who are assigned for care?
    A. Life and health are threatened if the wrong care is given.
    B. Visitors or doctors may ask for help to find someone.
    C. It is polite and professional to call a person by the right name.
    D. Care and work are doubled if care is given to the wrong person.
24. Which nursing assistant is not using a reliable way to identify the person?
    A. Nursing assistant A checks the person's identification bracelet.
    B. Nursing assistant B uses the person's picture and compares it to the person.
    C. Nursing assistant C follows the center's policy to identify the person.
    D. Nursing assistant D recognizes the person and greets them by name.
25. Which accidental injury or harm is the most likely to occur in children less than 4 years old and older persons who have trouble swallowing?
    A. Falls
    B. Burns
    C. Poisoning
    D. Suffocation
26. Which action would the supervising adult take when children are in the kitchen?
    A. Use the burners at the back of the stove
    B. Turn pot and pan handles so they point outward
    C. Supervise children to help cook at the stove
    D. Leave cooking utensils in pots and pans
27. What is the rationale for using dry oven mitts and pot holders to avoid burns?
    A. Dry material provides a thicker layer.
    B. Water conducts heat and can cause burns.
    C. Moisture allows bacteria to penetrate the cloth.
    D. Mitts and pot holders are not waterproof.
28. Which circumstance increases the risk of accidental poisoning of children?
    A. Harmful products are kept in their original containers.
    B. Harmful substances are labeled and stored in locked areas.
    C. Drugs are carried in purses, backpacks, and briefcases.
    D. Safety latches are used on cabinets and storage spaces.
29. Which item needs a "Mr. Yuk" sticker?
    A. A sealed box of dog biscuits
    B. An unopened bottle of red wine
    C. An opened jar of mayonnaise
    D. A spray bottle of bathroom cleaner
30. Which child has the greatest risk for lead poisoning?
    A. 6-month-old infant is being switched from breastfeeding to bottle feeding.
    B. 8-month old infant is crawling and likes to put objects in the mouth.
    C. 10-year old frequently plays with friends in a nearby forested area.
    D. 15-year old is learning to shoot guns and some bullets are made of lead.
31. Which action would the home health nursing assistant take if water is contaminated with lead from the interior plumbing?
    A. Use only bottled water until the plumbing is completely renovated
    B. Run the water until it is hot before drinking or using it for baby formula
    C. Boil all water for at least 20 minutes, cool, and then use in cooking
    D. Flush cold water through the faucets for several minutes before using it for cooking
32. Which gas is associated with accidental poisoning in the household?
    A. Oxygen
    B. Carbon dioxide
    C. Carbon monoxide
    D. Nitrogen
33. Which of these is a source of carbon monoxide?
    A. Computer
    B. Vacuum cleaner
    C. Furnace
    D. Electric heater
34. Which circumstance increases the risk of choking hazard for an older person?
    A. Loose dentures that fit poorly
    B. Sitting up in a wheelchair to eat
    C. Using supplemental oxygen
    D. Eating a snack after dinner time

35. Which toy would be the best to prevent accidental choking?
  A. Mobile hanging over the crib
  B. Stuffed toy with no removable parts
  C. Small plastic action figure
  D. Toy car with interchangeable parts
36. What is the universal sign for choking?
  A. Person begins to cough forcefully.
  B. Conscious person clutches at the throat.
  C. Person says he is choking.
  D. Person becomes unconscious.
37. For which person would the nursing assistant use abdominal thrusts for choking?
  A. Pregnant woman
  B. Obese older man
  C. 8-month-old infant
  D. 12-year-old child
38. What is the correct procedure for abdominal thrusts for a person who is choking?
  A. Make a fist, place the thumb side on the abdomen, and quickly thrust upward
  B. Press the fist against the abdomen and slowly push straight down
  C. Gently thrust upward on the abdomen with the palmar surface of the hand
  D. Lay the hands on top of each other over the abdomen and push down
39. Which action would the nursing assistant take upon observing a foreign object in the mouth of a conscious person?
  A. Turn the head to one side and pat the person's back
  B. Leave the object in place and do abdominal thrusts
  C. Remove the object if it is within easy reach
  D. Ask the person to forcefully cough out the object
40. Which action would the nursing assistant take if an infant is choking?
  A. Call 911 or take the infant to the nearest emergency room
  B. Give five abdominal thrusts using the same hand position and motions as for adults
  C. Hold the infant face down; give five forceful back slaps between the shoulder blades
  D. Reach in the mouth and try to retrieve the object or use finger sweeping motions
41. Which action would the nursing assistant take if emergency measures are unsuccessful and the choking person becomes unresponsive?
  A. Make sure Call Emergency Medical Services or Rapid Response was called
  B. Begin abdominal thrusts
  C. Give two rescue breaths
  D. Finger sweep mouth for foreign objects
42. Which occurrence suggests that there is a fault in the electrical item?
  A. The nursing assistant hears a sizzling or buzzing sound when the toaster oven is on.
  B. The lamp on the person's bedside table was left on overnight.
  C. The nursing assistant notices that a vacuum cleaner is not picking up dirt and dust.
  D. The light in the back of the refrigerator does not come on.
43. What is the primary purpose of the three-pronged plug?
  A. It acts as ground to carry leaking electricity away from the appliance.
  B. It stabilizes the contact with outlet so that the connection is more secure.
  C. It protects the function of the appliance if there is a power surge.
  D. It prevents fires by distributing the current if usage is prolonged.
44. An electrical shock is especially dangerous to which body system?
  A. Urinary system
  B. Circulatory system
  C. Lymphatic system
  D. Reproductive system
45. Which action would the nursing assistant take if shocked by electrical equipment?
  A. Report the shock at once
  B. Try to repair the equipment
  C. Make sure it has a ground prong
  D. Test the equipment in a different outlet
46. Which organization requires that health-care employees understand the risks of hazardous substances and how to handle them safely?
  A. Omnibus Budget Reconciliation of 1987 (OBRA)
  B. Occupational Safety and Health Administration (OSHA)
  C. Centers for Medicare and Medicaid Services (CMS)
  D. Centers for Disease Control and Prevention (CDC)
47. Which information is not included on the safety data sheet (SDS) of a hazardous chemical?
  A. Physical hazards and health hazards
  B. What protective equipment to wear
  C. Contact information for local resources
  D. Storage and disposal information
48. For which situation would the nursing assistant refer to the safety data sheets for hazardous materials?
  A. Trying to safely store the product
  B. Needing to order additional product
  C. Needing to replace the warning label
  D. Determining possibility of allergic reaction
49. For which circumstance is the nursing assistant most likely to don gloves for personal protection?
  A. A person is choking and requires abdominal thrusts.
  B. An electrical fan is sparking and needs to be unplugged.
  C. A cleaning solution is used to disinfect a bedpan.
  D. The nurse asks for help during an elopement situation.
50. Which of these is allowed in the room when a person is receiving oxygen?
  A. Visitors may smoke if they use caution.
  B. Wool or synthetic blankets in good condition
  C. Electrical items that are in good working order
  D. Alcohol-based aftershave in a glass container

51. Which action would the nursing assistant do first if a fire occurs?
    A. Rescue people in immediate danger
    B. Sound the nearest fire alarm
    C. Close doors and windows to confine the fire
    D. Use a fire extinguisher on a small fire
52. Which people would the nursing assistant help first if evacuation for a fire is necessary?
    A. Closest to the outside door are rescued first.
    B. Able to walk are rescued first.
    C. Closest to the fire are evacuated first.
    D. Helpless are rescued first.
53. What is a safety practice to use if a space heater is used in a home?
    A. Place the heater in doorways or in hallways, away from the bed.
    B. Keep the heater 3 feet away from curtains, drapes, and furniture.
    C. Use an extension cord and place the heater in a distant corner.
    D. Keep the heater on the lowest temperature throughout the night.
54. Which action would the nursing assistant take if there is a disaster?
    A. Immediately report to the agency's charge nurse for duty
    B. Follow the training for emergency procedures
    C. Stay away or leave to get out of the way
    D. Go home to check on family and friends
55. According to OSHA, which nursing assistant has the greatest risk for workplace violence?
    A. Nursing assistant A cares for elderly residents at a nursing center located in a farming community.
    B. Nursing assistant B works in an urban clinic that serves persons with a history of violence and substance abuse.
    C. Nursing assistant C has attended several training sessions for management of hostile and assaultive behaviors.
    D. Nursing assistant D is paired with a coworker, and they work together when transporting patients and residents.
56. What is the immediate action to use to prevent and control workplace violence when a person becomes angry and aggressive?
    A. Stand far enough away from the person to avoid being hit or kicked
    B. Call for help and then the staff stands together to create a defensive line
    C. Sit quietly with the person in his room and hold his hand
    D. Assume an authoritative posture, hands on hips, and chest thrust forward
57. Which nursing assistant is dressed to prevent workplace violence?
    A. Nursing assistant A has long hair up and off the collar.
    B. Nursing assistant B wears white shoes with leather soles.
    C. Nursing assistant C wears a long necklace and drop earrings.
    D. Nursing assistant D has a uniform that is loose and large.
58. Which action would the nursing assistant take if threatened in a home care setting?
    A. Call the agency for help, call the police, or leave the setting
    B. Refuse to go back and resolve the matter over the phone
    C. Confront the person who is making the threats
    D. Ignore the situation and continue to give care
59. What can cause a person to become agitated or aggressive?
    A. Daily exercise
    B. Confusion
    C. Morning hygiene routine
    D. Increased awareness of surroundings

Matching

Match each safety measure to the risk it prevents

A. Burns
B. Poisoning
C. Suffocation
D. Equipment accident
E. Hazardous substances
F. Fire

60. ________ Do not allow person to sleep with a heating pad.
61. ________ Apply sunscreen to children before they go outside.
62. ________ Keep child-resistant caps on all harmful products.
63. ________ Wear PPE to clean spills and leaks.
64. ________ Report loose teeth or dentures to the nurse.
65. ________ Turn off an electrical appliance when you are done using it.
66. ________ Attend to food cooking on the stove.
67. ________ Have water heaters set at 120°F or less.
68. ________ Never call drugs or vitamins "candy."
69. ________ Store flammable liquids outside in their original containers.

Fill in the Blanks

70. Write out the meaning of the abbreviations
    A. AED ____________________
    B. CO ____________________
    C. CPR ____________________
    D. EMS ____________________
    E. OSHA ____________________
    F. PPE ____________________
    G. RACE ____________________
    H. RRS ____________________
71. As part of the team, the nursing assistant can help provide a safe setting by correcting something that is unsafe. What would the nursing assistant do if
    A. There is a water spill on the floor ____________
    B. A person has risk for sliding out of a wheelchair ____________________
    C. A person is having problems holding a cup of coffee ____________________
    D. Food is left unattended in a microwave ____________________
    E. A grab bar is loose in the bathroom ____________ ____________________
72. When checking for safety issues, a survey team will observe ____________________.
73. A yellow color–coded wristband may indicate that the person has ____________________.
74. A red wristband warns of allergies to items, such as ____________________ ____________________.
75. The word PASS is used to remember how to use a ____________________.
    What action is taken for each of these steps?
    A. P ____________________
    B. A ____________________
    C. S ____________________
    D. S ____________________
76. Older persons are at risk for choking. Common causes include weakness, dentures that fit poorly, ____________________ and chronic illness
77. When giving ____________________, the rescuer is trying to dislodge a foreign body to relieve choking in an infant.

Short Answer

78. Identify the steps of RACE as depicted in the figure.

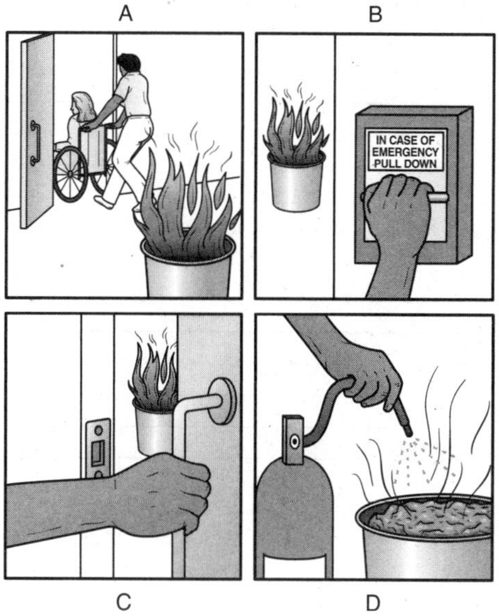

A. ____________________
B. ____________________
C. ____________________
D. ____________________

What should you do in these situations related to hazardous chemicals? (Box 14.8, p. 194)

79. When cleaning up a hazardous chemical, how do you know what equipment to wear? ____________________
80. When a spill occurs, what is the correct way to wipe it up? ____________________ ____________________
81. The nurse tells you that the person is having an X-ray done in her room. ____________________

What measures to prevent or control workplace violence are being used or should be used in these examples? (Box 14.10, p. 201)

82. What types of jewelry can serve as a weapon? ____________________ ____________________
83. Why is long hair worn up? ____________________ ____________________
84. Why are pictures, vases, and other items removed from certain areas? ____________________ ____________________
85. What clothing items should be worn by staff to safely manage aggressive persons? ____________________

Optional Learning Exercises

86. You have permission from the nurse and patient to discard outdated medication in the household trash. List four steps that you would take.
    A. ______________________________
    B. ______________________________
    C. ______________________________
    D. ______________________________
87. List at least six reasons why hoarding increases danger for the person, others in the home, and firefighters.
    A. ______________________________
    B. ______________________________
    C. ______________________________
    D. ______________________________
    E. ______________________________
    F. ______________________________

Use the FOCUS ON PRIDE section to complete these statements then use the critical thinking and discussion question to develop your ideas

88. What can you do to ensure the safety of self and other staff when arriving and leaving the agency?
    A. ______________________________
    B. ______________________________
    C. ______________________________
    D. ______________________________
    E. ______________________________

Critical Thinking and Discussion Question

89. You are caring for an older person who has dementia and occasionally, he is combative during morning hygiene. Today, he suddenly strikes out at you and bumps his arm on a side rail and sustains a laceration.
    A. Discuss how you would feel.
    B. Explain why it would be important to complete an incident report.

15 Preventing Falls

Fill in the Blanks: Key Terms

Bed rail
Gait belt
Position change alarm
Transfer belt

1. A device used to support a person who is unsteady or disabled is a ________________.
2. A ________________ is a device that serves as a guard or barrier along the side of the bed.
3. Another name for a transfer belt is a ________________.
4. A physical or electronic device that monitors a person's movement and alerts staff of movement is a ________________.

Circle the Best Answer

5. What is the most common cause of falls in nursing centers?
   A. Confusion and dementia
   B. Weakness and walking problems
   C. Throw rugs and clutter on the floor
   D. Loose or missing handrails and grab bars
6. Which of these measures would the staff use to prevent falls?
   A. Answer call lights promptly
   B. Restrain people who have risk factors
   C. Always keep side rails up
   D. Wait for position change alarms to sound
7. Which safety measure would the nursing assistant use to help prevent falls?
   A. Have the person wear reading glasses when walking
   B. Assist the person with bedpan, urinal, commode, or bathroom
   C. Rearrange the furniture and personal belongings
   D. Dim lights or limit the use of night-lights at night
8. What is the advantage of using a position change alarm?
   A. Prevents the person from getting out of bed or the chair
   B. Can be turned off and on by the person
   C. Warns when the person is getting up unassisted
   D. Is a substitute for restraints
9. Which consideration is essential if bed rails are being used?
   A. All older persons benefit from bed rails.
   B. Usage must be in the person's best interest.
   C. Usage prevents falls and reduces risk for injury.
   D. Bed rails are never used when giving care.
10. Which piece of equipment would prompt the nursing assistant to check with the nurse before using it for a patient who has a gastrostomy tube?
    A. Position change alarm
    B. Bed side rail
    C. Transfer belt
    D. Bed wheel lock
11. Which nursing assistant has correctly used the wheel locks?
    A. Nursing assistant A transfers the person to the bed and then locks wheels.
    B. Nursing assistant B locks the wheelchair wheels before transferring the person.
    C. Nursing assistant C unlocks the wheels on the bed before giving care.
    D. Nursing assistant D unlocks the stretcher wheels and then transfers the person.
12. What is the nursing assistant's primary responsibility in preventing falls during shift change?
    A. Quickly give and get shift report
    B. Know role and duties for shift change
    C. Ask the nurse to provide supervision
    D. Stay with assigned patients/residents
13. Which patient's circumstance requires checking with the nurse before using a transfer belt?
    A. Patient A is unsteady when moving from a chair to the bed.
    B. Patient B has diabetes and a heart problem.
    C. Patient C has an abdominal incision.
    D. Patient D needs help to stand up and walk.
14. Which measure might help to calm an elderly person who is agitated and upset?
    A. Bright lights and cheerful music
    B. Warm drink and a back massage
    C. Card game or a jigsaw puzzle
    D. Walk the person up and down the hallways
15. Which action would the nursing assistant take if a bariatric person starts to fall?
    A. Grasp the gait belt and pull them close
    B. Ease the person to the floor
    C. Quickly move items that could cause injury
    D. Call for help and hold the person up
16. Which action would the nursing assistant take when working alone and the bed must be raised for care and the side rails are used according to the care plan?
    A. Leave side rails up and work around them
    B. Raise the far bed rail when working alone
    C. Delay giving care until help is available
    D. Tell the person to remain still unless instructed to move

17. How would the nursing assistant position the bed after completing the care?
    A. Lower the bed to its lowest position
    B. Elevate the head of the bed and raise all side rails
    C. Ask the person how which position is preferred
    D. Raise the bed to a comfortable working height for the nurse

18. Which nursing assistant is correctly applying the principles for safe use of a position change alarm?
    A. Nursing assistant A finishes lunch break before responding to alarm.
    B. Nursing assistant B tests the alarm to confirm function before leaving the resident.
    C. Nursing assistant C puts the alarm close to the resident to allow easy access.
    D. Nursing assistant D ensures that alarm works to reduce observation of the resident.

19. Where is the information located that guides the nursing assistant in the use the bed rails for a person?
    A. Safety data sheet
    B. Doctor's orders
    C. Manufacturers' instructions
    D. Care plan

20. Which nursing assistant is correctly applying the transfer belt to a resident?
    A. Nursing assistant A places the quick-release buckle over the spine.
    B. Nursing assistant B wraps the belt at chest level and over the breasts.
    C. Nursing assistant C allows excess strap to dangle at waist level.
    D. Nursing assistant D wraps the belt around the waist over the clothing.

Fill in the Blanks

21. Tubs and showers may be made safer if they have ______________________ surfaces.

22. Handrails in hallways and stairways give support to persons who are ______________________.

23. When a transfer belt is applied, you should be able to slide ______________________ under the belt.

24. When a person starts to fall, you should protect the person's ______________________ as you ease the person to the floor.

25. Flooring is one color because bold designs can cause ____________ in older persons.

Optional Learning Exercises

26. What kinds of equipment and safety measures help to make bathrooms and showers safer?
    A. ______________________
    B. ______________________
    C. ______________________
    D. ______________________

27. What kind of footwear and clothing will help to prevent falls?
    A. Footwear
    ____
    ____
    B. Clothing
    ____
    ____

28. Why is it important to answer call lights promptly?
    ____
    ____

29. If a person does not use bed rails and you are giving care, how do you protect them from falling?
    ____

30. Wheels are locked at all times except when ______________________.

31. If a bariatric person starts to fall, you should
    A. ______________________
    B. ______________________
    C. ______________________
    D. ______________________
    E. ______________________

32. What is depicted in the figure?
    ____

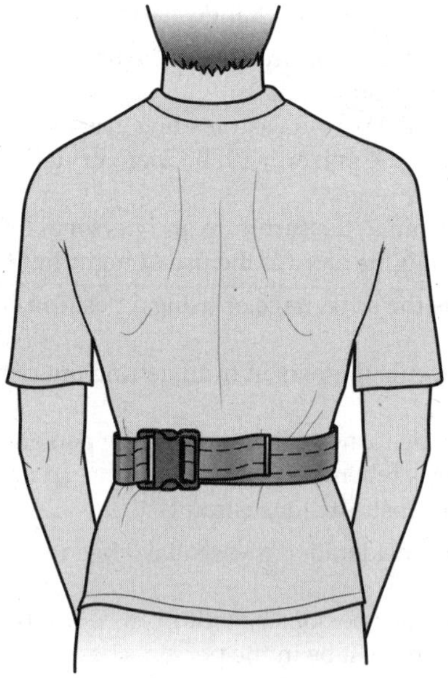

33. According to the documentation below, what safety measures were performed on 6/16 at 1415?

DATE: 06/16	TIME: 1415
ACTIVITY AND POSITIONING	
☐ Ambulate	☐ Chair
☐ Self	☒ Bed
☒ Assist of 1	☒ Right side
☐ Assist of 2	☐ Left side
☐ Mechanical lift	☐ Back

Turned Mr. Adams from his back to his right side. Placed pillows under his head, against his back, and under his left leg. He stated he was comfortable with needed items in reach (water mug, phone, tissues, urinal, call light). I told him that I will check on him every 15 minutes and to use the call light if he needs anything.

DATE: 06/16	TIME: 1415
SAFETY	
☐ Gait belt	☒ Belongings in reach
☐ Slip-resistant shoes	☒ Bed rails raised
☒ Call light in reach	☐ Bed rails lowered
☒ Bed in low position	☐ Bed/chair alarm

A. ____________________
B. ____________________
C. ____________________
D. ____________________

Use the FOCUS ON PRIDE Section to Complete These Statements and Then Use the Critical Thinking and Discussion Question to Develop Your Ideas

34. To show personal and professional responsibility, you do not take short cuts and take time to
A. ____________________
B. ____________________
C. ____________________
D. ____________________
E. ____________________

35. When assisting a coworker with a transfer, what information do you need?
A. ____________________
B. ____________________

Critical Thinking and Discussion Question

36. An elderly resident has frequent episodes of falling, despite everyone's best efforts to follow the care plan. There is no medical reason that warrants the use of restraints. The family is worried and upset. The charge nurse has called a care conference to elicit everyone's ideas about how to decrease falls for this resident. What suggestions could you offer?

16 Restraint Alternatives and Restraints

Fill in the Blanks: Key Terms

Physical restraint | Restraint alternative | Seclusion

1. Confining a person to a room or area and preventing the person from leaving is ________________________.
2. Any manual method or physical or mechanical device, material, or equipment that cannot be removed easily is a ________________________________.
3. ________________________ is a measure used instead of restraint to manage a potentially harmful situation.

Circle the Best Answer

4. Being in restraints increases the person's risk for which distressing physical condition?
   A. Fever
   B. Dehydration
   C. Vomiting
   D. Blurred vision
5. Which nursing assistant has failed, at the 2-hour interval, to meet the person's basic needs when the restraints are removed?
   A. Nursing assistant A assists the person to get up and go to the bathroom.
   B. Nursing assistant B looks underneath the restraint to see if the skin is intact.
   C. Nursing assistant C assists the person to sit up and offers food and fluids.
   D. Nursing assistant D gives emotional support and conversation while taking vital signs.
6. Which person would benefit from the application of a limb restraint?
   A. Person A occasionally strikes out at staff during care.
   B. Person B is continuously trying to stand up and is very weak.
   C. Person C is scratching and picking at a wound dressing.
   D. Person D wanders in the morning and tries to leave facility.
7. Which nursing assistant has correctly recorded a safety measure that was used for a person who is in restraints?
   A. Covered with warm blanket
   B. Applied restraints after breakfast
   C. Explained purpose of restraints
   D. Placed call light within reach
8. Which circumstance is an example of an appropriate use of restraints?
   A. Resident A is placed in seclusion for being argumentative with staff.
   B. Resident B is placed in a vest restraint to prevent continuous wandering.
   C. Resident C has a limb restraint on dominant arm to reduce pulling at a feeding tube.
   D. Resident D is put into mitt restraints for stealing property from other residents.
9. What is the purpose of restraints?
   A. To control aggression
   B. To treat a medical symptom
   C. To prevent falls
   D. To stop wandering
10. Which person is under chemical restraint?
    A. Person A is given a daily blood pressure medication.
    B. Person B is wearing a mitt restraint to prevent self-scratching.
    C. Person C is given a sleeping medication to prevent wandering.
    D. Person D is sitting in a chair that has a position change alarm.
11. Which potential cause for harmful behaviors is the most serious and needs to be reported immediately to the nurse?
    A. Person is scratching at their skin and blood is seeping out.
    B. Person is breathing fast, and loud wheezing is audible.
    C. Person walks toward the bathroom while struggling to get pants off.
    D. Person seems afraid and is anxiously looking around the room.
12. Which restraint alternative could the health care staff use to meet a person's love and belonging needs?
    A. Encourage family, friends, and volunteers to visit
    B. Pad the walls and corners of furniture
    C. Place knob guards on doors that go outside
    D. Make sure that sleep is not interrupted

13. Which person is displaying a physical need that could be relieved with a restraint alternative measure?
    A. Person A likes to talk about memories of friends and family.
    B. Person B is not sure who you are, what time it is, or where he is.
    C. Person C often talks to her dead husband and tries to touch him.
    D. Person D is always going to the bathroom to prevent incontinence.
14. Which of these is a type of restraint?
    A. A soft chair with a footstool to elevate the feet
    B. A bed that is in the lowest position
    C. A chair with a tray that prevents the person from rising
    D. A drug that helps a person function at the highest level
15. Which risks from restraints are the most common?
    A. Cuts, bruises, and fractures
    B. Death from strangulation
    C. Constipation or incontinence
    D. Depression, anger, and agitation
16. Which action would the nursing assistant take when assigned to care for a person who is in restraints, but the reason is unclear?
    A. Refuse to participate in possible false imprisonment
    B. Ask the nurse why the person is restrained
    C. Ask the person if he gave informed consent
    D. Follow the care plan for frequency of care
17. Which method would be considered the least restrictive?
    A. Vest restraint
    B. Elbow splint
    C. Positioning device
    D. Jacket restraint
18. For which person might the doctor order use of restraints?
    A. Obese person cannot fit into a wheelchair.
    B. Strong person is agitated and combative.
    C. Young person has risk for suicide
    D. Confused person has fallen out of bed several times.
19. Which action would the nursing assistant take if unsure how to apply a restraint?
    A. Ask the nurse to show the correct way to apply it
    B. Tell the nurse that someone else must apply the restraint
    C. Watch another nursing assistant apply it to a person
    D. Apply it to the person by using general safety principles
20. Which of these is a physical restraint?
    A. Raised bed rails
    B. Position change alarm
    C. Gait belt
    D. A sleeping pill
21. Which method will the health care team use when a combative and agitated person must be restrained?
    A. One staff member approaches slowly in a private area
    B. Restrain after explaining to the person what will be done
    C. Enough staff to complete the task safely and quickly
    D. In a public area so there are witnesses to the person's rights
22. How frequently must the person who is restrained be observed?
    A. Every 5 minutes
    B. Every 15 minutes
    C. Once an hour
    D. Once every 2 hours
23. Which nursing measure would the nursing assistant perform at least every 2 hours when caring for a person who is restrained?
    A. Look in on the person and make sure he is breathing
    B. Remove restraints, reposition the person, and meet basic needs
    C. Make sure the restraints are secure and person cannot get loose
    D. Change the restraints to a different type or a different position
24. For which person would wrist or limb restraints be used?
    A. Person A tries to get out of bed without calling for help.
    B. Person B moves the wheelchair without permission.
    C. Person C pulls at intravenous tube used to give fluids.
    D. Person D slides down or out of a chair easily.
25. What is the advantage of using a knob guard?
    A. It is more restrictive than other restraints but provides additional safety.
    B. It allows the residents to wander freely while preventing access to unsafe areas.
    C. It prevents confused residents from violating the personal space of others.
    D. It can only be used while the resident is being transported in a wheelchair.
26. What is the primary rationale for using a quick-release tie when securing restraints?
    A. Tie can be immediately released if there is an emergency.
    B. Person who is restrained cannot release the tie by themselves.
    C. Ensures that the restraint is snug but not restricting the person
    D. Is quick to tie if the person is struggling while being restrained

27. What is one reason to use elbow restraints?
    A. To remind adults not to pull on tubes
    B. To prevent children from touching incisions
    C. To limit use of the dominant hand
    D. To prevent injury to the staff by a confused person
28. Which action is used to correctly apply wrist restraints?
    A. Tie the straps to the bed rail.
    B. Tie firm knots in the straps.
    C. Place a warm blanket over restrained arm.
    D. Place the soft or foam part toward the skin.
29. Which nursing measure would the nursing assistant use when applying padded mitt restraints?
    A. Give the person a hand roll to hold
    B. Pad the mitt with soft material
    C. Make sure the person's hands are clean and dry
    D. Insert the hand into the restraint, palm upward
30. What would the nursing assistant check after applying a belt restraint?
    A. Person's understanding of informed consent
    B. Quick-release tie secured to the bed rail
    C. Comfort and good body alignment
    D. Pulses and skin temperature
31. Which action would the nursing assistant take to correctly apply a vest restraint for a person who is in bed?
    A. Ties are secured to the bed frame out of the person's reach.
    B. Ties are secured to the bed rail within the person's reach.
    C. Ensures that the vest crosses in the back and "V" is in the back
    D. Checks to see if the person can turn over or roll side to side
32. Which observation would the nursing assistant immediately report for a person in vest, jacket, or belt restraint?
    A. The skin is slightly reddened under the restraint.
    B. The person needs to urinate or have a bowel movement.
    C. The person is not breathing or is having difficulty breathing.
    D. The person needs to be repositioned.

Matching

Match the Laws and Safety Guidelines With the Correct Example

A. Restraints must protect the person.
B. Restraints require a written doctor's order.
C. The least restrictive method of restraint is used.
D. Restraints are used only after other methods fail to protect the person.
E. Unnecessary restraint is false imprisonment.
F. Informed consent is required for restraint use.
G. The manufacturer's instructions are followed.
H. Restraints are applied with enough help to protect the person and staff from injury.
I. Observe for increased confusion and agitation.
J. Quality of life must be protected.
K. The person is observed at least every 15 minutes or more often as required by the care plan.
L. The restraint is removed, the person repositioned, and basic needs are met at least every 2 hours.

33. ________ Injuries and deaths have occurred from improper restraint and poor observation.
34. ________ A restraint is used only when it is the best safety precaution for the person.
35. ________ You are provided the manufacturer's instructions for applying and securing restraints.
36. ________ Restrained persons need repeated explanations and reassurance.
37. ________ The doctor gives the reason for the restraint, what to use, and how long to use the restraint.
38. ________ Persons in immediate danger of harming themselves or others are restrained quickly.
39. ________ Positioning devices are used whenever possible, instead of vest or jacket restraints.
40. ________ Restraints are used only for a brief time.
41. ________ If told to apply a restraint, you must clearly understand the need for restraints and the risks.
42. ________ Restraint is removed. Person is ambulated or range-of-motion exercises are performed.
43. ________ The care plan must include measures to protect the person and to prevent the person from harming others.
44. ________ The person must understand the reason for the restraints.

Fill in the Blanks

45. The restriction of voluntary movement or the control of behavior is called ________________________.
46. Persons restrained in a supine position must be monitored constantly because they are at great risk for ________________________ if vomiting occurs.
47. You should carry scissors with you because in an emergency ________________________.
48. A ________________________ is any drug or drug dosage that is used for discipline or convenience that is not required to treat medical symptoms.

Optional Learning Exercises

49. When using restraints, what information is reported and recorded?
    A. ______
    B. ______
    C. ______
    D. ______
    E. ______
    F. ______
    G. ______
    H. ______
    I. ______
    J. ______
50. The nursing assistant is checking the patient who is in restraints at least every 2 hours. Which observations must be immediately reported to the nurse?
    A. ______
    B. ______
    C. ______
    D. ______
51. When you check a mitt, wrist, or ankle restraint every 15 minutes, tell the nurse at once if you observe these signs or symptoms.
    A. ______
    B. ______
    C. ______
    D. ______
52. When you remove the restraints every 2 hours, what are the basic needs that should be met?
    A. ______
    B. ______
    C. ______
    D. ______
    E. ______
    F. ______
    G. ______
53. When you are delegated to apply restraints, what information do you need from the nurse and the care plan?
    A. ______
    B. ______
    C. ______
    D. ______
    E. ______
    F. ______
    G. ______
    H. ______
    I. ______
    J. ______
    K. ______
    L. ______
    M. ______
    N. ______

Use the FOCUS ON PRIDE Section to Complete These Statements and Then Use the Critical Thinking and Discussion Question to Develop Your Ideas

54. When a person has restraints in place, what are your professional responsibilities?
    A. ______
    B. ______
    C. ______
    D. ______
    E. ______

Critical Thinking and Discussion Question

55. You are assigned to take over the care of a person who has been in restraints for the past 8 hours. As you are checking the person, you find that the person has urinated and defecated in the bed, the skin underneath the restraints is red and a small sore is noted in one area. The person immediately begs you for water and food. What will you do?

17 Preventing Infection

Fill in the Blanks: Key Terms

Antibiotic	Contamination	Infection control	Vaccination
Antiseptic	Cross-contamination	Nonpathogen	Vaccine
Antisepsis	Disinfectant	Normal flora	
Asepsis	Disinfection	Pathogen	
Biohazardous waste	Health care–associated infection (HAI)	Spore	
Carrier	Immunity	Sterile	
Communicable disease (contagious disease)	Infection	Sterile field	
		Sterilization	

1. ____________________ is passing microbes from person to person by contaminated hands, equipment, or supplies.
2. ____ are items contaminated with blood or other potentially infectious materials (OPIM), regulated medical waste, and infectious waste.
3. A microbe that is harmful and can cause an infection is a ____.
4. A human or animal that is a reservoir for microbes but does not have signs and symptoms of infection is a ____.
5. Protection against a certain disease is _____________.
6. A preparation containing dead or weakened microbes is a ____.
7. A work area free of all pathogens and nonpathogens is a ____.
8. Practices and procedures that prevent the spread of disease are ________________________________.
9. The administration of a vaccine to produce immunity against an infectious disease is __________________.
10. An _______________ is a drug that kills bacteria.
11. An ___________ is a disease state resulting from the invasion and growth of microorganisms in the body.
12. ____________________ is a disease caused by a pathogen that can spread to others.
13. A bacterium protected by a hard shell is a _________.
14. The process of destroying pathogens is ____________ _________________.
15. The processes, procedures, and chemical treatments that kill microbes or prevent them from causing an infection are ___________________.
16. A ___________________________ is an infection that develops in a person cared for in any setting where health care is given.
17. _________________ is being free of disease-producing microbes.
18. ________________________________ is the process of destroying all microbes.
19. A __________________ is a liquid chemical that can kill many or all pathogens except spores.
20. A microbe that does not usually cause an infection is a ____.
21. The process of becoming unclean is _______________.
22. The absence of all microbes is __________________.
23. __________________________ are microbes that usually live and grow in a certain area.
24. A substance applied to living tissue that prevents or stops the growth or action of microbes is an ___________________________.

Circle the Best Answer

25. Which nursing assistant is correctly performing one of the steps in hand hygiene?
    - A. Nursing assistant A rests hips against the sink to reach soap on a high shelf.
    - B. Nursing assistant B uses a dry towel to turn on and adjust water until it is hot.
    - C. Nursing assistant C uses a clean, dry paper towel to turn off the water.
    - D. Nursing assistant D touches the inside of the sink to clear the drain.
26. How long should the hands be rubbed together when using an alcohol-based hand sanitizer?
    - A. 10 seconds
    - B. 20 seconds
    - C. 1 minute
    - D. 2 minutes
27. Which action would the nursing assistant take if a sterile package becomes wet after the outer wrapper is removed?
    - A. Check the manufacturer's instructions for guidance
    - B. Discard the package because it is considered contaminated
    - C. Get a sterile drape and carefully relocate sterile contents to the new drape
    - D. Rely on the inner wrapper to maintain sterility and proceed

28. Which member of the health-care team is correctly maintaining the sterile field?
    A. Nursing assistant dons a mask before approaching the sterile field.
    B. Nurse turns on fan which causes a draft that moves across the sterile field.
    C. Doctor reaches across sterile field to pick up the patient's medical record.
    D. Student nurse is occasionally coughing and sneezing near the sterile field.
29. Which factor related to aging increases the risk for infection?
    A. Diet preferences related to dental problems
    B. Changes in the immune system
    C. Decreased muscle strength to perform exercise
    D. Less medical resources due to poverty
30. Health care–associated infections often occur when
    A. Insects are present.
    B. Handwashing is poor.
    C. Items are left on the floor.
    D. A person is in isolation.
31. Which action should the nursing assistant take first after getting accidentally stuck in the finger with a used needle?
    A. Report it at once to the supervising nurse
    B. Wash hands thoroughly with soap and water
    C. Save the needle in a puncture proof container for testing
    D. Observe self for any symptoms of the disease
32. Which nursing assistant has made an error in using personal protective equipment (PPE)?
    A. Nursing assistant A removes PPE when it becomes contaminated.
    B. Nursing assistant B removes PPE in the staff locker room.
    C. Nursing assistant C places used PPE in marked containers for discard.
    D. Nursing assistant D wears PPE with gloves when contact with blood is likely.
33. *Escherichia coli* is considered normal flora in the colon but is a pathogen if it enters the urinary system. How does this knowledge impact the nursing assistant's duties?
    A. Do not sit on the person's bed.
    B. Raw fruits and vegetables are washed.
    C. Attention is given to perineal care.
    D. Hand hygiene is performed.
34. Why are multidrug-resistant organisms (MDROs) a concern?
    A. The medications for MDROs have side effects.
    B. Infections caused by MDROs are hard to treat.
    C. MDROs are easily spread by coughing or sneezing.
    D. Health-care staff are more susceptible to MDROs.
35. Which of these is a sign or symptom of infection?
    A. Weight gain
    B. Constipation
    C. Confusion
    D. Increased appetite
36. Which nursing assistant has made an error in maintaining the sterile field?
    A. Nursing assistant A keeps all sterile items in sight.
    B. Nursing assistant B keeps sterile items above waist.
    C. Nursing assistant C keeps sterile-gloved hands above waist and in sight.
    D. Nursing assistant D leaves sterile field to get additional supplies.
37. Which care measure breaks the chain of infection at the portal of entry?
    A. Giving a person a tissue to cover the mouth while coughing
    B. Asking a visitor with a cold to defer a visit to a vulnerable person
    C. Washing your hands between caring for different people
    D. Helping a vulnerable person perform good oral hygiene
38. Which care measure breaks the chain of infection at the portal of exit?
    A. Putting a mask on a patient who has a cough
    B. Putting a susceptible host in a private room
    C. Helping a person wash his hands before eating
    D. Checking a child, who played outside for ticks
39. Which nursing assistant has performed an action that included a vehicle that could transmit microbes?
    A. Nursing assistant A assists a patient to ambulate in the hallway.
    B. Nursing assistant B washes hands and unwraps packaged food for patient.
    C. Nursing assistant C washes hands and dons gloves before assisting a patient.
    D. Nursing assistant D uses a stethoscope without cleaning it between patients.
40. Which situation requires surgical asepsis?
    A. Person vomited and you are helping her clean up.
    B. You are assisting the nurse with a sterile dressing change.
    C. You are caring for person with an MDRO infection.
    D. Person has a urine infection and needs help to the bathroom.
41. Which information does the nursing assistant need when directed to assist with a sterile procedure?
    A. Actions that the doctor will perform
    B. Expected outcomes of the procedure
    C. Whether or not the patient gave informed consent
    D. Whether to don sterile gloves or disposable gloves
42. Which action should the nursing assistant take while washing the hands?
    A. Use hot water
    B. Keep hands lower than the elbows
    C. Turn off faucets after lathering
    D. Use a disinfectant
43. Which routine would the nursing assistant use to clean under the fingernails by rubbing the fingers against the palms?
    A. Perform each time the hands are visibly soiled
    B. Use method if the fingernails are long or polished
    C. Perform only for the first handwashing of the day
    D. Use friction for at least 10 seconds

44. Which action should the nursing assistant take to avoid contaminating hands?
    A. Turn off the faucets after soap is applied
    B. Turn off the faucets before drying hands
    C. Turn off the faucets with clean paper towels
    D. Turn off the faucets by using the elbows

45. In which situation could the nursing assistant use an alcohol-based hand sanitizer to decontaminate the hands?
    A. Gloves are covered with blood after changing a person's peri-pad.
    B. Gloves are soiled while disposing of emesis from basin.
    C. Blood pressure was taken and the person's skin is intact.
    D. Person with infectious diarrhea needed help going to the bathroom.

46. Which common aseptic practice prevents the spread of microbes in the home care setting?
    A. Clean the tub or shower if the person has a cold
    B. Use a disinfectant to clean surfaces in the bathroom
    C. Wash bath and hand towels if they look soiled
    D. Keep the bathroom door closed to reduce odors

47. For older persons with dementia, what would the nursing assistant do to protect them from infection?
    A. Gently explain the need for aseptic practices
    B. Repeatedly tell them to wash their hands
    C. Frequently check and clean their hands and nails
    D. Ask the nurse what to do about their hygiene practices

48. Which action should the nursing assistant take when cleaning contaminated equipment?
    A. Wear PPE
    B. Rinse it in hot water first
    C. Use the clean utility room
    D. Remove organic materials with a paper towel

49. What is the best way to remove organic material from reusable items?
    A. Soap and hot water
    B. An autoclave
    C. Cold water rinse
    D. A disinfectant

50. Which option would the home health nursing assistant use for disinfecting surfaces, such as the floor or the toilet?
    A. Bleach solution
    B. Boiled water
    C. Vinegar and bleach solution
    D. Soap and hot water

51. What would the home health nursing assistant do upon finding out that the family is sterilizing needed items, by boiling them for 10 minutes?
    A. Check to see if organic material is being removed before boiling
    B. Discuss observations and family behaviors with supervising nurse
    C. Tell family that sterile items need to be purchased
    D. Advise family to increase boiling time to 20 minutes

52. Which infectious microorganisms are viruses that are considered blood-borne pathogens?
    A. Influenza and pneumococcus
    B. Measles and chicken pox
    C. Human immunodeficiency virus and hepatitis B virus (HBV)
    D. *Staphylococcus* and *Streptococcus*

53. Which item has the greatest risk for transmitting blood-borne pathogens?
    A. Blood pressure cuff
    B. Computer keyboard
    C. Needle used to draw body fluid
    D. Shirt with perspiration stains

54. Which information is included in the training for health-care staff who are at risk for exposure to blood-borne pathogens?
    A. Which tasks or circumstances might cause exposure?
    B. Which patients/residents have pathogens?
    C. How to respond to patients/residents with pathogens?
    D. How to differentiate pathogens from nonpathogens?

55. The nursing assistant is offered HBV vaccine by the agency. What is the routine for vaccination?
    A. Requires only 1 vaccination
    B. Must be given every year
    C. Involves three injections
    D. Is only effective if given before exposure

56. Which nursing assistant is using a work practice control to reduce exposure risks?
    A. Nursing assistant A discards a broken glass in the bedside trash can.
    B. Nursing assistant B puts her lunch in the unit's specimen refrigerator.
    C. Nursing assistant C breaks a contaminated needle and puts it in the sharps box.
    D. Nursing assistant D wash her hands after removing her gloves.

57. Which situation would prompt the nursing assistant to obtain PPE?
    A. Person is elderly, and the nurse says that a urinary tract infection is suspected.
    B. Person has a health care–associated infection and needs help getting out of bed.
    C. Person had an organ transplant last month and needs to be transported to X-ray.
    D. Person has diarrhea, and the nurse says *Clostridium difficile* is suspected.

58. Which action would the nursing assistant take to clean up broken glass?
    A. Pick it up carefully with gloved hands
    B. Use a brush and dustpan or tongs
    C. Alert the biohazardous material team
    D. Wipe it up with wet paper towels

59. Which waste would need to be treated and disposed of as regulated waste, in containers that are closable, puncture-resistant, leak-proof, and labeled with the *biohazard* symbol?
    A. Paper towels used for handwashing
    B. Tissues used for sneezing or coughing
    C. Leftover food and fluids
    D. Contaminated sharps or needles
60. Which action would the home health nursing assistant take to dispose of sharps?
    A. Place needles and other sharp items into hard plastic containers
    B. Rinse off organic materials and flush them down the toilet
    C. Place them in a plastic bag labeled with the *biohazard* symbol
    D. Discard them with the regular trash each day
61. Which nursing assistant has made an error in using gloves for infection control?
    A. Nursing assistant A wears gloves when handling contaminated items.
    B. Nursing assistant B washes or decontaminates disposable gloves for reuse.
    C. Nursing assistant C replaces worn, punctured, or contaminated gloves.
    D. Nursing assistant D discards utility gloves that show signs of cracking or tearing.
62. What is the rule if a sterile item touches a clean item?
    A. Sterile item is still sterile if there is no visible contamination.
    B. Sterile item is contaminated and should not be used.
    C. Sterile item should be handled with sterile gloves.
    D. Sterile item may still be used, but it depends on the purpose.
63. Which action would the nursing assistant take when working with a sterile field?
    A. Always wear a mask and sterile gloves
    B. Keep items within vision and above the waist
    C. Keep the door open or use a fan for good ventilation
    D. Wash hands before and after donning clean gloves
64. What would the nursing assistant do when arranging the inner package of sterile gloves?
    A. Arrange the gloves so they are in the middle of the package.
    B. Have the fingers pointing toward the body.
    C. Have the right glove on the right and the left glove on the left.
    D. Straighten the gloves to remove the cuff.
65. Which action should the nursing assistant perform when picking up the first sterile glove?
    A. Pick it up by the cuff and touch only the inside
    B. Reach under the cuff with the fingers
    C. Grasp the edge of the glove with the hand
    D. Unfold the cuff carefully before picking up the glove

Fill in the Blanks

66. Write out the meaning of the abbreviations
    A. EPA ____________________
    B. GI ____________________
    C. HAI ____________________
    D. HBV ____________________
    E. HIV ____________________
    F. MDRO ____________________
    G. MRSA ____________________
    H. OPIM ____________________
    I. OSHA ____________________
    J. PPE ____________________
    K. VRE ____________________
    L. AIDS ____________________
    M. *C. difficile* ____________________

Matching

Match the kind of asepsis being used with each example

A. Medical asepsis (clean technique)
B. Surgical asepsis (sterile technique)

67. ________ An item is placed in an autoclave.
68. ________ Each person has their own toothbrush, towel, washcloth, and other personal care items.
69. ________ Hands are washed before preparing food.
70. ________ Plastic bed ban is cleaned and disinfected.
71. ________ Disposable single-use item, such as a plastic syringe, is discarded.
72. ________ Liquid or gas chemicals are used to destroy microbes.
73. ________ Hands are washed every time you use the bathroom.

Match the aseptic measures which are the practices used to remove or reduce pathogens and to prevent their spread from one person or place to another person or place. These measures are used to control the related chain of infection with the step in the chain

A. Reservoir (host)
B. Portal of exit
C. Transmission
D. Portal of entry
E. Susceptible host

74. ________ Provide the person with tissues to use when coughing or sneezing
75. ________ Ask the nurse for instructions when caring for a person who had a transplant
76. ________ Assist the person with handwashing before eating
77. ________ Do not take equipment from one person to use on another person
78. ________ Hold equipment and linens away from your uniform
79. ________ Assist with cleaning or clean the genital area after a bowel movement
80. ________ Clean from cleanest area to the dirtiest
81. ________ Label bottles with the person's name and the date it was opened
82. ________ Follow the care plan to meet the person's nutritional and fluid needs
83. ________ Ensure that drainage containers are below drainage site
84. ________ Do not use items that are on the floor
85. ________ Assist the person with cough and deep-breathing exercises as directed
86. ________ Do not sit on a person's bed. You will pick up microorganisms and transfer them

Match the practices with the correct principles for surgical asepsis which is the practices that keep equipment and supplies free of all microbes

A. A sterile item can only touch another sterile item.
B. Sterile items or a sterile field is always kept within your vision and above your waist.
C. Airborne microbes can contaminate sterile items or a sterile field.
D. Fluid flows down in the direction of gravity.
E. The sterile field is kept dry unless the area below it is sterile.
F. The edges of a sterile field are contaminated.
G. Honesty is essential to sterile technique.

87. ________ Consider any item as contaminated if it touches a clean item
88. ________ Wear a mask if you need to talk during the procedure
89. ________ Place all sterile items inside the 1-inch margin of the sterile field
90. ________ Do not turn your back on a sterile field
91. ________ Prevent drafts by closing the door and avoiding extra movements
92. ________ Avoid spilling and splashing when pouring sterile fluids into sterile containers
93. ________ If you cannot see an item, then it is contaminated
94. ________ You report to the nurse that you contaminated an item or a field
95. ________ Point sterile forceps downward if holding a wet item

Optional Learning Exercises

96. A carrier (animal, insect) that transmits disease is a ________________________.
97. Microbes that are present in blood and can cause infection are considered to be ________________.
98. A ________________ is a small living plant or animal seen only with a microscope; a microbe.
99. Why are hands and forearms kept lower than elbows in handwashing?
____
____
100. Why is lotion applied after handwashing?
____
101. What information is included in training about bloodborne pathogens?
A. ________________________________
B. ________________________________
C. ________________________________
D. ________________________________
E. ________________________________
F. ________________________________
G. ________________________________
102. List the five moments when hand hygiene is essential as identified by the World Health Organization.
A. Moment 1 ________________________
B. Moment 2 ________________________
C. Moment 3 ________________________
D. Moment 4 ________________________
E. Moment 5 ________________________

Use the FOCUS ON PRIDE section to complete these statements and then use the critical thinking and discussion question to develop your ideas

103. You show personal and professional responsibility when you prevent infections. ________________ is the most important way to prevent the spread of microbes.
104. According to the Centers for Disease Control and Prevention, list six important times when hand hygiene should be performed.
A. ________________________________
B. ________________________________
C. ________________________________
D. ________________________________
E. ________________________________
F. ________________________________

Critical Thinking and Discussion Question

105. You observe another nursing assistant delivering meal trays to bedridden patients. The assistant is kind and prepares the trays by opening containers and cutting up food. However, you notice that the assistant is not offering to assist patients with hand hygiene before they start eating. What could you do or say to improve the quality of care?

18 Isolation Precautions

Fill in the Blanks: Key Terms

Infection control | Personal protective equipment (PPE)

1. ________________________ is the practices and procedures that prevent the spread of infection.
2. The clothing or equipment worn by the staff for protection against a hazard is ________________________

Circle the Best Answer

3. Which nursing assistant is correctly handling used laundry?
   A. Nursing assistant A wears gloves if blood or body fluids are likely to be on the soiled laundry.
   B. Nursing assistant B carries a large load of used laundry close to the body and uniform.
   C. Nursing assistant C gently shakes crumbs from bed linens and puts them in the laundry bag.
   D. Nursing assistant D puts used bed lines on the floor and picks them up after care is completed.
4. Which piece of equipment will need to be disinfected after it is used for a patient who is in an isolation room?
   A. Thermometer
   B. Blood pressure cuff
   C. Mechanical lift
   D. Disposable lunch tray
5. In which care setting is the nursing assistant most likely to encounter the need for *Enhanced Barrier Precautions (EBP)*?
   A. In a clinic for a patient who is being treated for a dog bite.
   B. In an acute care hospital for a patient who had surgery.
   C. In a nursing home for a resident who has a pressure wound.
   D. In the home setting for a person who needs assistance with bathing.
6. For which circumstance is standard precautions appropriate to use?
   A. Person A has a respiratory infection.
   B. Person B has a large wound infection.
   C. Person C is newly diagnosed with tuberculosis.
   D. Anytime care is given to any person.
7. What is the correct way to use gloves during standard precautions?
   A. Are worn for all tasks for the same person
   B. Can be worn until they tear or are punctured
   C. Are changed before caring for another person
   D. Are worn only if the person has an infection
8. When would the nursing assistant use clean and dry paper towels when working in a room with isolation precautions?
   A. To push contaminated sharps into container
   B. To clean the person's face and hands
   C. To handle contaminated items
   D. To clean up spills on the floor
9. What will surveyors observe about nursing assistants' actions when a person requires transmission-based precautions?
   A. Are nursing assistants changing gloves after providing personal care?
   B. Are nursing assistants making statements that make patients feel dirty or ashamed?
   C. How are nursing assistants performing care when PPE is not available?
   D. Do nursing assistants talk to the patients and meet their self-esteem needs?
10. Which piece of equipment does the nursing assistant need when asked to assist the nurse and the patient is actively coughing and having episodes of projectile vomiting?
    A. Eyeglasses
    B. Surgical mask
    C. Face shield
    D. Goggles
11. Which principle does the nursing assistant need to remember about the use of gloves when giving care?
    A. The inside of the gloves is always considered contaminated.
    B. Changing gloves is not necessary if caring for the same person.
    C. More than one pair of gloves may be needed for a task.
    D. Gloves are easier to put on when the hands are slightly damp.
12. Which action is included in the correct way to remove gloves?
    A. Make sure that glove touches only glove
    B. Pull the gloves off by the fingers
    C. Reach inside the glove with the gloved hand to pull it off
    D. Hold the discarded gloves tightly in your ungloved hand
13. Which areas are considered contaminated when wearing a gown for isolation precautions?
    A. The ties at the neck and waist
    B. The gown front and sleeves
    C. The gown back and sleeves
    D. Only the areas that touch the patient
14. Which step is first when removing the gown and gloves worn for isolation precautions?
    A. Untie the neck and waist strings
    B. Remove and discard your gloves
    C. Turn the gown inside out as it is removed
    D. Pull the gown down from each shoulder toward the same hand
15. For which circumstance would it be most important to make sure that a box of tissues is within the person's reach?
    A. Person has a wound infection and is on contact precautions.
    B. Person has respiratory symptoms and is on droplet precautions.
    C. Person had knee surgery and is on standard precautions.
    D. Person has measles and is on airborne precautions.

16. What is the rationale for only touching the ties or elastic bands when removing a mask?
    A. Front of the mask is contaminated.
    B. Front of the mask is sterile.
    C. Gloves are contaminated.
    D. Hands are contaminated.
17. Which step is performed first when donning a gown?
    A. Tie the strings at the back of the neck
    B. Tie the waist strings at the back
    C. Put on the gloves
    D. Overlap the back of the gown
18. Which step is done first when removing personal protective equipment?
    A. Remove the face mask
    B. Remove and discard the gloves
    C. Remove the gown
    D. Untie the waist strings of the gown
19. For which circumstance would the nursing assistant anticipate the need to wear an eye shield?
    A. Doctor needs assistance to irrigate a contaminated wound.
    B. Person in contact precautions needs help to walk around the room.
    C. Nurse suggests that a person with mild dementia needs coaching to put on clothes.
    D. Person who needs standard precautions needs to have vital signs taken.
20. Which nursing assistant is correctly following the double-bagging procedure for waste from an isolation room?
    A. Nursing assistant A places waste in a dirty bag, seals it, and then coworker places dirty bag in a clean bag.
    B. Nursing assistant B stands in the room and a coworker stands outside holding a wide cuff on a clean bag.
    C. Nursing assistant C places the dirty inner bag inside the clean outer bag and secures it.
    D. Nursing assistant D puts one bag inside a second bag and then loads waste into the double-bag.
21. Which nursing assistant has correctly collected a specimen from a person who is on transmission-based precautions?
    A. Nursing assistant A avoids contaminating the outside of the specimen container and the biohazard specimen bag.
    B. Nursing assistant B uses a paper towel to place the specimen inside the container, seals container, and puts it outside the room.
    C. Nursing assistant C puts the specimen inside the biohazard specimen bag and puts the bag in the specimen container.
    D. Nursing assistant D double bags the specimen and applies the warning labels according to agency policy.
22. Which question is the most important to ask the nurse when a patient who has transmission-based precautions needs to be transported to the X-ray department?
    A. How long does the patient have to stay in X-ray?
    B. What kind of infection does the patient have?
    C. What type of PPE does the patient need to wear?
    D. Does the stretcher need to be disinfected before use?
23. Which nursing care measure would the nursing assistant use to help meet love, belonging, and self-esteem needs for a person who is in isolation?
    A. Talk a lot while giving care
    B. Open the door so the person can see others
    C. Visit and interact pleasantly with the person
    D. Explain why people are avoiding the room
24. Which nursing care measure would help a 7-year-old child who is in isolation?
    A. Favorite toys or blankets are brought from home.
    B. PPE is put on before entering the room.
    C. Let child can hold and touch PPE (e.g., mask, eyewear).
    D. Avoid using PPE so the child is not scared.
25. Which action would you use to help a person to tolerate isolation if poor vision, confusion, or dementia are present?
    A. Let the person touch your face and hold your gloved hand
    B. Keep the door open so they can see people in the hall
    C. Tell the person who you are and what you need to do
    D. Avoid wearing a mask or face shield when in the room
26. Which type of transmission-based precautions would be used for a person with measles, chicken pox, or tuberculosis?
    A. Contact precautions
    B. Blood-borne Pathogen Standard
    C. Droplet precautions
    D. Airborne precautions
27. Which resident is at risk for transmission of multidrug-resistant organisms (MDROs) and therefore needs *Enhanced barrier precautions?*
    A. Resident A has been at the nursing center for several years.
    B. Resident B has an indwelling urinary catheter.
    C. Resident C has been sneezing and has a runny nose.
    D. Resident D is recently admitted and mildly confused.
28. For contact precautions, gloves are worn
    A. Upon entering the room or care setting
    B. Only if the skin has open lesions
    C. If you must touch the patient
    D. Only when the patient has symptoms
29. Which transmission-based precaution is specific to caring for a person who has tuberculosis?
    A. Placing reusable dishes and drinking vessels in a leakproof bag
    B. Removing the approved respirator after leaving the room
    C. Washing hands after removing all PPE and before leaving the room
    D. Wearing gloves to touch the person's intact skin or items near the person

Fill in the Blanks

30. Standard precautions are used to prevent the spread of infection from:
    A. ______
    B. ______
    C. ______
    D. ______
31. What is commonly needed in the setup for an isolation room?
    A. ______
    B. ______
    C. ______
    D. ______
32. According to the CDC, what is the correct order for donning PPE?
    A. ______
    B. ______
    C. ______
    D. ______

Labeling

33. The figure shows how to remove gloves. List the steps of the procedure shown in each drawing.

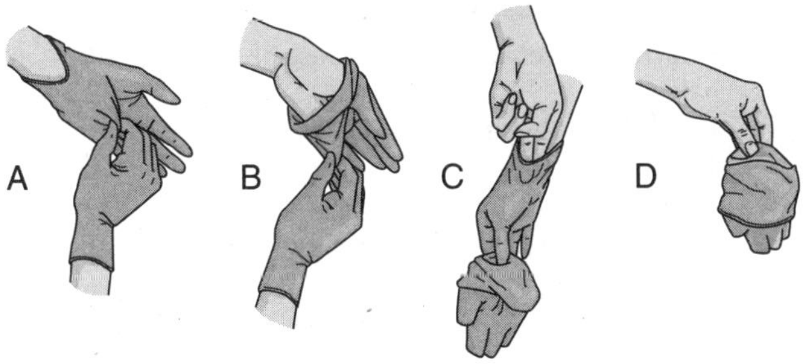

A. ______
B. ______
C. ______
D. ______

Optional Learning Exercises

34. When are the following worn for standard precautions?
    A. Gloves ______
    B. Masks, eye protection, and face shield ______
35. If a person has measles and you are susceptible, what should you do? ______
36. If a person in airborne precautions must leave the room, the person must wear a ______
37. Why is a gown turned inside out as you remove it? ______
38. Why is a moist mask or gown changed? ______
39. PPE may scare infants or children. Depending on age, the nurse may give the child a ______ or ______ to touch and play with.

Use the FOCUS ON PRIDE section to complete these statements and then use the critical thinking and discussion questions to develop your ideas

40. What can you do to help the person on transmission-based precautions from feeling lonely and isolated?
    A. ______
    B. ______
    C. ______
    D. ______

Critical Thinking and Discussion Question

41. Caring for people who need transmission-based precautions is very time-consuming. Consider the needs and circumstances of the four people and then discuss the following questions.
    Person A needs contact precautions and is likely to require frequent linen changes and help with perineal hygiene during the shift for infectious diarrhea
    Person B needs standard precautions and requires assistance to ambulate in the hallway several times during the shift
    Person C needs airborne precautions and is self-care, but is unable to leave the room for meals, socialization, or any other activities.
    Person D needs standard precautions and must be transported in the early morning for a procedure that will take approximately 6 hours.
    A. Which person is going to require the most time to complete care?
    B. Which person is going to require the least amount of your time?
    C. Discuss how you would organize and accomplish care for these four people.

19 Safe Handling and Positioning

Fill in the Blanks: Key Terms

Base of support	Dorsal recumbent position (supine position)	Fowler's position	Musculoskeletal disorders (MSDs)
Body alignment (posture)	Ergonomics	High Fowler's position	Prone position
Body mechanics		Semi-Fowler's position	

1. ____________________ is the science of designing the job to fit the worker.
2. The way in which the head, trunk, arms, and legs align with one another is ____________________.
3. ____________________ is using the body in an efficient and careful way.
4. The ____________________ is lying on the back.
5. The area on which an object rests is the ____________________.
6. ____________________ are injuries and disorders of the muscles, tendons, ligaments, joints, and cartilage.
7. Lying on the abdomen with the head turned to one side is ____________________.
8. A semi-sitting position with the head of the bed elevated 45 to 60 degrees is ____________________.
9. A variation of Fowler's position, the head of the bed is raised 30 degrees is ____________________.
10. A variation of Fowler's position, the head of the bed is raised 60 to 90 degrees is ____________________.

Circle the Best Answer

11. Which member of the health-care team is correctly applying the rules of body mechanics?
    A. Charge nurse is hunched over the computer for several hours.
    B. Doctor stands with feet apart for support during a long procedure.
    C. Nursing assistant holds a heavy laundry bag at arms length to protect uniform.
    D. Physical therapist leans over suddenly to catch a patient who is falling.
12. According to the Occupational Safety and Health Administration (OSHA) which element of an effective *Safe Handling Program* would a newly hired nursing assistant expect to find at the new job?
    A. Management guarantees that adequate staffing and functional equipment is always available for patient or resident handling.
    B. Residents and patients are included in the planning and share responsibilities for safe moving and transfer procedures.
    C. Paid time-off for recovery is ensured if a work-related injury or disability occurs during patient or resident handling.
    D. Training which includes hazard awareness, safe use of transfer and lift equipment, and safe practices for patient or resident handling.
13. Which device or assistive appliance may the nurse instruct the nursing assistant to use when a person is continuously leaning forward or to the side while seated in a chair?
    A. A vest restraint may be used.
    B. Postural supports help maintain alignment.
    C. A geriatric chair with a tray provides support.
    D. A belt restraint can be applied.
14. Which nursing assistant has made an error in using pillows to maintain good body alignment?
    A. Nursing assistant A uses a pillow to position the wrists slightly upward for a person with weak arms.
    B. Nursing assistant B places a pillow under the lower legs of a person who is in a supine position to lift the heels.
    C. Nursing assistant C places a small pillow under the head of a person who is in a high Fowler's position.
    D. Nursing assistant D places pillows behind the back of a person who is sitting in a chair and wearing a vest restraint.
15. What is the best rationale for using good body mechanics?
    A. Complies with facility policies
    B. Strengthens the back muscles
    C. Reduces the risk of injury
    D. Reduces muscle fatigue
16. Which action creates a wider base of support and balance?
    A. Keeping the knees slightly bent
    B. Aligning the head, trunk, arms, and legs
    C. Standing with the feet apart
    D. Maintaining physical condition
17. Which principle is the nursing assistant using when bending the knees and squatting to lift a heavy object?
    A. Using good body alignment
    B. Using good ergonomics
    C. Using strong back muscles
    D. Using good body mechanics
18. Which nursing assistant is using the rules of good body mechanics to move a heavy object?
    A. Nursing assistant A pushes, slides, or pulls the object.
    B. Nursing assistant B reaches upward to grab the object.
    C. Nursing assistant bends forward to lift the object.
    D. Nursing assistant D works alone to control the object.

19. Which factor creates the biggest risk for musculoskeletal disorders (MSDs)?
   A. Worker does not exercise regularly or eat healthy foods.
   B. Worker is small framed and lacks upper body strength.
   C. Worker uses force or repetitive action when moving objects.
   D. Worker has not memorized the rules of good body mechanics.
20. Which nursing assistant is correctly using the principles of body mechanics to prevent a back injury?
   A. Nursing assistant A maintains physical condition by routinely exercising.
   B. Nursing assistant B often tries to lift patients without asking for help.
   C. Nursing assistant C always leans across the bed while changing the linens.
   D. Nursing assistant D reaches upward to place a heavy box on the top shelf.
21. According to the OSHA, which of these behaviors can lead to musculoskeletal disorders (MSDs)?
   A. Resting between repetitive tasks
   B. Getting help to lift a heavy object
   C. Anticipating sudden movements
   D. Lifting with forceful movement
22. Which of these activities will help to prevent back injury?
   A. Reach across the bed to give care
   B. Bend at the waist to pick up an object
   C. Lift an object above your shoulder
   D. Carry objects close to your body
23. Which benefit is provided when the nursing assistant frequently changes the patient's position and helps the patient to maintain good body alignment?
   A. This is a good substitute for exercise.
   B. Pressure injuries and contractures are prevented.
   C. Helps to meet love and belonging needs
   D. Fulfills the criteria in the patient's care plan
24. What is the frequency for position changes for a resident who depends on the nursing team to be repositioned?
   A. At least every 2 hours
   B. Once an hour
   C. Every 15 minutes
   D. Once a shift
25. Ensuring that linens are clean, dry, and wrinkle-free is a nursing measure that helps to prevent which problem?
   A. Pressure injuries
   B. Contractures
   C. Breathing problems
   D. Need for frequent repositioning
26. Which position can help patients with heart and respiratory disorders to breathe more easily?
   A. Fowler's position
   B. Semi-Fowler's position
   C. Supine position
   D. Prone position
27. Which question would the nursing assistant ask an older patient who appears uncomfortable in the prone position, but the doctor has ordered the position as part of a medical treatment?
   A. "Do you want to talk to the doctor about the treatment plan?
   B. "Do you think you can endure this position for the treatment time?"
   C. "Would you like to sit up and do some range-of-motion exercises?"
   D. "Are you having pain or discomfort?"
28. Which benefit occurs when a person is in a supine position and a pillow is placed under the lower legs?
   A. Improves the circulation to feet
   B. Assists the person to breathe easier
   C. Prevents heels from rubbing on sheets
   D. Prevents swelling of the legs and feet
29. In which position is a pillow positioned against the person's back?
   A. Lateral position
   B. Prone position
   C. Supine position
   D. Semi-Fowler's position

Fill in the Blanks

30. ________________ help to reduce the risk of injury to staff and patients or residents from transferring, lifting, repositioning, and other moving activities.
31. ________________ refer to procedures that involve the movement and alignment of another person's body.
32. What are the four sets of strong, large muscles that are used to lift and move heavy objects?
   A. ________________
   B. ________________
   C. ________________
   D. ________________
33. The amount of physical effort needed to perform a task is ________________.
34. Performing the same motion or series of motions continually or frequently is ________________.
35. Assuming positions that place stress on the body is ________________.
36. Manually lifting people who cannot move themselves is ________________.

37. Name 17 nursing tasks that are known to be high risk for musculoskeletal disorders (MSDs).
    A. ______
    B. ______
    C. ______
    D. ______
    E. ______
    F. ______
    G. ______
    H. ______
    I. ______
    J. ______
    K. ______
    L. ______
    M. ______
    N. ______
    O. ______
    P. ______
    Q. ______
38. If you are delegated the task of positioning the person, which 11 items of information do you need?
    A. ______
    B. ______
    C. ______
    D. ______
    E. ______
    F. ______
    G. ______
    H. ______
    I. ______
    J. ______
    K. ______

In the following questions, list the measures needed for good alignment in each position

39. What measures are needed for good alignment when the person is in Fowler's position?
    A. ______
    B. ______
    C. ______
40. For supine position?
    A. ______
    B. ______
    C. ______
41. For prone position?
    A. ______
    B. ______
    C. ______
42. For lateral position?
    A. ______
    B. ______
    C. ______
    D. ______
    E. ______
43. For semiprone position?
    A. ______
    B. ______
    C. ______
    D. ______
    E. ______
44. For chair position?
    A. ______
    B. ______
    C. ______

Labeling

45. Label the positions in each of the drawings.

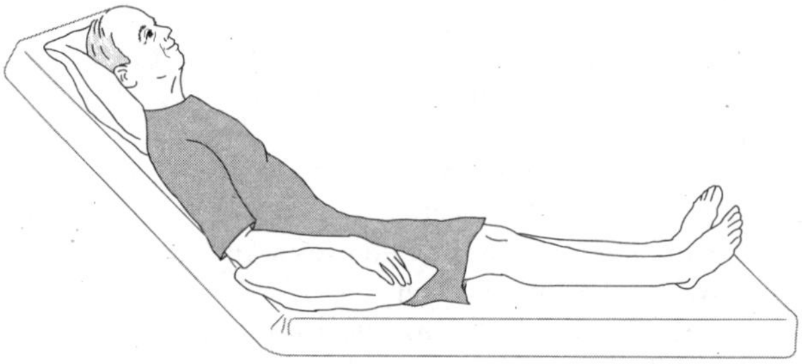

A. ______

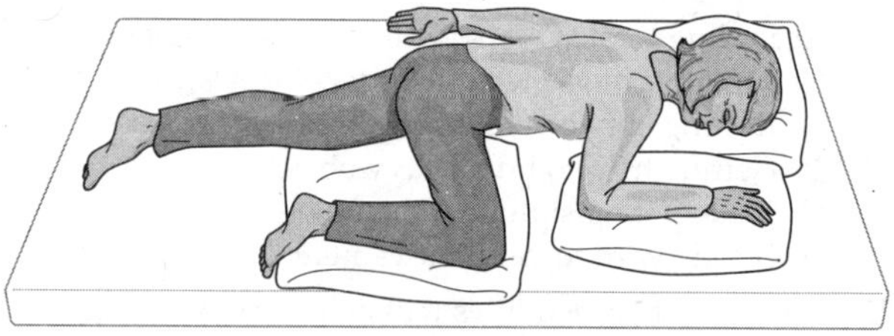

B. ______

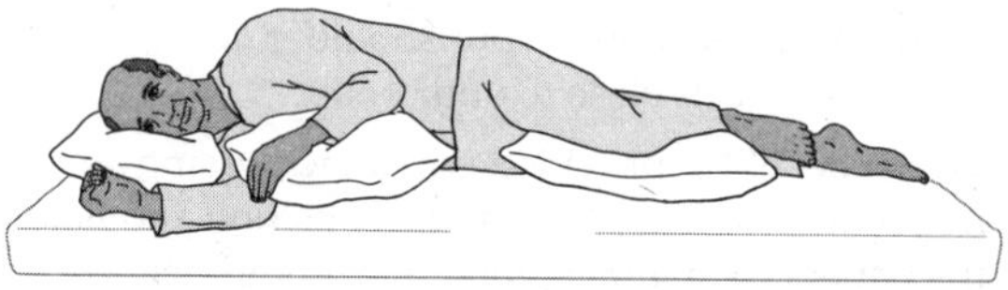

C. ______

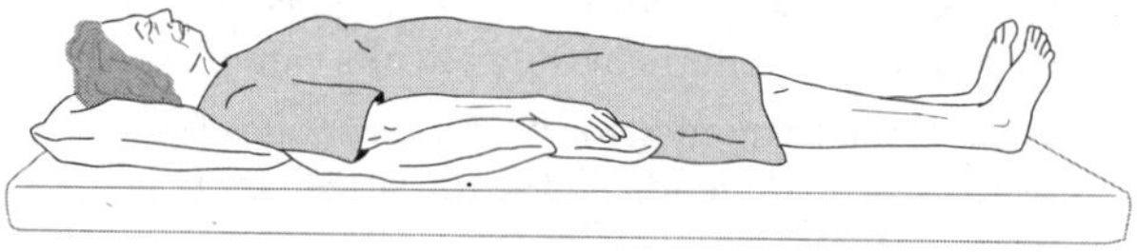

D. ______

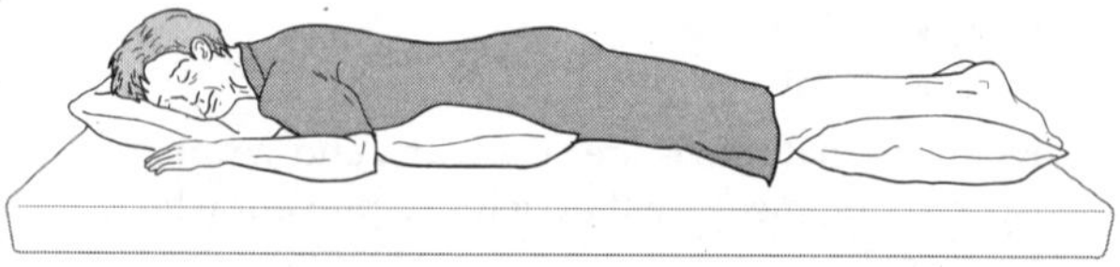

E. ______

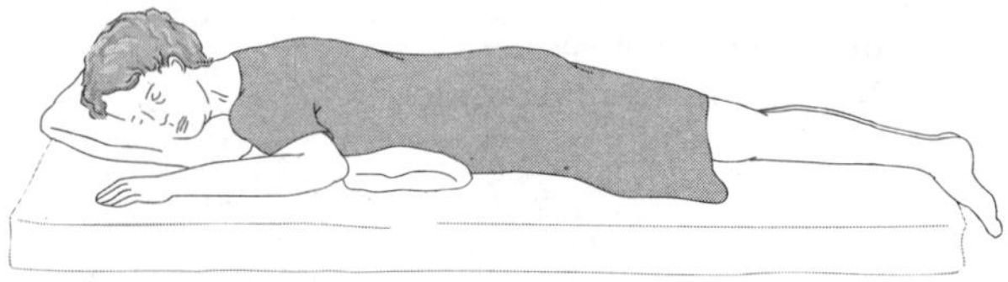

F. ______

Optional Learning Exercises

46. According to the OSHA, there are four risk factors (force, repeating action, awkward postures, heavy lifting) that contribute to musculoskeletal disorders (MSDs). Read the examples and identify the risk factor that could cause MSD in each scenario.
    A. The nursing assistant does not raise the level of the bed when changing linens. ______________________
    B. While you are walking with Mr. Smith, he slips and starts to fall. ______________________
    C. Mrs. Tippett often slides down in bed and always looks uncomfortable. ______________________
    D. You assist Mrs. Miller, who is a large and heavy woman, to use the toilet in her small bathroom. ______________________
    E. Mr. Thomas is confused and incontinent and you frequently clean and reposition him. ______________________
    F. You lean across the bed to hold the person while the nurse washes his back. ______________________
47. Regular position changes and good alignment promote
    A. ______________________
    B. ______________________
    C. ______________________
    D. ______________________
48. When you properly position and reposition a person, you help prevent a lack of joint or mobility or ______________________.

Use the FOCUS ON PRIDE section to complete these statements then use the critical thinking and discussion question to develop your ideas

49. You take responsibility for protecting yourself from harm when moving patients. What decisions do you make about protecting yourself?
    A. ______________________
    B. ______________________
    C. ______________________
    D. ______________________
    E. ______________________
50. How can you promote comfort, independence, and social interaction for a person you are caring for?
    A. ______________________
    B. ______________________

Critical Thinking and Discussion Question

51. Are you a strong young male? A slender petite female? Are you older with a history of back problems? Are you stronger than you appear? Consider your own stature, strength, and physical condition and discuss how you will protect yourself and your coworkers from sustaining MSDs.

20 Moving the Person

Fill in the Blanks: Key Terms

Bed mobility	Logrolling
Friction	Shearing

1. Turning the person as a unit, in alignment, with one motion is ________________________________.
2. ____________________ occurs when skin sticks to a surface and muscles slide in the direction the body is moving.
3. How a person moves to and from a lying position, turns from side to side, and repositions in bed or other furniture is ____________________________.
4. The rubbing of one surface against another is ____.

Circle the Best Answer

5. Which nursing measure could the nursing assistant and a coworker use to distract an elderly person with dementia who is grabbing and hitting while being turned?
   A. Firmly hold his hands and arms, while the coworker turns him
   B. Talk very cheerfully and ask him questions about his family
   C. Give him something soft to hold, such as a washcloth or stuffed animal
   D. Turn up the volume on the television and instruct him to watch the program
6. Which nursing measure would the nursing assistant use to prevent injuries when moving an older person?
   A. Do not move the person unless it is necessary
   B. Grasp a body part where there is no pain or injury
   C. Allow the person to move themselves
   D. Use a friction-reducing device
7. Which action would the nursing assistant take to prevent hitting the person's head on the headboard when moving the person up in bed?
   A. Place the person's hand against the headboard
   B. Place the pillow upright against the headboard
   C. Place dominant hand on the person's head
   D. Ask the person to bend their neck forward
8. What is the best strategy for moving a patient?
   A. Move only if the patient is very small
   B. Move patient with at least two staff members
   C. Move patient using a drawsheet
   D. Move patient only if totally dependent
9. Which recommendation comes from the Occupational Safety and Health Administration (OSHA) to prevent work-related injuries?
   A. Manual lifting be minimized or eliminated when possible
   B. Manual lifting be used at all times with three staff members
   C. Health-care workers never lift any person or object alone
   D. Mechanical lifts are always used for every lifting task
10. Which term describes the level of help that is needed if a person requires help to turn, reposition, sit up, and move in bed?
    A. Total dependence
    B. Extensive assistance
    C. Limited assistance
    D. Supervision
11. Why is the bed raised before moving the person?
    A. It prevents the person from falling out of bed.
    B. It reduces friction and shearing.
    C. It prevents pulling on drainage tubes.
    D. It reduces bending and reaching for staff members.
12. Which action would the nursing assistant take to reduce friction and shearing?
    A. Raise the head of the bed before moving the person
    B. Use a drawsheet or large reusable waterproof underpad
    C. Grasp the person under the arms and pull them up
    D. Massage the skin before and after moving
13. Which nursing measure would the nursing assistant use if a person with dementia resists being moved?
    A. Nurse should move the person to control confusion
    B. Get help, proceed slowly, and use a calm voice
    C. Leave the person alone and do not reposition
    D. Firmly tell the person that moving is necessary
14. Which information does the nursing assistant need when nurse delegates moving a resident in bed?
    A. Resident's level of knowledge about assist devices
    B. Previous work-related injuries of other staff members
    C. Resident's medical history and diagnosis
    D. Limits in the resident's ability to move or be repositioned
15. Which action would the nursing assistant take when raising a heavy older person's head and shoulders?
    A. Ask a coworker to help this reduces pain and injury
    B. Use a mechanical lift
    C. First try to accomplish the task without assistance
    D. Obtain and apply a transfer belt

16. Which action would be used to correctly raise the patient's head and shoulders?
    A. Both of the hands are placed under the back as the patient moves forward.
    B. Lock arms with the patient and support the neck and shoulders.
    C. Use a slide sheet to raise or drag the patient upward toward the head of the bed.
    D. Nursing assistant's free arm braces on the edge of the bed and the patient is pulled up.
17. In which circumstance could the nursing assistant independently move a smaller person up in bed?
    A. Person can assist using a trapeze.
    B. Rest of the staff is busy and cannot help.
    C. Nurse says to use a drawsheet or slide sheet.
    D. Nurse says to move the person without help.
18. What is the position of the bed when the nursing assistant is moving a person up in bed?
    A. Fowler's if the person is having a hard time breathing
    B. Flat, even if the person can only tolerate it temporarily
    C. As flat as possible for the person's condition
    D. Semi-Fowler's if the person can help by pushing with feet
19. For which patient will the nursing assistant need to get help from at least one coworker to safely move the patient?
    A. Patient A has mild dementia and needs supervision for activities of daily living.
    B. Patient B has a chronic disorder but is consider independent and mobile.
    C. Patient C has weakness in the lower extremities and needs limited assistance.
    D. Patient D has quadriplegia sustained in an accident and is to totally dependent.
20. Which nursing measure would the nursing assistance perform for a person who had a stroke and needs limited assistance?
    A. Remind and encourage the person to brush his teeth
    B. Guide the person's weaker arm while he puts on a shirt
    C. Ask a coworker to assist in bathing and total hygienic care
    D. Provide privacy for the person to independently take a bath
21. How is the turning sheet positioned?
    A. Under the head and shoulders
    B. Under the hips and buttocks
    C. From the head to above the knees or lower
    D. From the hips to below the knees
22. When using a turning sheet as a friction-reducing device, how do the members of the health-care team hold the device?
    A. Hold the sheet near the shoulders and hips
    B. Grasp the sheet at the four corners
    C. Hold and pull one side of the sheet at a time
    D. Grasp the sheet only at the top edge
23. What is the rationale for moving a patient to the side of the bed before turning?
    A. After turning, the person will not be in the middle of the bed.
    B. It makes it easier to turn the person if they are closer to you.
    C. Turning to the side reduces the need for side rails.
    D. Friction and shearing are reduced.
24. Which part of the body is supported when using a drawsheet to move the patient to the side of the bed?
    A. Back
    B. Knees
    C. Head
    D. Hips
25. Which action would the nursing assistant take after the person is turned?
    A. Put up all the side rails
    B. Position the person in good body alignment
    C. Elevate the head of the bed
    D. Raise the bed to its highest position
26. Which information does the nursing assistant need from the nurse and the care plan when delegated to turn a person?
    A. Whether the person has given informed consent?
    B. Which staff helped when the person was last turned?
    C. Whether the doctor has ordered turning?
    D. Which friction-reduction devices are needed?
27. Which instruction would the nursing assistant give to a patient who can use a trapeze for moving up in the bed?
    A. "Lift your buttocks and pull on the trapeze."
    B. "Grasp the trapeze and flex both of your knees"
    C. "Hold onto the trapeze while I adjust the bed."
    D. "Use your dominant hand and hang from the trapeze."
28. Which person will need the most assistance to move because of limited bed mobility?
    A. Person A is thin and elderly and has fragile skin.
    B. Person B is permanently paralyzed due to a car accident.
    C. Person C depends on assistance to maintain balance.
    D. Person D has arthritis, which causes joint stiffness.
29. Why are two or three staff members needed to logroll a person?
    A. A person who is being logrolled is usually in pain.
    B. It is important to keep the spine straight and in alignment.
    C. The person is probably totally dependent and needs extra help.
    D. No friction-reduction devices are used when a person is logrolled.
30. Where is the pillow placed when preparing to logroll a person?
    A. At the head of the bed
    B. Between the legs
    C. Under the head
    D. Under the shoulders

31. What information does the nursing assistant need before dangling a person?
    A. The person's medical diagnosis
    B. When the person ate last?
    C. The person's areas of weakness
    D. What kind of medication the person takes?
32. Which action would the nursing assistant take if a patient becomes faint or dizzy while dangling?
    A. Lay the patient down and tell the nurse
    B. Report this at the end of the shift
    C. Tell the patient to take deep breaths
    D. Have the patient move the legs around in circles
33. How is the head of the bed adjusted when preparing to dangle a patient?
    A. Flat
    B. Semi-sitting position
    C. Upright sitting position
    D. Comfortable for the patient
34. Which resident needs to be repositioned while sitting in a wheelchair?
    A. Resident A is in good alignment but is motioning for assistance.
    B. Resident B's back and buttocks are against the back of the chair.
    C. Resident C has slid downward and lacks strength to move self.
    D. Resident D is bored after sitting in the same position all day.
35. Which patient needs to be logrolled?
    A. Patient A is recovering from spinal surgery.
    B. Patient B has a chronic respiratory disorder.
    C. Patient C requires assistance to walk to the bathroom.
    D. Patient D recently delivered a healthy baby.
36. Which nursing assistant has made an error in repositioning a person in a wheelchair?
    A. Nursing assistant A applies a transfer belt around the person's waist.
    B. Nursing assistant B positions the person's feet flat on the floor.
    C. Nursing assistant C locks the wheels of the chair before repositioning.
    D. Nursing assistant D pulls at the person from behind the wheelchair.

Fill in the Blanks

37. Older persons are at great risk for skin damage from ______________________________.
38. To promote mental comfort when handling, moving, or transferring the person, you should ____________________ the person for privacy.
39. The level of assistance required for a person who is comatose would be defined as ______________________________.
40. When a person is logrolled, the head, neck, and spine are kept ______________________________.
41. When a person is dangling, the circulation can be stimulated by having the person move ______________________________.
42. The number of staff required to move a person depends on the person's ______________________________.
43. What simple hygiene measures can be performed while the person is dangling?
    ____
44. To prevent work-related injuries when moving a person, what should be done?
    A. ____________________
    B. ____________________
    C. ____________________
    D. ____________________
45. When you move a person in bed, report and record the following:
    A. ____________________
    B. ____________________
    C. ____________________
    D. ____________________
    E. ____________________
    F. ____________________
46. When you move a person, you move the body in segments. List the three steps in the correct order.
    A. ____________________
    B. ____________________
    C. ____________________
47. Identify five friction-reduction devices that are used to move persons to the side of the bed.
    A. ____________________
    B. ____________________
    C. ____________________
    D. ____________________
    E. ____________________
48. Before turning and repositioning a person, what information do you need from the nurse and care plan?
    A. ____________________
    B. ____________________
    C. ____________________
    D. ____________________
    E. ____________________
    F. ____________________
    G. ____________________
    H. ____________________
49. What should you report and record after you turn or move a person?
    A. ____________________
    B. ____________________
    C. ____________________
    D. ____________________
    E. ____________________

50. What observations should be reported and recorded after dangling a person?
A. ____________________
B. ____________________
C. ____________________
D. ____________________
E. ____________________
F. ____________________
G. ____________________

Optional Learning Exercises

51. If you need to move a person with dementia, they may resist because they may not ____________________ ____________________. What care measures will help you give safe care?
A. ____________________
B. ____________________
C. ____________________

52. If you must work alone, it is safer to move a person up in bed if
A. ____________________
B. ____________________
C. ____________________
D. ____________________
E. ____________________
F. ____________________
G. ____________________

53. What three features must an underpad or drawsheet have to accomplish a safe lift?
A. ____________________
B. ____________________
C. ____________________

54. Explain how moving a person to the side of the bed helps to avoid work-related injuries.
____

55. When you are delegated to turn a person, how will you know whether to turn them alone, with help, or by using logrolling?
____

56. When you turn a person and reposition them, what must be done to the bed level before you leave the room? ____________________

57. When two staff members are logrolling a person without a turning sheet, where does each staff member place the hands?
A. Staff member at head ____________________
B. Staff member at legs ____________________

58. Why should a person dangle for 1 to 5 minutes before walking or transferring? ____________________

59. What additional benefit is provided by moving the legs back and forth while dangling?
____

60. Refer to the charting sample below and answer the following questions:

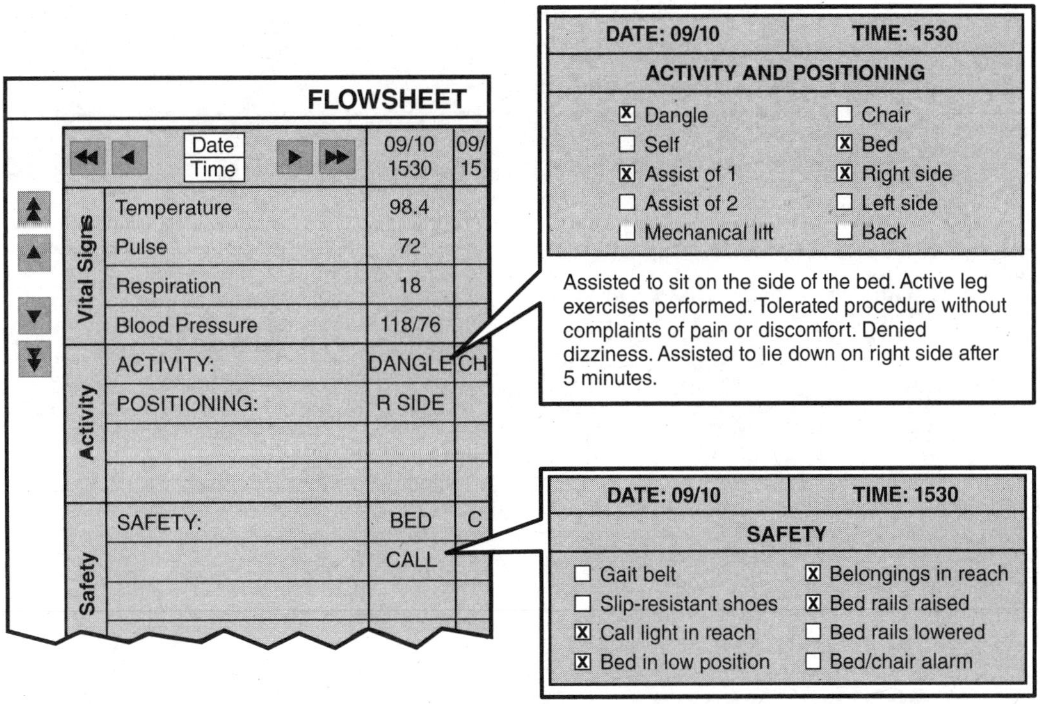
FLOWSHEET
Date
Time
09/10
1530
09/
15
Vital Signs
Temperature 98.4
Pulse 72
Respiration 18
Blood Pressure 118/76
Activity
ACTIVITY: DANGLE CH
POSITIONING: R SIDE
Safety
SAFETY: BED CALL C
DATE: 09/10
TIME: 1530
ACTIVITY AND POSITIONING
☒ Dangle
☐ Self
☒ Assist of 1
☐ Assist of 2
☐ Mechanical lift
☐ Chair
☒ Bed
☒ Right side
☐ Left side
☐ Back
Assisted to sit on the side of the bed. Active leg exercises performed. Tolerated procedure without complaints of pain or discomfort. Denied dizziness. Assisted to lie down on right side after 5 minutes.
DATE: 09/10
TIME: 1530
SAFETY
☐ Gait belt
☐ Slip-resistant shoes
☒ Call light in reach
☒ Bed in low position
☒ Belongings in reach
☒ Bed rails raised
☐ Bed rails lowered
☐ Bed/chair alarm

A. What activity and positioning were performed on 9/10 at 1530?
____

B. How did the person tolerate the activity?
____

C. How long did the activity last?
____

Use the FOCUS ON PRIDE section to complete these statements and then use the critical thinking and discussion question to develop your ideas

61. When moving a person, you promote pride, independence, and social interaction when you
    A. ______________________________
    B. ______________________________
    C. ______________________________
    D. ______________________________

Critical Thinking and Discussion Question

62. You are newly hired at a long-term care center. You notice that the other nursing assistants are always pairing up to help each other when moving and turning people. You can get help if you ask around, but no one seems overly eager to offer you help, and you feel a little awkward and left out. What could you do?

63. Caring for patients who have dementia is often challenging and simple tasks can be more difficult. The textbook offers one example of using distraction, *letting the person hold a washcloth or other soft object*. During your clinical rotations observe methods that experienced nursing assistants are using and then discuss with your classmates and share other ideas about how to distract patients with dementia.

21 Transferring the Person

Fill in the Blanks: Key Terms

Lateral transfer
Transfer
Pivot

1. ________________ is how a person moves to and from a surface.
2. When a person moves between two horizontal surfaces, it is a ________________________________.
3. To turn one's body from a set standing position is to ____.

Circle the Best Answer

4. What information would the nursing assistant give to a coworker when asking for help in performing a patient transfer using a mechanical lift?
   A. When informed consent was obtained?
   B. Patient's preference for type of mechanical lift
   C. What time the help is needed and for how long?
   D. Patient's medical diagnosis and history
5. Which action would the nursing assistant perform when preparing to transfer a person?
   A. Arrange the furniture for a safe transfer.
   B. Keep furniture in the position the resident likes.
   C. Remove all furniture from the room
   D. Shift all furniture away from the door
6. Which person could transfer from the bed to the chair with a stand and pivot transfer?
   A. Person A is strong enough to bear some or all of his own weight.
   B. Person B has upper body strength, but his legs are partially paralyzed.
   C. Person C can usually stand and walk by himself, but today refuses to try.
   D. Person D can independently walk, but is current agitated and combative.
7. Why would the nursing assistant lock the bed and wheelchair wheels when transferring the patient from the bed to the wheelchair?
   A. To follow the manufacturer's instructions
   B. To avoid damaging the bed or other equipment
   C. To prevent the bed and the wheelchair from moving
   D. To discourage the person from moving the equipment
8. How would the nursing assistant help the person out of bed when transferring from the bed to a wheelchair?
   A. Move the wheelchair to the right side of the bed
   B. Lead movement with the person's strong side
   C. Place the wheelchair on the person's weak side
   D. Orient the person and wheelchair toward the door
9. Which of these is the preferred method for chair or wheelchair transfers if not using a mechanical lift?
   A. Use a gait/transfer belt
   B. Ask the person to grasp your neck
   C. Perform a two-person manual lift
   D. Have the person use a trapeze
10. Which action would the nursing assistant take to increase the person's comfort when seated in a wheelchair?
    A. Place pillows around the person
    B. Ensure that nothing covers the vinyl seat and back
    C. Cover the back and seat with a folded bath blanket
    D. Remove any cushions or positioning devices
11. Which information would the nursing assistant expect to report before and after the transfer for a patient who frequently experiences dizziness and shortness of breath during transfers?
    A. Blood pressure, pulse, and respirations
    B. Height and weight
    C. Muscular strength and balance
    D. Level of confusion and ability to cooperate
12. Which action would the nursing assistant perform when using a transfer belt to prevent the person from sliding or falling?
    A. Bracing the knees against the person's knees
    B. Holding the person close to the body
    C. Having another staff member hold the person's feet in place
    D. Grasping the belt in the back to give better balance
13. Which patient may need an abdominal binder prior to a lateral transfer from the bed to the stretcher?
    A. Older patient with hip and knee pain related to arthritis
    B. Bariatric patient has excessive tissue in the abdominal area
    C. Frail elderly confused patient is picking at abdominal area
    D. Young female recently had a vaginal delivery of a healthy baby
14. How would the nursing assistant position the person when they need to be transferred back to bed from a chair or wheelchair?
    A. With the patient's weak side near the bed
    B. With the patient's strong side near the bed
    C. In the same position as getting out of bed
    D. At the foot of the bed, facing the head of the bed
15. Which potential injury is associated with a lateral transfer, such as moving a person from a bed to a stretcher?
    A. Fractures
    B. Shearing injuries
    C. Back injuries
    D. Head injuries

16. Which action would the nursing assistant take when moving a person to a stretcher?
    A. Position the stretcher to an equal level of the assist device
    B. Position the stretcher so it is 2 inches lower than the bed
    C. Position the stretcher so it is ½ inch lower than the bed
    D. Position the stretcher so it is 1 inch higher than the bed
17. Which patient is a candidate for the stand-assist mechanical lift?
    A. Patient A is too heavy for the staff to move.
    B. Patient B can bear or support some weight.
    C. Patient C is considered independent.
    D. Patient D has dementia and cannot follow instructions.
18. Which question would the nursing assistant ask that is specific to the use of the mechanical sling lift?
    A. "Is person strong enough to stand and pivot?"
    B. "Which type of sling should I use for this person?"
    C. "How much help is needed to use the sling lift?"
    D. "Which type of friction reducing device should I use?"
19. Which instruction would the nursing assistant give to the person who will be lifted in the sling of the mechanical lift?
    A. "Hold onto the swivel bar."
    B. "Hold the straps or chains."
    C. "Cross your arms across the chest."
    D. "Hold my hand while moving."
20. Which action would the nursing assistant use when transferring a person from a wheelchair to the toilet?
    A. The toilet should have a raised seat.
    B. The toilet seat should be removed.
    C. The wheelchair should be removed.
    D. The wheelchair should be unlocked
21. For which patient would the nursing assistant use a sliding board for a seated lateral transfer?
    A. Patient A can independently stand and pivot.
    B. Patient B has difficulty understanding and following instructions.
    C. Person C has upper body strength and good sitting balance.
    D. Patient D is overweight and has weakness in arms and legs.
22. Which nursing measure would the nursing assistant use when moving a person who weighs more than 200 pounds from the bed to a stretcher?
    A. Use a lateral sliding aid and at least three staff members.
    B. Use a transfer belt and three staff members.
    C. Use a friction-reducing device and one staff member.
    D. Use a stand-assist mechanical lift and two staff members.
23. Which nursing assistant has made an error in moving a patient from the bed to a stretcher?
    A. Nursing assistant A makes sure that the team has enough help.
    B. Nursing assistant B ensures that the bed and stretcher wheels are locked.
    C. Nursing assistant C positions the stretcher and bed as close as possible.
    D. Nursing assistant D uses an extended reach and bends toward the patient.
24. What is the rationale for asking the person to avoid putting their arms around your neck during a chair or wheelchair transfer?
    A. Person will have poor body alignment during the transfer.
    B. Person's hands and arms will contaminate your uniform.
    C. Person can pull you forward or cause you to lose your balance.
    D. Person may be too weak to maintain an adequate hold.

Fill in the Blanks

25. Locking the wheels on a wheelchair may be considered ____________________.
26. When using a transfer belt to transfer a person to a chair or wheelchair, your hands grasp the belt on either side and are in an __________ position.
27. If you transfer a person to a chair without a transfer belt, place your hands ____________________ and around the person's ____________________.
28. What is the purpose of each type of sling?
    A. Standard full sling ____________________
    B. Bathing sling ____________________
    C. Toileting sling ____________________
    D. Amputee sling ____________________
    E. Bariatric sling ____________________
29. What information do you need when you are delegated to use a mechanical lift?
    A. ____________________
    B. ____________________
    C. ____________________
    D. ____________________
    E. ____________________
    F. ____________________
30. To promote mental comfort when using a mechanical lift, you should explain the procedure before you begin and show the person ____________________.

Optional Learning Exercises

31. When transferring a person to and from the toilet, the toilet seat and the wheelchair should be at the ______________________________ level.
32. What safety measures are important when transferring a bariatric person to and from the toilet?
    A. ______________________________
    B. ______________________________
    C. ______________________________
33. When moving a person to a stretcher for a safe transfer at least ____________________ staff are needed
34. When moving a person to a stretcher if a person weighs more than 200 pounds, what are two devices that may be used?
    A. ______________________________
    B. ______________________________
35. What should you do after using a shared device, such as a mechanical lift, to be considerate of other staff members?
    A. ______________________________
    B. ______________________________
36. List the three transfer procedures that are routine nursing tasks.
    A. ______________________________
    B. ______________________________
    C. ______________________________
37. Why should you know the person's weight before using a mechanical lift?
    ____
38. What should you do if the mechanical lift available is different from the one you have used before?
    ____

Use the FOCUS ON PRIDE section to complete these statements and then use the critical thinking and discussion questions to develop your ideas

39. When transferring a person, you respect the person's privacy when you
    A. ______________________________
    B. ______________________________
40. When giving directions about transferring, what should you do to encourage independence and social interaction?
    A. ______________________________
    B. ______________________________
    C. ______________________________
    D. ______________________________
    E. ______________________________
    F. ______________________________
    G. ______________________________

Critical Thinking and Discussion Questions

41. The nurse tells you that an elderly resident, who is newly admitted, is at the "supervision" level for transfers and that the long-term goal is independence in mobility. However, when you give the resident the cues to transfer to the chair, she says, "You have to lift me up, my daughter says so."
    A. What would you do first?
    B. If the resident is newly admitted and you are unfamiliar with the resident's usual behavior, how would this affect your approach?

22 Bedmaking

Fill in the Blanks: Key Terms

Bath blanket
Waterproof underpad
Drawsheet

1. An absorbent pad with a quilted top layer and a waterproof bottom layer is a ____________________.
2. A ______________________________ is a small sheet placed over the middle of the bottom sheet to keep the mattress and bottom linens clean.
3. A covering used for privacy and warmth during bathing, hygiene, and other care measures is a ____.

Circle the Best Answer

4. In nursing centers, when are complete linen changes usually done?
   A. Once a week
   B. Every day
   C. On the bath or shower day
   D. On family visiting days
5. What is the primary purpose of keeping beds clean, dry, and wrinkle-free?
   A. To promote good posture and body alignment
   B. To meet the expectations of surveyors and visitors
   C. To promote comfort and prevent skin breakdown
   D. To provide a home-like atmosphere for residents
6. In which circumstance is the nursing assistant likely to use the closed bed procedure?
   A. Home care patient is weak, unable to move, and stays in bed.
   B. Resident in a nursing center left today to live in the family home.
   C. Acute care hospitalized patient is confined to bed for treatment purposes.
   D. Nursing center resident is up for activities most or all of the day.
7. Which patient would benefit the most from having a toe pleat across the foot of the bed?
   A. Patient A is independently ambulatory but has trouble lying flat in bed.
   B. Patient C has been unable to move extremities for several months.
   C. Patient B prefers to get up early, take a shower, and then get back in bed.
   D. Patient D needs to be transferred from the bed to a stretcher to go to surgery.
8. Which nursing assistant is adhering to the principles of medical asepsis while making a bed?
   A. Nursing assistant A places used or heavily soiled linens on the floor.
   B. Nursing assistant shakes clean linens out as they are placed on the bed.
   C. Nursing assistant places clean linens on the bed for easy access.
   D. Nursing assistant holds soiled linens away from body and uniform.
9. Which action would the nursing assistant take if extra clean linens are brought to a person's room?
   A. Return the unused linens to the linen room
   B. Use the linens for the person's roommate
   C. Put the unused linens in the laundry hamper
   D. Use the linens for a person in the next room
10. Which of these linens will be collected first when making a bed?
    A. Bath towel
    B. Bath blanket
    C. Mattress pad
    D. Top sheet
11. Which action would the nursing assistant use when removing used linens from the bed?
    A. Gather all used linens in one large roll and double-bag them.
    B. Wear gloves and roll each piece of soiled linen toward self.
    C. Top sheet, and drawsheets may be reused if not visibly soiled.
    D. Bedspread may be reused for the same person if not visibly soiled.
12. Which nursing measure allows the resident the right of personal choice?
    A. Nursing assistant asks the resident to choose the time when the bed is made.
    B. Nursing assistant decides which bedspread would look best in the room.
    C. Charge nurse tells the resident that the beds are made at 9 AM.
    D. LPN chooses the pillows and blanket the resident needs for comfort.
13. How often are the linens usually changed when caring for a person in the home?
    A. Once a day
    B. One or two times per week
    C. Depends on the doctor's orders
    D. Only if the person gives you permission

14. What purpose does a waterproof underpad serve?
    A. Protects against skin breakdown and pressure injuries
    B. Protects the blankets and bedspread from moisture and soil
    C. Protects the mattress and bottom linens from dampness and soiling
    D. Protects the person from getting wet or soiled
15. Which observation would prompt the home health nursing assistant to speak to the caregiver or the supervising nurse?
    A. A flat sheet is folded in half and is being used as a drawsheet.
    B. A plastic trash bag is placed between the mattress and linens.
    C. A drawsheet is in the middle of the bottom sheet on the bed.
    D. A waterproof underpad is in the middle of the bed under the patient.
16. Why does the nursing assistant need to know the person's schedule for treatments, therapies, and activities?
    A. To ensure that the bed is flat and that bed rails and frame are clean.
    B. It is best to change linens after the treatment or when the person is out of the room.
    C. Beds that may have been unlocked need to be checked and relocked, as needed.
    D. So that nursing assistant will know the type of bed to make and what type of linen to obtain.
17. Which nursing assistant is correctly handling used linens?
    A. Nursing assistant A stores foul smelling linens in the person's laundry hamper.
    B. Nursing assistant B carries used linens unbagged outside of the person's room.
    C. Nursing assistant C empties soiled laundry containers as needed.
    D. Nursing assistant D rinses a soiled waterproof underpad in the person's bathroom.
18. Which nursing assistant is using good body mechanics while making a bed?
    A. Nursing assistant A bends from the waist to remove and replace linens.
    B. Nursing assistant B stretches across the bed to smooth linens.
    C. Nursing assistant C raises the bed to a comfortable height to work.
    D. Nursing assistant D locks the wheels and raises the head of the bed.
19. Which nursing measure is done when a patient is discharged, in addition to changing the bed?
    A. New pillows are placed on the bed.
    B. The bed system is cleaned and disinfected.
    C. The bed system and all linens are sterilized.
    D. The bedspread and blanket are reused.
20. How does the nursing assistant position the bottom flat sheet when making a bed?
    A. The lower edge is even with the top of the mattress.
    B. The hemstitching faces away from the person.
    C. The large hem is at the bottom and the small hem is at the top.
    D. The crease is crosswise on the bed.
21. Which nursing assistant has correctly handled the top sheet, blanket, and bedspread on the bed?
    A. Nursing assistant A tucks top linens together under the foot of the bed and around the sides.
    B. Nursing assistant B tucks the sheet; the blanket and bedspread hang loosely around the bed.
    C. Nursing assistant C tucks top linens together under the foot of the bed and the corners are mitered.
    D. Nursing assistant D allows top sheet, blanket, and bedspread to hang loose over the foot of the bed.
22. What is the rationale for placing the pillow with the open end away from the door?
    A. For a neat appearance
    B. For infection control
    C. For safety
    D. For good hygiene
23. Which nursing assistant has correctly used one of the steps for making an open bed?
    A. Nursing assistant A fanfolds the linens to one side of the bed.
    B. Nursing assistant B fanfolds the top linens to the foot of the bed.
    C. Nursing assistant C changes the linens while the person is in bed.
    D. Nursing assistant D makes the bed when the room is vacated.
24. Which nursing measure would the nursing assistant use when changing the linens for a person who is comatose?
    A. Keep the bed in the lowest position
    B. Work alone and move slowly and quietly
    C. Keep the bed rails up at all times
    D. Ask a coworker to help and explain each step
25. What is the purpose of using a bath blanket when making an occupied bed?
    A. Protect the skin while being bathed
    B. Cover the person for warmth and privacy
    C. Protect the bed linens and mattress
    D. Protect the person from soiled linens
26. Which action would the nursing assistant take when making an occupied bed for a person who does not use bed rails?
    A. Have a coworker work on the other side of the bed
    B. Push the bed against the wall
    C. Always keep a hand on the person while making the bed
    D. Change linens only when the person is out of the bed for tests or therapies

27. Which nursing assistant is using a correct step to remove linens in making an occupied bed?
    A. Nursing assistant A removes all used linens from the bed first.
    B. Nursing assistant B has the person roll from side to side for each piece of the bottom linens.
    C. Nursing assistant C tucks the used bottom linens and the clean bottom linens under the person.
    D. Nursing assistant D asks the person to raise the hips and then pushes the linens under the buttocks.
28. Which nursing assistant needs a reminder about how to make a surgical bed?
    A. Nursing assistant A tucks the sides and bottom of top linens under the mattress.
    B. Nursing assistant B removes and discards soiled linens in a used laundry receptacle.
    C. Nursing assistant C positions a clean mattress pad on the mattress.
    D. Nursing assistant D smooths the wrinkles from the bottom flat sheet.
29. For which circumstance would it be the most advantageous for the nursing assistant to ask a coworker for assistance?
    A. Needs to make an open bed for a newly admitted patient who will arrive by wheelchair
    B. Needs to make a surgical bed for a patient who will return from surgery toward the end of the shift
    C. Needs to make an occupied bed for a patient who is overweight, and linens are heavily soiled
    D. Needs to make a closed bed after patient is discharged and bed system needs to be cleaned and disinfected

Fill in the Blanks

30. Number this list from 1 to 8 in the order you would collect the linens to make a bed.
    ________ Pillowcase(s)
    ________ Top sheet
    ________ Drawsheet (if needed)
    ________ Bottom sheet (flat or fitted)
    ________ Mattress pad (if needed)
    ________ Bedspread
    ________ Waterproof underpad (if needed)
    ________ Blanket (if needed)
31. Beds are made every day to
    A. Promote ________________________
    B. Prevent ________________________
    C. Prevent ________________________
32. When doing home care, list four guidelines that you should follow for doing the laundry.
    A. ________________________
    B. ________________________
    C. ________________________
    D. ________________________
33. List at least three circumstances where the nursing assistant would be assigned to make a surgical bed.
    A. ________________________
    B. ________________________
    C. ________________________

Optional Learning Exercises

34. Compare how often linen changes are made in a hospital and nursing center.
    A. How often is a complete linen change made in a nursing center? ________________________
    ____
    B. How often are linens changed in a hospital?
    ____
35. Even when a complete linen change is not scheduled, you should do the following to keep beds neat and clean.
    A. ________________________
    B. ________________________
    C. ________________________
    D. ________________________
    E. ________________________
36. The mattress pad, blanket, and bedspread are reused when making a bed in a home setting unless they are ________________________.
37. If you were making a bed in a home, how would you use a twin sheet for a drawsheet? ________________________
    ____
38. When a family member suggests using a plastic trash bag to protect the linens and mattress, the nursing assistant would inform family that there is a risk for __________ if the bag accidentally shifts and covers the person's nose and mouth.
39. Remember to wear ________________________ when you are handling used linen.

Use the FOCUS ON PRIDE section to complete these statements and then use the critical thinking and discussion question to develop your ideas

40. When making a bed in the home, you should follow the person's wishes unless the request is ________________________.
41. Leaving a person to lie on wet or soiled linens has legal implications because it would be considered a form of ________________________.

Critical Thinking and Discussion Question

42. You are caring for a woman in a nursing center who has been bedridden for several years. She is alert and conversant but is very frail and has limited mobility. Discuss how a clean and tidy bed could contribute to the woman's quality of life and her physical health.

23 Oral Hygiene

Fill in the Blanks: Key Terms

Aspiration
Dentures
Hygiene
Oral hygiene (mouth care)
Plaque
Tartar

1. ______________________ is the set of practices that promote healthy tissues and structures of the mouth.
2. Hardened plaque on teeth is ____________________.
3. ____________________________ occurs when breathing fluid, food, vomitus, or an object into the lungs.
4. ____________________ is a thin film that sticks to the teeth. It contains saliva, microbes, and other substances.
5. ________________ are a removable replacement for missing teeth.
6. ________________ is the cleanliness practices that promote health and prevent disease.

Circle the Best Answer

7. Which action would the nursing assistant take when preparing to assist with oral hygiene and the patient says, "I have gingivitis"?
   A. Don gloves and wear a face shield
   B. Observe the patient's teeth and gums
   C. Instruct the patient to brush their own teeth
   D. Ask the nurse if gingivitis requires special care
8. Which error is occurring when a new nursing assistant is performing oral hygiene for patients, and they are repeatedly gagging?
   A. Mouthwash is not being offered.
   B. Toothbrush is being inserted too far.
   C. Gums are being brushed too hard.
   D. Crowns are being brushed in the wrong direction.
9. Which activity is most likely to cause a dry mouth?
   A. Walking
   B. Sleeping
   C. Smoking
   D. Eating
10. In addition to the nurse, which health team member will assess the person's need for mouth care?
    A. Speech-language pathologist
    B. Nursing assistant
    C. Physical therapist
    D. Occupational therapist
11. Which child has increased risk for baby bottle tooth decay?
    A. 3-year old is drinking whole milk from a baby bottle.
    B. 4-month-old infant is being breastfed.
    C. 1-year-old child is being bottle-fed.
    D. 6-month-old infant is put to bed with a bottle.
12. Which method of oral hygiene would the nursing assistant use for a 3-month-old baby?
    A. Gently brush with a soft toothbrush
    B. Use a sponge swab and a smear of toothpaste
    C. Use a clean damp washcloth and wipe the gums
    D. Gently massage the gums with a fingertip
13. What is the frequency of flossing teeth, according to the American Dental Association?
    A. When teeth cannot be brushed
    B. Once or twice a week
    C. At least once a day
    D. When food is caught between teeth
14. For which patient would the nursing assistant use sponge swabs for oral hygiene?
    A. Person has sore, tender mouths
    B. Older person needs dentures to be cleaned
    C. 6-year-old child needs oral care
    D. Older person just finished eating
15. What is the rationale for using Standard Precautions and the Blood-borne Pathogen Standard when giving oral hygiene?
    A. Mouth care creates aerosol droplets.
    B. Bad breath indicates the presence of microbes.
    C. Gums may bleed during mouth care.
    D. Teeth and dentures are considered aseptic.
16. Where would the nursing assistant arrange supplies when the patient is able to perform oral hygiene in bed?
    A. On the overbed table
    B. On the closest bedside table
    C. On the patient's lap
    D. On a towel protecting the bedspread
17. Which of these steps would the nursing assistant use when brushing a person's teeth?
    A. Let the person rinse the mouth with water
    B. Use a sponge swab to clean the teeth
    C. Wipe the gums with a damp gauze
    D. Floss the teeth that are easily reached
18. What is the most serious complication of using a sponge swab to clean the mouth of an unconscious person?
    A. The sponge swab is uncomfortable in the person's mouth.
    B. The person could bite down on the swab stick.
    C. The person could choke on the foam pad if it comes off.
    D. The sponge swab does not remove plaque as well as a toothbrush.

19. Which action would the nursing assistant take when assisting a person who performs their own oral hygiene?
    A. Position the person for oral hygiene
    B. Coach the person to brush gently
    C. Move floss up and down between the teeth
    D. Apply lubricant to the lips if needed
20. Which nursing assistant needs a reminder about the steps to use when flossing a person's teeth?
    A. Nursing assistant A starts at the back side of an upper back tooth.
    B. Nursing assistant B holds the floss between the middle fingers.
    C. Nursing assistant C moves the floss gently up and down between the teeth and gums.
    D. Nursing assistant D moves to a new section of floss after every second tooth.
21. What is the rationale for positioning an unconscious person on their side with the head turned well to the side when providing mouth care?
    A. It is easier to brush the teeth.
    B. The person is more comfortable.
    C. Risk for aspiration is reduced.
    D. It is easier for the person to breathe.
22. Which nursing measure would the nursing assistant use when giving oral hygiene to an unconscious person who wears dentures?
    A. Remove the dentures, clean them, and replace them in the mouth
    B. Remove the dentures; they are not worn when the person is unconscious
    C. Clean the dentures in the mouth without removing them
    D. Use a sponge swab and gauze to clean the dentures
23. When is mouth care given to an unconscious person?
    A. After each meal
    B. When AM and PM care is given
    C. At least every 2 hours
    D. Once a day
24. Which patient is able to perform oral hygiene with minimal assistance?
    A. Patient A can independently sit up in bed and use handheld items.
    B. Patient B can keep the mouth open but cannot move the arms.
    C. Patient C can walk to the sink but is too confused to brush the teeth.
    D. Patient D is alert and cooperative but is very weak and frail.
25. What is the rationale for lining the sink with a towel prior to cleaning the dentures at a sink?
    A. To prevent infection and illnesses
    B. To prevent damage to the dentures if they are dropped
    C. To dry the dentures after they are cleaned
    D. To avoid contamination if dentures slip from the hand
26. How are dentures stored when they are not worn after cleaning?
    A. In cool water in a denture cup
    B. In hot water in an unbreakable container
    C. Wrapped in a soft towel and stored in a drawer
    D. Covered with soft tissues and placed on a clean surface
27. When should flossing of the teeth be initiated, according to the American Dental Association?
    A. When child starts brushing own teeth
    B. When baby starts chewing solid food
    C. When two baby teeth touch
    D. When the first permanent tooth appears
28. Which action would the nursing assistant take upon observing white patches on the tongue?
    A. Gently brush the tongue with a soft-bristle toothbrush
    B. Report the appearance of the tongue to the nurse
    C. Gently scrap the white patches off using a sponge swab
    D. Have the patient swish warm water in mouth and then spit

Fill in the Blanks

29. List five benefits of good oral hygiene.
    A. ______________________________
    B. ______________________________
    C. ______________________________
    D. ______________________________
    E. ______________________________
30. List four unpleasant signs or symptoms that may occur in the patient's mouth due to illness, disease, and some drugs.
    A. ______________________________
    B. ______________________________
    C. ______________________________
    D. ______________________________
31. List at least six changes related to aging that have an impact on the health of teeth and the oral cavity.
    A. ______________________________
    B. ______________________________
    C. ______________________________
    D. ______________________________
    E. ______________________________
    F. ______________________________
32. What observations related to oral hygiene should be reported and recorded?
    A. ______________________________
    B. ______________________________
    C. ______________________________
    D. ______________________________
    E. ______________________________
    F. ______________________________

Labeling

33. Look at the figure and answer these questions.

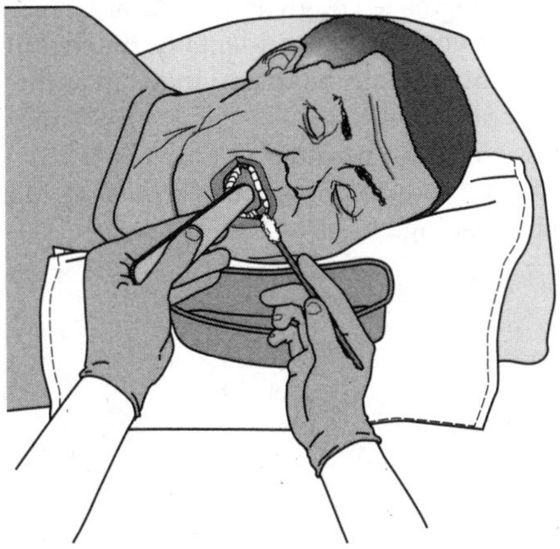

A. Why is the person positioned on his side?

____

B. What is the purpose of the plastic tongue depressor?

____

34. In this figure, what is the staff member using to remove the upper denture?

____

Why? __________________________________

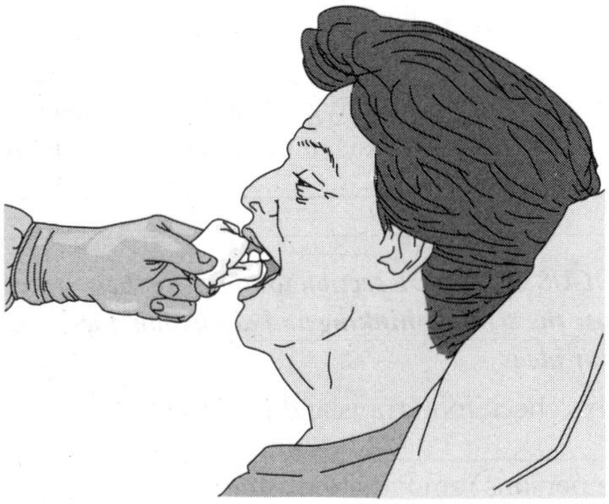

35. According to the charting sample, what observations were made and what care was performed?

____

____

ORAL HYGIENE

Observations

Lips
- ☒ Dry, cracked
- ☐ Swelling
- ☐ Blisters
- ☐ Pain
- ☐ Other:

Teeth
- ☒ Pain
- ☐ Loose teeth
- ☐ Other:

Gums
- ☐ Bleeding
- ☐ Swelling
- ☐ Redness
- ☐ Pain or irritation
- ☐ Other:

Dentures
- ☐ Rough or sharp area(s)
- ☐ Chipped area(s)
- ☐ Loose denture(s)

Mouth and tongue
- ☐ Mouth or breath odor
- ☐ Swelling
- ☐ Redness
- ☐ Pain or irritation
- ☐ Sores
- ☐ White patches
- ☐ Other:

Nurse notified: M. Rhodes, RN

Care Measures

Oral hygiene
- ☒ Teeth brushed
- ☒ Teeth flossed
- ☐ Mouth cleaned with sponge swabs
- ☒ Lip lubricant applied

Denture care
- ☐ Upper denture
- ☐ Lower denture
- ☐ Denture(s) cleaned
- ☐ Adhesive applied
- ☐ Denture(s) placed in mouth
- ☐ Denture(s) soaked in cleaning solution

Optional Learning Exercises

36. What factors cause mouth dryness for an unconscious person?
    A. ______________________________
    B. ______________________________
    C. ______________________________
37. When performing oral hygiene for an unconscious person, the nursing assistant may observe crusting on the ______________________________ and ______________________________.

Use the FOCUS ON PRIDE section to complete these statements and then use the critical thinking and discussion questions to develop your ideas

38. Always check food trays and place settings for ______________________________.
    Some persons remove them after meals or wrap them in ____________________ after eating.
39. A denture adhesive may be used to hold dentures in place and to keep ______________ out of the inner part of the denture.

Critical Thinking and Discussion Questions

40. You are assisting a person to remove his dentures before he goes to bed. As you are removing the dentures, he begins to cough and choke and reaches out and grabs your hand. Accidentally, the dentures are knocked out of your hand and they fall to the floor and break.
    A. Discuss what you would do.
    B. Discuss methods to prevent this type of incident from happening.

24 Daily Hygiene and Bathing

Fill in the Blanks: Key Terms

Circumcised
Diaphoresis
Early morning care (AM care)
Evening care (PM care)
Morning care
Perineal care (pericare)
Uncircumcised

1. The person is ____________________ when he has a foreskin covering the head of the penis.
2. Care given at bedtime is ____.
3. ____ is cleaning the genital and anal areas.
4. Profuse sweating is ____________________________.
5. Routine care given before breakfast is ____.
6. Care given after breakfast is called ____. Hygiene measures are more thorough at this time.
7. When the foreskin covering the glans of the penis was surgically removed, the man is __________________.

Circle the Best Answer

8. Which action would the nursing assistant take when the care plan indicates that the resident must shower in the morning but he says he has always taken his shower at night?
   A. Delay showering until the resident changes his mind
   B. Convince the resident that morning showers are refreshing
   C. Change the care plan to respect the resident's choice
   D. Report the resident's comment to the nurse
9. Which nursing assistant has made an error while assisting a resident with a tub bath?
   A. Nursing assistant A reminds the resident to use grab bars.
   B. Nursing assistant B leaves weak resident to answer a call light.
   C. Nursing assistant C places a rubber bathmat in the tub.
   D. Nursing assistant D provides the resident with warmth and privacy.
10. Which part of the body would the nursing assistant clean first based on the principle of the "head to toe" approach?
    A. Chest
    B. Hands
    C. Eyes
    D. Neck
11. Which action would the nursing assistant take upon noticing an unusual odor and brownish discharge on the perineal area?
    A. Ask the nurse to assess the patient's perineum
    B. Ask the person if there is itching or pain in the area
    C. Assist the person to take a bath or shower
    D. Make other observations based on personal experience
12. Which patient has a condition that would prompt the nursing assistant to verify the use of powder after bathing?
    A. Patient A has large pendulous breasts.
    B. Patient B perspires heavily in hot weather.
    C. Patient C has a respiratory disorder.
    D. Patient D takes medication for high blood pressure.
13. Which observation would the nursing assistant report to the nurse after assisting an older adult female to take a tub bath?
    A. Red rash underneath both breasts
    B. Fine white hair with streaks of graying
    C. Fine wrinkles and lines around the eyes
    D. Brown spots on the back of the hands
14. Which of these hygiene measures is done before breakfast?
    A. Assisting with washing the face and hand hygiene
    B. Providing back massage or other comfort measures
    C. Assisting with activity by providing range-of-motion exercises
    D. Storing eyeglasses, hearing aids, or other devices
15. Which nursing measure is done every time the nursing assistant is attending to a person's hygiene throughout the day?
    A. Offer to help with oral care
    B. Assist with elimination
    C. Encourage activity
    D. Change the person's clothes
16. What is the rationale for scheduling a complete bath or shower only twice a week for older persons?
    A. They are less active and perspire less.
    B. Illness and discomfort are common with aging.
    C. They are easily agitated and confused.
    D. Dry skin often occurs with aging.

17. Which products will the nursing assistant use to help soften the skin for a person who has dry skin?
    A. Soaps
    B. Creams and lotions
    C. Powders
    D. Deodorants and antiperspirants
18. Which nursing measure would the nursing assistant use for a person with dementia who resists bathing?
    A. Quickly perform the bath and limit the cleaning
    B. Speak firmly in a loud voice while giving clear instructions
    C. Try giving the bath during a time of day when the person is calmer
    D. Have a coworker hold the person so that no one is harmed
19. How would the nursing assistant choose the skin care products for bathing?
    A. A mild, low-cost soap or body wash is ideal.
    B. Use products the person prefers, whenever possible
    C. Use bath oils with a light fresh scent to soften the skin
    D. Select creams and lotions for moisturizers
20. Which factor would prompt the nursing assistant to ask the nurse about water temperature for a complete bed bath rather than relying on the standard temperature of between 110 °F and 115 °F (43.3°C and 46.1°C) for adults?
    A. Resident A is partially paralyzed but can move the arms.
    B. Resident B is 85 years old, weak, and has very fragile skin.
    C. Resident C is 70 years old and ate a large heavy meal.
    D. Resident D returns to nursing center after going to a park.
21. Which action would the nursing assistant use when applying powder?
    A. Shake or sprinkle the powder directly on the person
    B. Sprinkle a small amount of powder onto hands or a cloth
    C. Apply a thick and generous layer of powder
    D. Avoid putting powder on the feet or toes
22. Which action would the nursing assistant use when helping a bariatric person with hygiene?
    A. Use only water to prevent dry or irritated skin
    B. Dry under skin folds to prevent skin breakdown
    C. Work alone to protect the person's privacy
    D. Apply a thick layer of powder in skin folds
23. Which person needs a complete bed bath?
    A. Person A wants to experience a complete bed bath.
    B. Person B is ambulatory but is mildly confused.
    C. Person C is weak because of prolonged illness.
    D. Person D is newly admitted to the hospital.
24. When would the nursing assistant make the bed for a person who needs a complete bed bath?
    A. Change linens only if they get wet
    B. Make bed before the bath begins
    C. Make bed after the bath is completed
    D. Change linens according to the facility schedule
25. When would the nursing assistant offer the bedpan, urinal, commode, or assistance to the bathroom?
    A. Before the bath begins
    B. After the bath ends
    C. Elimination is unrelated to bath time
    D. When incontinence is anticipated
26. How would the nursing assistant deal with placing the bath blanket in preparation for a bed bath?
    A. Over the person after the top linens are removed
    B. Under the top linens
    C. Over the person before top linens are removed
    D. Under the person
27. For which area of the body would the nursing assistant avoid the use of soap?
    A. The face, ears, and neck
    B. Around the eyes
    C. The abdomen
    D. Around the perineal area
28. Which nursing measure would the nursing assistant use to avoid exposing the person when washing the chest?
    A. Keep the bath blanket over the area
    B. Keep the top linens over the chest
    C. Place a towel over the chest crosswise
    D. Make sure the curtains are closed
29. How frequently is the bath water changed?
    A. Every 5 minutes during the bath
    B. When it becomes cool and soapy
    C. Only once during the bath
    D. After washing the face, ears, and neck
30. Which person may respond well to a towel bath?
    A. Person A has mild dementia.
    B. Person B is frequently incontinent.
    C. Person C has skin breakdown.
    D. Person D needs a partial bath.
31. Which parts of the body would the nursing assistant clean and rinse for a patient who needs a partial bath?
    A. The body parts that are soiled
    B. The face, hands, underarms, back, buttocks, and perineal area
    C. The face and hands
    D. The perineal area
32. Which action would the nursing assistant use when giving any type of bath?
    A. Wash from the dirtiest to the cleanest areas
    B. Strive to remove all microbes
    C. Provide for privacy
    D. Decide what is best for the person
33. What is the maximum length of time that a person should be in a tub bath?
    A. 10 minutes
    B. 15 minutes
    C. 20 minutes
    D. 30 minutes
34. Which equipment would be used to safely accomplish bathing or showering if the person is weak or unsteady?
    A. Shower chair
    B. Vest restraint
    C. Wheelchair
    D. Stretcher

35. Which of these would be a time management strategy to use when giving a tub bath or shower?
    A. Take the person to the shower room and then collect your equipment
    B. Ask a coworker to give the bath or shower for you
    C. Ask a coworker to make the person's bed while you give the bath or shower
    D. Clean and disinfect the tub or shower before returning the person to the room
36. Which of these steps would the nursing assistant use first when assisting with a tub bath or shower?
    A. Help the person undress and remove footwear
    B. Assist or transport the person to the tub or shower room
    C. Put the occupied sign on the door
    D. Place a rubber bath math in the tub or on the shower floor
37. Which action would the nursing assistant use when cleaning the perineal area?
    A. Use a liberal amount of mild soap and flush with plenty of water
    B. Work from the anal area to the urethral area (back to front, bottom to top)
    C. Work from the urethral area to the anal area (front to back, top to bottom)
    D. Work from the dirtiest area to the cleanest area
38. Which equipment is needed for perineal care?
    A. One washcloth and toilet paper
    B. Two washcloths
    C. Three washcloths
    D. At least four washcloths
39. Which action would the nursing assistant use when giving perineal care to a male?
    A. Retract the foreskin if he is uncircumcised
    B. Wash from the scrotum to the tip of the penis
    C. Use one bag bath for the entire procedure
    D. Leave the foreskin retracted after finishing the care

Matching

Match the skin care product with the benefit or the problem that may occur if you use the product

A. Soaps
B. Bath oils
C. Creams and lotions
D. Powders
E. Deodorants and antiperspirants

40. ________ Absorbs moisture and prevents friction
41. ________ Makes showers and tubs slippery
42. ________ Protects skin from the drying effect of air and evaporation
43. ________ Excessive amounts can cause caking and crusts that can irritate the skin
44. ________ Masks and controls body odors or reduces perspiration
45. ________ Tends to dry and irritate skin
46. ________ Keeps skin soft and prevents drying of skin
47. ________ Removes dirt, dead skin, skin oil, some microbes, and perspiration

Fill in the Blanks

48. What water temperature is used for:
    A. Bed bath ________________
    B. Tub bath or shower ________________
    C. Perineal care ________________
49. The ________________ must be intact to prevent microbes from entering the body and causing an infection.
50. The religion of East Indian Hindus requires at least ________________ a day.
51. To prevent skin breakdown and odors in the perineal area, clean the skin any time ________________ are present.
52. List seven skin care products that the nursing assistant may use when assisting the person with bathing or showering
    A. ________________
    B. ________________
    C. ________________
    D. ________________
    E. ________________
    F. ________________
    G. ________________
53. What methods can be used to measure the water temperature for a bed bath?
    A. ________________
    B. ________________
54. When you place a person's hand in the basin during the bed bath, you may have the person ________________ the hands and fingers.
55. When assisting with partial baths, most people need help with washing the ________________.
56. A tub bath can cause a person to feel ________________, especially if the person has been on bed rest.
57. List two personal care products that may cause the bottom of the tub, shower, or floor to be slippery
    A. ________________
    B. ________________
58. When giving a tub bath or shower, you use safety measures to protect the person from ________________, ________________, and ________________.
59. When you are assisting a person with perineal care, what terms may help the person understand the anatomy and location of the care? ________________
60. What observations made while assisting with perineal care should be reported at once?
    A. ________________
    B. ________________
    C. ________________
    D. ________________
    E. ________________

Labeling

61. In this figure, explain what the staff member is doing.

____

Why is the towel positioned vertically on the person?

____

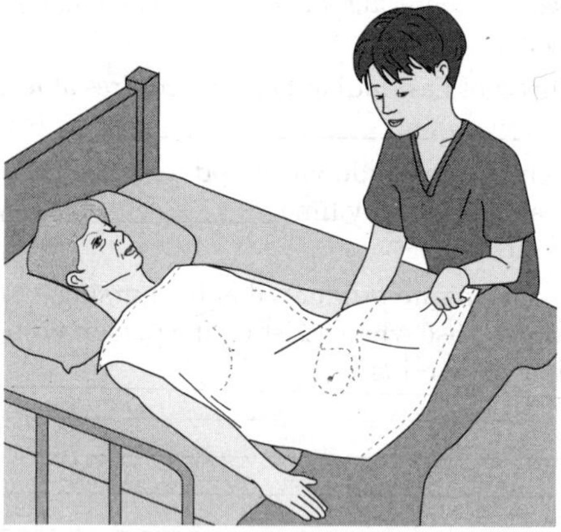

62. Refer to the charting sample below.

SKIN CARE

Abnormal Skin Observations

Problems:
- ☐ Blister
- ☐ Non-intact skin (open skin)
- ☐ Bruise
- ☐ Bleeding
- ☐ Drainage/discharge
- ☐ Swelling
- ☒ Rash
- ☒ Itching
- ☐ Odor

Color:
- ☒ Redness
- ☐ Pallor (pale skin)
- ☐ Gray
- ☐ Cyanosis (blue skin)
- ☐ Jaundice (yellow skin)

Texture:
- ☐ Rough
- ☐ Scaly/flaky

Temperature:
- ☐ Cold
- ☐ Cool
- ☐ Hot

Moisture:
- ☐ Dry
- ☐ Moist
- ☐ Diaphoresis (sweating)

Nurse notified: J. Anderson, RN

☐ No new skin issues

Bathing
- ☐ Shower
- ☐ Tub bath
- ☒ Complete bed bath
- ☐ Partial bath
- ☐ Bag/towel bath
- ☒ Perineal care

Click to mark affected area(s).

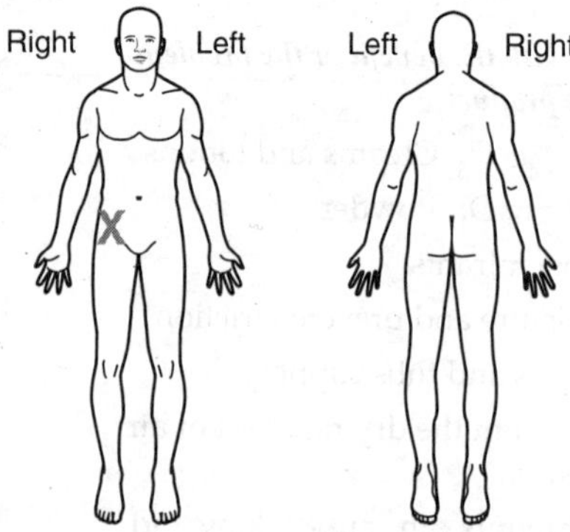

A. What abnormal skin observations were made?

____

B. What was the location on the person's body?

____

C. Which hygiene measures were performed?

____

Optional Learning Exercises

63. What does intact skin prevent? ____________________

64. What would you do if the foreskin that will not retract on an uncircumcised penis after completing male hygienic care? ____________________

65. When you are bathing a person with dementia, list five communication strategies that you can use.
    A. ____________________
    B. ____________________
    C. ____________________
    D. ____________________
    E. ____________________

66. You are preparing to give perineal care to a person. How many washcloths should you gather?
    ____________________ Why?
    ____
    ____
    ____

67. You are delegated to give an elderly person (Mrs. Johnson) a bath. Before beginning, what information do you need?
 A. ______________________
 B. ______________________
 C. ______________________
 D. ______________________
 E. ______________________
 F. ______________________
 G. ______________________
 H. ______________________

68. As you are bathing Mrs. Johnson, what observations should you make to report and record?
 A. ______________________
 B. ______________________
 C. ______________________
 D. ______________________
 E. ______________________
 F. ______________________
 G. ______________________
 H. ______________________
 I. ______________________
 J. ______________________
 K. ______________________
 L. ______________________

Use the FOCUS ON PRIDE section to complete these statements and then use the critical thinking and discussion question to develop your ideas

69. You can promote independence and social interaction when you allow
 A. Personal choice of ______________________
 B. Encourage the person to ______________________

Critical Thinking and Discussion Question

70. You are assigned to care for an elderly resident who has dementia. His regular shower days are Tuesday and Friday mornings. On Tuesday evening around 8:30 PM, he asks you to help him take a shower. You remind him that he had a shower this morning and that the next shower day is Friday. On Wednesday evening he asks you again to help him with a shower. He is easily redirected and you help him get ready for bed. On Thursday evening around 8:00 PM, you find him partially undressed and he is attempting to get into the shower.
 A. What do you think is happening with this resident?
 B. Why is it important to report this behavior to the nurse?

25 Grooming

Fill in the Blanks: Key Terms

Alopecia	Hirsutism	Pediculosis (lice)	Pediculosis pubis
Anticoagulant	Infestation	Pediculosis capitis	Scabies
Dandruff	Mite	Pediculosis corporis	

1. Being in or on a host is an ____________________.
2. The infestation with wingless insects (lice) that feed on blood is ____________________.
3. A very small spider-like organism is a ____________________.
4. ____________________ is an excessive amount of dry, white flakes from the scalp.
5. The infestation of the body with lice is ____________________.
6. Hair loss is ____________________.
7. ____________________ is the infestation of the pubic hair with lice.
8. Excessive body hair is ____________________.
9. The infestation of the scalp with lice is ____________________.
10. ____________________ is a skin disorder caused by the female mite.
11. A drug that prevents or slows down blood clotting is an ____________________.

Circle the Best Answer

12. Which nursing assistant is correctly focusing on communication related to the patient's skin and scalp condition?
    A. Nursing assistant A: "Ms. Smith you look really pale today and your hair is falling out. Are you feeling okay?"
    B. Nursing assistant B: "There is something disgusting in Ms. Smith's hair. I saw small, creepy, moving legs."
    C. Nursing assistant C: "Ms. Smith there are large red welts on your back with bloody specks! What's happening?"
    D. Nursing assistant D: "I saw small white specks in Ms. Smith's hair. Could you please look before I wash her hair?"
13. Which needs are most affected by having proper hair care, shaving, and nail and foot care?
    A. Safety and security needs
    B. Love, belonging, and self-esteem needs
    C. Physical needs
    D. Self-actualization needs
14. What is the rationale for reporting any signs of lice to the nurse?
    A. Lice bites can cause severe contagious infections.
    B. Lice spread to others through clothing, furniture, bed linens, and sexual contact.
    C. Lice can cause the person's hair to permanently fall out.
    D. The lice will cause the hair to mat and tangle.
15. What signs or symptoms may be present if a person has scabies?
    A. Visible lice that are small and tan to grayish white in color.
    B. A rash and intense itching on fingers, wrists, and underarms.
    C. Visible eggs (nits) attached to the hair shaft.
    D. An excessive amount of dry, white flakes on the scalp.
16. Who chooses how the nursing assistant will brush, comb, and style a person's hair?
    A. The person directs the assistant.
    B. Nursing assistant decides.
    C. The nurse explains what to do.
    D. The information is written in the care plan.
17. Which action should the nursing assistant take if long hair becomes matted or tangled?
    A. Braid the hair
    B. Cut the hair to remove the tangles and matting
    C. Tell the nurse and ask for directions
    D. Get the family's permission to change the hairstyle
18. Which of these measures could the nursing assistant use if hair is curly, coarse, and dry?
    A. Braid the hair
    B. Use a wide-toothed comb
    C. Comb downward
    D. Clip the dry ends
19. Which action should the nursing assistant use when assisting a person who has small braids?
    A. Undo the hair and rebraid it each time it is shampooed
    B. Leave the braids intact for shampooing
    C. Undo the braids only at night
    D. Comb out the braids once a week

20. Which nursing measure would the nursing assistant use if a woman's hair is done by the hairdresser in long-term care facility?
    A. Wash the hair only once a week
    B. Shampoo the hair after the beauty shop appointment
    C. Provide a shower cap during the tub bath or shower
    D. Wash the hair each time during the shower or tub bath
21. Which circumstance would be avoided if a person has limited range of motion in the neck and shoulders?
    A. Shampooing the hair at the sink or on a stretcher
    B. Rinsing the hair in the shower
    C. Washing the hair during a tub bath
    D. Combing and styling the hair while in bed
22. Which of these observations, noted while shampooing, should be reported to the nurse?
    A. Hair has been dyed and permed
    B. Amount of time it took to shampoo
    C. Hair is matted or tangled
    D. Amount of hair on the head
23. Which action should the nursing assistant take if a person receives anticoagulants and needs shaving?
    A. Use an electric razor
    B. Use disposable safety razors
    C. It is done by the nurse or barber
    D. It is done during the shower or bath
24. Which nursing measure would the nursing assistant use related to safety razors (blade razors)?
    A. The same razor can be used for several persons until it becomes dull.
    B. Use the resident's own razor as many times as possible
    C. Discard the disposable razor or razor blade in the sharps container
    D. Be careful when shaving a person who takes anticoagulants
25. What is the rationale for using an electric razor to shave a person with dementia?
    A. The person usually bleeds easily.
    B. The person may resist or move suddenly.
    C. It is faster than using a safety razor.
    D. The skin is tender and sensitive
26. What is the rationale for wearing gloves when shaving a person with a safety razor?
    A. To protect the person from infections
    B. To prevent contact with blood
    C. To apply shaving cream
    D. To maintain sterile technique
27. Which nursing measure should the nursing assistant use when grooming a person's mustache and beard?
    A. Trim the beard when it is obviously too long
    B. Shampoo the beard when the hair is shampooed
    C. Shave off the mustache if it interferes with eating
    D. Wash and comb the mustache or beard daily
28. What is the nursing assistant's responsibility related to cutting or trimming the toenails?
    A. Do toenail care whenever there is extra time
    B. Toenail care is required for assigned patients
    C. Follow the agency policy for toenail care
    D. Cut the toenails if the patient wants them cut
29. When caring for the fingernails or toenails, which action would you use?
    A. Shape the nails with an emery board or nail file
    B. Clean under the nails with a scrub brush
    C. Clip the nails in a curved shape to match the toe
    D. Cut the nails with small scissors
30. Which question about medication would the nursing assistant ask the nurse to provide safe care when shaving a person?
    A. "What time does the person take his blood pressure medication?"
    B. "Does the person take any anticoagulant medications?"
    C. "Will shaving interfere with medication administration today?"
    D. "Does the person take any medications that cause vomiting?"
31. Which person has a condition that would prompt the nursing assistant to check with the nurse before using an electric shaver?
    A. Person has mild dementia.
    B. Person B has a respiratory disorder.
    C. Person C has a pacemaker.
    D. Person D takes an anticoagulant.
32. Which action would the nursing assistant take first when the patient moves suddenly and the safety razor makes a small nick on the cheek?
    A. Apply direct pressure
    B. Report the nick to the nurse
    C. Write an incident report
    D. Instruct patient to hold still
33. Which additional nursing measure would the home health nursing assistant anticipate when the nurse says a family member is being treated with a medicated lotion for body lice?
    A. Infected family member should be isolated.
    B. Health-care staff need to wear personal protective equipment.
    C. Clothing and linens should be washed in hot water.
    D. The family's dog needs to stay outside.
34. Which nursing assistant has made an error while performing nail and foot care?
    A. Nursing assistant A reports observing a blister on the person's foot.
    B. Nursing assistant B clips toenails of person who has diabetes.
    C. Nursing assistant C asks the nurse how to position the person.
    D. Nursing assistant D soaks the person's feet for 15 minutes.

Fill in the Blanks

35. What should the nursing assistant report and record when brushing and combing the hair?
    A. ______
    B. ______
    C. ______
    D. ______
    E. ______
    F. ______
    G. ______
    H. ______
36. If you give hair care to a person in bed after a linen change, collect falling hair by ______ ______.
37. If hair is tangled or matted hair, divide the hair into small sections and start at the ______.
38. Grooming promotes self-esteem; therefore what will the surveyors observe about patients and residents?
    A. ______
    B. ______
    C. ______
    D. ______
39. You can protect the person's eyes during shampooing by asking the person to hold a ______.
40. What delegation guidelines does the nursing assistant need when shaving a person?
    A. ______
    B. ______
    C. ______
    D. ______
    E. ______
    F. ______
    G. ______
    H. ______
41. What should the nursing assistant immediately report when shaving a person?
    A. ______
    B. ______
    C. ______
    D. ______
42. When shaving legs with a safety razor, the nursing assistant would start shaving ______ ______, which is against the hair growth.
43. What delegation guidelines does the nursing assistant need when giving a person nail and foot care?
    A. ______
    B. ______
    C. ______
    D. ______
    E. ______
    F. ______
    G. ______
    H. ______
44. What does the nursing assistant report and record when delegated to give nail and foot care?
    A. ______
    B. ______
    C. ______
    D. ______
    E. ______
    F. ______
45. Foot care for persons with diabetes or poor circulation is provided by ______ or ______.

Optional Learning Exercises

46. You are caring for a person who is receiving cancer treatments. What effect could this treatment have on the person's hair? ______ ______
47. Dandruff not only occurs on the scalp but also may involve the ______.
48. Brushing the hair increases ______ to the scalp. It also brings ______ along the hair shaft.
49. Why do older persons usually have dry hair? ______ ______
50. What water temperature is usually used when shampooing the hair? ______
51. How can the beard be softened before shaving? ______ ______
52. After shaving, why do some people apply lotion or aftershave?
    A. Lotion ______
    B. Aftershave ______
53. Injuries to the feet of a person with poor circulation are serious because poor circulation prolongs ______.

Use the FOCUS ON PRIDE section to complete these statements and then use the critical thinking and discussion question to develop your ideas

54. Grooming promotes ______, ______, and ______. Clean hair and nails help mental well-being.
55. When a person allows family members to assist with giving personal care, this promotes ______.
56. If you cut a person's hair or shave a mustache or beard without permission, you have violated the person's right to be free from ______.

Critical Thinking and Discussion Question

57. You are assigned to help residents with morning hygiene and grooming. Resident A is usually alert, cheerful, and talkative, and she is very particular about how her hair is combed, how her makeup is applied, and the appearance of her nails. This morning when you offer to assist her with grooming, she seems tired and irritable. She turns away, refuses to acknowledge you and mumbles, "Leave me alone." Resident B has mild dementia and usually looks quite disheveled. He never wants your help with grooming. He does not like to change his clothes, and he usually pushes your hand away if you try to comb his hair or offer to file his nails. Both residents have refused your offers to help with hygiene. Discuss the difference between these two residents and discuss what you would do.

26 Changing Garments

Fill in the Blanks: Key Terms

Affected side	Unaffected side
Garment	Undergarment

1. An item of clothing is a ____________________.
2. The side of the body opposite the affected side; strong or "good" side is the __________ side.
3. The side of the body with weakness from illness or injury; weak side is the _________________ side.
4. An item of clothing worn next to the skin under clothing is an _____________________________.

Circle the Best Answer

5. Which action would the nursing assistant take when assisting a person to change clothing?
   A. Remove clothing from the weak side first
   B. Start with the lower limbs first
   C. Leave the right side until last
   D. Remove clothing from the strong side first
6. What does the nursing assistant need to obtain before assisting a person to undress while he is lying in bed?
   A. Washcloth
   B. Deodorant or antiperspirant
   C. Gloves
   D. Bath blanket
7. Which action would the nursing assistant always use when helping a person to dress or undress?
   A. Check for proper choice of undergarments
   B. Ask the person to dress themselves if able
   C. Provide for privacy. Do not expose the person
   D. Put clothing on the weak side first
8. Which nursing assistant is using good body mechanics when helping a person to undress?
   A. Nursing assistant A lowers the bed rail on the person's weak side.
   B. Nursing assistant B positions the person in a supine position.
   C. Nursing assistant C raises the bed to a good working level.
   D. Nursing assistant D turns the person toward the far side of bed.
9. Which action would the nursing assistant use for warmth and privacy when assisting a person to undress?
   A. Keep the top sheets in place
   B. Cover the person with a bath blanket
   C. Close the curtains
   D. Close the door
10. What is the best strategy to use when assisting a person with Alzheimer's to get dressed?
    A. Have the person put on the same clothes every day
    B. Take the person to the closet and show how to select clothes
    C. Stack clothes in the order they are to be put on
    D. Put the clothes selected for the day in an obvious place
11. Which action would the nursing assistant take first when assisting a person with weakness to remove a pullover garment?
    A. Remove the garment from the strong side
    B. Bring the garment over the person's head
    C. Undo any buttons, zippers, snaps, or ties
    D. Remove the garment from the weak side
12. What is the main role of the coworker who is asked to assist the nursing assistant with dressing a person?
    A. To help turn and position the person
    B. To select the person's clothing
    C. To undress the person
    D. To check the care plan for details
13. Which action would you use when assisting a person who is lying in bed and cannot sit up or lean forward to remove a garment that opens in the back?
    A. Turn the person away from you
    B. Put the garment on so the opening is in the front
    C. Use the bed mechanism to lower the head of the bed
    D. Cover the person with an extra bath blanket
14. Which nursing measure would the nursing assistant use when changing the gown of a person with an IV?
    A. Temporarily turn off the IV and later tell the nurse
    B. Lay the IV bag on the bed and remove the gown
    C. Slide the gathered sleeve over the tubing, hand, arm, and IV site
    D. Disconnect the IV where the tubing connects with the bag
15. Which action would the nursing assistant take after changing the gown of a person with an IV?
    A. Restart the pump
    B. Reconnect the IV
    C. Ask the nurse to check the flow rate
    D. Check the flow rate

16. In which circumstance, could the nursing assistant change the patient's gown without notifying the nurse?
    A. Patient has an IV that is attached to a pump and is wearing a standard gown.
    B. Patient has an IV that is attached to the pump, the bag is empty, and he is being discharged.
    C. Patient has an IV that is attached to a pump and is wearing a gown with snap fasteners on the sleeves.
    D. Patient has an IV that is not attached to a pump, but there is blood in the tubing and on the gown.
17. Which nursing assistant has made an error in adhering to the rules for dressing and undressing?
    A. Nursing assistant A lets a person select clothes and validates appropriate undergarments.
    B. Nursing assistant B puts the person's arm through the sleeve on the strong side first.
    C. Nursing assistant C encourages the person to do as much self-dressing as possible.
    D. Nursing assistant D makes sure that the selected garments belong to the person.
18. Which action would the nursing assistant use to remove pants for a person who has limits in raising the hips and buttocks off of the bed because of one-sided weakness?
    A. Check with the nurse to see if the person can go without wearing pants
    B. Pull the pants over the buttock and hip on the strong side first
    C. Have two coworkers on each side, they lift the hips while pants are pulled off
    D. Grab the pants by the cuffs and pull pants downward toward the feet
19. Which nurse has made an error in giving information after delegating dressing and undressing patients who are newly admitted to the facility?
    A. Nurse A says, "Patient can independently dress and undress, but needs help with small buttons."
    B. Nurse B says, "Patient is supposed to have weakness, but I'm not sure which side or how much it affects her mobility."
    C. Nurse C says, "Patient has special undergarments related to religious beliefs, be respectful and helpful as needed."
    D. Nurse D says, "Patient has limited range-of-motion in the right shoulder. Put the right sleeve on first and then the left."
20. Which nursing assistant is fulfilling personal and professional responsibility and demonstrating that the person is valued and cared for?
    A. Nursing assistant A efficiently does the task and leaves without speaking.
    B. Nursing assistant B smiles and chats but rushes the person to dress quickly.
    C. Nursing assistant C makes minimal effort to do a good job or help the person.
    D. Nursing assistant compliments the person's appearance after dressing is complete.
21. Which resident would benefit the most if the nursing assistant helped with dressing by handing the resident one item at a time and giving simple instructions?
    A. Patient A wears incontinence pants at night.
    B. Patient B has dementia with mild confusion.
    C. Patient C has arthritis with joint pain in hands.
    D. Patient D likes to wear a long-sleeved shirt every day.

Fill in the Blanks

22. List three questions you can ask to promote personal choice and independence.
    A. ______________________________
    B. ______________________________
    C. ______________________________
23. According to Alzheimer's and related Dementias Education and Referral Center (ADEAR), what are the six strategies that are useful when assisting people with dementia to get dressed?
    A. ______________________________
    B. ______________________________
    C. ______________________________
    D. ______________________________
    E. ______________________________
    F. ______________________________
24. Before changing a person's hospital gown who has an IV, what information do you need from the nurse and the care plan?
    A. ______________________________
    B. ______________________________
25. The nursing assistant has correctly performed the steps of assisting a person who had a stroke to remove his gown. Based on the figure, which side is the person's affected (weak) side?

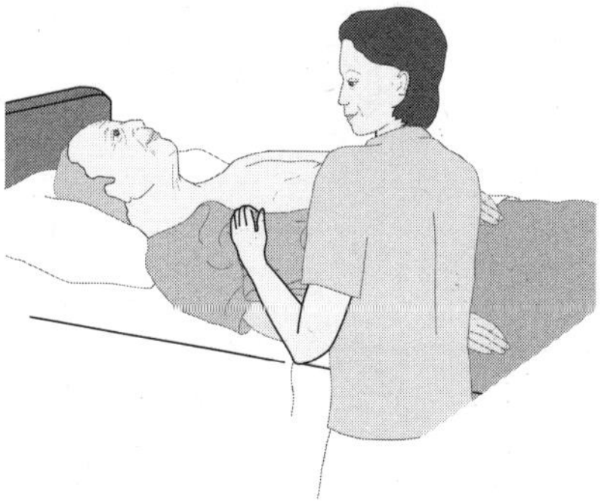

____

Optional Learning Exercises

Use the FOCUS ON PRIDE section to complete these statements and then use the critical thinking and discussion question to develop your ideas

26. Appearance affects ____________. Garments should be __________, not wrinkled, and comfortable.

Critical Thinking and Discussion Question

27. You are assigned to assist an elderly resident with daily hygiene and grooming. He performs most of the care by himself, which includes bathing, dental hygiene, and grooming. For the past week, he puts his dirty clothes, (including his underwear) back on. You informed the nurse who instructed you to "just keep trying" to get him to wear clean clothes. Discuss this situation:
    A. What do you think about this elderly resident's choices?
    B. What are the main reasons for trying to get him to wear clean clothes?
    C. What could you do?

27 Urinary Needs

Fill in the Blanks: Key Terms

Dysuria
Enuresis
Functional incontinence
Groin
Hematuria
Mixed incontinence
Nocturia
Oliguria
Overflow incontinence
Polyuria
Reflex incontinence
Stress incontinence
Transient incontinence
Urge incontinence
Urinary frequency
Urinary incontinence
Urinary retention
Urinary urgency
Urination (voiding)

1. Where the thigh and abdomen meet is called the ________________.
2. The production of abnormally large amounts of urine is ________________.
3. ________________ is the combination of stress incontinence and urge incontinence.
4. ________________ is the loss of bladder control.
5. Frequent urination at night is ________________.
6. The loss of small amounts of urine that leak from a bladder that is always full is ________________.
7. The lack of bladder control when past the usual age of toilet training is ________________.
8. ________________ occurs when the person has bladder control but cannot use the toilet in time.
9. The process of emptying urine from the bladder is ________________.
10. Blood in the urine is ________________.
11. Voiding at frequent intervals is ________________.
12. When urine leaks during exercise and certain movements that cause pressure on the bladder, it is called ________________.
13. Not being able to completely empty the bladder is ________________.
14. ________________ is the need to void at once.
15. The loss of urine in response to a sudden, urgent need to void is ________________.
16. Painful or difficult urination is ________________.
17. ________________ is when urine is lost at predictable intervals when a specific amount of urine is in the bladder.
18. A scant amount of urine, usually less than 500 mL in 24 hours, is ________________.
19. ________________ is temporary or occasional incontinence that is reversed when the cause is treated.

Circle the Best Answer

20. Which action would the nursing assistant take to mask urination sounds for a person who is embarrassed to void if others are nearby?
    A. Turn up the television volume
    B. Make noise outside of the bathroom
    C. Talk very loudly to the person
    D. Run water in the sink
21. Which substance is likely to increase urine production?
    A. Coffee
    B. Citrus fruits
    C. Tomatoes
    D. Spicy foods
22. How much urine does a healthy adult excrete in a day?
    A. 500 mL
    B. 1000 mL
    C. 1500 mL
    D. 2000 mL
23. Which voiding pattern is typical for most people?
    A. After bathing, eating, and exercise
    B. In the morning and in the evening
    C. Bedtime, after sleep, and before meals
    D. Goes only when there is complete privacy
24. Which nursing measure would the nursing assistant try if the person has difficulty starting the urine stream?
    A. Play music on the TV
    B. Provide perineal care
    C. Use a stainless steel bedpan
    D. Place the person's fingers in warm water
25. Which food would cause the urine to be bright yellow?
    A. Asparagus
    B. Carrots or sweet potatoes
    C. Beets or blackberries
    D. Rhubarb
26. Which of these observations should the nursing assistant report, at once, to the nurse when caring for an infant?
    A. The infant has had a wet diaper four times in 3 hours.
    B. The infant has not had a wet diaper for several hours.
    C. The urine in the diaper is pale yellow.
    D. The urine in the diaper has a faint odor.

27. Which action would the nursing assistant take when getting ready to give a person the bedpan?
   A. Raise the head of the bed slightly for the comfort
   B. Position the person in Fowler's position
   C. Warm the bedpan using hot water
   D. Place the bed in a flat position
28. Where would the nursing assistant put the urinal after the patient is done using it?
   A. Hang it on the bed rails
   B. Place it on the overbed table
   C. Put it on the bedside stand
   D. Store if on the floor under the bed
29. Which action would the nursing assistant take if a man is unable to stand and handle a urinal to void?
   A. Tell the nurse
   B. Ask a male coworker to help the man
   C. Place and hold the urinal for him
   D. Pad the bed with incontinence pads
30. For which situation would a commode chair be used?
   A. Person is unable to stand and pivot.
   B. Person is not allowed to get out of bed.
   C. Person needs a natural position for elimination.
   D. Bathroom is being used by another person.
31. Which action would the nursing assistant take when placing a commode over the toilet?
   A. Attach a transfer belt to the commode
   B. Stay in the room with the person
   C. Lock the wheels
   D. Make sure the container is in place
32. Which type of incontinence is aggravated when the nursing assistant does not answer call lights quickly or leave the call light within the person's reach?
   A. Overflow incontinence
   B. Mixed incontinence
   C. Reflex incontinence
   D. Functional incontinence
33. Which action would the nursing assistant take for an incontinent person who often wets right after the clothes and bedding have been changed?
   A. Wait 15 to 30 minutes before changing the person each time
   B. Place extra waterproof underpads over the wet bedding
   C. Talk to the nurse immediately if feeling impatient or frustrated
   D. Tell the person that the linens can only be changed once a shift
34. Which nursing measure would the nursing assistant use to keep a person who has dementia clean and dry?
   A. Tell the person to use the call light when there is a need to void
   B. Decrease fluid intake at breakfast, lunchtime, and bedtime
   C. Observe for signs that the person may need to void, such as pulling at the clothing
   D. Remove any incontinence garments and seat the person on a commode
35. Which nursing assistant needs a communication reminder related to assisting people with incontinence products?
   A. Nursing assistant A asks, "Would you like to try a different size of incontinence briefs."
   B. Nursing assistant B offers, "I want to help you change your wet underwear."
   C. Nursing assistant C says, "Don't be embarrassed, an adult diaper will keep you dry."
   D. Nursing assistant D says, "If the incontinence pad is uncomfortable, let me know."
36. Which nursing measure would the nursing assistant use when applying an incontinence product?
   A. Apply a new one when the old one has a strong odor
   B. Weigh the used product to determine the urine output
   C. Mark the date, time, and initials on the new product
   D. Clean the skin by rubbing it with dry paper towels
37. What is the primary goal of bladder training?
   A. To keep the person dry
   B. To control urination
   C. To prevent skin breakdown
   D. To prevent infection
38. Which nursing measure would the nursing assistant use when assisting the person with habit training to have normal elimination?
   A. Help the person to the bathroom every 15 or 20 minutes
   B. Voiding is scheduled at regular times to match the person's voiding habits
   C. Make sure the person drinks at least 1000 mL each shift
   D. Tell the person bathroom trips occur twice a shift
39. Which patient would benefit the most if a fracture pan is used for urination?
   A. Patient A has a respiratory disorder.
   B. Patient B recently had spinal cord surgery.
   C. Patient C weighs 450 pounds (204 kg).
   D. Patient D has a prostate problem.
40. Which change related to aging increases the risk for incontinence?
   A. Older people have trouble remembering to go to the bathroom.
   B. Older people are obese, and this increases pressure on the bladder.
   C. The aging bladder muscles lose strength and capacity decreases.
   D. The aging kidney system produces more concentrated urine.
41. Which information would the nursing assistant report to the nurse after assisting a person to void in a bedpan?
   A. The type of bedpan that was used.
   B. How many coworkers assisted?
   C. Color, clarity, and odor of the urine
   D. How the person was positioned on the bedpan?

42. Which nurse has made a delegation error when assigning a new nursing assistant to help a patient use the bedpan?
    A. Nurse A recommends that a standard bedpan is adequate.
    B. Nurse B explains the patient's position and activity limits.
    C. Nurse C instructs to stay with the patient at all times.
    D. Nurse D says to report anything abnormal about the urine.
43. Which chronic health condition is associated with polyuria?
    A. Diabetes
    B. Heart failure
    C. Respiratory disorder
    D. Chronic constipation
44. Which dietary item is most likely to be restricted if a patient has temporary urinary incontinence?
    A. Asparagus
    B. Milk
    C. Blackberries
    D. Diet soda
45. Which information does the nursing assistant need from the nurse and care plan to apply an incontinence product on a newly admitted resident?
    A. How to position the penis?
    B. Which product and size to use?
    C. Purpose of the incontinent product
    D. Whether the patient smokes or drinks alcohol?
46. Which nursing assistant has made an error in providing perineal care after a person is incontinent?
    A. Nursing assistant A uses a safe and comfortable water temperature.
    B. Nursing assistant B uses soap and water or a no-rinse incontinent cleanser.
    C. Nursing assistant C follows Standard Precautions and the Blood-borne Pathogen Standard.
    D. Nursing assistant D exposes chest and abdomen and covers the legs with a bath blanket.
47. Which outcome would the nursing assistant expect for a person who eats a diet high in salt and takes a drug that causes the body to retain water?
    A. Less urine is produced.
    B. Risk for incontinence is increased.
    C. Urination will be painful.
    D. Very large amounts of urine are voided.
48. What is the purpose of a bladder scanner?
    A. To empty the drainage bag every hour
    B. To detect the amount of urine in the bladder
    C. To alert staff when confused patients need to void
    D. To stimulate voiding for patients with urinary retention

Fill in the Blanks

49. Write out the abbreviations
    A. BM ____________________
    B. mL ____________________
    C. OAB ____________________
    D. UI ____________________
    E. UTI ____________________
50. A normal position for voiding for women is ____________________. For men, a normal position is ____________________.
51. A bariatric bedpan is placed with the ____________ end under the buttocks.
52. Most children achieve daytime bladder control (dryness) between ages ____________________. Nighttime bladder control comes later—usually by age ____________.
53. You should report if the person has urgency, burning, or ____________________ when voiding.
54. When you are handling bedpans, urinals, and commodes and their contents, you should follow ____________________ and ____________________.
55. When you transfer a person to a commode from bed, you must practice safe transfer procedures and use a ____________________ and lock the wheels.
56. For women, ____________, ____________________, and ____________________ are risk factors for incontinence.
57. Rewarding the child for ______________ the treatment plan for bed-wetting or daytime enuresis is important.

Optional Learning Exercises

58. An infant can have ____________________ wet diapers a day.
59. A fracture pan can be used with older persons who have fragile bones from ______________ or painful joints from ____________________.
60. Covering the lap and legs of a person using a commode provides warmth and promotes ____________________.
61. What patient rights are you protecting when you immediately talk to the nurse because you feel short-tempered and impatient with a patient who is incontinent?
    ____
62. When using incontinence products, it is important to use the correct size. If the product is too large, urine can ____________________. If it is too small, the product will cause ____________________ from being too tight.
63. When bladder retraining (bladder rehabilitation) is being done, the goal is to increase the ______________ between the urge to void and voiding.
64. What observations should you report and record when you are delegated to apply incontinence products?
    A. ____________________
    B. ____________________
    C. ____________________
    D. ____________________
    E. ____________________
    F. ____________________
    G. ____________________

Use the FOCUS ON PRIDE section to complete these statements and then use the critical thinking and discussion question to develop your ideas

65. If you notice a person is uncomfortable talking about urinary elimination, what can you do put the person at ease?
    A. ______________________________
    B. ______________________________
    C. ______________________________
66. Urine-filled devices in the person's room do not respect the person's right to ____________________.

Critical Thinking and Discussion Question

67. You are recently hired at a long-term care center. You observe that nursing assistant A, who has worked there a long time, is leaving the residents on the commode or the bedpan for prolonged periods without checking on them. You answer a call light and the resident asks you for help because nursing assistant A, "put me on the bedpan a long time ago and never came back." When you mention the incident to nursing assistant A, she says, "I told the person to call when she was finished. I believe that people need their privacy." What would you do?

Crossword

Fill in the crossword by answering the clues below with words from this list

Dysuria	Hematuria	Nocturia	Polyuria
Frequency	Incontinence	Oliguria	Urgency

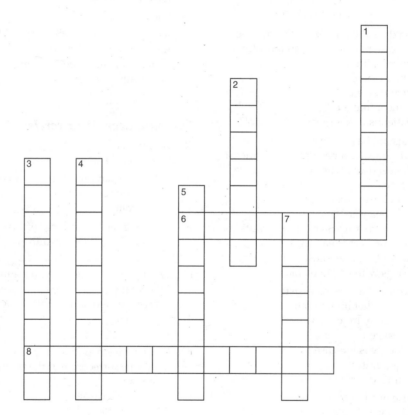

Across

7. Scant amount of urine, usually less than 500 mL in 24 hours
8. Inability to control the loss of urine from bladder

Down

1. Production of abnormally large amount of urine
2. Painful or difficult urination
3. Blood in the urine
4. Voiding at frequent intervals
5. Frequent urination at night
6. Need to void immediately

28 Urinary Catheters

Fill in the Blanks: Key Terms

Catheter
Catheterization
Condom catheter
Gravity
Indwelling catheter (Foley catheter, retention catheter)
Straight catheter
Suprapubic catheter

1. A soft sheath that slides over the penis and is used to drain urine is a ______________________.
2. A natural force that pulls things downward is ______________________.
3. The process of inserting a catheter is ______________________.
4. A catheter left in the bladder so urine drains constantly into a drainage bag is called an ______________________.
5. A ______________________ is a tube used to drain or inject fluid through a body opening.
6. A catheter that drains the bladder and then is removed is a ______________________.
7. A ______________ is surgically inserted into the bladder through an incision above (supra) the pubis bone (pubic).

Circle the Best Answer

8. Which observation would the nursing assistant report to the nurse that needs follow-up because of possible urinary tract infection (UTI)?
   A. Condom catheter is loose.
   B. Drainage bag is full.
   C. Report of flank pain.
   D. Increase in body weight.
9. Which person is most likely to have a catheter?
   A. Person A is scheduled to have surgery today.
   B. Person B cannot walk to the bathroom.
   C. Person C has frequent episodes of incontinence.
   D. Person D has a urinary tract infection.
10. Which action would the nursing assistant use when securing the drainage tubing?
    A. Clip the tubing to the person's gown.
    B. Pin the tubing so that it is tight and straight.
    C. Secure the tubing to the bottom linens.
    D. Attach the tubing to the bed rails.
11. Which action would the nursing assistant use when cleaning a catheter?
    A. Wipe the entire catheter and the tubing.
    B. Disconnect the tubing from the drainage bag.
    C. Clean from the meatus down the catheter about 4 inches.
    D. Wash the catheter by wiping up and down the tubing.
12. Where would the nursing assistant attach the urinary drainage bag?
    A. Hang it from the bed frame.
    B. Pin it to the bottom linens.
    C. Secure it to the person's gown.
    D. Loop it over the bed rail.
13. Which nursing measure would the nursing assistant use if a condom catheter accidentally loosens or leaks?
    A. Clean downward starting at the meatus and down the catheter for 4 inches.
    B. Clamp the catheter to prevent leakage and get permission to remove it.
    C. Perform perineal hygiene, inform the nurse, and reapply the catheter as directed.
    D. Wipe the connecting ends of the tube and catheter with clean antiseptic wipes.
14. Which action would the nursing assistant use if a person has a leg drainage bag?
    A. Switch it to a drainage bag when the person is in bed.
    B. Attach it to the person's clothing with tape or safety pins.
    C. Hang it from the bed frame when the person is in bed.
    D. Empty it frequently if the person wears it 24 hours a day.
15. What is the rationale for emptying a leg bag more frequently than a drainage bag?
    A. It holds less than 1000 mL and the drainage bag holds about 2000 mL.
    B. It is more likely to leak than the drainage bag.
    C. It holds about 250 mL and the drainage bag holds 1000 mL.
    D. It interferes with walking if it is full.
16. Which action would the nursing assistant use when emptying a drainage bag?
    A. Disconnect the bag from the tubing.
    B. Clamp the catheter to prevent leakage.
    C. Open the tubing clamp and let urine drain into a graduate.
    D. Take the bag into the bathroom to empty it.
17. What is the purpose of using a syringe when removing an indwelling catheter?
    A. To remove water from the balloon.
    B. To instill water into the drainage bag.
    C. To flush the catheter with water.
    D. To rinse the perineal area after catheter removal.

18. When is a condom catheter changed?
    A. Daily after perineal care.
    B. Once or twice a week on bath days.
    C. When the adhesive wears out.
    D. When a leg bag is switched to a large drainage bag.
19. Which nursing measure would the nursing assistant use when applying a condom catheter?
    A. Apply elastic tape in a spiral around the penis.
    B. Make sure the catheter tip is flush with the head of the penis.
    C. Apply adhesive tape securely in a snug circle around the penis.
    D. Clean the penis and reapply condom every shift.
20. Which equipment would be considered sterile when working with urinary drainage systems?
    A. Plug and cap.
    B. Graduate cylinder.
    C. Outside of connection tubing.
    D. Drainage bag.
21. Which nursing assistant is correctly managing the patient's urinary drainage system?
    A. Nursing assistant A puts the drainage bag on the floor while helping patient to stand.
    B. Nursing assistant B hangs the drainage bag from the patient's walker during ambulation.
    C. Nursing assistant C positions tubing so it will not get tangled in wheelchair wheels.
    D. Nursing assistant D allows tubing to loop below the drainage bag to decrease friction on meatus.
22. Which poor outcome is associated with positioning the drainage bag higher than the bladder?
    A. Increases pain and discomfort.
    B. Decreases urinary output.
    C. Increases risk for infection.
    D. Urine may leak out on the patient.
23. For which circumstance, is the nursing assistant likely to encounter a patient who needs catheterization using a straight catheter?
    A. Person A needs hourly urine output measurements.
    B. Person B does intermittent self-catheterization at home.
    C. Person C has dementia and has functional incontinence.
    D. Person D has a terminal illness and is weak and dying.
24. What is the nursing assistant's most important role in helping to prevent catheter-associated urinary tract infections (CAUTIs)?
    A. Remind patients to perform hand hygiene.
    B. Give proper patient and catheter care.
    C. Report patient concerns about the catheter.
    D. Assist patients to go to the bathroom.
25. Which nursing assistant has used a correct step in applying a condom catheter?
    A. Nursing assistant A puts a 1-inch space between the condom and penis tip.
    B. Nursing assistant B spirals plastic tape down the condom and penis.
    C. Nursing assistant C circles the penis and condom with adhesive tape.
    D. Nursing assistant D gently applies the condom to the erect penis.

Fill in the Blanks

26. A tube holder, tape, leg band, or other device is used to secure the catheter to the ______________ or ______________.
27. When you give catheter care, clean down from the meatus with one stroke; clean the catheter about ______________ inches.
28. A ______________ occurs when microbes enter the urinary tract through the catheter and cause an infection.
29. When a person has a catheter, what observations should you report and record?
    A. ______________
    B. ______________
    C. ______________
    D. ______________
    E. ______________
    F. ______________
    G. ______________
    H. ______________
30. Name two things you could do to make a person with a catheter feel less embarrassed and more comfortable when visitors are coming.
    A. ______________
    B. ______________
31. When you are allowed to remove a catheter, what information is needed from the nurse?
    A. ______________
    B. ______________
    C. ______________
    D. ______________
    E. ______________
    F. ______________

Optional Learning Exercises

32. What can happen if microbes enter a closed drainage system? ______________
33. What are the signs and symptoms of a urinary tract infection that must be reported at once to the nurse?
    A. ______________
    B. ______________
    C. ______________
    D. ______________
    E. ______________
    F. ______________

Labeling

34. Mark the places you would secure the catheter and drainage bag.

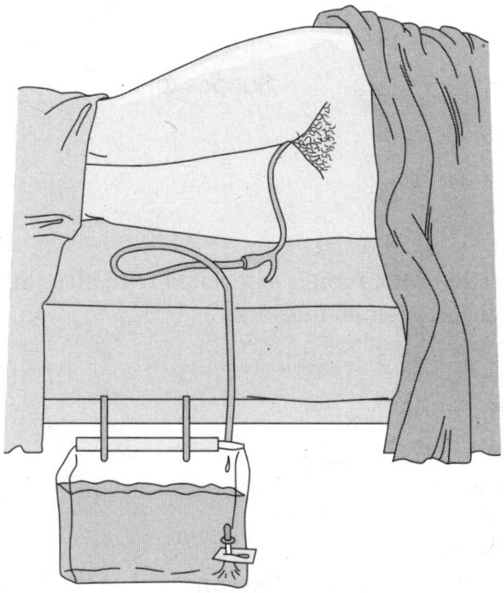

35. Mark the places you would secure the catheter.

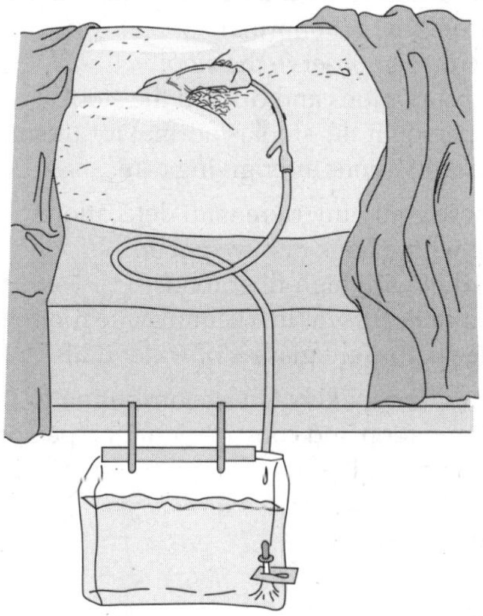

36. Why is it important to secure the catheters and drainage tubing as shown in the drawings?
____
____

Use the FOCUS ON PRIDE section to complete these statements and then use the critical thinking and discussion question to develop your ideas

37. With more training, some states and agencies allow nursing assistants to ________________ or remove indwelling catheters. Never perform a task outside your role limits.
38. When you need to transfer a person from the bed to the chair or move a drainage bag to the other side of the bed, list four things that you should do.
    A. ____
    B. ____
    C. ____
    D. ____

Critical Thinking and Discussion Question

39. The risk for urinary tract infection (UTI) increases when a person has a catheter. UTI can be life-threatening, especially for older people. There are many actions that you can perform to help prevent infection for people who must wear catheters. For example, using a clean area of the washcloth for each stroke during catheter care. Name at least six other actions that you could do.

29 Bowel Needs

Fill in the Blanks: Key Terms

Colostomy	Enema	Flatus	Stoma
Constipation	Fecal impaction	Ileostomy	Suppository
Defecation	Fecal incontinence	Melena	
Dehydration	Feces (stool)	Ostomy	
Diarrhea	Flatulence	Peristalsis	

1. A surgically created opening that connects an internal organ to the body's surface is a stoma or ______________________________.
2. The process of excreting feces from the rectum through the anus is a bowel movement or ______________________________.
3. The excessive formation of gas in the stomach and intestines is ______________________________.
4. A ____________________ is a cone-shaped solid drug that is inserted into a body opening.
5. The frequent passage of liquid stools is ______________________________.
6. ______________________________ is the prolonged retention and buildup of feces in the rectum.
7. ______________________________ is the excessive loss of water from tissues.
8. Gas or air passed through the anus is ______________________________.
9. The introduction of fluid into the rectum and lower colon is an ______________________________.
10. Black, tarry stool is ______________________________.
11. A surgically created opening between the colon and the body's surface is a ______________________________.
12. ______________________________ is the alternating contraction and relaxation of intestinal muscles.
13. The passage of a hard, dry stool is ______________________________.
14. ____________________ is the inability to control the passage of feces and gas through the anus.
15. A surgically created opening seen on the body's surface is an ostomy or a ______________________________.
16. The semisolid mass of waste products in the colon is ______________________________.
17. A surgically created opening between the ileum and the body's surface is an ______________________________.

Circle the Best Answer

18. Which bowel movement pattern might be considered abnormal for an adult?
    A. Every day.
    B. Every 2 to 3 days.
    C. Two or three times a day.
    D. Six or eight times a day.
19. Which stool coloration is associated with bleeding in the stomach or small intestines?
    A. Brown.
    B. Black.
    C. Red.
    D. Clay-colored.
20. What causes the characteristic odor of stool?
    A. Poor personal hygiene.
    B. Poor nutrition.
    C. Bacterial action in the intestines.
    D. Lack of fluid intake.
21. Which action would the nursing assistant take when observing stool that is abnormal?
    A. Ask the nurse to observe the stool.
    B. Report observations and discard the stool.
    C. Ask the person if the stool is normal for them.
    D. Record observations after giving care.
22. Which of these could interfere with defecation?
    A. Relaxing with a book or newspaper.
    B. Eating a diet with high-fiber foods.
    C. Having others present in a semiprivate room.
    D. Drinking six to eight glasses of water daily.
23. Which factor is most likely to be contributing to irregular elimination and constipation for a person who must stay in bed?
    A. Poor diet.
    B. Poor fluid intake.
    C. Inactivity.
    D. Lack of privacy.
24. Which of these would provide safety for the person during bowel elimination?
    A. Make sure the bedpan is warm.
    B. Place the call light and toilet paper within reach.
    C. Provide privacy by closing the door.
    D. Allow enough time for defecation.
25. Which nursing measure would help to relieve constipation?
    A. Encouraging a low-fiber diet.
    B. Helping patient to increase activity.
    C. Discouraging intake of extra fluids.
    D. Encouraging a delay of defecation.
26. Which condition is suspected when a person tries several times to have a bowel movement without success but liquid feces seep from the anus?
    A. Diarrhea.
    B. Constipation.
    C. Fecal impaction.
    D. Fecal incontinence.

27. Which nursing measure would the nurse use to help to relieve a fecal impaction?
    A. Ask the dietary staff to change the person's diet.
    B. Tell nursing assistant to offer more fluids.
    C. Remove the fecal mass manually with a gloved finger.
    D. Tell nursing assistant to help the person to ambulate.
28. Which observation would the nursing assistant immediately report when assisting the nurse to check for and remove a fecal impaction?
    A. Patient is sweating and appears anxious.
    B. Pulse is slowed to 45 beats/minute.
    C. Respirations are increased to 28/minute.
    D. Patient is grimacing but says he is okay.
29. What is the most important reason to give good skin care when a person has diarrhea?
    A. To prevent noxious odors.
    B. To prevent skin breakdown.
    C. To prevent the spread of microbes.
    D. To prevent fluid loss.
30. Why is diarrhea very serious in older persons?
    A. It causes skin breakdown.
    B. It causes odors.
    C. It can cause dehydration and death.
    D. It decreases activity.
31. Which action would the nursing assistant take if a person with diarrhea has *Clostridium difficile*?
    A. Wear sterile gloves and gown.
    B. Practice Standard Precautions and contact precautions.
    C. Restrict all visitors from visiting the person.
    D. Use alcohol hand rubs to clean the hands.
32. Which nursing action is the responsibility of the nursing assistant when fecal incontinence occurs?
    A. Reviewing diet and medications as contributing factors.
    B. Designing an individualized bowel training program.
    C. Assessing when the person needs help with elimination.
    D. Changing incontinence products to keep garments and linens clean.
33. Which sign or symptom is the person likely to experience if excessive flatus is not expelled?
    A. Abdominal cramping or pain.
    B. Diarrhea.
    C. Fecal incontinence.
    D. Nausea.
34. Which action could the nursing assistant take to help the person expel flatus?
    A. Assist the person to walk.
    B. Encourage the person to eat vegetables.
    C. Offer the person extra fluids.
    D. Gently massage the person's abdomen.
35. Which observation would be most useful to the nurse who must plan a bowel training program for a person?
    A. The amount and appearance of the stool the person expels.
    B. The person's response to perineal care following fecal incontinence.
    C. The usual time o f day the person has a bowel movement.
    D. The type of foods and fluids that cause flatus for the person.
36. Which solution would the nursing assistant prepare when delegated to give a soapsuds enema to an adult?
    A. Two teaspoons of salt in 1000 mL of tap water.
    B. 3 to 5 mL of castile soap in 500 to 1000 mL of tap water.
    C. 2 mL of mild dish soap in 200 mL of tap water.
    D. Mineral oil with sterile water.
37. What is the correct length of time for administering a cleansing enema?
    A. Over 5 to 6 minutes.
    B. Over 30 minutes.
    C. Over 10 to 15 minutes.
    D. Over 20 minutes.
38. Which position is the most suitable when a person must receive an enema?
    A. Supine position.
    B. Prone position.
    C. Semi-Fowler's position.
    D. Left side-lying position.
39. Which nursing assistant needs a reminder about preparing and giving cleansing enemas for adults?
    A. Nursing assistant A prepares the solution at 110 °F (43.3°C).
    B. Nursing assistant B inserts the tubing 2 to 4 inches into the rectum.
    C. Nursing assistant C holds the solution container about 12 inches above the bed.
    D. Nursing assistant D lubricates the enema tip before inserting it into the rectum.
40. Which action would the nursing assistant use when the doctor orders enemas until clear?
    A. Give one enema using a clear fluid.
    B. Give enemas until the return is clear.
    C. Ask the nurse how many enemas to give.
    D. Use clear tap water for repeated enemas.
41. Which action would the nursing assistant take when giving an enema and the person reports cramping?
    A. Tell the person that cramps are normal and continue the enema.
    B. Clamp the tube until the cramping subsides.
    C. Discontinue the enema immediately and tell the nurse.
    D. Raise the bag higher to increase the flow rate.

42. Which type of enema is used when giving a cleansing enema to a child?
    A. Soapsuds enema.
    B. Saline enema.
    C. Small-volume enema.
    D. Tap water enema.
43. What is the rationale for maintaining pressure on the bottle, rather than releasing it, when giving a small-volume enema?
    A. It will cause cramping if pressure is released.
    B. The fluid will leak from the rectum.
    C. Solution will be drawn back into the bottle.
    D. It will cause flatulence.
44. Which action would the nursing assistant take when giving a small-volume enema to an adult?
    A. Place the person in the prone position.
    B. Insert the enema tip 2 inches into the rectum.
    C. Heat the solution to 105 °F.
    D. Clamp the tubing if cramping occurs.
45. What is the purpose of an oil-retention enema?
    A. To cleanse the bowel to prepare for surgery.
    B. To regulate the person who is receiving bowel training.
    C. To relieve flatulence.
    D. To soften the feces and lubricate the rectum.
46. Which action would the nursing assistant take if resistance occurs when inserting an enema tube?
    A. Relubricate the tube.
    B. Push firmly to insert the tube.
    C. Stop tube insertion.
    D. Encourage deep breathing.
47. Which person is most likely to have skin irritation if the nursing assistant fails to give good care related to ostomies?
    A. Person has a permanent colostomy.
    B. Person has temporary colostomy.
    C. Person has ileostomy.
    D. Person's stoma bleeds slightly.
48. Which nursing measure would help a person with an ostomy pouch who is worried that the pouch will cause a bulge under the clothing?
    A. Assist the person to empty the pouch whenever it is 1/3 to 1/2 full.
    B. Suggest that wearing a snug pair of jeans will flatten the bulge.
    C. Make a small slit at the top of the pouch, so that flatus does not cause ballooning.
    D. Recommend that extra-large flowing clothes are loose at the waist.
49. What is the best rationale for notifying the nurse when a person with an ostomy requests a pouch change after every bowel movement?
    A. The person will run out of pouches and supplies.
    B. The care plan indicates that it should be changed once a day.
    C. Frequent pouch changes are damaging to the skin.
    D. Stool is continuously being expelled in small amounts.
50. When is best time to assist the person who has an ostomy and would like to shower with the pouch off?
    A. Before breakfast.
    B. Before going to bed.
    C. After lunch.
    D. After exercise.
51. When can the nursing assistant help the person to take a bath or a shower, after a new ostomy pouch has been applied?
    A. 15 to 20 minutes after pouch application.
    B. 1 to 2 hours after the new pouch has been applied.
    C. Later in the day, toward bedtime.
    D. The day after the pouch has been applied.
52. Which snack would be best for a person who needs high dietary fiber?
    A. Apple.
    B. Glass of milk.
    C. Saltine crackers.
    D. Small chocolate bar.
53. Which food item would the nursing assistant query upon seeing it on the lunch tray for a person who has an ostomy and wants to avoid gas-forming foods?
    A. Small orange.
    B. Plain bagel.
    C. Unsalted potato chips.
    D. Sauteed cabbage.
54. Which vital sign will the nurse ask the nursing assistant to frequently take and report while assisting with the removal a fecal impaction?
    A. Temperature.
    B. Pulse.
    C. Respirations.
    D. Blood pressure.
55. Which characteristics related to urine and urination would the nursing assistant report that indicate that the person may be dehydrated?
    A. Urine is a very pale yellow color.
    B. Urine is dark and amount is small.
    C. Urination is urgent and voiding is painful.
    D. Urination is frequent and amount is large.
56. How soon would the nursing assistant expect the person to defecate after the nurse inserts a suppository?
    A. 1 to 2 minutes.
    B. 5 minutes.
    C. 30 minutes.
    D. 1 to 2 hours.
57. Which nursing assistant has made an error prior to giving an enema?
    A. Nursing assistant A asks the nurse several relevant questions related to the procedure.
    B. Nursing assistant B verifies that giving an enema is included in the job description.
    C. Nursing assistant C received training related to enemas during orientation.
    D. Nursing assistant D is unfamiliar with state laws related to enema administration.

58. Which nursing measure would the nursing assistant use to prevent cramping during an cleansing enema?
   A. Hang the enema bag up high.
   B. Give the solution very slowly.
   C. Tell person that the cramping is temporary.
   D. Use a cool temperature for the solution.
59. How long does it usually take for a cleansing enema to take effect?
   A. Within 2 to 3 minutes.
   B. Within 10 minutes.
   C. At least 30 minutes.
   D. 1 to 2 hours.
60. The nursing assistant must give a 750 mL saline enema over 15 minutes. How many mL must be given each minute?
   A. 25 mL/minute.
   B. 50 mL/minute.
   C. 75 mL/minute.
   D. 750 mL/minute.
61. What is the risk to the patient if repeated tap water enemas are given?
   A. Excessive fluid absorption.
   B. Uncontrollable diarrhea.
   C. Infection to the intestine.
   D. Abdominal pain and distention.
62. What would the nursing assistant expect if touching the person's stoma while cleaning the surrounding skin?
   A. Person may look shocked or startled by the touch.
   B. Person may grimace because of slight pain or tenderness.
   C. Stoma will begin to slowly ooze blood or pink tinged fluid.
   D. Stoma has no sensation, so the person will not feel discomfort.
63. For which condition is a small-volume enema most likely to be given?
   A. Diarrhea.
   B. Constipation.
   C. Procedure preparation.
   D. Surgical preparation.
64. Which nursing assistant has made an error when assisting a patient with bowel elimination?
   A. Nursing assistant A reports that an infant had a large amount of watery stool.
   B. Nursing assistant B uses Standard Precautions when giving perineal care.
   C. Nursing assistant C leaves an elderly patient on a bedpan to answer call light.
   D. Nursing assistant D helps with elimination after meals and every 2 to 3 hours.

Fill in the Blanks

65. Write out the abbreviations
   A. BM ______________________________
   B. *C. difficile* ______________________________
   C. GI ______________________________
   D. IV ______________________________
   E. mL ______________________________
   F. SSE ______________________________
66. ____________ Precautions and______________ Precautions are required when caring for a person with *C. difficile* or norovirus.
67. Flatulence may be caused when a person __________________ while eating and drinking.
68. Drinking warm fluids such as coffee, tea, hot cider, and warm water will increase ____________________.
69. When the nursing assistant is inserting an enema tube or administering enema solution, asking the person to take slow, ________________________________ will help the person to relax.
70. An ostomy pouch is changed every _________ to _________days and when it leaks.
71. Showers and baths are delayed 1 or 2 hours after applying a new pouch to allow __________________ __________________________?
72. List four actions that will help the patient to expel flatus.
   A. ______________________________
   B. ______________________________
   C. ______________________________
   D. ______________________________
73. When observing stool, what should be reported to the nurse?
   A. ______________________________
   B. ______________________________
   C. ______________________________
   D. ______________________________
   E. ______________________________
   F. ______________________________
   G. ______________________________
   H. ______________________________
   I. ______________________________
74. After giving an enema, what should be reported and recorded?
   A. ______________________________
   B. ______________________________
   C. ______________________________
   D. ______________________________
   E. ______________________________
   F. ______________________________
   G. ______________________________

Labeling

Answer questions 75 to 77 using these figures.

75. Name the four colostomies shown.

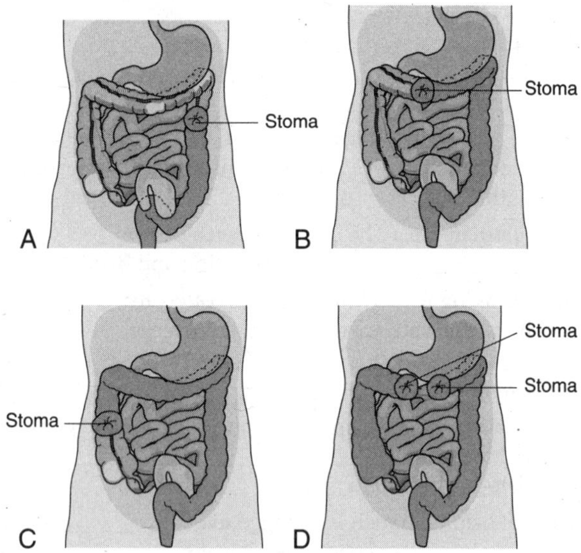

A. ____________________
B. ____________________
C. ____________________
D. ____________________

76. Why does would a sigmoid colostomy have the most solid and formed stool? ____________________

77. Which type of colostomy is usually a temporary colostomy?
____

Answer questions 78 to 80 using this figure.

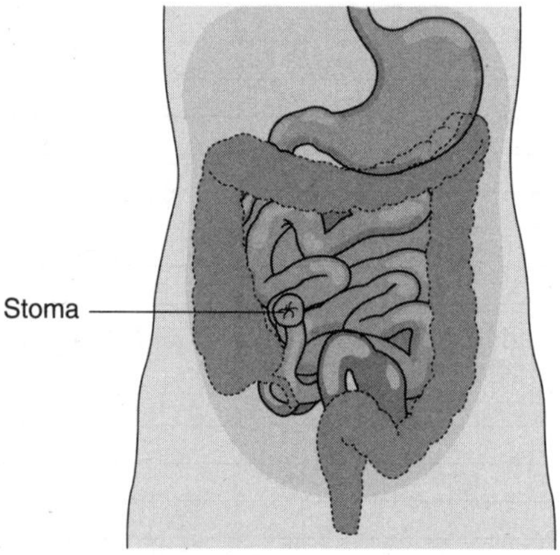

78. What type of ostomy is shown?
____

79. What part of the bowel has been removed?
____

80. Will the stool from the ostomy be liquid or formed?
____

Optional Learning Exercises

81. You are caring for Mr. Evans, who is in a semiprivate room. His roommate has a large family and many visitors. Mr. Evans has not had a bowel movement in 3 days, even though he is eating well and taking medications to assist elimination. What could be a reason he has not had a bowel movement?
____
____
____

82. Mrs. Weller usually has a bowel movement after breakfast. What are some activities that may assist her to defecate more easily?
____
____

83. The nurse tells you to make sure Mr. Johnson eats the high-fiber foods in his diet to assist in his elimination. What foods are high in fiber?
____
____

84. Mrs. Shaffer tells you she cannot digest fruits and vegetables and she refuses to eat them. With her permission, what may be added to her cereal and prune juice to provide fiber?
____

85. You offer Mr. Murphy ____________________ of water each day to promote normal bowel elimination.

86. Mr. Hernandez has been taking an antibiotic to treat his pneumonia and he has developed diarrhea. You think he may have diarrhea because
____________________.

87. You are caring for 83-year-old Mrs. Chen and you helped her to the bathroom 30 minutes ago where she had a bowel movement. When you enter her room to make her bed, she tells you she needs to use the bathroom for a bowel movement. You know that older people ____________________
____

Use the FOCUS ON PRIDE section to complete these statements and then use the critical thinking and discussion question to develop your ideas

88. Give one example of an action taken by a nursing assistant, related to bowel or bladder elimination, that would be considered abuse, mistreatment, and neglect. ____________________
____

89. When the person needs to have a bowel elimination, you can provide comfort and privacy when you
A. ____________________
B. ____________________
C. ____________________
D. ____________________
E. ____________________
F. ____________________
G. ____________________

Critical Thinking and Discussion Question

90. You overhear a coworker, who also happens to be your friend, tell a resident to "go ahead and just pee or have a bowel movement in the bed." You have cared for this resident and she is often incontinent, and she will also pull off dry and clean incontinence pants whenever she feels like it. You know that your coworker is frustrated. What would you do?

30 Nutrition

Fill in the Blanks: Key Terms

Calorie
Cholesterol
Dysphagia
Nutrient
Nutrition

1. A soft, waxy substance found in the bloodstream and all body cells is ______________________.
2. The amount of energy produced from the burning of food by the body is a ______________________.
3. ______________________ is difficulty or discomfort in swallowing.
4. The many processes involved in the ingestion, digestion, absorption, and use of food and fluids by the body is ______________________.
5. A substance that is ingested, digested, absorbed, and used by the body is a ______________________.

Circle the Best Answer

6. Which person is using MyPlate to improve healthy eating?
   A. Person A reviews eating routine and makes nutrient-rich choices.
   B. Person B develops an eating routine that matches preferred lifestyle.
   C. Person C primarily eats a variety of grains with added sugar.
   D. Person D eats unlimited amounts of healthy food from each food group.
7. How many calories are in 1 g of fat?
   A. 1 calorie
   B. 4 calories
   C. 8 calories
   D. 9 calories
8. Which type of diet will the doctor prescribe for a person who is constipated?
   A. Full-liquid diet
   B. Pureed diet
   C. High-fiber diet
   D. Bland diet
9. Which food item would supply a healthy fat?
   A. Fish fillet
   B. Croissant
   C. Pork chop
   D. Oatmeal cookie
10. Which food choice is aligned with the recommendations from MyPlate for a person who is ordering food at a restaurant?
    A. French fries with ketchup
    B. Steamed vegetables
    C. Double meat cheeseburger
    D. Orange soda with ice
11. Which factors affect the amount needed from each food group?
    A. The cultural and religious preferences of the person
    B. The age, sex, and physical activity of the person
    C. The likes and dislikes of the person
    D. The budget available to the person
12. Which foods are whole grains included in the grain group?
    A. Bulgur, oatmeal, and brown rice
    B. White flour and white rice
    C. Snack crackers and rice noodles
    D. Biscuits and cookies
13. Which protein foods may contribute to a higher risk for heart disease?
    A. Seafood, such as trout, salmon, or herring
    B. Nuts, such as almonds, walnuts, or pistachios
    C. Legumes, such as soybeans, pinto beans, or chickpeas
    D. Meats that are processed, such as deli meats and hot dogs
14. Which food would not be allowed on a full-liquid diet?
    A. Yogurt
    B. Ice cream
    C. Pudding
    D. Mashed potatoes
15. Which level of physical activity is recommended by the *Physical Activity Guidelines for Americans*?
    A. 2 hours and 30 minutes of moderate-intensity physical activity each week
    B. Muscle-strengthening activities at least 5 days a week.
    C. Vigorous-intensity activity, such as running once a week
    D. Walking and jogging every day for 60 minutes
16. Which nutrient is especially important for children because of tissue growth?
    A. Carbohydrates
    B. Fats
    C. Vitamins
    D. Protein
17. Which vitamin is important for wound healing?
    A. Vitamin K
    B. Vitamin C
    C. Vitamin A
    D. Vitamin B_{12}
18. Which food item has the most calories?
    A. 4 g butter
    B. 4 g white sugar
    C. 4 g chicken breast
    D. 4 g rice

19. Which person needs a pureed diet?
    A. Person A has dementia.
    B. Person B has diabetes.
    C. Person C is scheduled for surgery.
    D. Person D has trouble swallowing.
20. Which dietary instruction would the nursing assistant expect the nurse to give for a person who has a thyroid problem and needs a high-calorie intake?
    A. Offer large servings of high-fiber foods
    B. Encourage eating cake and candy
    C. Offer three between-meal snacks every day
    D. Use extra large amounts of butter and cream
21. Which snack would be best to supply vitamin C for a person who has decreased immunity?
    A. Hard-boiled egg
    B. Orange
    C. Green gelatin
    D. Glass of milk
22. Which person is likely to receive a general diet?
    A. Person A has chronic heart problems.
    B. Person B has no dietary limits or restrictions.
    C. Person C needs restricted amounts of sodium.
    D. Person D eats meat and produce, but no desserts.
23. How much sodium does the American Heart Association recommend each day?
    A. No more than 1500 mg
    B. Greater than 3400 mg
    C. More than 2300 mg/day
    D. Less than 5000 mg
24. Which effect on a body organ occurs when the body tissues swell with water?
    A. Kidneys are less effective.
    B. Liver function is unaffected.
    C. Heart works harder.
    D. Lungs tissue shrinks.
25. Which snack item should be offered to a person on a sodium-controlled diet?
    A. Bag of mini-pretzels
    B. Sardines on crackers
    C. Tomato juice and nuts
    D. Pear and plum slices
26. Which person may be given a mechanical soft diet?
    A. Person A is overweight.
    B. Person B has dental problems.
    C. Person C has diarrhea.
    D. Person D has constipation.
27. Which food item needs to be removed from the tray if a person is on a fiber- and residue-restricted diet?
    A. Raw plum
    B. Cottage cheese
    C. White toast
    D. Plain pasta
28. Which type of diet would the doctor prescribe for a person who has serious burns?
    A. Sodium-controlled diet
    B. Fat-controlled diet
    C. High-calorie diet
    D. High-protein diet
29. How many calories are in 1 g of protein?
    A. 1 calorie
    B. 4 calories
    C. 8 calories
    D. 9 calories
30. What are the three main purposes of *Dietary Guidelines for Americans*?
    A. Promote health, reduce the risk of chronic diseases, and meet nutrient needs.
    B. Research dietary habits, promote equity in food access, and improve food quality.
    C. Improve nutrition for seniors, reduce obesity in children, and reduce risk for cancer.
    D. Guide weight control, recommend calorie intake, and identify food nutrients.
31. Which snack would be offered to a patient who needs to have potassium sources in the diet?
    A. Crackers
    B. Banana
    C. Snack cake
    D. Sugar cookie
32. Which food group can help lower calorie intake?
    A. Grain group
    B. Dairy group
    C. Vegetable group
    D. Protein food group
33. Which food would be allowed for a person who needs a clear-liquid diet?
    A. Coffee without milk or cream
    B. Custard
    C. Strained soup
    D. Plain ice cream
34. Which mineral is necessary for nerve function, muscle contraction, and heart function?
    A. Iron
    B. Folate
    C. Iodine
    D. Potassium
35. Which snack would be offered to a patient who is prone to constipation?
    A. Yogurt
    B. Apple
    C. Bowl of cereal
    D. Graham crackers
36. Which diet would the doctor order to increase the amount of residue and fiber in the colon to stimulate peristalsis?
    A. Mechanical soft diet
    B. Fat-controlled diet
    C. Fiber- and residue-restricted diet
    D. High-fiber diet
37. Which person has selected food choices according to recommendations from MyPlate?
    A. Person A fills half of the plate with fruits and vegetables.
    B. Person B selects half proteins and half grain to fill the plate.
    C. Person C selects two-thirds with grains and one-third with fruit.
    D. Person D fills all of the plate with fruits and vegetables.

38. Which food group is most essential to build and maintain bone mass for an older woman who has risk for osteoporosis?
    A. Grain group
    B. Vegetable group
    C. Dairy group
    D. Fruit group
39. What is the most important nutrient for tissue growth and repair?
    A. Protein
    B. Carbohydrate
    C. Fat
    D. Minerals
40. Which vitamin must be ingested daily?
    A. Vitamin A
    B. Vitamin K
    C. Vitamin C
    D. Vitamin D
41. Which mineral is needed for red blood cell formation?
    A. Iodine
    B. Sodium
    C. Iron
    D. Potassium

Fill in the Blanks

42. Write out the abbreviations
    A. FDA ______
    B. GI ______
    C. mg ______
    D. oz ______
    E. USDA ______
43. ______ is a vitamin which is recommended for pregnant women to prevent birth defects.
44. If dietary fat is not needed by the body, it is stored as ______.
45. Which vitamins can be stored by the body?
    ______
46. Vitamin ______ is important for the formation of substances that hold tissues together, immune function, and wound healing and is also an *antioxidant* (substance that prevents cell damage).
47. If a person is receiving a high-calorie diet, the calorie intake is ______ daily.
48. What are the five food groups in MyPlate?
    A. ______
    B. ______
    C. ______
    D. ______
    E. ______
49. What is the function of each of these nutrients?
    A. Protein ______
    B. Carbohydrates ______
    C. Fats ______
    D. Vitamins ______
    E. Minerals ______
    F. Water ______

Optional Learning Exercises

50. This is a person's food intake for 1 day. Place the foods in the correct food groups on MyPlate.

BREAKFAST

¾ cup Orange juice
1 cup Oatmeal
2 slices Toast
¼ cup Milk
2 cups Black coffee

LUNCH

1 cup Tomato soup
Grilled cheese sandwich
½ cup Applesauce
Can of regular soda
Candy bar

DINNER

2–4 oz lean pork chops
Baked potato/butter
¼ cup Green beans
2 Brownies
2 cups Black coffee

SNACKS

1 Apple
One 4-oz bag Potato chips
⅓ cup Nuts
Can of regular soda
½ cup Ice cream

A. Grains ______
______
B. Vegetables ______
______
C. Fruits ______
______
D. Dairy ______
______
E. Proteins ______
______
F. Oils ______
______
G. Other ______
______

Figure

51. Based on the food label. What is the serving size? ___________ How many servings are in the container? _____________ How many calories are in one serving? ______________ How many calories would the person get if they ate all of the food in the container? _____________

Nutrition Facts

8 servings per container
Serving size 2/3 cup (55 g)

Amount per serving	
Calories	**230**
	% Daily Value*
Total Fat 8 g	**10%**
Saturated Fat 1 g	**5%**
Trans Fat 0 g	
Cholesterol 0 mg	**0%**
Sodium 160 mg	**7%**
Total Carbohydrate 37 g	**13%**
Dietary Fiber 4 g	**14%**
Total Sugars 12 g	
Includes 10 g Added Sugars	**20%**
Protein 3 g	
Vitamin D 2 mcg	10%
Calcium 260 mg	20%
Iron 8 mg	45%
Potassium 240 mg	6%

* The % Daily Value (DV) tells you how much a nutrient in a serving of food contributes to a daily diet. 2,000 calories a day is used for general nutrition advice.

Focus on math

Review the food label below and answer questions 52 to 54.

	Calories	Total Fat	Sodium
1 Serving = 1 cup	280 calories	9 g	850 mg
½ Serving = ½ cup (divide by 2)	140 calories	4 ½ g	425 mg
2 Servings = 2 cups (multiply by 2)	560 calories	18 g	1700 mg

52. How many calories should be recorded when a person eats 1½ cup servings?
    A. 140 calories
    B. 280 calories
    C. 420 calories
    D. 560 calories

53. What is the total fat intake when a person eats 1½ cup servings?
    A. 4½ g
    B. 9 g
    C. 13½ g
    D. 425 mg

54. Person is advised to restrict sodium intake to 1500 mg/day. If the person eats one serving of food, how many additional milligrams would the person be allowed for the day?
    A. 425 mg
    B. 650 mg
    C. 850 mg
    D. 1500 mg

Use the FOCUS ON PRIDE section to complete these statements

55. Learning the person's likes and dislikes of food can_________________ nutrition.

Critical Thinking and Discussion Question

56. After reading the nutritional information in this chapter, compare your own dietary habits to the MyPlate recommendations. What changes could you make to improve your own nutrition?
    ____
    ____
    ____

31 Meeting Nutrition Needs

Fill in the Blanks: Key Terms

Anorexia | Aspiration | Dysphagia

1. Difficulty swallowing is ______________________.
2. The loss of appetite is ______________________.
3. Breathing fluid, food, vomitus, or an object into the lungs is ______________________.

Circle the Best Answer

4. Which task could the nursing assistant perform to contribute to the requirements set by the Centers for Medicare and Medicaid Services (CMS) for assessment of the resident's nutritional status?
   A. Ask the person if their drugs are causing dry mouth or nausea
   B. Find out about factors that affect eating and nutrition
   C. Obtain and report the resident's height and weight
   D. Observe the resident for signs and symptoms of fluid imbalance
5. Which food represents the type of food that a person with a limited income is most likely to buy?
   A. Chicken
   B. Bread
   C. Lettuce
   D. Cheese
6. Which nutrient is likely to be lacking in the diet when people have fewer financial resources to buy foods?
   A. Fats
   B. Starch
   C. Vitamins
   D. Sugars
7. Which nursing measure could be used to stimulate a person's appetite?
   A. Increasing fluid intake
   B. Increasing portion size
   C. Controlling odors
   D. Talking about food
8. What would the nursing assistant expect when a person is ill?
   A. Appetite for carbohydrate food increases.
   B. Fewer nutrients and calories are needed.
   C. Nutritional needs increase to heal tissue.
   D. The person will prefer protein foods.
9. Which physiologic change is expected in older adults?
   A. Increased sensitivity to smells and odors
   B. Decreased secretion of digestive juices
   C. Decreased interest in food and fluids
   D. Increased need for calories for tissue repair
10. What is a requirement for food served in long-term care centers, according to the Centers for Medicare and Medicaid Services (CMS)?
    A. The center provides needed adaptive equipment and utensils.
    B. The person's diet should include whatever they want to eat.
    C. All food is served at room temperature and all liquids must be chilled.
    D. People with diabetes must receive three meals a day and unlimited snacks.
11. Who determines the thickness of the liquids and food when a person has dysphagia?
    A. Chef
    B. Dietician
    C. Nurse
    D. Speech therapist
12. Which observation would the nursing assistant report because it is a possible sign of dysphagia?
    A. Patient has frequent episodes of diarrhea.
    B. Patient prefers foods that are sweet or salty.
    C. Patient demonstrates excessive drooling of saliva.
    D. Patient eats well in the morning, but refuses dinner.
13. Which position is preferred for a person who is on aspiration precautions?
    A. Semi-Fowler's position
    B. Upright a position
    C. Side-lying position
    D. Supine position
14. What would the nursing assistant expect when residents are served meals in a family dining program?
    A. Residents serve themselves as at home.
    B. Residents can eat any time the buffet is open.
    C. Food is available in a common area refrigerator.
    D. Food is served as in a restaurant.
15. Which nursing measure must the nursing assistant perform before the person is served a meal?
    A. Give complete personal care
    B. Change all linens
    C. Check the person's position
    D. Ask if the visitors want food
16. Which action would the nursing assistant use to provide comfort for patients during meals?
    A. Ask visitors to leave until patient has finished eating
    B. Make sure dentures, eyeglasses, or hearing aids are in place
    C. Suggest different foods if the patient does not like what is served
    D. Give complete personal hygiene and a linen change

17. Which action would the nursing assistant take if a food tray has not been served within 15 minutes?
    A. Recheck the food temperatures
    B. Serve the tray immediately
    C. Throw the food away
    D. Serve only the cold items on the tray
18. How can the nursing assistant make sure that the food tray is complete?
    A. Ask the person being served
    B. Ask the nurse
    C. Call the dietary department
    D. Check items on the tray with the dietary card
19. Which action would the nursing assistant take when feeling impatient while feeding a resident with dementia?
    A. Take a break
    B. Give finger foods
    C. Talk to the nurse
    D. Feed the person later
20. Which nursing measure would the nursing assistant use when feeding a person?
    A. Allow the person to assist by holding their own coffee cup
    B. Offer a fork and knife and supervise the cutting of food
    C. Feed the person in a private area to maintain confidentiality
    D. Use a teaspoon because it is less likely to cause injury
21. How are liquid foods given when a person needs to be feed?
    A. Only at the start of feeding
    B. During the meal, alternating with solid foods
    C. At the end of the meal when all solids have been eaten
    D. Provide a straw if there is difficulty swallowing
22. What is the temperature that should be achieved when reheating cooked foods?
    A. 105°F
    B. 165°F
    C. According to agency policy
    D. Room temperature
23. Which action would the home health nursing assistant take in handling leftover food to help prevent foodborne illness?
    A. Examine leftover food for obvious signs of cross-contamination
    B. Ask the person how long they like to keep leftovers in the refrigerator
    C. Reheating cooked food to a temperature preferred by the person
    D. Refrigerate or freeze leftover food that can spoil within 2 hours
24. Which question would the home health nursing assistant ask to prevent foodborne illness when the person requests reheated leftovers for lunch?
    A. What type of leftover food would you like to eat?
    B. How long have the leftovers been in the refrigerator?
    C. How hot do you like your food?
    D. What time would you like to eat?
25. Which government agency sets requirements for the food served in nursing centers?
    A. United States Department of Health and Human Services
    B. United States Department of Agriculture (USDA)
    C. Food and Drug Administration (FDA)
    D. CMS
26. Which type of dining program would be best for a person who is confused?
    A. Social dining
    B. Restaurant-style menus
    C. Low-stimulation dining
    D. Family dining
27. Why do the diets of some older people lack protein?
    A. Protein foods are harder to digest.
    B. High-protein foods are often costly.
    C. Poor dentition makes proteins difficult to chew.
    D. Proteins smell different because of changes with aging.
28. Which nursing assistant has made an error in promoting comfort when preparing residents for meals?
    A. Nursing assistant A provides oral hygiene and ensures that dentures are in place.
    B. Nursing assistant B makes sure that eyeglasses and hearing aids are in place.
    C. Nursing assistant C tells incontinent person that hygienic care is done after lunch.
    D. Nursing assistant D positions the person in a comfortable, upright position.
29. Which nursing assistant is using the correct approach when feeding a person?
    A. Nursing assistant A raises bed to maintain body mechanics.
    B. Nursing assistant B positions self to meet the person's eye level.
    C. Nursing assistant C sits down and faces the person.
    D. Nursing assistant D bends over to offer each spoonful.
30. Which question might a surveyor ask you about meeting a person's nutrition needs?
    A. "Have you ever caused a person with dysphagia to choke?"
    B. "Do you think the goals for nutrition in the care plans are adequate?"
    C. "How are food and fluid intake observed and reported?"
    D. "How long does it take you to assist a person to eat?"
31. Which action would the nursing assistant take when the nurse advises that a patient tends to pocket food while eating?
    A. Ensure that dentures are cleaned and securely in place before feeding.
    B. Check inside the cheeks, under the tongue, and on the roof of the mouth.
    C. Offer honey-thickened liquids after every spoonful of solid foods
    D. Check inside the patient's pockets and underneath napkins or clothing

Fill in the Blanks

32. The person remains upright for at least __________ hour after eating.
33. Place food in the mouth on the ______________ side if there is weakness on one side.
34. Pathogens grow rapidly between ______________ and ________ (Fahrenheit). This range is called the __________________ by the United States Department of Agriculture (USDA).
35. When you are feeding a person, the spoon should be filled ______________________________.
36. If you are feeding a person a dysphagia diet, what observations should be reported to the nurse immediately?
    A. ______________________________
    B. ______________________________
    C. ______________________________
    D. ______________________________
37. When you are delegated to serve meal trays, what information do you need from the nurse or care plan?
    A. ______________________________
    B. ______________________________
    C. ______________________________
    D. ______________________________
    E. ______________________________
    F. ______________________________
38. What should be reported after you have fed a person?
    A. ______________________________
    B. ______________________________
    C. ______________________________
    D. ______________________________
39. Explain each of the concepts below that are recommended by the United States Department of Agriculture (USDA) to keep food safe.
    A. Clean ______________________________
    ____
    B. Separate ______________________________
    ____
    C. Cook ______________________________
    ____
    D. Chill ______________________________
    ____

Optional Learning Exercises

40. Label the plate in the figure with numbers so that you can describe the location of food to a blind person. What would you tell a visually impaired person who asks you where to find these food items on the plate?

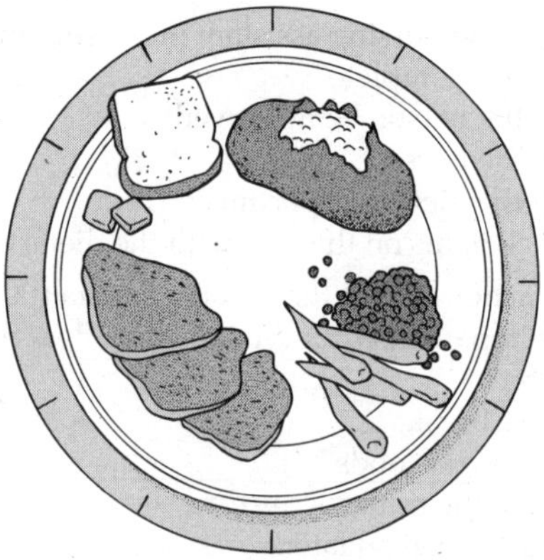

    A. Bread ______________________________
    B. Baked potato ______________________________
    C. Vegetables ______________________________
    D. Meat ______________________________

Use the FOCUS ON PRIDE section to complete these statements

41. When family members bring food to a resident, it is important that you tell ______________. The food must not interfere with the ______________.

Critical Thinking and Discussion Question

42. Think about a meal tray that you have seen being served in a hospital or nursing care center.
    A. If you had to eat that type of food, how would that food compare to what you normally eat?
    B. Think about people who have to eat institutional food every day for every meal. What could you talk about as you are feeding them or assisting them to eat?
    C. What can health-care staff do to help patients and residents who miss familiar foods?

32 Fluid Needs

Fill in the Blanks: Key Terms

Dehydration
Edema
Electrolyte
Graduate
Intake
Output

1. Minerals dissolved in water are ________________.
2. ________________ is the amount of fluid taken in.
3. A decrease in the amount of water in body tissues is ________________.
4. The amount of fluid lost is ________________.
5. A ________________ is a calibrated container used to measure fluid.
6. ________________ is the swelling of body tissues with water.

Circle the Best Answer

7. Which person has a high risk for dehydration?
   A. Person A refuses to drink tap water.
   B. Person B has dry skin.
   C. Person C has late-stage dementia.
   D. Person D has liver disease.
8. What would occur if a person's fluid intake exceeds fluid output?
   A. Person will have edema (swelling) in the tissues.
   B. Increased risk for urinary infection
   C. Vomiting and diarrhea will occur.
   D. Person will show signs of dehydration.
9. How much fluid is needed every day for normal fluid balance?
   A. 1500 mL
   B. 1000 to 1500 mL
   C. 2000 to 2500 mL
   D. 3000 to 4000 mL
10. Which action would the nursing assistant take first upon noting that a person is heavily perspiring, and pajamas and linens are damp with sweat?
    A. Help the person shower
    B. Tell the nurse
    C. Give the person drinking water
    D. Change the linens
11. What would the nursing assistant expect to observe when obtaining a urine sample from a person who is likely to be dehydrated?
    A. Moderate amount of normal urine
    B. Large amount or pale straw-colored urine
    C. Small amount of urine with blood
    D. Scant amount of dark amber urine
12. Which fluid imbalance is suspected when the nursing assistant reports to the nurse that the blood pressure is low and the pulse and respirations are high?
    A. Overhydration
    B. Edema
    C. Dehydration
    D. Low electrolytes
13. Which person is most likely to have increased fluid requirements?
    A. Person who works as a nursing assistant.
    B. Elderly person with nocturia
    C. Child who just woke up
    D. Woman who is breastfeeding.
14. Which person is most likely to have an order to "encourage fluids"?
    A. Person who has kidney stones.
    B. Person who has urinary retention.
    C. Person who has kidney failure.
    D. Person who has trouble swallowing.
15. What would the nursing assistant do when a person who is mildly confused keeps asking for water, but there is a preprocedure NPO order?
    A. Remind the person that water will be given after the procedure
    B. Place NPO signs above the bed, on the door, and in the bathroom
    C. Tell the nurse that the person is having difficulties complying with NPO
    D. Help the person with oral hygiene and offer a few ice chips
16. During the day shift a person drank 350 mL at breakfast, 390 mL at lunch, 225 mL as a snack, and 400 mL of water. What is the total fluid intake for the shift?
    A. 1315 mL
    B. 1325 mL
    C. 1350 mL
    D. 1365 mL
17. What was the total output for the shift, for a person who voided two times during the shift—350 mL and 150 mL; vomited once—100 mL and there was 125 mL in the wound drainage container?
    A. 705 mL
    B. 725 mL
    C. 825 mL
    D. 855 mL
18. Which nursing measure would the nursing assistant use if a patient has an order for restricted fluids?
    A. Offer a variety of liquids
    B. Thicken all fluids
    C. Remove the water mug or keep it out of sight
    D. Remind the person to spit out liquids during oral hygiene
19. Which nursing assistant needs a reminder about what is counted in Intake and Output (I&O) records?
    A. Nursing assistant A measures milk, water, coffee, and tea.
    B. Nursing assistant B records mashed potatoes and creamed vegetables.
    C. Nursing assistant C adds amounts of soups and gelatin.
    D. Nursing assistant D includes ice cream, custard, and pudding.

20. What is the milliliter equivalent for 1 ounce?
    A. 10 mL
    B. 30 mL
    C. 100 mL
    D. 500 mL
21. Which action would the nursing assistant take when reading the fluid level on a graduate to measure output?
    A. Hold the graduate and look down into the container
    B. Hold the graduate steady while looking at the fluid level
    C. Place the graduate on a flat surface at eye level to read it
    D. Set the graduate on the floor and bend down to read it
22. Which body substance is included in an I&O measurement?
    A. Mucous
    B. Solid stool
    C. Blood on a bandage
    D. Vomitus
23. Which information does the nursing assistant need from the nurse and the care plan when delegated to provide drinking water?
    A. What size of mug to use
    B. How much ice to add
    C. If the person prefers a personal mug
    D. How often to refill the mug
24. Which person needs frequent oral hygiene?
    A. Person A needs thickened liquids.
    B. Person B has an encourage fluids order.
    C. Person C is on restricted fluids.
    D. Person D needs I&O measurements.
25. Which person is likely to need thickened liquids?
    A. Person A has dehydration.
    B. Person B has edema.
    C. Person C has kidney disease.
    D. Person D has dysphagia.

Fill in the Blanks

26. Write out the abbreviations
    A. I&O ______
    B. mL ______
    C. NPO ______
    D. oz ______
27. Why is it important to frequently offer water to older persons?
    ______
28. What information do you need when you are delegated to measure I&O?
    A. ______
    B. ______
    C. ______
    D. ______
    E. ______
29. A person drank 1/2 of an 8 oz cup of juice. How many milliliters would be counted as intake?
    ______

Table Activity

30. Complete the table below by writing in the correct equivalent amounts in milliliter

Unit	Equivalent amount in mL
1 cubic centimeter	
1 teaspoon	
1 tablespoon	
1 ounce	
1 cup	
1 pint	
1 quart	
1 liter	

31. Examine the illustration of the urinal below. How much urine is in the urinal?

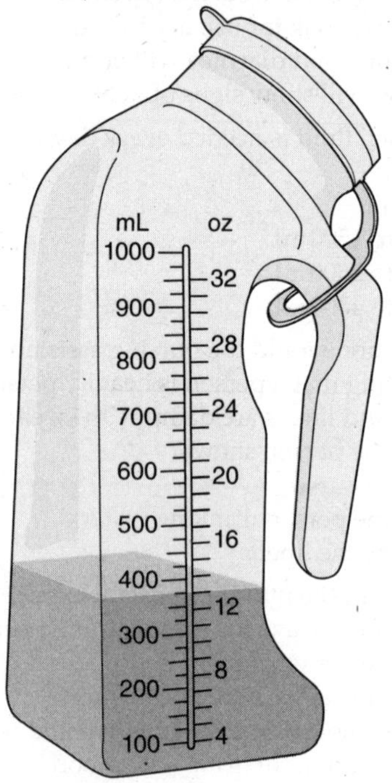

32. A. Use ***Milliliters for Standard Containers*** as shown on the I&O record and convert serving sizes to milliliters.

Milliliters for standard containers
Water glass 240 mL, Juice glass 120 mL, Milk carton 240 mL ,Coffee cup 240 mL,
Tea glass 180 mL, Gelatin 120 mL, Ice cream 90 mL, Soup bowl 180 mL

Time	*Intake*	*Conversion from standard containers to mL*	*Output*
0200			*Urine 300 mL*
0600			*Urine 500 mL*
0615	*Water (1 glass)*		
0730	***Breakfast***		
	Orange juice (whole glass)		
	Milk (1/2 carton)		
	Coffee (1 cup)		
0800			*Urine 300 mL*
1130	***Lunch***		
	Soup (whole bowl)		
	Milk (1/2 carton)		
	Tea (1 cup)		
	Gelatin (1 serving)		
1330			*Urine 450 mL*
1430	*Water (1 glass)*		
1530			*Urine 50 mL*
1730	***Dinner***		
	Soup (whole bowl)		
	Tea (1 cup)		
	Juice (whole glass)		
	Ice cream (all)		
1830			*Vomited 50 mL*
1845	*Water (1 glass)*		
1915			*Urine 500 mL*
2000	*Milk (1 carton)*		
2015			*Urine 300 mL*
2230			*Urine 200 mL*

B. Answer the following questions by referring to the I&O record above and calculate I&O for the 8-hour shift increments (2300–7000, 0700–1500, and 1500–2300) and calculate the total I&O for the 24-hour period.

Intake

1) What is the total intake for 2300–0700 in milliliters? ____________________
2) What is the total intake for 0700–1500 in milliliters? ____________________
3) What is the total intake for 1500–2300 in milliliters? ____________________
4) What is the total intake for 24 hours in milliliters? ____________________

Output

1) What is the total output for 2300–7000 in milliliters? ____________________
2) What is the total output for 0700–1500 in milliliters? ____________________
3) What is the total output for 1500–2300 in milliliters? ____________________
4) What is the total output for 24 hours in milliliters? ____________________

Optional Learning Exercises

Use the FOCUS ON PRIDE section to complete these statements and then use the critical thinking and discussion questions to develop your ideas

33. What are the three of your responsibilities that promote good fluid intake?
    A. ______________________________
    B. ______________________________
    C. ______________________________

Critical Thinking and Discussion Questions

34. Review the case of Caruso v Pine Manor Nursing Center, Ill., 1989, in the FOCUS ON PRIDE section of Chapter 32.
    A. What factors do you think may have contributed to Mr. Caruso's dehydration?
    B. If you had been a nursing assistant who had taken care of Mr. Caruso, what could you have done that might have prevented his death?

33 Nutritional Support and IV Therapy

Fill in the Blanks: Key Terms

Aspiration	Gavage	Nasogastric (NG) tube	Regurgitation
Enteral nutrition	Intravenous (IV) therapy	Parenteral nutrition	
Flow rate	Jejunostomy tube	Percutaneous endoscopic gastrostomy (PEG) tube	
Gastrostomy tube	Naso-enteral tube		

1. Giving nutrients into the gastrointestinal (GI) tract through a feeding tube is ______________________________.
2. A ______________________ is a tube inserted through a surgically created opening in the stomach.
3. ______________________ is the backward flow of stomach contents into the mouth.
4. A ______________________ is a feeding tube inserted into a surgically created opening in the jejunum of the small intestine.
5. The process of giving a tube feeding is called ______________________.
6. The ______________ is the number of drops per minute.
7. ______________________ is breathing fluid, food, vomitus, or an object into the lungs.
8. Giving nutrients through a catheter inserted into a vein is ______________________.
9. ______________________ is giving fluids through a needle or catheter inserted into a vein.
10. A feeding tube inserted through the nose into the stomach is a ______________________.
11. A ______________________ is a feeding tube inserted into the stomach through a small incision made through the skin.
12. A feeding tube inserted through the nose into the small bowel is a ______________________.

Circle the Best Answer

13. What is the most important thing for the nursing assistant to do before starting the delegated task of syringe feeding a patient?
    A. Make sure that the nurse is available to answer questions
    B. Ask the nurse about the type of formula and the rate
    C. Locate the correct equipment for the procedure
    D. Know the state laws related to doing the procedure
14. Which of these tubes is used for short-term nutritional support?
    A. Nasogastric (NG) tube
    B. Gastrostomy tube
    C. Jejunostomy tube
    D. Percutaneous endoscopic gastrostomy (PEG) tube
15. What would the nursing assistant do when the nurse instructs to warm the formula for a tube feeding?
    A. Take formula out of the refrigerator about 4 hours before the feeding
    B. Take formula out of the refrigerator about 30 minutes before the feeding
    C. Warm refrigerated formula in the microwave for several minutes
    D. Obtain an unopened can that has been stored at room temperature
16. Which person is most likely to need frequent cleaning of the nose and nostrils as a comfort measure related to a feeding tube?
    A. Person A has a jejunostomy tube.
    B. Person B has a gastrostomy tube.
    C. Person C has a percutaneous endoscopic gastrostomy (PEG) tube.
    D. Person D has a naso-enteral tube.
17. Which complication is a major risk with nasogastric (NG) tube feedings?
    A. Nausea
    B. Flatulence
    C. Aspiration
    D. Elevated temperature
18. Which sign/symptom would the nursing assistant immediately report for a person who is receiving a tube feeding?
    A. Fatigue
    B. Respiratory distress
    C. Loss of appetite
    D. Feeling of hunger
19. Which nursing measure would the nursing assistant use to prevent regurgitation when a person is receiving gavage feeding?
    A. Position the person in a left-side-lying position
    B. Maintain Fowler's or semi-Fowler's position after the feeding
    C. Assist the person to ambulate in the hallway
    D. Offer the person extra water or other clear fluid

20. Which rationale supports the need for oral hygiene when a person is nothing by mouth (NPO) and receiving nutrition through a tube?
    A. It stimulates peristalsis to aid digestion.
    B. It decreases dry mouth, dry lips, and sore throat.
    C. Formula feedings increase the risk for dental caries.
    D. Tube feedings give the person bad breath.
21. Which task can the nursing assistant perform if allowed by the state and agency?
    A. Insert a feeding tube
    B. Check tube for placement
    C. Remove a nasogastric (NG) tube
    D. Check for residual stomach contents
22. What would the nursing assistant do upon seeing a new and recently graduated nurse preparing to administer formula feeding through an intravenous (IV) line?
    A. Observe for signs and symptoms of distress
    B. Assist by positioning the patient and obtaining a pump
    C. Offer to provide frequent oral hygiene and other basic needs
    D. Tell her to stop and immediately find the charge nurse
23. What should the nursing assistant do upon noticing that the drip rate of the person's IV therapy seems to be very rapid?
    A. Adjust the flow to slow it down
    B. Tell the nurse about the observations
    C. Try changing the position of the person's arm
    D. Change the IV bag when it is empty
24. Which nursing assistant has made an error in offering a comfort measure every 2 hours while awake, to a person who reports a dry mouth and is nothing by mouth (NPO) with a feeding tube?
    A. Nursing assistant A assists with oral hygiene.
    B. Nursing assistant B applies lubricant for the lips.
    C. Nursing assistant C offers mouthwash or rinses.
    D. Nursing assistant D offers sips of preferred fluid.
25. Which action would the nursing assistant take first when observing that the person's intravenous (IV) has stopped flowing and the IV site is cool and puffy?
    A. Tell the person to keep the arm straight
    B. Ask the person if there is pain or itching
    C. Raise the height of the IV bag
    D. Tell the nurse about the site and the IV
26. Which nursing assistant has correctly prepared the formula to be given through a feeding tube?
    A. Nursing assistant A allows the formula to sit at to room temperature for 30 minutes.
    B. Nursing assistant B uses cold formula that has been stored in the refrigerator.
    C. Nursing assistant C warms the formula for 3 minutes in a pan of hot water.
    D. Nursing assistant D rewarms formula that was leftover from last week's feeding.
27. Which action, related to intravenous (IV) bag and IV tubing, would the nursing assistant take when assisting a person who has an IV to move and turn in bed?
    A. Turn off the IV pump
    B. Allow enough slack in the tubing
    C. Temporarily clamp the tubing
    D. Place the IV bag on the bed
28. Which patient has a condition that is likely to require a feeding tube?
    A. Patient A had a heart attack 4 days ago.
    B. Patient B is in bed because of a broken leg.
    C. Patient C has cancer of the neck.
    D. Patient D is nothing by mouth (NPO) for a procedure.
29. Which action would the nursing assistant take upon hearing the alarm of an IV pump?
    A. Immediately notify the nurse
    B. Observe for fluid flow blockage
    C. Note if the pump's battery is low
    D. Check for air in the tubing
30. What would the nursing assistant do when a person who has a nasogastric (NG) tube starts to cough and sneeze after a feeding?
    A. Check the position of the tube
    B. Offer tissues and assist with hygiene
    C. Alert the nurse about the symptoms
    D. Use a syringe and withdraw the secretions
31. Which nursing assistant has made an error related to the prevention of regurgitation and aspiration?
    A. Nursing assistant A positions the person in a semi-Fowler's position before the feeding.
    B. Nursing assistant B maintains Fowler's position after the feeding for at least 1 to 2 hours.
    C. Nursing assistant C positions the person in a left-side-lying position after the feeding.
    D. Nursing assistant D reports to the nurse when the flow rate of the feeding is too fast.
32. Why are older persons more at risk for regurgitation and aspiration?
    A. Stomach emptying slows with aging.
    B. Digestion accelerates with aging.
    C. Ability to detect choking is decreased.
    D. Capacity to understand instructions is limited.
33. Which communication measure would the nursing assistant use if a person with a feeding tube asks for something to eat or drink?
    A. Ask the person what they would prefer to eat and drink
    B. Suggest that eating and drinking is readily available at meal times
    C. Advise the person to contact the doctor or the nurse about the care plan
    D. Politely explain that eating or drinking with a feeding tube is usually not allowed

34. Which nursing assistant has made an error when assisting with tube feedings?
    A. Nursing assistant A traces the feeding tube back to the insertion site.
    B. Nursing assistant B checks the tube placement and measures the residual.
    C. Nursing assistant C asks the nurse to check and inspect the feeding tube and label.
    D. Nursing assistant D turns the lights on before beginning the procedure.
35. Which action would the nursing assistant take when observing that a person who is receiving total parenteral nutrition (TPN) is sweating profusely and reporting thirst?
    A. Provide oral hygiene and offer mouth rinse
    B. Offer the patient sips of water or clear juice
    C. Assist with hygiene and change clothing and linens
    D. Immediately report observations to the nurse

Fill in the Blanks

36. Write out the abbreviations
    A. GI ______
    B. gtt ______
    C. gtt/min ______
    D. IV ______
    E. mL ______
    F. mL/hr ______
    G. NG ______
    H. NPO ______
    I. oz ______
    J. PEG ______
    K. TPN ______
37. Gastrostomy, jejunostomy, and percutaneous endoscopic gastrostomy (PEG) tubes are used for long-term support, usually longer than ______.
38. The nose and nostrils are cleaned every 4 to 8 hours because a feeding tube can ______ and cause ______ on the nose.
39. You are caring for a person receiving continuous tube feeding. You note that the formula was hung 7¾ hours ago, so you tell the nurse. Why did you report this to the nurse?
    ______
    ______
    ______
40. How can you check the flow rate of an intravenous (IV) infusion?
    ______
41. When you check the intravenous (IV) flow rate, which abnormal findings would prompt you to immediately report to the RN?
    A. ______
    B. ______
    C. ______
    D. ______
42. When caring for a person who is receiving intravenous (IV) therapy, which signs or symptoms should be reported to the nurse to prevent complications that may occur at the IV site?
    A. ______
    B. ______
    C. ______
    D. ______
    E. ______
    F. ______
43. You are caring for a person who is receiving tube feedings. List 12 observations that need to be reported to the nurse that could be related to the enteral therapy.
    A. ______
    B. ______
    C. ______
    D. ______
    E. ______
    F. ______
    G. ______
    H. ______
    I. ______
    J. ______
    K. ______
    L. ______

Optional Learning Exercises

44. What type of feeding tube would be used for each of these persons?
    A. The nurse tells you Mr. S is expected to have a feeding tube to his stomach for 2 to 3 weeks.
       ______
    B. Mrs. G. has had a feeding tube inserted into her stomach for 9 months. ______ or ______
    C. The nurse tells you to observe Mr. H. for irritation of his nose and nostrils when you give care. ______ or ______
    D. The nurse tells you that Mrs. K. is at great risk for regurgitation from her feeding tube. ______ or ______
45. Mrs. H. has a feeding tube in her nose. Answer these questions about caring for her nose and nostrils.
    A. How often should the nose and nostrils be cleaned?
       ______
    B. How is the tube secured to the nose?
       ______
    C. Why is the tube secured to the person's garment at the shoulder?
       ______
       ______
    D. What are the two ways the tube can be secured at the shoulder?
       ______
       ______

Use the FOCUS ON PRIDE section to complete these statements and then use the critical thinking and discussion question to develop your ideas

46. A person receiving intravenous therapy needs a shower. The nurse may have you apply a ______________, ______________, or ______________ ______________.

47. A person receiving intravenous (IV) therapy needs to move from the bed to the chair. You must plan the move to avoid ______________.

Critical Thinking and Discussion Question

48. The nurse is very busy, so she tells you how to change the setting on the person's intravenous (IV) pump. You have watched how it is done and the task seems simple and the nurse's instructions are clear, but you were told in orientation that nursing assistants are not allowed to alter the settings on the pump. What would you do?

34 Vital Signs

Fill in the Blanks: Key Terms

Afebrile
Apical-radial pulse
Blood pressure
Body temperature
Bradycardia
Diastole
Diastolic pressure
Fever (febrile)
Hypertension
Hypotension
Pulse
Pulse deficit
Pulse rate
Respiration
Sphygmomanometer
Stethoscope
Systole
Systolic pressure
Tachycardia
Thermometer
Vital signs

1. Elevated body temperature is ______________________________.
2. A rapid heart rate is ______________________. The heart rate is over 100 beats per minute.
3. The ______________________________ is taking the apical and radial pulse at the same time.
4. An instrument used to listen to the sounds produced by the heart, lungs, and other body organs is a ______________________________.
5. Low blood pressure is called ___________________.
6. The ___________________ is the number of heartbeats or pulses felt in 1 minute.
7. The amount of heat in the body that is a balance between the amount of heat produced and the amount lost by the body is the ___________________.
8. ____________________________ is the period of heart muscle contraction; the heart is pumping blood.
9. High blood pressure is called ______________________________.
10. The cuff and measuring device used to measure blood pressure is a ______________________________.
11. The beat of the heart felt at an artery as a wave of blood passes through the artery is the ______________________________.
12. Without a fever is ______________________________.
13. Measurements of body function, temperature, pulse, respirations, and blood pressure are ___________; pulse oximetry and pain are included in some agencies.
14. ___________________ is a slow heart rate; the rate is less than 60 beats per minute.
15. The amount of force it takes to pump blood out of the heart into the arterial circulation is the ______________________________.
16. The period when the heart is at rest is ______________________________.
17. The difference between the apical and radial pulse rates is the ______________________________.
18. __________________________ is the amount of force exerted against the walls of an artery by the blood.
19. Breathing air into and out of the lungs is ______________________________.
20. __________________________ is the pressure in the arteries when the heart is at rest.
21. A ______________________ is a device used to measure temperature.

Circle the Best Answer

22. Which pulse rate would be described as bradycardia?
    A. 45 beats per minute
    B. 66 beats per minute
    C. 115 beats per minute
    D. 170 beats per minute
23. How frequently are vital signs usually taken in nursing centers?
    A. Once a shift
    B. Every 4 hours
    C. Once a month
    D. Weekly
24. In which situation would the nursing assistant usually take vital signs, unless otherwise ordered?
    A. With the person in a lying or sitting position
    B. After the person has been walking or exercising
    C. Just after the person has finished eating breakfast
    D. Just before the person is ready to take a shower or tub bath
25. Which time of the day is the body temperature usually lower?
    A. Afternoon
    B. Morning
    C. Evening
    D. Night
26. Which nursing measure would the nursing assistant use when taking vital signs on a person with dementia?
    A. Ask a coworker to hold the person so they do not move
    B. Take the vital signs when the person is asleep
    C. Pulse and respirations are done first
    D. Ask the nurse to take the vital signs
27. Which response would the nursing assistant give when a person asks about their vital sign measurements?
    A. Tell the person the measurements if the policy allows
    B. Tell the nurse that the person wants to know the measurements
    C. Tell the person that vital signs require professional interpretation
    D. Tell the person that information is private and cannot be shared

28. What is the normal range of a rectal temperature?
 A. 96.6°F to 98.6°F (35.9°C to 37.0°C)
 B. 97.6°F to 99.6°F (36.5°C to 37.5°C)
 C. 98.6°F to 100.4°F (37.0°C to 38°C)
 D. 98.6°F to 101°F (37°C to 38.3°C)
29. What would the nursing assistant expect to observe when taking the temperature of an older person?
 A. Lower than the normal range
 B. Higher than the normal range
 C. Always in the normal range
 D. The same as in a younger adult
30. Which equipment would the nursing assistant use to ensure safety and to get the most accurate temperature when taking the temperature of a 1-year-old child with an ear infection?
 A. Tympanic thermometer with probe cover
 B. Glass mercury thermometer with a red stem
 C. Digital thermometer at the axillary site
 D. Electronic probe with a red stem
31. Which technique would the nursing assistant use to read a glass thermometer?
 A. Hold it at the stem above eye level and look up to read it
 B. Hold it in the middle and bring it to eye level to read it
 C. Hold it at the stem and bring it to eye level to read it
 D. Hold it at waist level and look down to read it
32. Which instruction would the nursing assistant give to the person prior to taking an oral temperature?
 A. Do not eat or chew gum for at least 15 to 20 minutes
 B. Shower or bathe right before the temperature is taken
 C. If you exercise, wait 30 minutes before temperature is taken
 D. Do not eat, drink, or smoke for at least 5 to 10 minutes
33. How far into the rectum would the nursing assistant insert an electronic thermometer?
 A. 1 inch
 B. 2 inches
 C. ½ inch
 D. 3 inches
34. Which choice would be best when taking a temperature for a person who is confused and resists care?
 A. Take a rectal temperature
 B. Use a glass oral thermometer
 C. Take an axillary temperature
 D. Use a tympanic or temporal artery thermometer
35. Which site is most commonly used to check the pulse?
 A. Carotid
 B. Brachial
 C. Radial
 D. Popliteal
36. Which site is used to take a pulse during cardiopulmonary resuscitation (CPR)?
 A. Carotid
 B. Temporal
 C. Femoral
 D. Radial
37. Which action would the nursing assistant use to prevent cross-infection when using a stethoscope?
 A. Cover the earpieces and diaphragm with a disposable plastic cover
 B. Wipe the earpieces and diaphragm with antiseptic wipes before and after use
 C. Soak and wash the stethoscope in a disinfectant solution
 D. Place a clean paper towel between the person's skin and the diaphragm
38. Which term describes a pulse rate of 120 beats per minute?
 A. Bradycardia
 B. Bounding
 C. Tachycardia
 D. Irregular
39. Which pulse rate would the nursing assistant record after counting 40 heartbeats in 30 seconds?
 A. 40 beats per minute
 B. 60 beats per minute
 C. 70 beats per minute
 D. 80 beats per minute
40. Which finding would the nursing assistant expect when checking a person's pulse if the nurse says that the pulse was thready on the previous shift?
 A. Decreased force
 B. Rapid rate
 C. Regular rhythm
 D. Increased strength
41. Which action would the nursing assistant use when taking a radial pulse?
 A. Place the thumb over the pulse site
 B. Lay the index finger on the middle of the wrist
 C. Put two fingers on the thumb side of the wrist
 D. Hold the stethoscope on the chest wall
42. In which circumstance would it be acceptable for the nursing assistant to count the radial pulse for 30 seconds and multiple by 2?
 A. The pulse is easy to locate.
 B. Count is interrupted at 30 seconds.
 C. The pulse is regular.
 D. The person is restless.
43. The apical pulse is taken
 A. For a full minute
 B. For 2 minutes if there is a pulse deficit
 C. For 15 seconds and multiplied by 4
 D. For 30 seconds and multiplied by 2
44. Which notation would the nursing assistant use to record an apical pulse of 72?
 A. Pulse 72
 B. 72—Apical pulse
 C. 72Ap
 D. P 72
45. Which technique would the nursing assistant use to take an apical-radial pulse?
 A. Count the radial pulse for 1 minute and then count the apical pulse for 1 minute
 B. Count each pulse then subtract the apical pulse from the radial pulse
 C. One staff member counts the apical pulse, and another staff member simultaneously counts the radial pulse.
 D. Two staff members simultaneously take the apical pulse; then the two staff members simultaneously take the radial pulse.

46. Where is the pedal pulse located?
    A. On the medial side of the elbow
    B. Over a foot bone
    C. On the thumb side of the wrist
    D. At the apex of the heart, just to the left of the sternum
47. Which technique is the best way to count respirations?
    A. Place a hand on the person's chest and watch the chest rise and fall
    B. Keep the fingers on the pulse site while counting the respirations
    C. Tell the person to breathe normally while respirations are counted
    D. Use a stethoscope to hear the respirations clearly and count for 1 full minute
48. What does each respiration involve?
    A. 1 inhalation
    B. 1 exhalation
    C. 1 inhalation and 1 exhalation
    D. Breathing slowly and deeply in and out
49. Which rationale supports the observation that blood pressure may be higher in older persons?
    A. They have orthostatic hypotension.
    B. Their diet is higher in sodium.
    C. Blood pressure increases with age.
    D. They are usually overweight.
50. Which person should not have the blood pressure taken in the left arm?
    A. Person A has a dialysis access site in the left arm.
    B. Person B has been sleeping on their left side.
    C. Person C is very obese and both arms are large.
    D. Person D plays sports and is left-handed.
51. Which action would the nursing assistant take to find out the correct size of blood pressure cuff?
    A. Ask the nurse
    B. Measure the person's arm
    C. Look at the equipment
    D. Ask the person
52. Where would the nursing assistant place the stethoscope diaphragm when taking a blood pressure with an aneroid manometer?
    A. Over the radial artery on the thumb side of the wrist
    B. Over the brachial artery at the inner aspect of the elbow
    C. Over the carotid during CPR
    D. Over the apical pulse site just left of the sternum
53. Where would the nursing assistant position the person's arm when getting ready to take a blood pressure?
    A. Anatomical position beside the body
    B. At the level with the heart
    C. Below the level of the heart
    D. Abducted from the body
54. The blood pressure cuff is inflated ________________ beyond point where you last felt the radial pulse.
    A. 10 mm Hg
    B. 20 mm Hg
    C. 30 mm Hg
    D. 40 mm Hg
55. Which nursing assistant has made an error in deciding to immediately report or to record vital signs?
    A. Nursing assistant A reports a blood pressure of 160 mm Hg/90 mm Hg.
    B. Nursing assistant B reports a pulse of 50 beats per minute.
    C. Nursing assistant C records a temperature of 95.8°F (35.44°C).
    D. Nursing assistant D records a temperature of 98.8°F (37.11°C).
56. Which site has the highest normal range temperature?
    A. Oral
    B. Rectum
    C. Axilla
    D. Tympanic membrane
57. Which nursing assistant has correctly placed the tip of the thermometer to take an oral temperature?
    A. Toward the back of the throat
    B. Under the tongue and to one side
    C. Between lower molars and cheek
    D. Position for comfort of the patient
58. Which site for taking a patient's temperature is the least reliable?
    A. Axilla
    B. Rectal
    C. Temporal arterial
    D. Oral
59. Which action would the nursing assistant take when taking a tympanic membrane temperature on an adult to straighten the ear canal?
    A. Pull up and back on the ear
    B. Tip patient's head forward
    C. Pull straight back at the middle
    D. Pull down and out on the ear
60. Which person has a pulse rate that the nursing assistant would report, at once, to the nurse?
    A. Person A has a pulse of 60 beats per minute.
    B. Person B has a pulse of 75 beats per minute.
    C. Person C has a pulse of 90 beats per minute.
    D. Person D has a pulse of 140 beats per minute.
61. How long would the nursing assistant leave an oral glass thermometer in place when taking a person's temperature?
    A. 1 minute
    B. 2 minutes
    C. 2 to 3 minutes
    D. 5 to 10 minutes
62. Which person needs to have the pulse counted for 1 full minute?
    A. Person A has a weak pedal pulse.
    B. Person B has a bounding pulse.
    C. Person C has an irregular pulse.
    D. Person D has an elevated temperature.

63. For which person would it better to use a tympanic membrane or temporal artery thermometer to take the temperature?
    A. Person A has dental problems and bad breath.
    B. Person B is confused and has trouble following instructions.
    C. Person C has a high fever and is profusely sweating.
    D. Person D is diabetic and just finished taking a shower.
64. Which nursing assistant has made an error when taking a person's pulse?
    A. Nursing assistant A asks the person to sit or lie down.
    B. Nursing assistant B positions the person's arm, so it is supported.
    C. Nursing assistant C places a thumb over the radial pulse.
    D. Nursing assistant D uses first two or three fingertips to take the pulse.
65. Which adult patient has a respiratory rate that the nursing assistant would report, at once, to the nurse?
    A. Patient A has a respiratory rate of 10 breaths per minute.
    B. Patient B has a respiratory rate of 12 breaths per minute.
    C. Patient C has a respiratory rate of 18 breaths per minute.
    D. Patient D has a respiratory rate of 20 breaths per minute.
66. Which action would the nursing assistant take upon observing an X marked on the patient's foot?
    A. Wash it off with soap and water
    B. Check the brachial pulse
    C. Ask the patient about the mark
    D. Check the pedal pulse

Fill in the Blanks

67. Write out the abbreviations
    A. BP ____________________
    B. C ____________________
    C. F ____________________
    D. Hg ____________________
    E. IV ____________________
    F. mm ____________________
    G. mm Hg ____________________
    H. TPR ____________________
68. You count 9 breaths in 30 seconds. What would you record for the respiratory rate?
    ____
69. The nurse instructs you and a coworker to take an apical-radial pulse and report the pulse deficit. You count the apical pulse and obtain 82 beats per minute. Your coworker counts the radial pulse and obtains 79 beats per minute. What is the pulse deficit that you will report to the nurse? ____________________
70. If a glass thermometer breaks, report it to the nurse at once because it may contain ____________________, which is a hazardous substance.
71. When you read a Fahrenheit thermometer, the short lines mean ____________________.
72. When taking an axillary temperature, the axilla must be ____________________.
73. When using an electronic thermometer, what does the color of the probe mean?
    A. Blue ____________________
    B. Red ____________________
74. Sites for measuring temperature are the
    A. ____________________
    B. ____________________
    C. ____________________
    D. ____________________
    E. ____________________
75. List words used to describe:
    A. Forceful pulse ____________________
    B. Hard-to-feel pulse ____________________
76. When taking an apical pulse, each *lub-dub* sound is counted as ____________________.
77. When you take a pulse, what observations should be reported and recorded?
    A. ____________________
    B. ____________________
    C. ____________________
    D. ____________________
    E. ____________________
78. Respirations are counted for ____________________ ____________________ if they are abnormal or irregular.
79. What observations should be reported and recorded when counting respirations?
    A. ____________________
    B. ____________________
    C. ____________________
    D. ____________________
    E. ____________________
    F. ____________________
80. Blood pressure is controlled by
    A. ____________________
    B. ____________________
    C. ____________________
81. Report blood pressures that have these readings
    A. Systolic over ____________________; systolic below ____________________
    B. Diastolic over ____________________; diastolic below ____________________

82. Let the person rest for ______________________ before taking the blood pressure.

83. When you are taking a blood pressure, the person should be in a ______________________ or ______________________ position.

84. What information do you need from the nurse or the care plan before you take a person's blood pressure?
A. ______________________
B. ______________________
C. ______________________
D. ______________________
E. ______________________
F. ______________________
G. ______________________
H. ______________________
I. ______________________
J. ______________________

Optional Learning Exercises

Taking Temperatures

85. The home health nursing assistant is preparing to take Mrs. Harrison's temperature with an oral thermometer and she says that she just brushed her teeth. What would the home health nursing assistant do? ______________________.

Taking Pulses and Respirations

86. You are assigned to take Mrs. Sanchez's pulse and respirations. You note that the pulse rate and respirations are regular, so you take each one for ______________________. When you complete counting the pulse, you keep your ______________________ and count respirations. This is done so that Mrs. Sanchez will assume you are taking the pulse.

87. When you finish counting Mrs. Sanchez's pulse and respirations, your numbers are pulse 36 and respirations 9. What would you record?
Pulse ______________________
Respirations ______________________

88. The nurse tells you to take an apical-radial pulse on Mrs. Hellman. Why do you ask a coworker to help you? ______________________

89. How long is an apical-radial pulse counted? ______________________ After you have taken the apical-radial pulse, how do you calculate the pulse deficit? ______________________
____

Taking Blood Pressures

90. You are assigned to take Mr. Hardaway's blood pressure. You know that he goes for dialysis three times a week. What do you need to know before you take his blood pressure? ______________________
____
____
Why? ______________________
____

91. When you inflate the cuff, you cannot feel the pulse after you pump the cuff to 130 mm Hg. How high will you inflate the cuff to take his blood pressure?
____

92. You should deflate the cuff at an even rate of ______________________ per second.

Labeling

93. Fill in the drawings so that the thermometers read correctly.

A 95.8° F

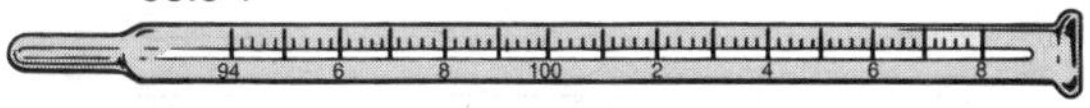

B 98.4° F

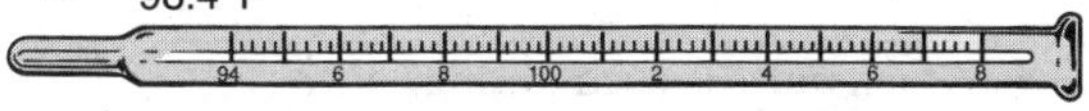

C 100.2° F

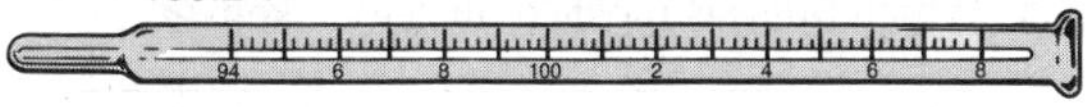

D 35.5° C

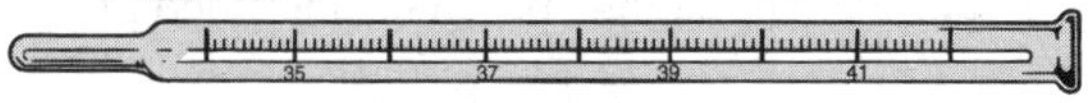

E 36.5° C

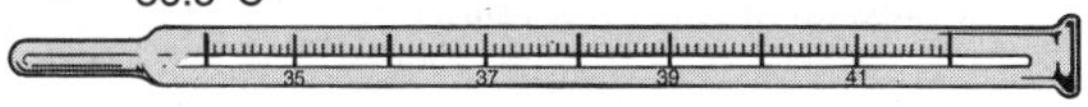

F 37° C

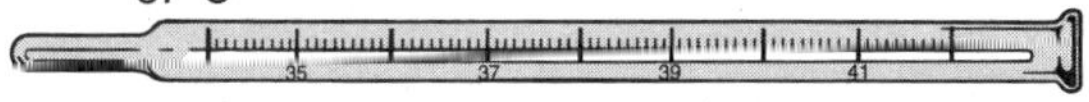

94. Name the pulse sites shown.

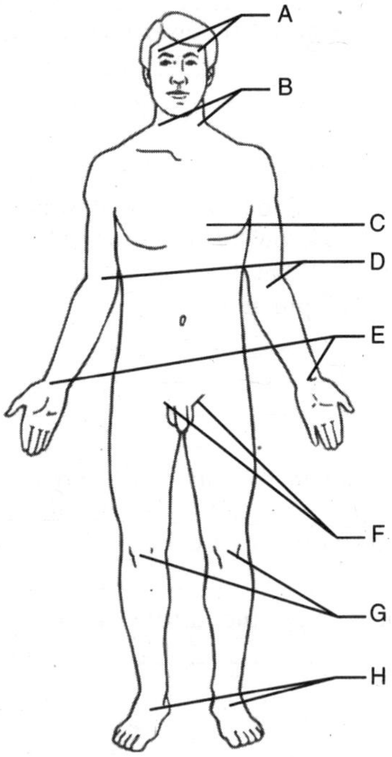

A. ______________________________
B. ______________________________
C. ______________________________
D. ______________________________
E. ______________________________
F. ______________________________
G. ______________________________
H. ______________________________
I. Which pulse is used during CPR?
____
J. Which pulse is most commonly taken?
____
K. Which pulse is most commonly used when placing the stethoscope to take the blood pressure?
____
L. Which pulse is found with a stethoscope when taking an apical-radial pulse? ______________
____

95. Fill in the drawings so that the dials show the correct blood pressures.

A 168/102

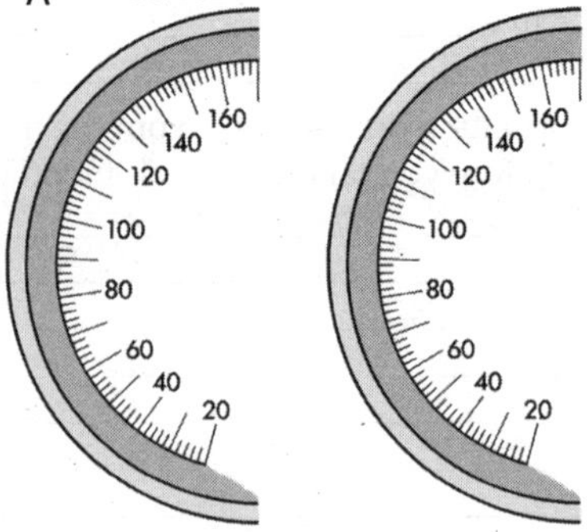

B 104/68

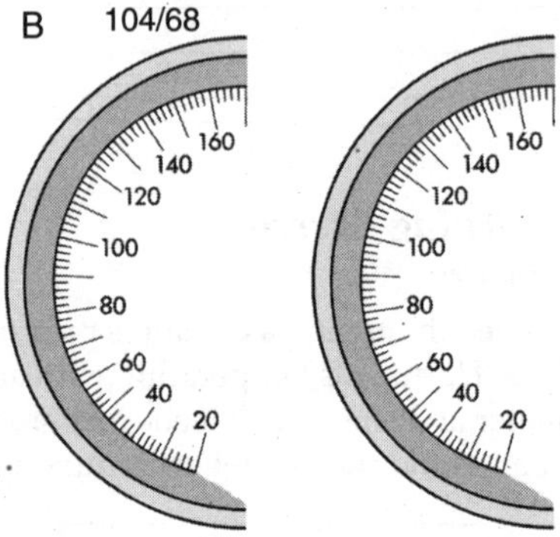

96. Which step, for taking a blood pressure, is depicted in the figure?

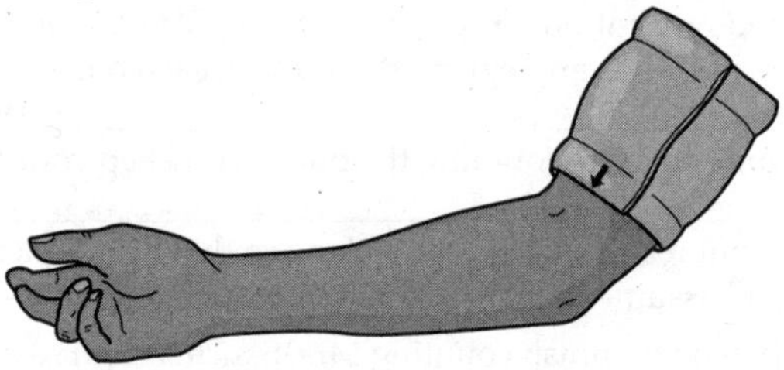

Use the FOCUS ON PRIDE section to complete the statement

97. If the person is on transmission-based precautions, the isolation cart with the vital sign equipment must be ______________________________.

Critical Thinking and Discussion Question

98. A friend is in the nursing assistants' program with you. She is unable to master the skill of taking a blood pressure using a stethoscope and an aneroid manometer. Suggest ways to help her.

35 Exercise and Activity

Fill in the Blanks: Key Terms

Abduction
Adduction
Ambulation
Atrophy
Bed rest
Contracture
Deconditioning
Dorsiflexion
Extension
External rotation
Flexion
Foot drop
Hyperextension
Internal rotation
Opposition
Orthostatic hypotension (postural hypotension)
Orthotic device
Plantar flexion
Pronation
Range of motion (ROM)
Rotation
Supination
Syncope

1. Touching the opposite finger with the thumb is ______________________.
2. The foot is bent down at the ankle when ______________________ is present.
3. A brief loss of consciousness or fainting is ______________________.
4. Bending a body part is ______________________.
5. Moving a body part away from the midline of the body is ______________________.
6. ______________________ is the movement of a joint to the extent possible without causing pain.
7. Turning the joint outward is ______________________.
8. A drop in blood pressure when the person suddenly stands up is ______________________.
9. ______________________ occurs when moving a body part toward the midline of the body.
10. Turning the joint upward is called ______________________.
11. Bending the toes and foot up at the ankle is ______________________.
12. Excessive straightening of a body part is ______________________.
13. A decrease in size or a wasting away of tissue is ______________________.
14. Turning the joint is ______________________.
15. ______________________ is straightening of a body part.
16. Restricting a person to bed and limiting activity for health reasons is ______________________.
17. ______________________ is permanent plantar flexion; the foot falls down at the ankle.
18. The act of walking is ______________________.
19. ______________________ is turning the joint downward.
20. The loss of muscle strength from inactivity is ______________________.
21. ______________________ is turning the joint inward.
22. The lack of joint mobility caused by abnormal shortening of a muscle is a ______________________.
23. An ______________________ is used to support a muscle, promote a certain motion, or correct a deformity.

Circle the Best Answer

24. Which device would be prescribed for a home care patient who has back pain?
    A. Splint
    B. Trochanter roll
    C. Bed cradle
    D. Bed board
25. Which complication of bed rest will result in loss of function and deformity of the joint?
    A. Contracture
    B. Pressure injury
    C. Blood clot
    D. Postural hypotension
26. Which outcome is likely if a contracture develops?
    A. It will require extra range-of-motion (ROM) exercises to correct it.
    B. Good body alignment and positioning will relieve the complication.
    C. The contracted muscle is fixed into position and cannot stretch.
    D. It will resolve as soon as the person is able to walk and exercise.
27. Which nursing measure should the nursing assistant use when caring for a person who has orthostatic hypotension?
    A. Raise the head of the bed slowly to Fowler's position
    B. Have the person stand up and pause while the dizziness passes
    C. Keep the bed flat when getting the person out of bed
    D. Have the person slowly walk around to decrease dizziness
28. Which nursing care prevents complications from bed rest?
    A. Using Fowler's position
    B. Taking frequent vital signs
    C. Maintaining good body alignment
    D. Encouraging deconditioning

29. Which action should the nursing assistant take if a person sitting on the edge of the bed reports weakness, dizziness, or spots before the eyes?
    A. Assist the person to slowly stand
    B. Help the person to sit in a chair or walk around
    C. Have the person return to Fowler's position
    D. Tell the person that the symptoms are a normal response
30. What is the purpose of a bed board?
    A. Maintain alignment by preventing the mattress from sagging
    B. Prevent plantar flexion that can lead to foot drop
    C. Keep the hips abducted
    D. Keep the weight of top linens off the feet
31. Which equipment does the nursing assistant need to obtain to position the person and prevent plantar flexion?
    A. Footboard
    B. Bed cradle
    C. Foam rubber sponge
    D. Abduction wedge
32. Which equipment would the nursing assistant use to prevent the hips and legs from turning outward?
    A. Bed cradles
    B. Hip abduction wedges
    C. Trochanter rolls
    D. Splints
33. Which action would be the best to help the person, who has decreased arm strength, to exercise?
    A. Give the person a schedule of activities
    B. Talk about the benefits of exercise
    C. Encourage the person to use a trapeze to move
    D. Leave the person alone to do self-care
34. Which action would the nursing assistant perform when the nurse delegates passive range of motion (ROM) exercises?
    A. Supervise person during active ROM exercises
    B. Assists the person with passive activities of daily living
    C. Assists the person to perform ROM exercises
    D. Moves the person's joints through the ROM
35. Which person is most likely to have an order for bed rest?
    A. Person A prefers to sleep in every morning.
    B. Person B recently delivered a healthy baby boy.
    C. Person C has had trouble breathing for past several days.
    D. Person D is confused and expects to get breakfast in bed.
36. With the nurse's approval, which play activity would be the best for a child who needs shoulder range of motion (ROM)?
    A. Pretending to fly like a bird
    B. Drawing a picture of a bird
    C. Making a bird out of clay
    D. Playing a video game with birds
37. Which body part would the nursing assistant pronate and supinate during the ROM exercises?
    A. Hands
    B. Elbows
    C. Knees
    D. Fingers
38. Which of these joints can be adducted and abducted?
    A. Neck
    B. Hip
    C. Forearm
    D. Knee
39. Which nursing measure should the nursing assistant use when helping a person who is weak and unsteady to walk?
    A. Apply a gait (transfer) belt
    B. Have the person lean on furniture for balance
    C. Put the person in a wheelchair
    D. Get the person a pair of crutches
40. Which clothing would the nursing assistant suggest for the person who is walking with crutches?
    A. Soft slippers on the feet
    B. Clothes that fit well
    C. Clothes that are padded
    D. Exercise pants
41. How should the person hold a cane while walking?
    A. On the strong side of the body
    B. On the weak side of the body
    C. In the right hand
    D. On the left side of the body
42. Which motion would the nursing assistant suggest to a person who is using a walker?
    A. Pick it up and move it 1 to 2 inches in front of self
    B. Move it forward with a rocking motion
    C. Move it first on the left side and then on the right
    D. Push and move it 6 to 8 inches in front of self
43. Which observation would the nursing assistant immediately report when caring for a person who wears a brace?
    A. How far the person can walk without assistance
    B. Progress the person has made in independently donning the brace
    C. The amount of mobility in joints when doing range of motion (ROM) exercises
    D. Any redness or signs of skin breakdown noted when brace is removed.
44. Which resident is likely to require the most assistance during the morning shift?
    A. Resident A is on bed rest, but can use the bathroom.
    B. Resident B is on strict (complete) bed rest.
    C. Resident C is on bed rest and does some self-care.
    D. Resident D is on bed rest with commode privileges.
45. How many times, unless otherwise noted in the care plan, is each movement generally repeated when performing range of motion (ROM) exercises?
    A. Once
    B. Twice
    C. 5 times
    D. 20 times
46. Which patient will benefit the most from a trapeze bar?
    A. Patient A has a fractured leg.
    B. Patient B has risk for foot drop.
    C. Patient C needs to strengthen arm muscles.
    D. Patient D needs assistance with activities of daily living.

47. Which device would the nursing assistant use to keep a person's hips apart after hip replacement surgery?
    A. Hip abduction wedge
    B. Splint
    C. Brace
    D. Footboard
48. Which vital sign change would the nursing assistant expect to observe when the nurse advises that the person experiences orthostatic hypotension?
    A. Blood pressure is normal during the day and low at night.
    B. Blood pressure increases when the person is dizzy.
    C. Blood pressure drops when the person is lying down.
    D. Blood pressure drops when the person stands up suddenly.
49. Which complication is related to immobility and the heavy weight of top linens?
    A. Urinary tract infection
    B. Constipation
    C. Postural hypotension
    D. Foot drop
50. Which action would the nursing assistant use when helping a person to walk?
    A. Stand at the side and slightly behind the person on the weak side
    B. Stand back and allow the person to freely move at their own pace
    C. Stand directly behind the person and firmly hold gait belt with both hands
    D. Stand in front of the person and hold forearms as they walk forward

Fill in the Blanks

51. Write out the abbreviations
    A. ADL ______________________________
    B. PROM ______________________________
    C. ROM ______________________________
52. A nursing assistant can perform range of motion (ROM) exercises on the ____________________ only if allowed by center policy.
53. When using a footboard, the nursing assistant ensures that the soles of the feet are ____________________ against the footboard to prevent foot drop.
54. Hand rolls or grips prevent ____________________ of the thumb, fingers, and wrists.
55. A splint is used to keep these joints in their normal positions.
    A. ______________________________
    B. ______________________________
    C. ______________________________
    D. ______________________________
    E. ______________________________
    F. ______________________________
56. When a person does exercises with some help, they are doing ____________________ range of motion (ROM) exercises.
57. When range of motion (ROM) exercises are done, what should be reported or recorded?
    A. ______________________________
    B. ______________________________
    C. ______________________________
    D. ______________________________
    E. ______________________________
58. List the safety measures to follow when performing range of motion (ROM) exercises.
    A. ______________________________
    B. ______________________________
    C. ______________________________
    D. ______________________________
    E. ______________________________
    F. ______________________________
    G. ______________________________
    H. ______________________________
    I. ______________________________

Optional Learning Exercises

59. What kind of range of motion (ROM) would be used with each of these residents?
    A. The resident needs complete care for bathing, grooming, and feeding.
    ____
    B. The resident takes part in many activities in the center. She walks to most activities independently.
    ____
    C. The resident has weakness on his left side. He is able to feed himself but needs help with bathing and dressing.
    ____
60. As you plan to help a person out of bed, you are concerned about orthostatic hypotension. To make sure the person is able to stand and get up safely, you plan to take the blood pressure, pulse, and respirations several times. When would you take the blood pressure?
    A. ______________________________
    B. ______________________________
    C. ______________________________
    D. ______________________________
    E. ______________________________
61. When doing range of motion (ROM) exercises, you should ask the person if they
    A. ______________________________
    B. ______________________________
    C. ______________________________
62. When you are going to assist a person to ambulate, you can promote comfort and reduce fears when you explain
    A. ______________________________
    B. ______________________________
    C. ______________________________
    D. ______________________________
    E. ______________________________

63. When you help a person to walk, what observations are reported and recorded?
A. ______________________________
B. ______________________________
C. ______________________________
D. ______________________________
E. ______________________________

64. When using a cane, the person walks as follows:
A. Step A: ______________________________
B. Step B: ______________________________
C. Step C: ______________________________

65. What should be immediately reported if observed when a brace is removed?
____

Use the FOCUS ON PRIDE section to complete these statements

66. You assist the nurse in promoting ______________ and ______________ for all persons to the extent possible.

67. You can promote activity, exercise, and well-being when you
A. ______________________________
B. ______________________________
C. ______________________________
D. ______________________________

Critical Thinking and Discussion Question

68. If an elderly person can slowly ambulate, pushing them in a wheelchair to the dining room is contributing to that person's deconditioning. What other examples can you think of that contribute to deconditioning?

Labeling

69. ROM exercises for the ______________ joint are shown in these drawings. Name the movements shown in each drawing.

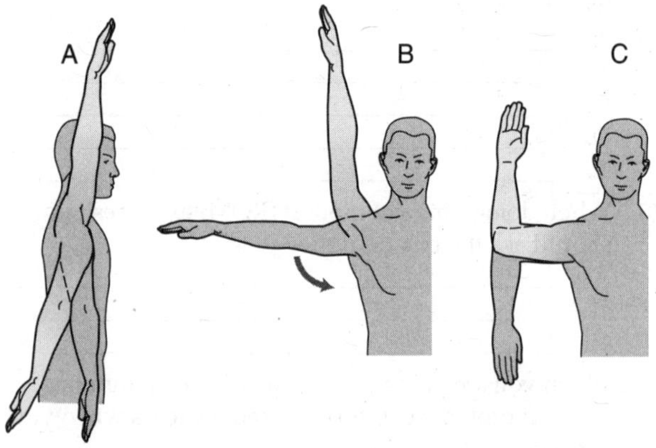

A. ______________________________
B. ______________________________
C. ______________________________

70. ROM exercises for the ______________ are shown in these drawings. Name the movements shown in each drawing.

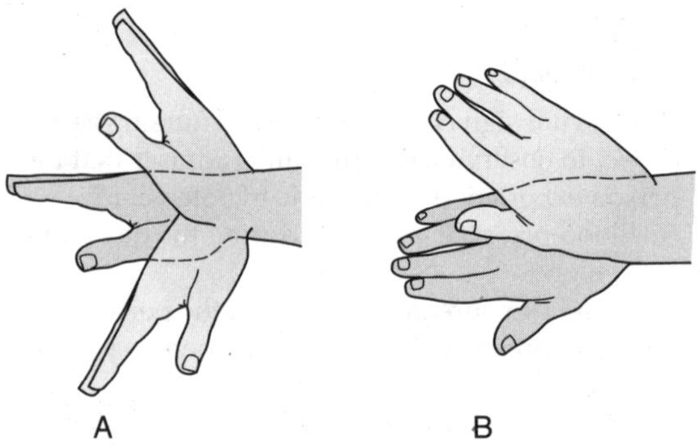

A. ______________________________
B. ______________________________

71. ROM exercises for the ______________ are shown in these drawings. Name the movements shown in each drawing.

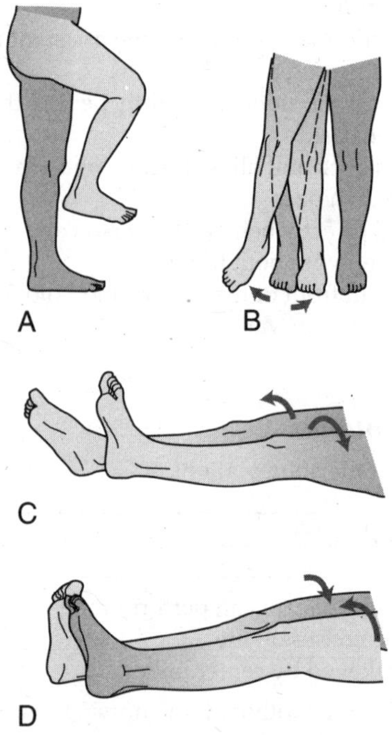

A. ______________________________
B. ______________________________
C. ______________________________
D. ______________________________

Crossword

Fill in the crossword by answering the clues below with the words from this list

Abduction	Flexion	Rotation	Plantar flexion
Adduction	Hyperextension	Internal rotation	Pronation
Extension	Dorsiflexion	External rotation	Supination

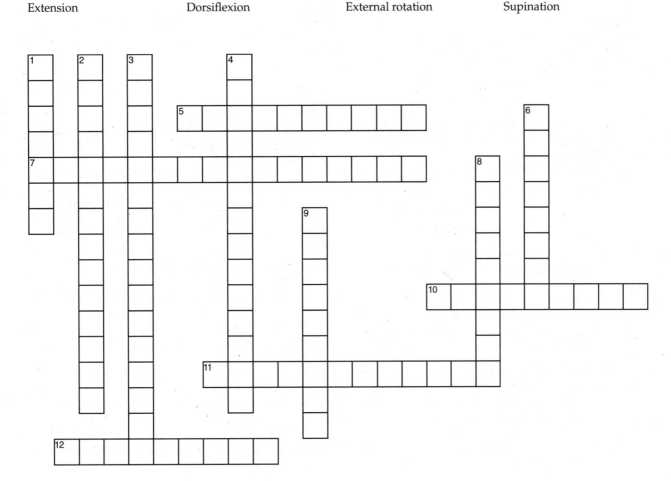

Across

5. Turning the joint upward
7. Turning the joint inward
10. Straightening a body part
11 Bending the toes and foot up at the ankle
12. Turning the joint downward

Down

1. Bending a body part
2. Bending the foot down at the ankle
3. Turning the joint outward
4. Excessive straightening of a body part
6. Turning the joint
8. Moving a body part away from the midline of the body
9. Moving a body part toward the midline of the body

36 Comfort, Rest, and Sleep

Fill in the Blanks: Key Terms

Acute pain
Chronic pain
Circadian rhythm
Comfort
Distraction
Guided imagery
Insomnia
Pain (discomfort)
Phantom pain
Radiating pain
Referred pain
Relaxation
Rest
Sleep
Sleep apnea
Sleep deprivation
Sleepwalking

1. ____________________ occurs when the amount and quality of sleep are not adequate, and this causes reduced function and alertness.
2. To hurt, ache or be sore is ____________________.
3. ____________________ is pain that is felt suddenly from injury, disease, trauma, or surgery.
4. ____________________ is a way to focus a person's attention on something unrelated to the pain.
5. ____________ is a state of unconsciousness, reduced voluntary muscle activity, and lowered metabolism.
6. Pain lasting longer than 12 weeks is____________. It is constant or occurs off and on.
7. ____________________ is to be free from mental or physical stress.
8. ____________________ is a state of well-being. The person has no physical or emotional pain and is calm and at peace.
9. To be calm, at ease, and relaxed is to ____________. The person is free of anxiety and stress.
10. Creating and focusing on an image is ____________________.
11. Pain from a body part that is felt in another body part is ____________________.
12. ____________________ is a chronic condition in which the person cannot sleep or stay asleep all night.
13. The day-night cycle or body rhythm is also called ____________________. This daily rhythm is based on a 24-hour cycle.
14. ____________________ is felt at the site of tissue damage and spreads to other areas.
15. A pause in breathing that occur during sleep is ____________________.
16. Pain felt in a body part that is no longer there is ____________________.
17. When the person leaves the bed and walks about while sleeping, they are ____________________.

Circle the Best Answer

18. Which nursing measure would the nursing assistant use for an elderly person who is sleepwalking?
    A. Alert the nurse, so that the person can be medicated
    B. Walk around with the person until he wakes up
    C. Wake the person and ask him where he is going
    D. Protect the person from injury, especially falling
19. Which question indicates that the nursing assistant wants the person to be comfortable?
    A. "What do you want to drink for lunch?"
    B. "Did you have a nice visit with your family?"
    C. "What time do you like to go to bed?"
    D. "Should I adjust your pillow?"
20. Which question, related to pain, is a surveyor most likely to ask?
    A. "What would you do to restore a person's well-being?"
    B. "What kind of medications are given for pain?"
    C. "What are the signs and symptoms of pain?"
    D. "How would you teach a person to relax?"
21. What is the primary purpose of rest and sleep?
    A. Restore well-being and energy
    B. Prevent anxiety
    C. Increase muscle strength
    D. Prevent pain
22. What is included in the Centers for Medicare and Medicaid Services (CMS) requirements related to comfort, rest, and sleep?
    A. Only two people in a room
    B. Bright lighting in all areas
    C. Room temperature between 65°F and 71°F
    D. Adequate ventilation and room humidity
23. What would the nursing assistant do when a person reports pain or discomfort?
    A. Rely on what the person says about the pain
    B. Measure the pain to determine the reality
    C. Compare the person's pain with others' pain
    D. Watch the person for obvious signs of pain

24. Which kind of pain is the person describing when there is pain near an area of tissue damage?
A. Acute
B. Chronic
C. Radiating
D. Phantom

25. Which behavior is a person most likely to display if there is a belief that pain is a sign of weakness?
A. Cries quietly and softly
B. Enjoys being pampered
C. Denies or ignores pain
D. Seeks support from others

26. Which factor is frequently associated with a stoic reaction to pain?
A. Illness
B. Culture
C. Anxiety
D. Attention

27. How does a feeling of anxiety affect the person's experience of pain?
A. May feel increased pain
B. Will usually feel less pain
C. May deny having pain
D. Will usually refuse pain medication

28. Which information can be obtained by asking the person to rate the pain on a scale of 0 to 10?
A. Description of the pain
B. The location of the pain
C. Onset and duration of the pain
D. The intensity of the pain

29. Which behavior may an older child use to deal with pain?
A. Restrict play or school activities
B. Describe pain to an adult
C. Ask for pain medications
D. Read or play very quietly

30. Which rationale explains why older persons may ignore new pain?
A. They cannot verbally communicate pain.
B. They believe it is part of a known health problem.
C. They usually have increased anxiety.
D. They are used to being in pain.

31. Which information is obtained when a person reports pain during coughing or deep breathing?
A. A factor causing pain
B. A measurement of the onset of pain
C. Words used to describe the pain
D. The location of the pain

32. Which nursing measure uses distraction to promote comfort and relieve pain?
A. Asking the person to focus on an image
B. Learning to breathe deeply and slowly
C. Listening to music or playing games
D. Contracting and relaxing muscle groups

33. Which action would the nursing assistant use if the nurse has just given a person a dose of pain medication?
A. Give the person a bath
B. Walk the person according to the care plan
C. Wait 30 minutes before giving care
D. Give care before the medication makes the person sleepy

34. Which time of day is pain most likely to seem worse for the person?
A. Upon waking
B. Just before meals
C. Late afternoon
D. Nighttime

35. Which nursing measure promotes comfort and helps to relieve pain?
A. Perform passive range-of-motion exercises
B. Provide blankets for warmth and to prevent chilling
C. Make sure the person ambulates every 2 hours
D. Keep the person in the supine position

36. What is the purpose of using lotion during a back massage?
A. Stimulates circulation
B. Heals any skin breakdown
C. Reduces friction during the massage
D. Refreshes the skin

37. Which condition could be a dangerous contraindication for giving a back massage?
A. Sleep deprivation
B. Lung disorder
C. Arthritis
D. Insomnia

38. What is the best position for a back massage?
A. Prone position
B. Supine position
C. Semi-Fowler's position
D. Fowler's position

39. Which action would the nursing assistant use to maximize the strokes when giving a back massage?
A. Start at the shoulders and go up toward the neck
B. Use circular motions over the buttocks and up and down on the arms
C. Start at the lower back and go up to the shoulders
D. Continue the stroking for at least 10 minutes

40. Which action promotes rest?
A. Helping with elimination needs
B. Making sure the person feels happy
C. Allowing the person to sleep through breakfast
D. Giving care whenever there is extra time

41. Which action would help an ill or injured person to get the extra rest needed for healing?
A. Provide range-of-motion exercises on a set schedule
B. Provide rest periods during or after a procedure
C. Give complete hygiene and grooming measures
D. Spend time talking with the person to distract from the pain

42. Which of these occurs during sleep?
A. The person cannot respond to stimuli.
B. Metabolism is reduced during sleep.
C. Vital signs are higher.
D. Arm or leg movements are voluntary.

43. Which personal factor would the nursing assistant consider if taking a night shift job?
A. Circadian rhythm
B. Bedtime rituals
C. Ability to relax
D. Preference for job tasks

44. What is an elderly resident most likely to be experiencing when he frequently gets up at 3:00 a.m. and comes to the nursing station to visit with the staff?
    A. Sleepwalking
    B. Agitation
    C. Disorientation
    D. Insomnia
45. Which food would help to induce sleep if given as a snack before bedtime?
    A. Apple slices
    B. Low-fat milk
    C. Tomato juice
    D. Chocolate cookie
46. Which age-group requires the least amount of sleep?
    A. Newborns
    B. Preschoolers
    C. Teenagers
    D. Adults, including the elderly
47. Which person is most likely to have an increased need for sleep?
    A. Person A who started a new exercise program.
    B. Person B who was seriously injured in a car accident.
    C. Person C who started an extreme weight loss diet.
    D. Person D who was transferred to night shift.
48. When is an increase in vital signs expected?
    A. When a person naps during the day.
    B. When a person experiences insomnia.
    C. When a person is sleeping soundly.
    D. When a person is having acute pain.
49. Which pain report is the most serious and requires that the nurse be immediately notified?
    A. Person A is having referred pain that is felt in the left arm and shoulder.
    B. Person B is having phantom pain that is felt in the amputated leg.
    C. Person C is having chronic pain related to joint stiffness and arthritis.
    D. Person D is having radiating pain that starts in the lower back and goes to buttocks.
50. Which sleep disturbance is a risk for persons who are ill, in pain, or receiving hospital care?
    A. Sleep deprivation
    B. Sleepwalking
    C. Insomnia
    D. Oversedation
51. Which person would normally need the most sleep?
    A. A 3-month-old infant
    B. An 8-year-old child
    C. A 17-year-old person
    D. A 78-year-old person
52. Which of these nursing measures help to promote sleep?
    A. Provide extra blankets and turn down the room temperatures
    B. Help persons to void or make sure incontinent persons are clean and dry.
    C. Follow bedtime routines to make sure everyone is in bed at the scheduled time
    D. Offer everyone a cup of coffee or tea with crackers at bedtime.
53. Which nursing measure would the nursing assistant use to assist a person with Alzheimer disease who wanders at night?
    A. Give her a cup of coffee or tea
    B. Turn on the TV in the room to distract her
    C. Be calm and quiet and help her back to her room
    D. Explain that it is night and time to go to bed
54. Which nursing measures would be best to promote sleep for a 9-year-old child having trouble falling asleep in the strange hospital environment?
    A. Hold the child and rock her
    B. Help her take a warm bath
    C. Darken the room and close the door
    D. Read a favorite story to her
55. Which room temperature setting is in accordance with Centers for Medicare & Medicaid Services (CMS) requirements?
    A. Room temperature is between 71°F and 81°F (Fahrenheit).
    B. Room temperature is determined by agreement between roommates.
    C. Room temperature is set according to the season and weather conditions.
    D. Room temperature is between 61°F and 81°F (Fahrenheit).
56. Which behavior suggests that the patient may be experiencing pain?
    A. Frequently shifts body or changes position
    B. Changes position while asleep, without waking
    C. Uses cane as instructed by physical therapy
    D. Walks three times a day in hallway
57. Which observation would the nursing assistant report to the nurse because the child may be having pain?
    A. Child is hopping around the nurses' station.
    B. Child wanted cookies and candy before dinner.
    C. Child is playing, but is guarding the dominant hand.
    D. Child did routine bedtime rituals and fell asleep.
58. Which person is most likely to ignore or deny new pain?
    A. A 62-year-old person has an active sex life.
    B. A 55-year-old person likes to babysit a grandchild.
    C. A 70-year-old person has a fear of reoccurring cancer.
    D. A 58-year-old person wants to keep working.

Fill in the Blanks

59. Name the type of pain described.
    A. A person with an amputated leg may still sense leg pain. ______________________
    B. There is tissue damage. The pain decreases with healing.
    ____
    C. Pain from a heart attack is often felt in the left chest, left jaw, left shoulder, and left arm.
    ____
    D. The pain remains for a long time. Common causes are arthritis and cancer.
    ____

E. Person has gallbladder disease, but experiences pain in the right shoulder ______

60. When gathering information about a person in pain, you can use a scale of 1 to 10. Which end of the scale is the most severe pain? ______
61. What happens to vital signs when the person has acute pain? ______
62. What happens to vital signs when the person has chronic pain? ______
63. What body responses that you can see or measure (objective signs) may mean the person has pain?
A. ______
B. ______
C. ______
D. ______
E. ______
64. List nursing measures to promote comfort and relieve pain related to these clues.
A. Position of the person ______
B. Linens ______
C. Blankets ______
D. Pain medications ______
E. Family members ______
65. If a person is receiving strong pain medication or sedatives, what safety measures are important?
A. ______
B. ______
C. ______
D. ______
66. For persons with dementia who cannot verbally express pain, list five examples of changes in mood or behavior that the nursing assistant would report as possible signals for pain.
A. ______
B. ______
C. ______
D. ______
E. ______
67. When giving a back massage, what is the effect of
A. Fast movements ______
B. Slow movements ______
68. When you are delegated to give a back massage, what observations should you report and record?
A. ______
B. ______
C. ______
D. ______
69. If work hours change, it can affect the normal ______ cycle or ______ rhythm.
70. Alcohol tends to cause ______ and sleep. However, after drinking alcohol the person may ______ and have difficulty falling back to sleep.
71. List six questions you could ask the person to see if they need additional nursing measures to promote comfort.
A. ______
B. ______
C. ______
D. ______
E. ______
F. ______
72. A person reports pain. List the eight things that the nurse needs to know about the person's pain.
A. ______
B. ______
C. ______
D. ______
E. ______
F. ______
G. ______
H. ______

Optional Learning Exercises

73. You are caring for two residents who both have arthritis. Mr. Forman tells you this is the first time he has had any health problems. Mrs. Wegman tells you she has had several surgeries and has had three children. Who is likely to be more anxious about the pain and to be unable to handle the pain well, Mr. Forman or Mrs. Wegman? ______ Why? ______
74. Mr. Forman tells you his pain seems much worse at night. What could be the reason for this reaction? ______
75. You are caring for Mrs. Reynolds. She tells you she misses her children who have moved to another state. Today, Mrs. Reynolds is reporting pain in her abdomen. Despite providing nursing comfort measures, she still rates her pain at 7. What is a possible reason that Mrs. Reynolds is not getting relief of her pain? ______
76. When a person is ill, how do these affect sleep?
A. Treatments and therapies ______.
B. Care devices such as traction or a cast ______.
C. Emotions that affect sleep include ______.
77. Certain foods affect sleep. Tell how these foods affect sleep and list foods that contain the substances.
A. Caffeine ______ sleep. It is found in ______.
B. Trytophan ______ sleep. It is found in ______.

78. List at least eight signs and symptoms of sleep disorders
    A. ______________________________
    B. ______________________________
    C. ______________________________
    D. ______________________________
    E. ______________________________
    F. ______________________________
    G. ______________________________
    H. ______________________________

Labeling

79. Complete the Wong-Baker FACES Pain Scale by writing the number and the description of the pain under each face.

(From Hockenberry MJ, Wilson D. *Wong's Nursing Care of Infants and Children*. 11th ed. Elsevier; 2019.)

Use the FOCUS ON PRIDE section to complete these statements

80. When you are caring for persons who have pain, what is your responsibility?
    A. Report ______________ and ______________
    ______________________________.
    B. Report what the person ______________
    and what you ______________________.
81. It is important to report signs and symptoms of pain because the nurse uses this information to
    ______________________________.
82. Avoid making ______________ about the person's pain.

Critical Thinking and Discussion Question

83. You are assigned to help a person with hygiene and ADLs in a home setting. You notice that the person frequently reports pain when certain family members are present. You suspect that the person may enjoy the extra attention and pampering from family members. What would you do?

37 Admissions, Transfers, and Discharges

Fill in the Blanks: Key Terms

Admission   Discharge   Transfer

1. Moving the person to another health-care setting or moving the person to a new room within the agency is a ______________________________
2. The official entry of a person into a healthcare setting is ______________________________.
3. ______________________ occurs with the official departure of a person from a healthcare setting.

Circle the Best Answer

4. Which information does the nursing assistant need to get from the nurse when instructed to assist with the admission of a person to a healthcare facility?
   A. Reason for admission and anticipated the length of stay
   B. What to say about who gives care and how care is given
   C. If the person if being separated from family and friends
   D. How the person will move about: walk, wheelchair, or stretcher
5. Which event would most likely be viewed as a happy time for the person?
   A. Admission from home to a long-term care facility
   B. Discharge from the hospital to the home setting
   C. Transfer from a hospital to a rehabilitation center
   D. Transfer from a long-term care facility to the hospital
6. Which response is most likely to occur when a person with dementia is admitted to a nursing center?
   A. Sudden onset of depression
   B. An increase in confusion
   C. An interest in the environment
   D. A display of aggression
7. Which action would the nursing assistant take when a person who is being admitted arrives by stretcher?
   A. Raise the bed to the level of the stretcher
   B. Place the stretcher perpendicular to the bed
   C. Raise the head of the bed to Fowler's position
   D. Assist the person to get off of the stretcher
8. Which information does the nursing assistant need to get from the nurse when asked to weigh a newly admitted person?
   A. Where to record the weight?
   B. What the person should wear?
   C. Person's normal weight
   D. What type of scale to use?
9. What would the nursing assistant do first if the nurse instructs to get the person's weight using a wheelchair scale?
   A. Weigh the person in the wheelchair
   B. Weigh the wheelchair
   C. Subtract the weight of wheelchair
   D. Add the weight of the person
10. You measure a person's height using the standing scale and obtain a reading of 61 inches. You must record the height in feet and inches. What will you record?
    A. 5 ft
    B. 5 ft 1 in
    C. 5 ft 11 in
    D. 6 ft 1 in
11. What would the nursing assistant ask a resident to do before obtaining a weight?
    A. Put on socks and shoes and a bathrobe
    B. Remove regular clothes and wear a gown or sleepwear
    C. Wear regular street clothes and usual shoes
    D. Remove clothing after weighing and then weigh the clothes
12. Which person would need to be weighed on a chair scale?
    A. Person A cannot transfer from a wheelchair.
    B. Person B cannot stand.
    C. Person C can sit with support.
    D. Person D is in the supine position.
13. Which action would the nursing assistant take when a person cannot stand on the scale to have height measured?
    A. Ask the person or the family the height of the person at the last known measurement
    B. Have the person sit in a chair and measure from head to toe with a tape measure
    C. Position the person in the supine position, if allowed, and measure with a tape measure
    D. Have the person roll to the side while you measure the height along the person's back
14. Which action would the nursing assistant use to show support and reassurance when a person is being moved to a new room?
    A. Promise to come and visit the person
    B. Introduce the person to the staff and roommates
    C. Pat the person on the head and say, "You're okay."
    D. Sit with the person until the end of your shift

15. Which statement typifies the nursing assistant's reporting responsibilities to the receiving nurse when transferring a person?
    A. "The person is difficult to take care of and is argumentative."
    B. "The person is being transferred because the condition has changed."
    C. "The person is being transferred after a disagreement with a roommate."
    D. "The person vomited a small amount during the transfer."
16. Which action would the nursing assistant take if a person wishes to leave the center without the doctor's permission?
    A. Tell the person this is not allowed
    B. Prevent the person from leaving
    C. Tell the nurse at once
    D. Try to convince the person to stay
17. Which task is the nursing assistant's responsibility when assisting a person who is being discharged?
    A. Give the prescriptions to the person or family
    B. Help with the clothing and personal belongings
    C. Give the valuables to the person or the family
    D. Provide discharge and follow-up instructions
18. Which person would not meet the criteria standards established by Centers for Medicare and Medicaid Services for a transfer or discharge from a long-term care center?
    A. Person A has needs that cannot be met in the center.
    B. Person B had a disagreement with a roommate.
    C. Person C has improved and services are no longer needed.
    D. Person D has behaviors that are a danger to self and others.
19. Which identifying information is the nursing assistant responsible to obtain when a person is being admitted?
    A. Full name
    B. Mailing address
    C. Driver license number
    D. Social security number
20. In which healthcare setting is the person likely to have a photo identification (ID) taken?
    A. Emergency department
    B. Outpatient surgical center
    C. Acute care hospital
    D. Long-term care center
21. Which nursing assistant needs a reminder about making a good first impression when asked to admit a person?
    A. Nursing assistant A makes roommate introductions.
    B. Nursing assistant B greets the person by name and title.
    C. Nursing assistant C introduces self by name and title.
    D. Nursing assistant D talks about personal plans after work.
22. Why is it important to have a person void before being weighed?
    A. A full bladder adds weight.
    B. Person will feel more relaxed.
    C. Doctor will want a specimen.
    D. It is part of the procedure.
23. Which nursing assistant needs a reminder about how to prepare the balance scale before having the person step on it?
    A. Nursing assistant A places paper towels on the scale platform.
    B. Nursing assistant B raises the height rod.
    C. Nursing assistant C balances the scale by moving the weights to zero.
    D. Nursing assistant D adjusts the pointer to rest at lowest point.
24. Which nursing measure can be performed by the nursing assistant when a person is being transferred or discharged?
    A. Give medical records as needed
    B. Provide discharge instructions
    C. Get valuables from the safe
    D. Assist the person to move to the wheelchair

Fill in the Blanks

25. Write out the abbreviations
    A. ft ________________
    B. in ________________
    C. lb ________________
26. When you are delegated to assist with admissions, transfers, or discharges, what information do you need from the nurse?
    A. ________________
    B. ________________
    C. ________________
    D. ________________
    E. ________________
    F. ________________
    G. ________________
    H. ________________
    I. ________________
    J. ________________
27. During admission, what is the person given to allow the staff to identify the person?
    ________________ and ________________
    ____
28. When measuring a person in the supine position, the ruler is placed ________________.
29. When you assist with a discharge, you should report and record
    A. ________________
    B. ________________
    C. ________________
    D. ________________
    E. ________________
    F. ________________

Optional Learning Exercises

Answer the questions about the following resident and situation: Rosa Romirez, 65, had a stroke (CVA) last week and is being admitted to a rehabilitation unit in the nursing care center where you work

30. Since you know Mrs. Romirez is arriving by wheelchair, you leave the bed ____________ and ________________ the bed to its ________________.
31. Which necessary equipment would the nursing assistant obtain for Mrs. Romirez as a newly admitted resident?
 A. ____________________
 B. ____________________
 C. ____________________
 D. ____________________
 E. ____________________
 F. ____________________
 G. ____________________
 H. ____________________
 I. ____________________
 J. ____________________
32. When Mrs. Romirez arrives with her husband, it may help them feel more comfortable if you offer them ____________________.
33. You greet Mrs. Romirez by name and ask her if a certain ____________________.
34. Mrs. Romirez has some weakness on her left side and cannot stand alone but can safely transfer from the wheelchair to chairs or the bed. The nurse tells you to weigh Mrs. Romirez with the ______________ scale.

When you arrive at work one day, you are told Mrs. Romirez is being transferred to another nursing unit and you are asked to assist. Answer these questions about transferring her

35. When you transport Mrs. Romirez in a wheelchair, she is covered with a ____________________.
36. What items are taken with Mrs. Romirez to the new unit? ____________________
37. What information is recorded and reported about the transfer?
 A. ____________________
 B. ____________________
 C. ____________________
 D. ____________________
 E. ____________________
 F. ____________________
 G. ____________________

Several weeks later, you are sent to the nursing unit where Mrs. Romirez is living and find she is going home. Answer these questions about her discharge

38. Mrs. Romirez tells you she and her family have been taught about her _______, ____________, ____________, ____________, and ______________.
39. Good communication skills should be used when assisting with the discharge. When Mrs. Romirez and her family leave, you should ____________________.

Use the FOCUS ON PRIDE section to complete these statements and then use the critical thinking and discussion question to develop your ideas

40. When you admit, transfer, or discharge a person, it is your professional responsibility to help the person adjust by
 A. ____________________
 B. ____________________
 C. ____________________
 D. ____________________
 E. ____________________
41. List five ways that you can show care and concern for the family if the person needs privacy during the admission process.
 A. ____________________
 B. ____________________
 C. ____________________
 D. ____________________
 E. ____________________

Critical Thinking and Discussion Question

42. A resident who is newly admitted to a long-term care facility is quiet and seems depressed. She frequently sits by herself and looks out the window. When you ask how she is doing, she says, "I was watching to see if my daughter is coming to take me home." What would you do?

38 Assisting With the Physical Examination

Fill in the Blanks: Key Terms

Dorsal recumbent position (horizontal recumbent position)
Knee-chest position (genupectoral position)
Laryngeal mirror
Lithotomy position
Nasal speculum
Ophthalmoscope
Otoscope
Percussion hammer
Tuning fork
Vaginal speculum

1. An instrument vibrated to test hearing is a ______________________________.
2. In the ______________________, the woman lies on her back with her hips at the edge of the exam table, her knees are flexed, her hips are externally rotated, and her feet are in stirrups.
3. The supine position with the legs together is called the ______________________________.
4. An ______________________ is a lighted instrument used to examine the external ear and the eardrum (tympanic membrane).
5. A ______________________ is an instrument used to open the vagina for examination of the vagina and the cervix.
6. When a person kneels and rests the body on the knees and chest, the head is turned to one side, the arms are above the head or flexed at the elbows, the back is straight, and the body is flexed about 90 degrees at the hip, the person is in the ______________________________.
7. A ______________________ is an instrument used to tap body parts to test reflexes.
8. An instrument used to examine the mouth, teeth, and throat is called a ______________________.
9. An instrument used to examine the inside of the nose is a ______________________________.
10. An ______________________ is a lighted instrument used to examine the internal structures of the eye.

Circle the Best Answer

11. Which nursing assistant needs a reminder about the equipment that should be collected when the nose, mouth, and throat are being examined?
    A. Nursing assistant A hands the doctor a tongue bladder.
    B. Nursing assistant B obtains a nasal speculum.
    C. Nursing assistant C prepares a vaginal speculum.
    D. Nursing assistant D cleans the laryngeal mirror.
12. Which position would be best for an older person who needs to have a rectal examination?
    A. Knee-chest position
    B. Supine position
    C. Side-lying position
    D. Genupectoral position
13. When would residents have a physical examination in a nursing center?
    A. Only when the person is admitted
    B. Once a month
    C. At least once a year
    D. Only when the person is ill
14. Which task would be a nursing assistant responsibility when a person is having a physical examination?
    A. Restraining a person who is confused or struggling
    B. Asking if the person wants a same gender examiner
    C. Explaining why the examination is being done
    D. Positioning and draping the person
15. Which instrument would the doctor need when examining the person's mouth, teeth, and throat?
    A. Ophthalmoscope
    B. Percussion hammer
    C. Tuning fork
    D. Laryngeal mirror
16. Which piece of equipment is most essential in providing privacy for a person who is undergoing a physical examination?
    A. Towel
    B. Waterproof underpad
    C. Drape
    D. Undergarments
17. What are the parents generally encouraged to do when a child is examined?
    A. Leave during painful procedures
    B. Stay and provide support for child
    C. Assist the examiner if staying in the room
    D. Stay if the examiner has questions
18. Which rationale supports the importance of having a person empty the bladder before an examination?
    A. An empty bladder allows the examiner to feel the abdominal organs.
    B. A full bladder may cause the person to be incontinent.
    C. A urine specimen is always collected before an examination.
    D. A full bladder will cause the person to have intense pain.
19. Which action would promote safety during an exam?
    A. Tell the person how to put on the gown
    B. Have an extra bath blanket
    C. Screen the person or close the door
    D. Stay with the person
20. Which action would the nursing assistant use after escorting the person to the exam room and positioning the person?
    A. Put on the call light for the examiner
    B. Leave the room so the person has privacy
    C. Go to the examiner to report that the person is ready
    D. Open the door to alert the examiner

21. Which position will the nursing assistant place the person in when the abdomen, chest, and breasts need to be examined?
    A. Lithotomy position
    B. Genupectoral position
    C. Dorsal recumbent position
    D. Knee-chest position
22. Which action would the nursing assistant perform if a person has to stand on the floor during an exam?
    A. Assist the person to put on shoes
    B. Place paper towels on the floor
    C. Place a clean sheet on the floor
    D. Wipe the floor with antiseptic cleaner
23. Which piece of equipment would the nursing assistant need to collect when the ears are being examined?
    A. Snellen chart
    B. Otoscope
    C. Percussion hammer
    D. Laryngeal mirror
24. Which piece of equipment is needed to examine the eyes?
    A. Ophthalmoscope
    B. Nasal speculum
    C. Pulse oximeter
    D. Tuning fork
25. Which person should be in the examination room when a male doctor needs to exam a female patient?
    A. First available staff member
    B. Patient's partner
    C. Female nursing assistant
    D. Male nurse
26. Which action would the nursing assistant take when instructed by the nurse to prepare the patient for a vaginal examination, but the patient declines the procedure because he identifies as a male?
    A. Ask the patient what type of examination he prefers
    B. Tell the patient that the doctor has ordered this examination
    C. Report the patient's comments and decision to the nurse
    D. Respect the patient's wishes and allow him to rest

Fill in the Blanks

27. What are the three purposes of physical examination?
    A. ______________________________
    B. ______________________________
    C. ______________________________
28. What concerns may the person have about the physical examination?
    A. ______________________________
    B. ______________________________
    C. ______________________________
29. When you are delegated the job of preparing a person for an exam, what information do you need from the nurse and the care plan?
    A. ______________________________
    B. ______________________________
    C. ______________________________
    D. ______________________________
    E. ______________________________
    F. ______________________________
30. When you are delegated the job of preparing a person for an exam, why do you need the following information?
    A. The time of the examination. ______________________________
    B. What are the two reasons it would be helpful to know which examinations will be done?
    ____
    C. What equipment will you need if you are assigned to take vital signs? ______________________________

Labeling

Look at the instruments and answer the questions

31. Name the instruments.

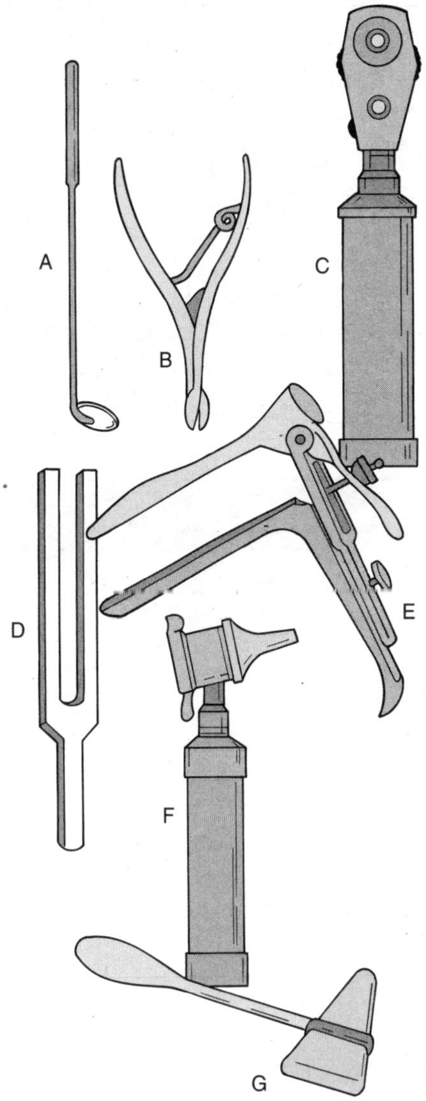

A. ______________________________
B. ______________________________
C. ______________________________
D. ______________________________
E. ______________________________
F. ______________________________
G. ______________________________

32. Which instrument is used to examine the nose? ________________________________

33. When the eye is examined, the examiner uses the ________________________________.

34. If a person has a sore throat, the examiner will look at the throat with the ________________________________.

35. The reflexes are examined by using the ____________.

Look at the positions and answer these questions.

A

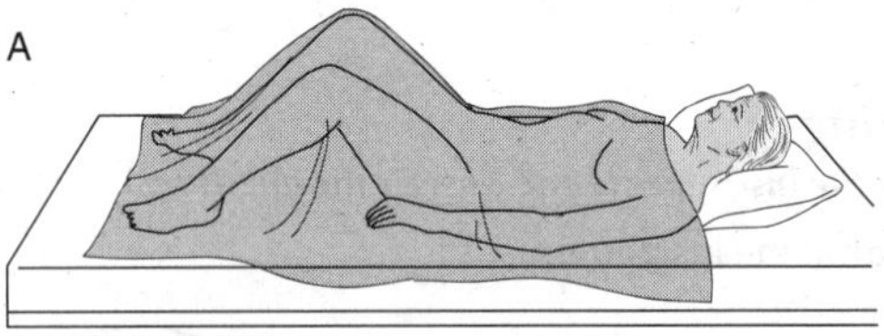

B

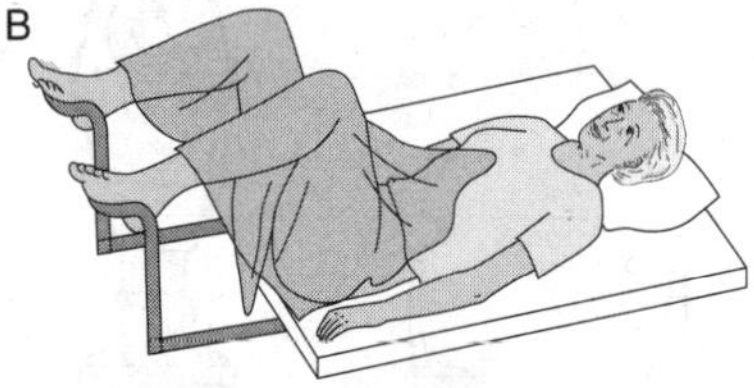

C

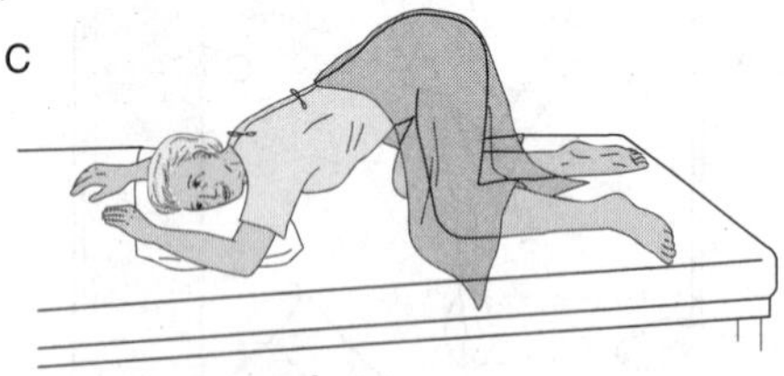

D

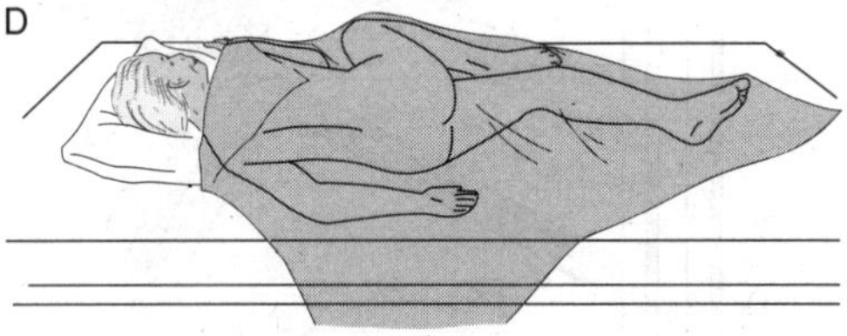

36. Name the positions.
    A. ________________________________
    B. ________________________________
    C. ________________________________
    D. ________________________________

37. Which positions may be used when a rectal examination is done?
    A. ________________________________
    B. ________________________________

38. When the abdomen, chest, and breasts are examined, the person is placed in ________________________________.

39. The ________________________________ position is used for a vaginal exam.

Use the FOCUS ON PRIDE section to complete these statements and then use the critical thinking and discussion questions to develop your ideas

40. Fears about the exam affect the person's well-being. List at least four common questions that the person might have or wonder about.
    A. ________________________________
    B. ________________________________
    C. ________________________________
    D. ________________________________

41. What could you do to ease a person's fears about examination?
    A. ________________________________
    B. ________________________________
    C. ________________________________

Critical Thinking and Discussion Questions

42. A nursing assistant that you work with tells you to check out her social media posting. In the posting she describes helping an examiner with a vaginal examination. She does not reveal any names or dates but gives explicit details about the examiner's findings and observations. Discuss this situation, from different viewpoints:
    A. The nursing assistant who posted
    B. The unnamed person who had the vaginal examination
    C. What would you do if your friends and coworkers told you they are posting stories about work on social media?

39 Collecting and Testing Specimens

Fill in the Blanks: Key Terms

Glucometer	Hemoptysis	Sputum
Glucosuria	Ketone (acetone, ketone body)	
Hematoma	Melena	
Hematuria		

1. Bloody sputum is ______________________________.
2. A swelling that contains blood is a _______________.
3. A black, tarry stool is __________________________.
4. ____________ is sugar in the urine.
5. ____________ is mucus from the respiratory system that is expectorated through the mouth.
6. ____________ is a substance that appears in urine from the rapid breakdown of fat for energy.
7. ____________ is blood in the urine.
8. A device for measuring blood glucose is a _________.

Circle the Best Answer

9. Which nursing measure would the nursing assistant use to clean the female perineum for a midstream specimen?
   A. Use a peri-bottle and flush the perineum
   B. Assist the patient to take a shower
   C. Use a towelette and wipe from front to back
   D. Ask patient to wipe perineum with toilet paper
10. How much urine is usually collected for a random urine specimen?
   A. 2 mL
   B. 10 mL
   C. 120 mL
   D. 500 mL
11. Which piece of equipment, in addition to the test kit, does the nursing assistant need for an occult blood test on a stool specimen?
   A. Glucometer
   B. Tongue blades
   C. Gauze sponges
   D. Lancet
12. When would the nursing assistant apply the label to the specimen container for a midstream urine specimen?
   A. At the nurses' station in the presence of the nurse
   B. Before the specimen is collected in the presence of the person
   C. After putting the specimen container in the biohazard bag
   D. After the specimen is collected in the presence of the person
13. Which part of the collection system can the nursing assistant touch with a nonsterile gloved hand when collecting a specimen?
   A. It depends on the type of specimen being collected.
   B. The inside of the lid
   C. The inside of the container
   D. The outside of the biohazard bag
14. In which circumstance would the nursing assistant need to wear a respirator when collecting the specimen?
   A. Sputum specimen from a person who might have tuberculosis
   B. Random urine specimen from a person who might have a urinary tract infection
   C. Stool specimen from a person who might have infectious diarrhea
   D. Blood glucose from a person who might have acquired immunodeficiency syndrome
15. When is a random urine specimen collected?
   A. First thing in the morning
   B. After meals
   C. At any time
   D. At bedtime
16. Which instruction would the nursing assistant give to the person who is collecting a random urine specimen?
   A. Dispose of the toilet paper in the toilet
   B. Add the toilet paper to the specimen container
   C. Put the toilet paper in the specimen pan
   D. Place used toilet paper in the bedpan
17. Why is it important to carefully clean the perineal area when obtaining a midstream specimen?
   A. To remove all microbes from the perineal area
   B. To reduce the number of microbes in the urethral area
   C. To follow Standard Precautions and the Bloodborne Pathogen Standard
   D. To reduce patient's risk for urinary tract infection
18. Which nursing measure would the nursing assistant use when collecting a midstream specimen?
   A. Collect the entire amount of urine voided just before bedtime
   B. Collect about 4 oz (120 mL) of urine from the first morning void
   C. Have the person void, then stop, position the sterile specimen cup, and void into the cup
   D. Collect several specimens and add them to the specimen cup, until the cup is filled

19. Where is the urine kept when collecting a 24-hour urine specimen?
    A. Chilled on ice or refrigerated
    B. At room temperature in the bathroom
    C. In a sterile container at the nurses' station
    D. In a drainage collection bag at the bedside
20. When is a 24-hour urine specimen collection started?
    A. At the beginning of a shift
    B. After breakfast before showering
    C. At night just before going to bed
    D. After the person voids and that urine is discarded
21. Which action would the nursing assistant use at the end of 24-hour specimen collection?
    A. Ask the person to void and save the urine
    B. Report and record any missed or spilled urine
    C. Report and record the amount of urine collected
    D. Ask the person to void and discard that urine
22. How is a urine specimen obtained from infants or very young children?
    A. Inserting a straight catheter
    B. Using a collection bag applied over the urethra
    C. Having the parent hold the child on a potty chair until the child voids
    D. Applying a diaper and then squeezing the urine out of the diaper
23. When would the nursing assistant offer oral fluids to help the child to void a urine specimen?
    A. 5 to 10 minutes before the test
    B. 30 minutes before the test
    C. 1 hour before the test
    D. While obtaining the specimen
24. Which action would the nursing assistant use when testing urine with a reagent strip?
    A. Follow the manufacturer's instructions
    B. Use a sterile urine specimen
    C. Wear sterile gloves
    D. Make sure the urine is cold
25. Which nursing measure would the nursing assistant use when assigned to strain a person's urine?
    A. Have the person void directly into the strainer and then measure the urine
    B. Collect all urine and save it so that it can be sent to the laboratory
    C. Have the person void into the voiding device and then pour the urine through the strainer
    D. Discard the strainer if it contains stones and obtain a new one for the next voiding
26. Which action would the nursing assistant use if a warm stool specimen is required?
    A. Place specimen in an insulated container
    B. Store specimen on the nursing unit until the end of the shift
    C. Test the sample at once on the nursing unit
    D. Take the sample at once to the laboratory or the storage area
27. Which nursing measure would the nursing assistant use when collecting a stool specimen?
    A. Ask the person to void and have a bowel movement in a bedpan
    B. Offer only a bedpan or commode to collect the specimen
    C. Ask the person to urinate into the toilet and collect the stool in the specimen pan
    D. Have the person place the toilet tissue in the bedpan with the stool
28. Which nursing measure would the nursing assistant use when collecting the stool specimen?
    A. Pour it into the specimen container and use a tongue blade to collect remaining stool from collection device
    B. Use gloved hand to obtain a specimen, place the stool in the container, remove gloves, and perform hand hygiene
    C. Use a tongue blade to take about 2 tablespoons of stool from the middle of the formed stool
    D. Use a tongue blade to scoop the entire stool specimen from the collection device into the specimen container
29. Which action would the nursing assistant use when testing a stool specimen for occult blood?
    A. It must be sent to the laboratory.
    B. The specimen must be sterile.
    C. Test the entire stool specimen
    D. Use a tongue blade to make a thin smear of stool on the test card
30. When is the best time for the nursing assistant to collect a sputum specimen?
    A. Upon awakening
    B. After eating
    C. At bedtime
    D. After activity
31. Which instruction would the nursing assistant give the patient before obtaining a sputum specimen?
    A. Rinse the mouth with clear water
    B. Brush the teeth and use mouthwash
    C. Cough and discard the first sputum expectorated
    D. Walk around for a short time to stimulate secretions
32. What is the purpose of performing postural drainage before collecting a sputum specimen?
    A. To ensure sterile specimens
    B. To liquefy the sputum specimen
    C. To stimulate coughing
    D. To help secretions drain by gravity
33. Which task would the nursing assistant be assigned to perform if a sputum specimen is needed from an infant or small child?
    A. Position the child for postural drainage
    B. Hold the child's head and arms still
    C. Suction the sputum from the trachea
    D. Give the child a breathing treatment

34. What is the most common site for testing blood glucose?
    A. The earlobe
    B. A fingertip
    C. The forearm
    D. The abdomen
35. Which rationale supports doing glucose testing at correct times?
    A. The results are needed before certain drugs are given.
    B. The results determine how much the person is allowed to eat.
    C. A low blood glucose in the morning is a danger sign.
    D. It must be done at a time when the person is not sleeping.
36. Where would the nursing assistant start when cleaning the penis and perineum for a male patient who needs a midstream specimen?
    A. Around the foreskin
    B. Around the groin
    C. At the meatus
    D. At the base of the shaft
37. Which information is marked on the room and bathroom container labels for a 24-hour urine collection?
    A. Name of the doctor who ordered the test
    B. Initials of nursing assistant collecting the urine
    C. Amount of urine collected each time
    D. The time the test began and the time it ended.
38. Which nursing assistant has used the correct method to read a reagent strip?
    A. Nursing assistant A gives the reagent strip to the nurse.
    B. Nursing assistant B compares the strip to the color chart on the bottle.
    C. Nursing assistant C places a drop of developer on the strip.
    D. Nursing assistant D inserts the strip into the lancet device.
39. Which nursing assistant needs a reminder about observations related to using a strainer in the urine specimen container?
    A. Nursing assistant A looks for and reports crystals.
    B. Nursing assistant B observes for and records stones.
    C. Nursing assistant C reports patient's refusal to strain urine.
    D. Nursing assistant D strains only the first morning void.
40. What is the probable source of bleeding when stools are black and tarry?
    A. Perineal area
    B. Rectum
    C. Urinary bladder
    D. Upper gastrointestinal tract
41. Which nursing assistant has performed a correct step in obtaining a sputum specimen?
    A. Nursing assistant A instructs patient to rinse with mouthwash before giving sputum.
    B. Nursing assistant B tells patient to spit saliva into the specimen container.
    C. Nursing assistant C has the patient rinse the mouth with water before giving sputum.
    D. Nursing assistant D has patient put on a respirator mask before producing sputum.
42. Which nursing assistant has correctly chosen a site to test for blood glucose?
    A. Nursing assistant A punctures an index finger that is swollen.
    B. Nursing assistant B uses a side toward the tip of the ring finger.
    C. Nursing assistant C selects a site on a finger with a thick callous.
    D. Nursing assistant D uses the center, fleshy part of the fingertip.
43. Which patient is most likely to need a test for ketones?
    A. Patient A has diabetes.
    B. Patient B has a kidney stone.
    C. Patient C has tarry stool.
    D. Patient D had a breathing treatment.
44. Which stool characteristics would the nursing assistant expect to observe in a stool specimen when the nurse instructs to test for occult blood?
    A. Bright red blood around stool
    B. Large blood clots mixed in stool
    C. Normal brown color of stool
    D. Deep red stool with red mucus

Fill in the Blanks

45. Write out the abbreviations
    A. BM ________________
    B. I&O ________________
    C. mL ________________
    D. oz ________________
    E. U/A ________________
46. When collecting a midstream urine specimen, the person may not be able to stop voiding. If so, you will pass the specimen container into the ________________.
47. When you are obtaining a midstream specimen from a female, spread the labia with your thumb and index finger with your ________________ hand.
48. Urine pH measures if the urine is ________________ or ________________.
49. When you strain urine, you are looking for stones that can develop in the ________________.

50. When collecting urine specimens, what observations are reported and recorded?
A. ____________________
B. ____________________
C. ____________________
D. ____________________
E. ____________________
F. ____________________

51. List five substances that may be detected in a stool specimen.
A. ____________________
B. ____________________
C. ____________________
D. ____________________
E. ____________________

52. When you are delegated to collect a stool specimen, what observations are reported and recorded?
A. ____________________
B. ____________________
C. ____________________
D. ____________________
E. ____________________

53. When you are assisting a person to collect a sputum specimen, ask the person to take two or three ____________ and ____________ the sputum.

54. What would the nursing assistant report and record when delegated to collect a sputum specimen?
A. ____________________
B. ____________________
C. ____________________
D. ____________________
E. ____________________
F. ____________________
G. ____________________
H. ____________________
I. ____________________

55. What would the nursing assistant report and record when testing for blood glucose?
A. ____________________
B. ____________________
C. ____________________
D. ____________________
E. ____________________
F. ____________________
G. ____________________

Optional Learning Exercises

56. If you are collecting a midstream specimen, what should you do if it is hard for the person to stop the stream of urine? ____________________

57. You are caring for a person who is having a 24-hour urine specimen test. He tells you he forgot to save a specimen an hour ago. What should you do and why?
____

58. What is normal pH for urine? ____________ What can cause changes in the normal pH? ____________

59. When the body cannot use sugar for energy, it uses fat. When this happens ____________________
____________________ appear in the urine.

60. Why is privacy important when collecting a sputum specimen? ____________________
____

Use the FOCUS ON PRIDE section to complete these statements

61. When collecting a specimen, you are responsible to correctly ____________ the person.

62. What can you do respect the person's right to privacy when collecting specimens?
A. ____________________
B. ____________________
C. ____________________

Critical Thinking and Discussion Questions

63. The nurse instructed you to get a midstream urine specimen from an older overweight woman. You explained how to collect the specimen, but she was not able to spread the labia and clean and maintain the hand position. You tried to assist her, but cleaning and maintaining the hand position was still not achieved.
A. What would you tell the nurse? ____________________
____
B. Why is it important to report this to the nurse? ____
____

Crossword

Fill in the crossword by answering the clues below with the words from this list

Calculi	Expectorated	Midstream	Postural	Specimens
Dysuria	Labia	Occult	Random	Suctioning

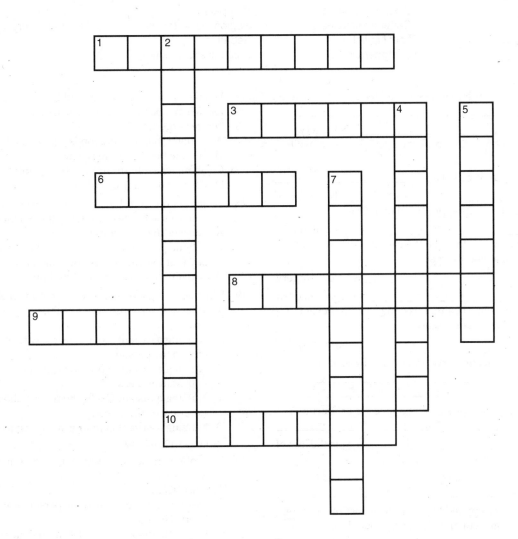

Across

1. Samples
3. Urine specimen that can be collected at any time
6. Hidden, as in blood in stool
8. Drainage position with head lower than body used to cause fluid to flow downward
9. Folds of tissue on each side of the vagina
10. Pain when urinating

Down

2. Expelled, as in sputum through the mouth
4. Urine specimen that is collected after the person starts to void
5. Stones that develop in kidneys, ureters, or bladder
7. Nurse may withdraw or suck out sputum from a child's trachea to obtain a specimen

40 The Person Having Surgery

Fill in the Blanks: Key Terms

Anesthesia	Emergency surgery	Preoperative	Thrombus
Antiseptic	General anesthesia	Regional anesthesia	Urgent surgery
Elective surgery	Local anesthesia	Sedation	
Embolus	Postoperative	Surgical site infection	

1. The loss of consciousness and all feeling or sensation is ______________________________.
2. ______________________________ is surgery done by choice to improve the person's life or well-being.
3. A blood clot is called a ______________________________.
4. ______________________________ is the loss of feeling or sensation produced by a drug.
5. An ______________________________ is a blood clot that travels through the vascular system until it lodges in a blood vessel.
6. ______________________________ is before surgery.
7. ______________________________ is surgery needed for the person's health. It is done soon to prevent further damage or disease.
8. ______________________________ is after surgery.
9. The loss of feeling or sensation in a large area of the body is ______________________________.
10. Surgery done immediately to save life or function is ______________________________.
11. ______________________________ is the loss of feeling or sensation in a small area.
12. A state of quiet, calmness, or sleep produced by a drug is ______________________________.
13. A substance applied to living tissue that prevents or stops the growth or action of microbes is an ______________________________.
14. An infection that occurs after surgery in the body part where the surgery took place is a ______________________________.

Circle the Best Answer

15. Which type of surgery can be delayed for a few days?
    A. Emergency surgery
    B. Elective surgery
    C. Urgent surgery
    D. Outpatient surgery
16. Which person would require emergency surgery?
    A. Person A desires a cosmetic facial procedure.
    B. Person B was in a serious motor vehicle accident.
    C. Person C needs knee replacement.
    D. Person D fell and broke her wrist.
17. Which nursing measure would the nursing assistant use when a person expresses fears and concerns before surgery?
    A. Explain that the surgeon is very skilled
    B. Tell the person not to worry
    C. Show warmth, sensitivity, and caring
    D. Change the subject and talk about something else
18. Which action would the nursing assistant take when a patient asks about test results or the diagnosis?
    A. Answer the questions honestly
    B. Tell the person that the nurse can explain
    C. Say that information is not available
    D. Explain that someone will find out
19. Which nursing assistant needs a reminder about the roles and responsibilities of caring for a surgical patient?
    A. Nursing assistant A explains the care that she will give to the person.
    B. Nursing assistant B provides preoperative care with skill and ease.
    C. Nursing assistant C tells the person about her own experience with surgery.
    D. Nursing assistant D reports a request to see the clergy to the nurse.
20. How often are deep breathing and coughing exercises done after surgery?
    A. Once a shift
    B. Every 1 or 2 hours when the person is awake
    C. Every 4 hours
    D. Every 2 hours for the first 48 hours after surgery
21. How is a child prepared for surgery?
    A. The parents are responsible for explaining the surgery to the child.
    B. A doll may be used to show the site of the surgery.
    C. Children are told an imaginary story about the surgery.
    D. The child is introduced to another child who had the same surgery.
22. Which test is done preoperatively if blood loss is expected during surgery?
    A. Type and crossmatch
    B. Complete blood count
    C. Urinalysis
    D. Electrocardiogram

23. Why does the doctor order the patient to have nothing by mouth (NPO) for 6 to 8 hours before surgery?
    A. To reduce breathing problems after surgery
    B. To eliminate pain postoperatively
    C. To decrease diarrhea and flatulence postoperatively
    D. To prevent vomiting and aspiration during and after surgery
24. What is the purpose of giving a cleansing enema to the patient before surgery?
    A. To reduce contamination of the abdominal cavity during surgery
    B. To reduce incontinence during and after surgery
    C. To decrease the risk for infectious diarrhea after surgery
    D. To avoid abdominal pain and constipation after surgery
25. When does the person who is being prepared for surgery need to void?
    A. Right before going to the operating room
    B. The morning of surgery
    C. Before the nurse gives the preoperative drugs
    D. Before an enema is given
26. Why are makeup, nail polish, and fake nails removed before surgery?
    A. These artificial substances are sources of infection
    B. It reduces the number of microbes on the body
    C. Skin, lips, and nail beds are observed for color during and after surgery
    D. A baseline appearance needs to be established before surgery
27. What is the most important observation for the nursing assistant to report when preparing a child for surgery?
    A. A dry mouth
    B. Any loose teeth
    C. Any missing teeth
    D. Last oral hygiene
28. Which action would the nursing assistant use if a person is allowed to wear a wedding ring during surgery?
    A. Record this information on the chart
    B. Secure it according to agency policy
    C. Make sure it fits well and will not come off
    D. Put a clean glove on the person's hand
29. Which task is the nursing assistant most likely to be assigned related to the preoperative skin preparation for a person who will have surgery in the perineal area?
    A. Clean the perineum and surrounding area with antiseptic
    B. Use a razor and carefully shave away the pubic hair
    C. Mark the surgical site with a waterproof ink pen
    D. Assist the person to take a shower with special soap
30. What would the nursing assistant do when patient says, "I didn't understand what the surgeon said about the risks and complications"?
    A. Check to see if the surgical consent was signed by the patient
    B. Report the patient's concerns to the nurse
    C. Call the surgeon and explain what the person said
    D. Reassure the patient that the surgeon is experienced
31. When are preoperative medications given?
    A. After the person gets up to void
    B. At a time specified by the checklist
    C. Before the person takes a shower
    D. After the person is assisted to the stretcher
32. When must the nursing assistant's portion of the preoperative checklist be completed?
    A. Before the nurse gives the preoperative drugs
    B. Before the consent form is signed and completed
    C. Just before the patient leaves the unit for surgery
    D. The night before the surgery
33. Which preoperative action helps to reduce the incidence of surgical site infection?
    A. Assisting with a complete bath with special cleanser
    B. Helping the person to follow nil per os (NPO) instructions
    C. Removing, cleaning, and storing dentures
    D. Correctly applying antiembolic stockings
34. Which equipment will the nursing assistant obtain when preparing the room for a person who will soon be transferred from post-anesthesia care unit (PACU)?
    A. Kidney basin
    B. Elastic bandage
    C. Gauze sponges
    D. Extra pillow
35. Which nursing measure will the nursing assistant perform when preparing a room for a person to return from surgery?
    A. Raise the head of the bed and the side rails
    B. Put the bed in the lowest position
    C. Raise the bed for a transfer from a stretcher
    D. Make the bed using sterile sheets and blankets
36. When are the vital signs usually measured for postoperative patients?
    A. Once a shift
    B. Every 15 minutes until the person is stable
    C. Every 2 hours
    D. Every 5 minutes for the first hour
37. Which goal is the priority when positioning the person who is postoperative?
    A. To meet the preference of the person
    B. To allow for easy and comfortable breathing
    C. To allow for independence of movement
    D. To provide for easy turning and repositioning
38. What is the purpose of the coughing and deep breathing exercises that are done after surgery?
    A. To decrease hemorrhage and hypovolemia
    B. To prevent pneumonia and atelectasis
    C. To alleviate pain and discomfort
    D. To decrease the risk for nausea and vomiting
39. What is the main purpose of assisting a postsurgical patient with leg exercises?
    A. To discourage staying in bed
    B. To prevent thrombus and embolus (blood clots)
    C. To decrease pain at the surgical site
    D. To counteract low blood pressure

40. How often would the nursing assistant assist with leg exercises?
    A. At least every 1 to 2 hours while the person is awake
    B. Once in the morning and once in the evening
    C. When the person has leg cramps or discomfort
    D. After the person begins to independently ambulate
41. What is the purpose of elastic stockings?
    A. Prevent weakness and discomfort in the legs
    B. Prevent hypertension and dizziness
    C. Promote blood return to the heart and prevent blood clots
    D. Give support to the legs when ambulation begins
42. Which instruction will the nursing assistant give to the patient when applying elastic stockings?
    A. "Please lie in a supine position."
    B. "Please sit down in the chair."
    C. "Please lean slightly forward."
    D. "Please walk around the room before we start."
43. Which action will the nursing assistant use when applying elastic bandages?
    A. Start at the proximal part of the extremity
    B. Completely cover the fingers or toes
    C. Use a figure-eight pattern
    D. Expose the fingers and toes if possible
44. Which measurement would the nursing assistant perform before assisting a person to walk after surgery?
    A. The person's temperature
    B. The blood pressure and pulse
    C. The distance from the bed to the door
    D. The person's weight
45. Which comfort and hygiene measure would the nursing assistant offer if a patient is nil per os (NPO) after surgery?
    A. Give frequent oral hygiene
    B. Offer ice chips frequently
    C. Offer sips of cool water
    D. Give a complete bed bath
46. When must the person void after surgery?
    A. Within 2 hours after surgery
    B. During the first 24 hours after surgery
    C. Within 8 hours after surgery
    D. At least 1000 mL within the first 4 hours after surgery
47. What can the nursing assistant do to promote dignity and self-esteem when dentures must be removed before surgery?
    A. Compliment appearance after dentures are removed
    B. Let them wear dentures for as long as possible
    C. Talk about how long they have been wearing dentures
    D. Help them brush and clean dentures after removal
48. Which patient activity is discouraged after the preoperative drugs are given?
    A. Talking about the surgery
    B. Calling friends or family
    C. Getting out of bed
    D. Asking to see the doctor
49. Which postsurgical patient may the nursing assistant be able to turn without assistance from a coworker?
    A. Patient A has always been very independent.
    B. Patient B says the other nursing assistant never needs help.
    C. Patient C is stable and the care is simple.
    D. Patient D is very anxious to be repositioned.
50. Why are older persons at risk for respiratory complications?
    A. Lung tissue is less elastic.
    B. Respiratory muscles are stronger.
    C. Older people cannot follow postoperative instructions.
    D. Older people are confused.
51. How many repetitions for each type of leg exercise does the nursing assistant usually perform?
    A. 2 times
    B. 5 times
    C. 10 times
    D. 20 times
52. Which nursing assistant needs retraining related to leg exercises that are done postoperatively to promote venous blood flow and to prevent thrombi?
    A. Nursing assistant A suggests that the patient circle with the toes to rotate the ankles.
    B. Nursing assistant B helps the patient to do low squats at the bedside.
    C. Nursing assistant C has the patient to dorsiflex and plantar flex the feet.
    D. Nursing assistant D asks the patient to flex and extend one knee and then the other.
53. Which complication can occur if the nursing assistant fails to smooth out the creases and wrinkles when applying elastic stockings?
    A. Can cause embarrassment
    B. Interferes with toileting
    C. Increases risk for falls
    D. Can cause skin breakdown
54. What is the purpose of sequential compression devices?
    A. Meets the standard of care for postsurgical patients
    B. Stimulates the circulation to promote rapid healing
    C. Massages the lower extremities to decrease pain and stiffness
    D. Promotes venous blood flow to the heart by causing pressure on the veins
55. Why is it important to make sure that the sequential compression device is plugged in and functioning?
    A. Risk for blood clots increases if the pump is not working.
    B. Patient does not know how to monitor or use the device.
    C. This is included in the nursing assistant's job description.
    D. Pain and discomfort increase when the pump is off.

Fill in the Blanks

56. Write out the abbreviations
    A. AE ______
    B. ASC ______
    C. CBC ______
    D. ECG; EKG ______
    E. IV ______
    F. NG ______
    G. NPO ______
    H. OR ______
    I. PACU ______
    J. Pre-op ______
    K. Post-op ______
    L. SCD ______
    M. SSI ______
    N. TED ______
57. If a person has outpatient, 1-day, or ambulatory surgery, the person is admitted in the morning and ______.
58. Before surgery, special personal care is done. Describe the care given and the reasons it is important.
    A. Baths ______
    B. Removing makeup, nail polish, and fake nails ______
    C. Hair care ______
    D. Oral hygiene ______
59. When you are delegated to apply elastic stockings, what information do you need from the nurse?
    A. ______
    B. ______
    C. ______
    D. ______
60. Which vital signs are recorded on the preoperative checklist ______
61. List the sequence and frequency for how often vital signs are usually done for postoperative patients when the patient returns to the unit after surgery.
    A. ______
    B. ______
    C. ______
    D. ______
62. What postoperative observations of the vital signs should be reported to the nurse?
    A. Temperature ______
    B. Pulse
       i. ______
       ii. ______
       iii. ______
       iv. ______
    C. Respirations
       i. ______
       ii. ______
       iii. ______
       iv. ______
       v. ______
       vi. ______
       vii. ______
    D. Blood pressure ______
63. When you apply elastic bandages, what observations are reported and recorded?
    A. ______
    B. ______
    C. ______
    D. ______
    E. ______
    F. ______
    G. ______
    H. ______
64. What complications can be prevented with early ambulation?
    A. ______
    B. ______
    C. ______
    D. ______
    E. ______

Optional Learning Exercises

Mr. Shafer is an 82-year-old man admitted for knee replacement surgery. Answer the following questions about Mr. Shafer and his preoperative care

65. This surgery is done by choice and is an ______ surgery.
66. When you are in the room, you listen quietly while Mr. Shafer talks about his fears and concerns. By sitting quietly and showing concern for his feelings, you can assist in Mr. Shafer's ______ care.

67. The nurse teaches Mr. Shafer about what to expect. What preoperative topics will the nurse cover?
A. ____________________
B. ____________________
C. ____________________
D. ____________________
E. ____________________
F. ____________________
G. ____________________
H. ____________________
I. ____________________
J. ____________________

68. The nurse tells you she will give Mr. Shafer his preoperative drugs in 10 minutes. What should you do?
____

Mrs. Johnson is a 70-year-old woman who is scheduled for abdominal surgery. Answer the following questions about her care

69. The nurse tells you she is busy and asks you to have Mrs. Johnson sign the surgery consent. What should you do? ____________________
____

70. Mrs. Johnson returns to her room 2 hours after the surgery is completed. What patient conditions must be present before she is transported to her room?
A. ____________________
B. ____________________
C. ____________________

71. How is the room prepared for Mrs. Johnson's return?
A. ____________________
B. ____________________
C. ____________________

72. You are caring for Mrs. Johnson 3 days after her surgery. She tells you she has not had a bowel movement since before surgery. You know that one reason for constipation can be drugs given for
____________________.

Matching

Instructions: Match the postoperative complication with the observation that is most likely to signal the complication.

Complication	Observation
73. _____ Pneumonia	a. Increased temperature
74. _____ Hypovolemic shock	b. Cannot void
75. _____ Thrombus	c. Weak rapid pulse
76. _____ Urinary retention	d. Shortness of breath
77. _____ Wound infection	e. Discomfort and swelling in calf

Labeling

78. Describe the correct application of an elastic bandage as depicted in the figure.

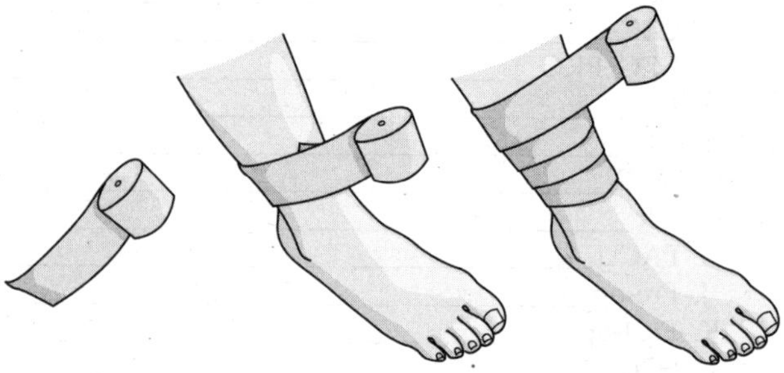

____
____
____
____
____

Use the FOCUS ON PRIDE section to complete these statements and then use the critical thinking and discussion questions to develop your ideas

79. How can you ease a person's fears and concerns related to an upcoming surgery?
A. ____________________
B. ____________________
C. ____________________
D. ____________________

80. What questions can you answer when caring for a person having surgery? ____________________
____
____

81. When you are delegated to take postoperative vital signs, what should you report at once to the nurse?
A. ____________________
B. ____________________
C. ____________________

Critical Thinking and Discussion Questions

82. You and the nurse are very busy. You are assigned to assist the nurse with three patients who need postoperative care.
Patient A had surgery on her leg 2 days ago. Today the surgical site is red and painful. The drainage has a foul odor. She appears flushed and her skin is hot to the touch.
Patient B had abdominal surgery this morning. She is confused and disoriented. Her skin is pale and cool. Her abdomen is distended and she says it hurts.
Patient C had surgery for a broken wrist this morning. She says the pain was relieved by the pain medication. She tells you she is "ready to eat and drink something, take a brief nap and go home as soon as possible."
A. Which patient needs attention from you and the nurse first?
B. Discuss your decision and what you think might be happening to each patient.

41 Wound Care

Fill in the Blanks: Key Terms

Abrasion
Arterial ulcer (ischemic ulcer)
Avulsion
Chronic wound
Circulatory ulcer (vascular ulcer)
Diabetic foot ulcer
Excoriation
Incision
Laceration
Penetrating wound
Puncture wound
Purulent drainage
Sanguineous drainage
Serosanguineous drainage
Serous drainage
Skin tear
Stasis ulcer (venous ulcer)
Ulcer
Wound

1. A ________________ is a break or rip in the skin that separates the epidermis from underlying tissues.
2. An open wound with clean, straight edges, usually intentional from a sharp instrument, is an ________________.
3. A shallow or deep craterlike sore of the skin or mucous membrane is an ________________.
4. ________________ is thick green, yellow, or brown drainage.
5. A ________________ is damage to the skin or mucous membrane.
6. An ________________ is a partial thickness wound caused by the scraping away or rubbing of the skin from friction or trauma.
7. A ________________ is an open wound on the foot caused by complications from diabetes.
8. Thin, watery drainage that is blood-tinged is called ________________.
9. An open sore on the lower legs or feet caused by decreased blood flow through arteries or veins is a ________________.
10. A ________________ is a wound with torn tissues and jagged edges caused by trauma.
11. An ________________ is an open wound on the lower legs and feet caused by poor arterial blood flow.
12. Clear, watery fluid is ________________.
13. A ________________ is a wound that does not heal easily.
14. An open sore on the lower legs or feet caused by poor blood flow through the veins is a ________________.
15. A wound caused by a piercing from a pointed object is a ________________.
16. A ________________ is a wound caused by an object that breaks the skin and enters a body area, organ, or cavity.
17. A wound that occurs when skin or tissue is torn away is an ________________.
18. ________________ is damage to the epidermis (top skin layer) caused by scratching.
19. Bloody drainage is called ________________.

Circle the Best Answer

20. Which action would the nursing assistant use to prevent skin tears when lifting and turning the person?
    A. Ask the nurse for help
    B. Roll the person
    C. Use an assist device
    D. Ask person to turn self
21. Which skin condition would the nursing assistant report and record upon observing that the skin on the elbow appears rubbed away?
    A. A laceration
    B. An abrasion
    C. An ulcer
    D. An incision
22. Which skin condition would the nursing assistant report and record when a resident's arm is caught on the chair and the tissue is torn with jagged edges?
    A. Puncture wound
    B. Abrasion
    C. Penetrating wound
    D. Laceration
23. Which person has the greatest risk for skin tears?
    A. Person A is obese and requires help with bathing.
    B. Person B is thin, confused, and requires total help to move.
    C. Person C needs help to eat and drink.
    D. Person D has episodic confusion but is ambulatory
24. Which rationale supports applying lotion to help prevent skin breakdown or skin tears?
    A. Inhibits loss of fatty layer
    B. Reverses thinning of the skin
    C. Decreases dryness of the skin
    D. Prevents excoriation of the skin
25. What causes ulcers of the feet and legs?
    A. Poor hygiene and poor nutrition
    B. Decreased blood flow through arteries or veins
    C. Walking on concrete or paved surfaces
    D. Obesity and lack of exercise

26. Which nursing measure would the nursing assistant use to help prevent venous (stasis) ulcers?
    A. Secure the person's socks tightly in place
    B. Remind the person not to sit with the legs crossed
    C. Dry the skin vigorously to stimulate circulation
    D. Massage the legs and feet after bathing
27. Which action would be best for the prevention of arterial ulcers?
    A. Encourage the person to wear warm socks
    B. Support the person's efforts to stop smoking
    C. Assist the person to stand up and walk
    D. Help to the person to prepare for rest and sleep
28. Which rationale supports checking the feet of a person with diabetes every day?
    A. Diabetes can mask sensation of an injury to the foot.
    B. People with diabetes cannot check their own feet.
    C. Diabetes makes is difficult to achieve good hygiene.
    D. People with diabetes have poor nutrition.
29. Which suggestion would the nursing assistant give to a person with diabetes?
    A. Apply cream or petroleum jelly to toes
    B. Use a heating pad to stimulate circulation
    C. Wear athletic or walking shoes
    D. Soak feet in water to keep skin moisturized
30. When would signs and symptoms of inflammation: redness, swelling, heat or warmth, and pain be considered normal and expected?
    A. During phase 1 of wound healing
    B. During phase 3 of wound healing
    C. Recently discovered diabetic foot ulcer
    D. Skin tear that is not healing
31. Which action would the nursing assistant take in caring for a patient with a surgical wound that is supposed to heal by first intention?
    A. Take vital signs frequently as directed by the nurse
    B. Alert the nurse if the sutures or staples are not intact
    C. Alert the nurse when the infected wound drainage is excessive
    D. Give emotional support to the person for prolonged wound healing
32. Which observation would the nursing assistant report as a sign of hemorrhage?
    A. Dressings that are soaked with blood
    B. Warmth at the surgical site
    C. An increase in the blood pressure
    D. Watery drainage from the wound
33. Which action would the nursing assistant take upon observing signs of shock or hemorrhage?
    A. Report it to the nurse at once
    B. Place the person in Fowler's position
    C. Record observations on the flow sheet
    D. Hold pressure on the wound site
34. Which reminder would the nursing assistant give to the patient to protect against dehiscence?
    A. Use call bell for assistance as needed
    B. Remember to ask for pain medication, as needed
    C. Wash your hands after going to the bathroom
    D. Support the abdominal wound when coughing
35. Which type of drainage would be reported immediately because it indicates hemorrhage?
    A. Thick purulent drainage
    B. Watery serosanguineous drainage
    C. Clear thin serous drainage
    D. Bright red sanguineous drainage
36. Which nursing measure would the nursing assistant use when removing an old, soiled dressing from a wound?
    A. Don sterile gloves and grasp the center of the dressing
    B. Perform hand hygiene and use forceps to grasp edge of the dressing
    C. Don clean nonsterile gloves, grasp dressing edge, and gently lift
    D. Pour sterile water on the dressing and then pull it off
37. For which patient would plastic and paper tape be used to secure a dressing?
    A. Patient A needs to move the body part.
    B. Patient B needs to have frequent dressing changes.
    C. Patient C is allergic to adhesive tape.
    D. Patient D requires a tape that sticks well to the skin.
38. Which nursing assistant has correctly handled materials when performing a dressing change?
    A. Touches the dressing surface that contacts the wound.
    B. Touches only the outer edges of the dressing
    C. Applies the dressing with clean hands
    D. Places clean gauze over existing gauze layer
39. Which information does the nursing assistant need when assigned to change a dressing?
    A. What kind of medication the person receives
    B. The person's medical diagnosis
    C. How long to wait for pain medication to take effect
    D. When the dressing was last changed
40. Which nursing measure would the nursing assistant use to make the patient more comfortable when changing the dressing?
    A. Talk about topics that are not related to the wound
    B. Remove tape by pulling it toward the wound
    C. Encourage the patient to look at the wound and ask questions
    D. Tell the patient that the wound site is normal and healing
41. What would the nursing assistant do when gentle removal of an old dressing, causes a tiny skin tear and the person says, "My skin tears easily. The nurses always smooth it down and cover it"?
    A. Do as the person suggests
    B. Report the incident to the nurse
    C. Gently clean it with an antiseptic
    D. Document what the person told you to do
42. What is the purpose of a binder?
    A. To prevent infection which would delay healing
    B. To reduce drainage and prevent bleeding
    C. To reduce swelling, promote comfort, and prevent injury
    D. To limit movements that may cause wound dehiscence

43. How should a binder be applied?
    A. With firm, even pressure over the area
    B. Tightly secured with cloth straps
    C. Very loosely to allow breathing and movement
    D. During AM care and removed during PM care
44. Which food would the nursing assistant encourage an elderly person to order and eat because it contains the nutrient that is most important for wound healing?
    A. Oatmeal with cinnamon
    B. Orange and apple slices
    C. Tossed salad with croutons
    D. Grilled chicken breast
45. What kind of clothing would be helpful to prevent skin tears?
    A. Soft clothing with long sleeves and long pants
    B. Standard patient hospital gown with cloth ties
    C. Soft loose flowing clothing without belts or buttons
    D. Stiff protective clothing with snug closures
46. Which nursing assistant needs a reminder about decreasing the risk for skin tears while caring for patients with fragile skin?
    A. Nursing assistant A pads the wheelchair arms.
    B. Nursing assistant B wears clean dry gloves.
    C. Nursing assistant C wears a ring with a raised stone.
    D. Nursing assistant D keeps fingernails short and smooth.
47. Which action would the nursing assistant take for a person who has problems with venous circulation and the person's toenails are long and sharp?
    A. Ask the family to do the nail care
    B. Report the observations to the nurse
    C. Carefully clip and shorten the toenails
    D. Use a file and smooth the nail edges
48. Which person has a health condition that is a risk factor for circulatory ulcers?
    A. Person A has diabetes.
    B. Person B has a stomach ulcer.
    C. Person C has seasonal allergies.
    D. Person D has a urinary tract infection.
49. Which action would the nursing assistant take upon finding a person's wound has dehisced or eviscerated?
    A. Call the doctor at once and ask for instructions
    B. Apply firm but gentle pressure with a dry dressing
    C. Check underneath the person for bleeding
    D. Tell the nurse at once and help prepare the person for surgery
50. Which nursing measure would the nursing assistant use when the old dressings stick to the wound during a dressing change?
    A. Ask the nurse to perform the task
    B. Wet the dressing with a saline solution
    C. Assist the person to soak in the bathtub
    D. Gently pull on the dressing toward the wound
51. What is the advantage of a transparent dressing?
    A. Allows for wound observation
    B. Easier to change the dressing
    C. Remains intact during bathing
    D. It seals the wound and prevents bleeding
52. Which question would the nursing assistant ask the patient before applying tape?
    A. "Do you know where the nurse put the tape?"
    B. "Do you have any allergies to tape?"
    C. "What did the doctor tell you about tape?"
    D. "Do you care what kind of tape is used?"

Fill in the Blanks

53. What are common causes of skin tears?
    A. ______________________
    B. ______________________
    C. ______________________
    D. ______________________
    E. ______________________
    F. ______________________
    G. ______________________
    H. ______________________
54. Skin tears are portals of entry for ______________________.
55. When a person has diabetes, they may not be able to feel ____________, ____________, or ____________.
56. Explain what can happen if a person with diabetes has these foot problems.
    A. Athlete's foot ______________________
    B. Ingrown toenails ______________________
    C. Hammer toes ______________________
    D. Dry and cracked skin ______________________
57. With first intention healing, the wound edges are held together with ______________________.
58. Second intention healing is used for ______________________ wounds. Because healing takes longer, the threat of ______________________ is great.
59. Where would the nursing assistant check for drainage, for a suspicion of external hemorrhage? ______________________.
60. What observations would you make about wound appearance?
    A. ______________________
    B. ______________________
    C. ______________________
    D. ______________________
    E. ______________________
61. List four types of drainage that you might observe at a wound site.
    A. ______________________
    B. ______________________
    C. ______________________
    D. ______________________
62. When large amounts of drainage are expected, the doctor inserts a ______________________ into the wound.
63. Name two closed drainage systems that prevent microbes from entering a wound.
    ____

64. When you are changing a nonsterile dressing, why do you need two pairs of gloves?
____
____

65. When taping a dressing in place, the tape should not encircle the entire body part because ______________
____.

66. When delegated to apply dressings, list what observations should be reported and recorded.
A. ____
B. ____
C. ____
D. ____
E. ____
F. ____
G. ____
H. ____
I. ____
J. ____
K. ____
L. ____

Optional Learning Exercises

You are assigned to care for Mrs. Stevens. She is 87 years old and has diabetes and high blood pressure. She walks with difficulty and spends most of her day sitting in her chair. She is somewhat overweight and tells you she had a knee replacement 5 years ago and had phlebitis after surgery. The nurse tells you to watch carefully for signs of circulatory ulcers.

67. Identify seven risk factors that Mrs. Stevens has that place her at risk for circulatory ulcers.
A. ____
B. ____
C. ____
D. ____
E. ____
F. ____
G. ____

Mr. Hawkins, age 74, was in an automobile accident and has a wound on his leg that is large and open. It has become infected and he is being treated with antibiotics. When you are talking with him, he tells you he has smoked for 55 years and has poor circulation in his legs. He lives alone and generally eats takeout foods or eats cereal when he is at home.

68. Identify four factors that increase Mr. Hawkins' risk for complications.
A. ____
B. ____
C. ____
D. ____

69. What is missing in Mr. Hawkins' diet that is needed to help in healing the wound?
____

70. When a wound is infected and has poor circulation, the wound may be left open at first and then closed later. This type of wound healing is called healing through ______________________________.
This type of healing combines ______________ and ______________ intention healing.

You are assisting the nurse with wound care. Mr. Wendel has a drain in his wound that is attached to suction

71. How does the nurse find out the amount of drainage from Mr. Wendel's wound? ______________________
____

Use the FOCUS ON PRIDE section to complete these statements and then use the critical thinking and discussion questions to develop your ideas

72. When you are giving care, you are responsible for protecting the person's safety and well-being. What are your responsibilities regarding wound care in these situations?
A. If you are careless during a transfer, you can cause a ____.
B. If you rush during a bath, you may not notice a ______________ between skin folds on a bariatric person.
C. If you do not apply shoes properly on a diabetic person, __________ can develop.

73. To promote comfort and interaction with family and friends for a person with a wound, you may
A. ____
B. ____
C. ____
D. ____
E. ____

Critical Thinking and Discussion Questions

74. Review the care measures in Box 41.3 (p. 640) and discuss your professional responsibilities in helping people with diabetes take good care of their feet.

42 Pressure Injuries

Fill in the Blanks: Key Terms

Avoidable pressure injury	Chairfast	Pressure injury
Bedfast	Epidermal stripping	Shear
Blanch	Erythema	Skin breakdown
Bony prominence (pressure point)	Eschar	Slough
	Intact skin	Unavoidable pressure injury

1. Skin that is not broken is ______________________.
2. To become white is to ______________________.
3. Dead tissue that is shed from the skin is ______________________.
4. A pressure injury that develops from the improper use of the nursing process is an ______________________.
5. A ______________________ is an area where the bone sticks out or projects from the flat surface of the body.
6. Thick, leathery dead tissue that may be loose or adhered to the skin is ______________________.
7. Redness is ______________________.
8. ______________________ occurs when layers of the skin rub against each other; when the skin remains in place and underlying tissues move and stretch and tear underlying capillaries and blood vessels causing tissue damage.
9. ______________________ means confined to bed.
10. An ______________________ is a pressure injury that occurs despite efforts to prevent one through proper use of the nursing process.
11. Localized damage to the skin and/or underlying tissue, usually over a bony prominence, resulting from pressure or pressure in combination with shear is a ______________________.
12. ______________________ means confined to a chair.
13. Removing the epidermis as tape is removed from the skin is ______________________.
14. Changes or damage to intact skin is ______________________.

Circle the Best Answer

15. Which piece of equipment is most likely to provide a surface that is involved in a pressure injury?
    A. Commode chair
    B. Mattress
    C. Blood pressure cuff
    D. Mechanical lift
16. Which occurrence is most likely to result in a pressure injury?
    A. Dizziness causes the person to stumble and fall.
    B. Sharp edges can cause skin lacerations.
    C. Laying in same position for too long.
    D. Repositioning is done too frequently.
17. Which factor increases the risk for pressure injuries for older persons?
    A. They have acute illnesses that are not properly treated.
    B. Their physical needs cannot be met.
    C. Presence of thin and fragile skin that is easily injured.
    D. They lose interest in performing daily hygiene.
18. Which person's behavior creates the greatest risk factor for a pressure injury?
    A. Often paces back and forth, and nursing assistant has to redirect
    B. Frequently slumps in bed and is pulled up by nursing assistant
    C. Continually asks nursing assistant for help with hygienic care
    D. Repeatedly asks nursing assistant for help to go to the bathroom
19. What is an early sign of a pressure injury?
    A. Erythema over a bony prominence
    B. Small wound that is pink and moist
    C. A skin flap over a bony prominence
    D. Exposed tissue and some drainage
20. Which type of tissue damage can be prevented by raising the head of the bed no more than 30 degrees?
    A. Eschar
    B. Shearing
    C. Slough
    D. Ulcer
21. Where do pressure injuries commonly occur in children and infants?
    A. Over bony areas such as the hips
    B. Underneath the buttocks
    C. Between abdominal folds
    D. On the back of the head
22. Which action is the nurse assistant most likely to perform for a person who has a Kennedy terminal injury?
    A. Increase turning frequency to every 30 minutes to relieve pressure
    B. Give comfort measures because death will occur in 2 to 3 days
    C. Assist the person to drink extra fluids and eat high-protein foods
    D. Avoid using soap because person is having an allergic reaction

23. Which person has a risk for developing a pressure injury on the ears?
    A. Person A is obese and sits all day in a recliner chair.
    B. Person B has fragile, thin skin, but is alert and mobile.
    C. Person C cannot walk, but is able to move self in a wheelchair.
    D. Person D is bedridden and prefers to lie on the left side.
24. What is the most common site for a pressure injury?
    A. Elbow
    B. Sacrum
    C. Thighs
    D. Ears
25. How frequently would the nursing assistant reposition a person when following a repositioning schedule?
    A. Every 15 minutes
    B. Every 60 minutes
    C. Every 2 hours
    D. According to the individualized plan
26. Which factor increases friction when moving people in the bed?
    A. Decreased ability to sense pain
    B. Supine position and flat surface
    C. Pillow placement to prevent skin on skin contact
    D. Moisture on the skin and bed linens
27. What is the purpose of a bed cradle?
    A. To maintain good body alignment
    B. To prevent pressure on the legs, feet, and toes
    C. To keep the heels off the bed
    D. To distribute body weight evenly
28. What is the advantage of a special bed for persons who are at risk for pressure injuries?
    A. The person can move around easily.
    B. Changes where pressure is placed on the body.
    C. One staff member can move the person every 2 hours.
    D. Bed automatically aligns the body position.
29. How often should a bedfast person be repositioned?
    A. Every 30 to 60 minutes
    B. At least every 1 to 2 hours
    C. Three to four times per shift
    D. After every toileting and hygiene
30. Which nursing assistant needs a reminder about using the information from the care plan related to raising the head of the bed?
    A. Nursing assistant A confirms when to raise the head of the bed.
    B. Nursing assistant B asks the patient about raising the head of the bed.
    C. Nursing assistant C looks to see how far to raise the head of the bed.
    D. Nursing assistant D checks to see how long (in minutes) to raise the head of the bed.
31. Which nursing assistant needs a reminder about prevention of shearing injuries?
    A. Nursing assistant A uses an assistive device when moving a patient.
    B. Nursing assistant B raises the head of the bed to a high Fowler's position.
    C. Nursing assistant C cleans skin and dries moisture before repositioning a patient.
    D. Nursing assistant D asks several coworkers to help move a bariatric patient.
32. Which person has a factor that protects against developing pressure injuries?
    A. Person A has fecal incontinence.
    B. Person B has poor nutrition.
    C. Person C is significantly underweight.
    D. Person D is independently ambulatory.
33. How often should a chairfast person be repositioned?
    A. Every hour
    B. Every 2 hours
    C. Whenever the person looks uncomfortable
    D. Whenever the person asks for help
34. How quickly can a person develop a pressure injury after the onset of pressure?
    A. 1 to 2 hours
    B. 2 to 6 hours
    C. 1 to 2 days
    D. 1 week
35. Which resident has the greatest risk for a shearing injury?
    A. Resident A frequently gets up to urinate.
    B. Resident B can walk, but has dementia.
    C. Resident C is thin and keeps sliding down in bed.
    D. Resident D can eat, but lacks protein in diet.

Fill in the Blanks

36. Write out the abbreviation
    A. NPIAP ______________________________
37. You can help prevent shearing by raising the head of the bed only ____________.
38. Explain how the following conditions place a person at risk for pressure injuries.
    A. Urinary or fecal incontinence ______________________________
    B. Poor nutrition ______________________________
    C. Limited mental awareness ______________________________
    D. Circulatory problems ______________________________
    E. Have weight loss or are very thin ______________________________
39. Explain how these protective devices help prevent pressure injuries.
    A. Bed cradle prevents pressure on______________________________.
    B. Heel and elbow protectors promote ______________________________ and reduce ______________ and ______________.
    C. Heel and foot elevators raise ______________________________.
    D. Gel or fluid-filled pads have ______________________________.
    E. Special beds are particularly useful for patients who have ______________________ injuries.

Labeling

Answer questions 40 and 41 using the following illustration.

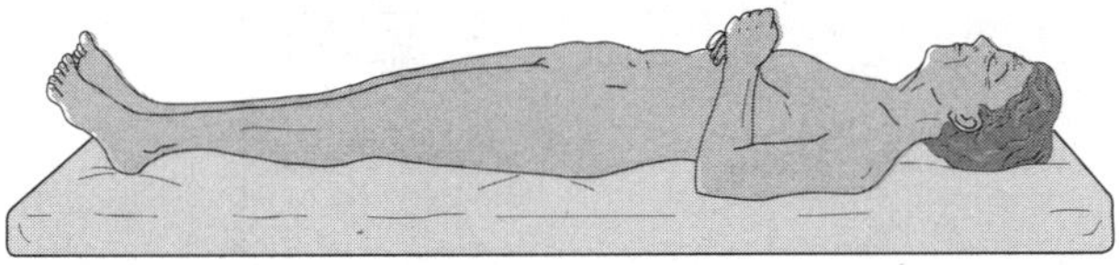

40. Name this position. ______________________
41. Place an "X" on each of the five pressure points. Name the bony point for each one.
    A. ______________________
    B. ______________________
    C. ______________________
    D. ______________________
    E. ______________________

Answer questions 42 and 43 using the following illustration.

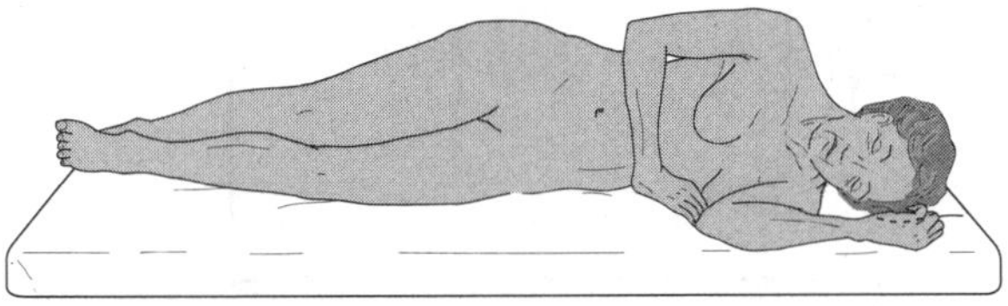

42. Name this position. ______________________
43. Place an "X" on each of the 10 pressure points. Name the bony point for each one.
    A. ______________________
    B. ______________________
    C. ______________________
    D. ______________________
    E. ______________________
    F. ______________________
    G. ______________________
    H. ______________________
    I. ______________________
    J. ______________________

Answer questions 44 and 45 using the following illustration.

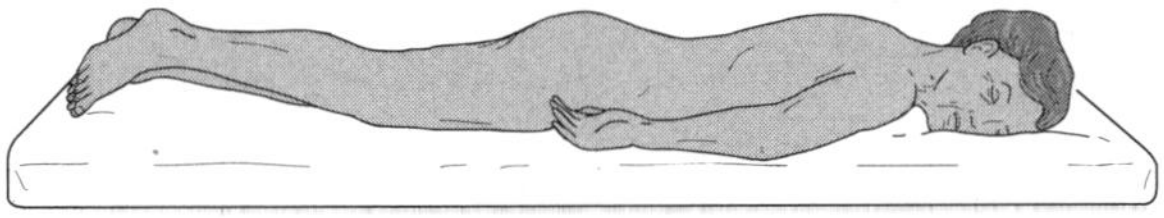

44. Name this position. ______________________
45. Place an "X" on each of the 10 pressure points. Name the bony point for each one.
    A. ______________________
    B. ______________________
    C. ______________________
    D. ______________________
    E. ______________________
    F. ______________________
    G. ______________________
    H. ______________________
    I. ______________________
    J. ______________________

Answer questions 46 and 47 using the following illustration.

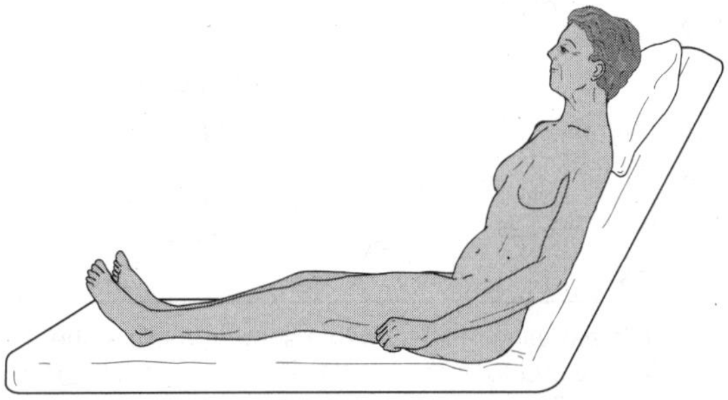

46. Name this position. ______________________
47. Place an "X" on each of the six pressure points. Name the bony point for each one.
    A. ______________________
    B. ______________________
    C. ______________________
    D. ______________________
    E. ______________________
    F. ______________________

Answer questions 48 and 49 using the following illustration.

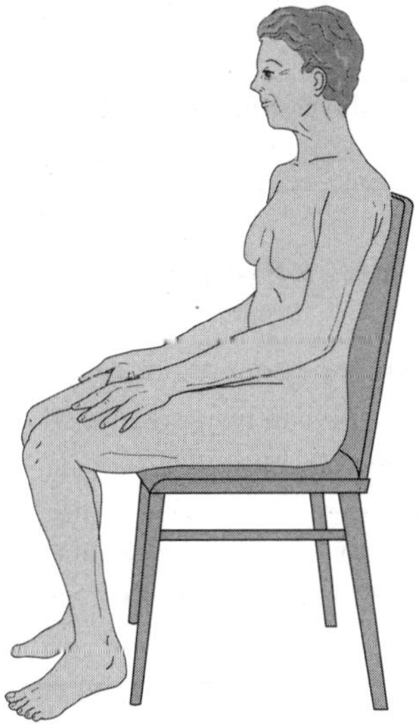

48. Name this position. ______________________
49. Place an "X" on each of the five pressure points. Name the bony point for each one.
    A. ______________________
    B. ______________________
    C. ______________________
    D. ______________________
    E. ______________________

50. Examine the documentation sample below and answer the following questions.

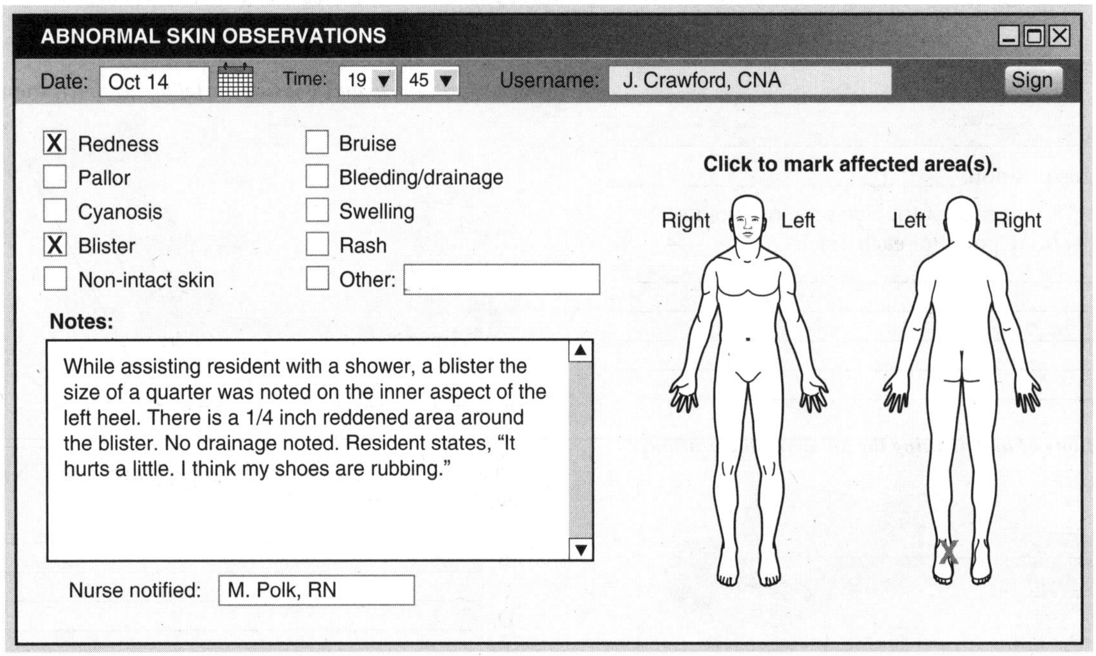
ABNORMAL SKIN OBSERVATIONS

Date: Oct 14 Time: 19 45 Username: J. Crawford, CNA Sign

- [X] Redness
- [ ] Pallor
- [ ] Cyanosis
- [X] Blister
- [ ] Non-intact skin
- [ ] Bruise
- [ ] Bleeding/drainage
- [ ] Swelling
- [ ] Rash
- [ ] Other:

Click to mark affected area(s).

Right Left Left Right

Notes:

While assisting resident with a shower, a blister the size of a quarter was noted on the inner aspect of the left heel. There is a 1/4 inch reddened area around the blister. No drainage noted. Resident states, "It hurts a little. I think my shoes are rubbing."

Nurse notified: M. Polk, RN

A. The nursing assistant observed a problem with the patient's skin. Which body part was affected? ____________________

B. How did the nursing assistant describe the area? ____________________

C. What did the resident say about the wound? ____________________

Optional Learning Exercises

51. The ____________________ requires that nursing centers identify persons at risk for pressure injuries.

52. Why would a person be repositioned more frequently (as often as every 15 minutes)? ____________________

53. If you are interviewed during a survey, what questions may be asked about pressure injuries?
    A. ____________________
    B. ____________________
    C. ____________________
    D. ____________________
    E. ____________________

Use the FOCUS ON PRIDE section to complete these statements

54. When you observe and report skin problems to the nurse, it can prevent ____________________.

55. When you speak up for your patients and residents, this is called being an ____________________.

Critical Thinking and Discussion Question

56. Discuss reasons why the nursing assistant may be the first member of the healthcare team to notice a problem with a person's skin.

43 Heat and Cold Applications

Fill in the Blanks: Key Terms

Compress
Constrict
Cyanosis
Dilate
Pack

1. A bluish color is ______________________________.
2. ______________________________ means to narrow.
3. A commercial application for heat or cold therapy is a ______________________________.
4. A ______________________ is a soft pad applied over a body area.
5. ______________________________ means to expand or open wider.

Circle the Best Answer

6. Which person is most likely to have an order for a heat application?
   A. Person reports straining back muscles after bending forward.
   B. Pregnant woman would like relief from mild abdominal cramps.
   C. Older person with metal wrist implant reports mild swelling.
   D. Older confused person has swelling in knee and lower leg.
7. Which observation would be considered normal and expected when the nursing assistant applies a warm moist pack to a person's arm according to the nurse's instructions?
   A. Skin is pale and numb.
   B. Skin is warm and red.
   C. Skin is moist and painful.
   D. Skin is hot and blistered.
8. What occurs when heat is applied to the skin?
   A. Blood vessels in the area dilate.
   B. Tissues have less oxygen.
   C. Blood flow decreases.
   D. Skin and muscle constrict.
9. Which observation would accompany the blood vessel constriction if heat is applied too long?
   A. Skin becomes excessively red.
   B. Skin becomes pale and damaged.
   C. Skin becomes thin and fragile.
   D. Skin becomes moist with sweat.
10. Which nursing assistant needs a reminder about securing an aquathermia pad?
    A. Nursing assistant A uses ties to keep the aquathermia pad in place.
    B. Nursing assistant B tapes the aquathermia pad to keep it from slipping.
    C. Nursing assistant C uses a safety pin to secure the device to the bed linens.
    D. Nursing assistant D wraps roller gauze around the pad and body part.
11. Which nursing assistant is using the best time management after applying a heat application to a person's arm and that must be frequently checked?
    A. Nursing assistant A helps a person in the next room to take a shower.
    B. Nursing assistant B makes the person's bed and straightens the room.
    C. Nursing assistant C tells the nurse about tasks for the next 5 minutes.
    D. Nursing assistant D tells the person to push the call bell in 5 minutes.
12. Which safety measure would the nursing assistant use when the care plan states that the person must receive a heat application?
    A. Cleans the skin before applying the heat pack
    B. Avoids applying an application that is above 106°F
    C. Asks the person if the application is too warm
    D. Applies the pack and reminds the person not to remove it
13. How long are heat and cold applications applied?
    A. 15 to 20 minutes
    B. 30 to 45 minutes
    C. 1 hour
    D. 2 hours
14. How often would the nursing assistant check the area when a hot or cold application is in place?
    A. Every 5 minutes
    B. Every 15 to 20 minutes
    C. About every 30 minutes
    D. Once an hour
15. What is the purpose of applying an aquathermia pad over the compress when hot compresses are in place?
    A. To keep the compress wet
    B. To protect the area from injury
    C. To measure the temperature of the compress
    D. To maintain the correct temperature of the compress
16. Which action would the nursing assistant use when helping the person with a hot soak?
    A. Put the body part into water
    B. Apply a soft pad to a body part
    C. Cover body part with plastic wrap
    D. Wait until the water temperature cools down
17. Which safety measure would the nursing assistant use when giving a sitz bath?
    A. Check the person often to assess for weakness, fainting, or fatigue
    B. Keep the door open so the person is visible from the hallway
    C. Give privacy by closing the door and leaving the person alone
    D. Make sure the water temperature is hot and deep enough to sit in

18. Which nursing measure would the nursing assistant use when applying an aquathermia pad?
    A. Wrap the pad in a moist towel and place it over the body part
    B. Instruct the person how to use the temperature setting key
    C. Place the pad underneath the person's body part
    D. Check the hoses for kinks and bubbles; water must flow freely
19. Which patient condition would commonly be treated with an ice pack application?
    A. Sprained ankle
    B. Hypothermia
    C. Mild headache
    D. Sore throat
20. What is the main advantage of the numbing effect when a cold application is applied?
    A. Helps to reduce or relieve pain in the part
    B. Increases the constriction of blood vessels
    C. Rapidly decreases the blood flow
    D. Helps to cool the body part
21. Which of these cold applications is moist?
    A. Ice bag
    B. Ice collar
    C. Ice glove
    D. Cold compress
22. When should the nursing assistant remove the cold application?
    A. The skin is red, moist, and cool to the touch.
    B. The person says the area feels numb and pain has decreased.
    C. The skin appears pale, white, gray, or bluish in color.
    D. The person is slightly chilled and asks for another blanket.
23. Which piece of equipment is the nurse most likely to ask the nursing assistant to obtain when a person has hypothermia?
    A. Ice glove
    B. Sitz bath
    C. Aquathermia pad
    D. Warming blanket
24. What is the main advantage of dry heat applications?
    A. Dry heat applications stay at the desired temperature longer.
    B. Patients will not get wet and linens stay dry.
    C. Patients get more effective relief from pain.
    D. Dry heat applications are cheaper and easier to use.
25. What is the correct temperature range for a warm soak?
    A. 65°F to 79°F (18°C to 26°C)
    B. 80°F to 92°F (26°C to 34°C)
    C. 93°F to 98°F (34°C to 37°C)
    D. 99°F to 106°F (37°C to 41°C)
26. Which person would benefit from a cold application?
    A. Person A has a sprained wrist.
    B. Person B has hemorrhoids.
    C. Person C had pelvic surgery.
    D. Person D has an anal wound.
27. Which task would the nursing assistant frequently perform when a cooling blanket is being used?
    A. Take and report vital signs
    B. Check for urinary incontinence
    C. Help the patient to eat and drink
    D. Change the fluid in the blanket

Fill in the Blanks

28. Write out the abbreviations
    A. F ______________________
    B. C ______________________
29. What are the effects of heat applications?
    A. ______________________
    B. ______________________
    C. ______________________
    D. ______________________
    E. ______________________
30. In applying heat or cold applications for infants or children, crying can communicate ______________________.
31. An aquathermia pad is an example of a ______________________ application.
32. Moist heat applications should have ______________ temperatures than dry heat applications because heat penetrates ______________ with a moist application.
33. What observations should the nursing assistant report to the nurse when giving a sitz bath?
    A. ______________________
    B. ______________________
    C. ______________________
    D. ______________________
34. List three questions that you should ask the person when you are applying heat or cold.
    A. ______________________
    B. ______________________
    C. ______________________
35. How can you manage your time to stay in or near the person's room during a heat or cold application?
    A. ______________________
    B. ______________________
    C. ______________________
    D. ______________________
    E. ______________________
    F. ______________________

Optional Learning Exercises

Situation: The nurse instructs you to apply a cold pack to a resident who has twisted her ankle. Use the information you learned in this chapter to answer these questions about carrying out this treatment.

36. What is the purpose of the cold application for this injury? ______________________
37. What can you use to make a cool dry application to the ankle if no commercial packs are available?
    ____

38. Why do you squeeze the application tightly after filling it with ice?

____

39. How will you protect the person's skin?

____

40. How often do you check the application?

____

41. When you check the area where the cold pack was applied, what signs and symptoms should be reported?
A. _______________
B. _______________
C. _______________
D. _______________
E. _______________
F. _______________
G. _______________

42. What should you do if any of these signs or symptoms are present?

____

43. How long should you leave the application in place?

____

44. What happens if you leave the cold pack in place for too long?

____

Table Activity

45. Instructions: Complete the table below by filling in the missing temperature or temperature ranges

Heat and Cold Temperature Ranges

Temperature	Fahrenheit (F) Range	Centigrade (C) Range
Hot		37°C to 41°C
Warm		34°C to 37°C
Tepid	80°F to 92°F	26°C to 34°C
Cool	65°F to 79°F	
Cold		10°C to 18°C

Use the FOCUS ON PRIDE section to complete these statements and then use the critical thinking and discussion question to develop your ideas

46. When applying heat or cold, you must allow time for
A. _______________
B. _______________
C. _______________
D. _______________
E. _______________

47. When applying heat and cold, harm and legal action can result if you
A. _______________
B. _______________
C. _______________
D. _______________
E. _______________
F. _______________
G. _______________

Critical Thinking and Discussion Question

48. You are assigned to assist a person in the home setting with hygienic care and activities of daily living. The person asks you to prepare a hot water bottle and place it on her stomach. You tell her that this is not in her care plan, but she says, "Please get it for me. I have been doing this since I was a little girl and it makes me feel so much better." What would you do?

44 Oxygen Needs

Fill in the Blanks: Key Terms

Allergy	Cyanosis	Hypoxia	Pulse oximetry
Apnea	Dyspnea	Kussmaul respirations	Respiratory arrest
Atelectasis	Hemoptysis	Orthopnea	Respiratory depression
Biot's respirations	Hyperventilation	Orthopneic position	Sputum
Bradypnea	Hypoventilation	Oxygen concentration	Tachypnea
Cheyne-Stokes respirations	Hypoxemia	Pollutant	

1. ________________________ are respirations that are rapid and deep followed by 10 to 30 seconds of apnea.
2. Bloody sputum is called ________________________.
3. Rapid breathing where respirations are usually greater than 20 per minute is called ________________________.
4. An __________________ is a sensitivity to a substance that causes the body to react with signs and symptoms.
5. Difficult, labored, or painful breathing is ________________________.
6. Mucus from the respiratory system that is expectorated through the mouth is ________________________.
7. Being able to breathe deeply and comfortably only while sitting is ________________________.
8. Respirations that are less than 12 per minute is slow breathing or ________________________.
9. A reduced amount of oxygen in the blood is ________________________.
10. ________________________ describes slow, weak respirations that occur at a rate of fewer than 12 per minute.
11. The lack or absence of breathing is ________________________.
12. ________________________ is a pattern of respirations that is rapid and deeper than normal.
13. A harmful chemical or substance in the air or water is a ________________________.
14. ________________________ are respirations that gradually increase in rate and depth and then become shallow and slow. Breathing may stop for 10 to 20 seconds.
15. The ________________________ is sitting up and leaning over a table to breathe.
16. When breathing stops, it is ________________________.
17. Very deep and rapid respirations (can occur with diabetic acidosis) are ________________________.
18. ________________________ is the amount (percentage) of hemoglobin containing oxygen.
19. When cells do not have enough oxygen, it is called ________________________.
20. Respirations that are slow, shallow, and sometimes irregular is ________________________.
21. The collapse of a portion of the lung is ________________________.
22. ____________ is a bluish color to the skin, lips, mucous membrane, and nail beds.
23. ________________________ measures the oxygen concentration in arterial blood.

Circle the Best Answer

24. Which respiratory condition becomes more of a risk for an elderly person because respiratory muscles weaken with aging?
    A. Tachypnea
    B. Hemoptysis
    C. Allergic reactions
    D. Pneumonia
25. What causes an increased need for oxygen?
    A. Aging
    B. Pain medication
    C. Fever
    D. Digestion
26. Which circumstance is associated with respiratory depression or arrest?
    A. The person exercises too strenuously.
    B. Iron and vitamins are excluded from the diet.
    C. Morphine is taken in excessively large doses.
    D. The person smokes or uses tobacco products.
27. Which respiratory state is associated with restlessness as an early sign?
    A. Hypoxia
    B. Kussmaul respiration
    C. Hyperventilation
    D. Eupnea
28. Which of these is a sign of hypoxia?
    A. Sputum production
    B. Decrease in pulse rate
    C. Apprehension and anxiety
    D. Red, flushed skin
29. Which site would the nursing assistant select for a pulse oximeter measurement if the person has tremors or poor circulation in the extremities?
    A. A toe
    B. A finger
    C. Palm of the hand
    D. An earlobe

30. Which information would the nursing assistant report to the nurse when delegated to place a pulse oximeter on a person?
    A. How to use the equipment
    B. Pulse rate below the alarm limit
    C. The person's normal SpO_2 range
    D. Type of tape used to secure the oximeter
31. Which position is usually better when the person is having difficulty with breathing?
    A. Supine position
    B. Side-lying position
    C. Semi-Fowler's or Fowler's position
    D. Prone position
32. What is the purpose of deep breathing and coughing exercises?
    A. Helps to prevent pneumonia and atelectasis
    B. Acts to decrease pain after surgery or injury
    C. Replaces the person's need for supplemental oxygen
    D. Used to reverse and treat a collapsed lung
33. Which instruction would the nursing assistant give to the patient when assisting with coughing and deep breathing?
    A. Inhale through the mouth
    B. Hold the breath for 30 seconds
    C. Exhale slowly through pursed lips
    D. Repeat the exercise one or two times
34. What is the goal when using an incentive spirometer?
    A. Teach the person how to use oxygen
    B. Increase the number of respirations
    C. Improve lung function and prevent complications
    D. Help the person stop smoking
35. Which task related to oxygen administration is within the nursing assistant's role?
    A. Set the flow rate
    B. Adjust the flow rate
    C. Set up the system
    D. Turn on the oxygen
36. Which task can the nursing assistant perform when caring for a person who has oxygen therapy?
    A. Remove the person's mask for eating and drinking
    B. Stop the oxygen if the person wants to walk
    C. Tell the person if the rate is too high or too low
    D. Check for skin irritation from the oxygen device
37. Which action would the nursing assistant take when a home care patient who uses oxygen requests that an electric space heater be placed close to the bed for warmth?
    A. Tell the person that the space heater is too dangerous
    B. Place the heater 10 feet from the oxygen and tell the nurse
    C. Turn off the oxygen whenever the heater is running
    D. Turn off the heater whenever you leave the house
38. Where would the nursing assistant check for irritation if a person receives oxygen through a nasal cannula?
    A. On the nose, ears, and cheekbones
    B. Under the mask
    C. In the throat
    D. In the oral cavity
39. Which task can the nursing assistant perform when delegated to set up for oxygen administration?
    A. Determine which device and tubing are needed
    B. Attach the flowmeter to the wall outlet or tank
    C. Apply the oxygen device to the person
    D. Ask the person if the oxygen is helping
40. Which observation related to the humidifier would the nursing assistant report for a person who is receiving oxygen?
    A. Water vapor is coming from the device.
    B. Humidifier has water in it.
    C. Gentle bubbling is occurring within the device.
    D. Humidifier has a low water level.
41. What happens to lung tissue as a person ages?
    A. Pollutants fill the lungs.
    B. Tissue becomes less elastic.
    C. Tissue is withered and fragile.
    D. Fat deposits replace lung tissue.
42. Which disease is least likely to be associated with smoking?
    A. Coronary artery disease
    B. Chronic bronchitis
    C. Emphysema
    D. Diabetes
43. Which adverse effect on the respiratory system can be caused by drinking excessive alcohol?
    A. Increases risk of aspiration
    B. Decreases body's ability to use oxygen
    C. Increases chance for lung collapse
    D. Decreases lung capacity
44. What is the normal range for oxygen concentration?
    A. 85% to 90%
    B. 90% to 93%
    C. 95% to 98%
    D. 95% to 100%
45. Which nursing assistant needs a reminder about reporting to the nurse for a patient who has a pulse oximeter is in place?
    A. Nursing assistant A reports an SpO_2 below the alarm limit.
    B. Nursing assistant B reports a pulse rate goes above the alarm limit.
    C. Nursing assistant C reports disorientation and confusion.
    D. Nursing assistant D reports eupnea and SpO_2 of 98%.
46. Which equipment will the nursing assistant obtain when assisting the patient to achieve the orthopneic position?
    A. Pillow
    B. Nasal cannula
    C. Incentive spirometer
    D. Pulse oximeter
47. Which patient needs a reminder about respiratory hygiene and cough etiquette?
    A. Patient A covers the nose and mouth when coughing or sneezing.
    B. Patient B uses tissues to contain respiratory secretions.
    C. Patient C puts used tissues in a coat pocket for later disposal.
    D. Patient D washes hands after coughing or contact with respiratory secretions.

48. How long should a person who is using an incentive spirometer hold their breath to keep the piston floating?
    A. 2 to 3 seconds
    B. 3 to 5 seconds
    C. 10 to 20 seconds
    D. For several seconds
49. What would the nursing assistant do when the person needs to eat but is wearing a mask to receive oxygen?
    A. Inform the nurse
    B. Remove the mask
    C. Place a nasal cannula
    D. Turn off the oxygen

Fill in the Blanks

50. Write out the meaning of the abbreviations
    A. CO_2 ______
    B. L/min ______
    C. O_2 ______
    D. RBC ______
    E. SpO_2 ______
51. With aging the person's strength for coughing ______.
52. Alcohol reduces the ______ reflex, which is needed to reduce risk for aspiration.
53. Normal breathing is ______.
54. What terms can be used to describe sputum when reporting and recording?
    A. Color: ______
    B. Odor: ______
    C. Consistency: ______
    D. Hemoptysis: ______
55. If you are caring for a person with a pulse oximeter, what observations should be reported and recorded?
    A. ______
    B. ______
    C. ______
    D. ______
    E. ______
    F. ______
56. What observations should be reported after a person uses an incentive spirometer?
    A. ______
    B. ______
    C. ______
    D. ______

Optional Learning Exercises

Situation: You are caring for Mr. R., age 84, who has chronic obstructive pulmonary disease. Answer questions 57 and 58 about caring for Mr. R

57. What position would make it easier for Mr. R. to breathe when he is in bed?
    ______
    ______
58. How can you increase his comfort when he is sitting up?
    ______
    ______
    What is this position called?
    ______

Situation: Mrs. F. is receiving nonhumidified oxygen through a nasal cannula at 2 L/min. Her respirations are unlabored at 16 per minute unless she is walking about or doing personal care. Then her respirations are 32 and dyspneic. Answer questions 59 to 62 about her care

59. Why is there no humidifier with the oxygen setup for Mrs. F.?
    ______
60. Where should you check for signs of irritation from the cannula?
    ______
    ______
61. You should make sure that there are ______ in the tubing and that Mrs. F. does not lie on any part of the tubing.
62. What are the abnormal respirations that Mrs. F has with activity called?
    ______

Use the FOCUS ON PRIDE section to complete these statements and then use the critical thinking and discussion question to develop your ideas

63. When you remind the person or visitors not to smoke when NO SMOKING signs are used, you are protecting the person's right to a ______.
64. You do not adjust the oxygen flow rate unless allowed by your ______ and ______ and instructed ______.

Critical Thinking and Discussion Question

65. You are caring for a person in the home setting. He uses oxygen occasionally. You catch him smoking while the oxygen is on. When you remind him about the "no smoking" rule for safety, he just smiles and tells you he forgets, because, "I've smoked all my life, but just lately started to need this oxygen. I'll try to remember." What should you do?

Crossword

Fill in the crossword puzzle by answering the clues below with the words from this list

Apnea	Bradypnea	Dyspnea	Hypoventilation	Orthopnea
Biot's	Cheyne-Stokes	Hyperventilation	Kussmaul	Tachypnea

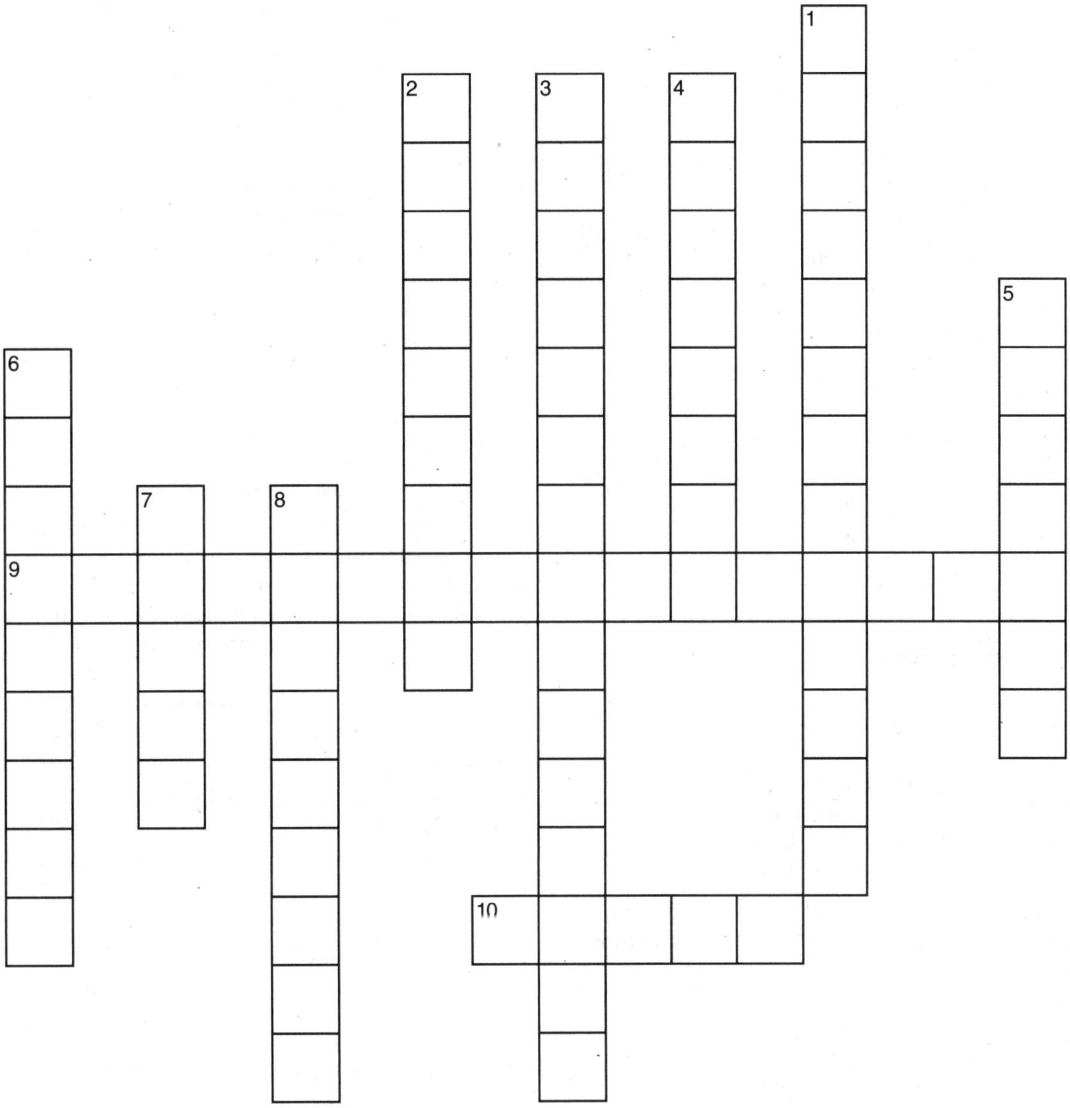

Across

9. Respirations are rapid and deeper than normal
10. Rapid and deep respirations followed by 10 to 30 seconds of apnea; occur with nervous disorders

Down

1. Respirations gradually increase in rate and depth; common when death is near
2. Respirations are 20 or more per minute
3. Respirations are slow, shallow, and sometimes irregular
4. Very deep and rapid respirations; signal diabetic coma
5. Difficult, labored, or painful breathing
6. Breathing deeply and comfortably only when sitting
7. Lack or absence of breathing
8. Respirations are fewer than 12 per minute

45 Respiratory Support and Therapies

Fill in the Blanks: Key Terms

Hemothorax	Mechanical ventilation	Pleural effusion	Suction
Intubation	Patent	Pneumothorax	Tracheostomy

1. The escape and collection of fluid in the pleural space is ________________.
2. ________________ is blood in the pleural space.
3. A ________________ is a surgically created opening into the trachea.
4. ________________ is the process of withdrawing or sucking up fluid.
5. Inserting an artificial airway is ________________.
6. ________________ is air in the pleural space.
7. ________________ is using a machine to move air into and out of the lungs.
8. ________________ is open or unblocked.

Circle the Best Answer

9. Which observation needs to be reported to the nurse at once when caring for a person with an artificial airway?
   A. The airway interferes with speaking.
   B. The person needs frequent oral hygiene.
   C. The airway comes out or is dislodged.
   D. The person feels uncomfortable.
10. Which communication method would the nursing assistant use for a person with an endotracheal tube (ET) who cannot speak?
    A. Never ask questions
    B. Speak clearly and loudly
    C. Always keep the call light within reach
    D. Use simple language during explanations
11. Which equipment will the nurse ask the nursing assistant to obtain to assist the person with communication for a person with an endotracheal tube (ET)?
    A. Headphones
    B. Paper and pencil
    C. Hearing aid
    D. Self-help device
12. Which task will the nursing assistant perform when assisting the nurse to change the ties that secure the outer cannula in place?
    A. Cut the soiled ties and then assist the nurse to insert clean ties
    B. Hold the outer cannula in place until the nurse secures the new ties
    C. Clean the inner and outer cannulas while the nurse inserts the new ties
    D. Remove the soiled ties; clean the stoma and cannulas; replace the ties
13. Which nursing measure would the nursing assistant use to protect a person's stoma or tube while giving care?
    A. Cover when shaving
    B. Cover with plastic when outdoors
    C. Cover with a loose gauze dressing when bathing
    D. Uncover when the person goes swimming
14. Which task would the nursing assistant be allowed to perform when delegated to assist with tracheostomy care?
    A. Remove the ties and wash them
    B. Suction the tube before and after meals
    C. Clean around the stoma to prevent skin breakdown
    D. Remove the inner and outer cannulas to clean them
15. Which position would the nursing assistant help the patient to achieve when assisting the nurse with suctioning the airway?
    A. Prone position with head turned to the side
    B. Semi-Fowler's position with head turned to the side
    C. Supine position with head elevated on small pillow
    D. Dorsal recumbent with head in a neutral position
16. When is suctioning usually performed?
    A. In the morning
    B. As needed
    C. Every 2 hours
    D. After meals
17. Which action would the nursing assistant perform first when the alarm sounds on a machine used for mechanical ventilation?
    A. Report to the nurse at once
    B. Reset the alarms
    C. Reassure the person that the alarm is normal
    D. Check to see if the tube is attached to the ventilator
18. Which observation needs to be reported to the nurse at once when caring for a person with chest tubes?
    A. The person is reluctant to do the deep breathing exercises.
    B. There is a small amount of drainage in the chest tube.
    C. The bubbling in the drainage system has increased.
    D. The person indicates that there is a need for suctioning.
19. What is the purpose of keeping petrolatum gauze is kept at the bedside of a person with chest tubes?
    A. To cover the insertion site if the chest tube comes out
    B. To lubricate the site of the chest tube
    C. To protect the skin around the chest tube
    D. To cover the insertion site to prevent drainage

20. Which observation needs to be immediately reported to the nurse when assisting with suctioning?
   A. Pulse of 80 beats/min
   B. An irregular pulse rhythm
   C. Oxygen saturation of 98%
   D. Signs and symptoms of eupnea
21. Which part of the tracheostomy tube is removed for cleaning and mucus removal?
   A. Obdurator
   B. Outer cannula
   C. Inner cannula
   D. Oxygen tubing
22. Who would perform hyperoxygenation before and after suctioning the lower airways?
   A. Patient
   B. Nurse
   C. Nursing assistant
   D. Doctor
23. Which part of the tracheostomy tube is not removed?
   A. Obturator
   B. Outer cannula
   C. Inner cannula
   D. Stoma covering
24. How many seconds should it take to complete suctioning?
   A. 1 to 3 seconds
   B. 10 to 15 seconds
   C. 1 to 2 minutes
   D. 5 to 10 minutes
25. Why is the obturator kept at the bedside?
   A. The patient may desire to perform tracheostomy care.
   B. The doctor may need it to change the inner cannula.
   C. In case the tracheostomy tube falls out and needs insertion.
   D. In case the person stops breathing or has severe distress.
26. Which communication method would the nursing assistant use when entering the room of a person who has mechanical ventilation?
   A. Explain who you are and what you are going to do
   B. Pantomime or use gestures to communicate nursing care
   C. Quickly and quietly take vital signs without waking the person
   D. Direct comments to the family and explain what needs to be done
27. Which nursing assistant needs a reminder about what should be done each time when leaving the room of a person who is on mechanical ventilation?
   A. Nursing assistant A informs the person when leaving the room.
   B. Nursing assistant B tells the person when to expect a return visit.
   C. Nursing assistant C completes a safety check before leaving the room.
   D. Nursing assistant D finishes tasks and waves goodbye from the doorway.
28. Which piece of equipment would the nursing assistant need to obtain when assisting the nurse who needs to quickly insert an artificial airway to keep the patient's airway patent?
   A. Oropharyngeal airway
   B. Endotracheal tube
   C. Nasogastric tube
   D. Tracheostomy tube

Fill in the Blanks

29. Write out the meaning of the abbreviations
   A. CO_2 ______________________
   B. ET ______________________
   C. O_2 ______________________
   D. RT ______________________
30. What are the three parts of a tracheostomy tube?
   A. ______________________
   B. ______________________
   C. ______________________
31. Before, during, and after suctioning, what is checked and observed?
   A. ______________________
   B. ______________________
   C. ______________________
   D. ______________________
32. If chest tubes are in place, what should be reported to the nurse at once?
   A. ______________________
   B. ______________________
   C. ______________________
   D. ______________________
   E. ______________________
   F. ______________________

Optional Learning Exercises

33. If you are caring for a person with a tracheostomy, why is the tracheostomy covered when the person is outdoors? ______________; ______________
34. If a person with a tracheostomy is outdoors, what is used to cover the tracheostomy? ______________________
35. What is done to protect the stoma in the following situations?
   A. Showers ______________________
   B. Shaving ______________________
   C. Shampooing ______________________
36. The stoma is never covered with ______________________
   Why? ______________________
37. If a person has mechanical ventilation, where do you find the methods for communication? ______________
   All healthcare team members must use the ______________ signals for communication.

38. If a person has chest tubes, why is it important to prevent kinks in the tubing? ____________________
____

39. Which step of tracheostomy care is depicted in the figure? ______________________________________
____
____

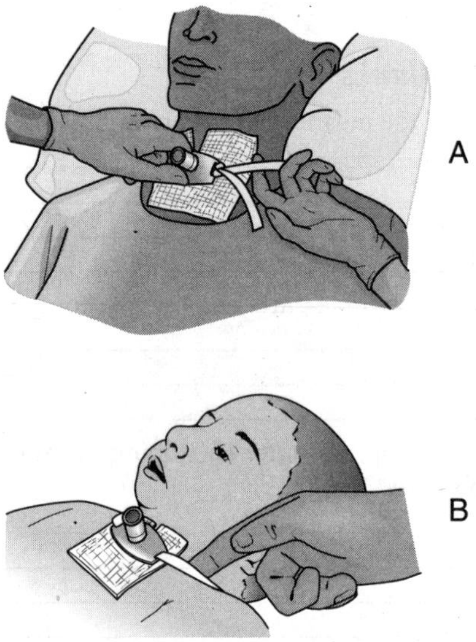

Use the FOCUS ON PRIDE section to complete these statements and then use the critical thinking and discussion question to develop your ideas

40. Tell the nurse at once if you suspect a problem. Delay can cause _____________ or _____________.

41. When a person has an endotracheal tube (ET), you can provide social support by
    A. ____
    B. ____
    C. ____
    D. ____
    E. ____

Critical Thinking and Discussion Question

42. You are caring for a woman who has a tracheostomy; she is currently living in a long-term care facility. Her daughter says, "Mom was always very chatty and social before having the tracheostomy, but now she can't talk like she used to. She's so withdrawn. I wished we could do something to help her." Discuss ways that the healthcare team could assist this person and her family.

46 Rehabilitation Needs

Fill in the Blanks: Key Terms

Activities of daily living
Disability
Prosthesis
Rehabilitation
Restorative aide
Restorative nursing care

1. A nursing assistant with special training in restorative nursing and rehabilitation skills is a ________________________________.
2. __________________ are activities usually done during a normal day in a person's life.
3. An artificial replacement for a missing body part is a ________________________________.
4. Nursing care that helps persons regain their health and strength for safe and independent living is ________________________________.
5. A __________________ is any lost, absent, or impaired physical or mental function.
6. The process of restoring the disabled person to the highest possible level of physical, psychological, social, and economic functioning is ________________________________.

Circle the Best Answer

7. Which person is acting to fulfill one of the goals of rehabilitation?
   A. Athlete is training to improve his endurance.
   B. Person takes prescribed antibiotics as directed.
   C. Person does physical therapy exercises after knee surgery.
   D. Older person practices yoga for better balance and strength.
8. Which nursing goals would be included in restorative nursing programs?
   A. Teaching management of self-care, elimination, and positioning
   B. Providing total care to persons who are incapacitated
   C. Assisting with curing disease and restoring normal function
   D. Giving good nursing care for rapid postsurgical recovery
9. Which question is a surveyor most likely to ask the nursing assistant about caring for people with rehabilitation needs?
   A. What kinds of rehabilitation programs are offered?
   B. How long does it take for people to complete therapy?
   C. How much do you for the person when you assist with hygiene?
   D. Have you experienced hostility when caring for people with disabilities?
10. Which action would the nursing assistant perform during mealtime when assisting patients who need rehabilitation and restorative care?
    A. Put the food tray in front of person and let the person figure how to eat
    B. Cut the food into small pieces and put assistive eating devices within reach
    C. Suggest that eating should be done in the dining room for socialization
    D. Feed the person with a spoon, give sips of fluid, and wipe the face
11. Which of these would be most helpful for a person receiving rehabilitative care?
    A. Give the person pity or sympathy when tasks are difficult
    B. Remind the person not to try new skills or those that are difficult
    C. Give praise when even a little progress is made
    D. Tell the person to do the task like everything is normal
12. Which aspect of rehabilitation and restorative care is addressed by good alignment, turning and repositioning, and range-of-motion exercises?
    A. Psychological
    B. Economic
    C. Social
    D. Physical
13. When does rehabilitation begin?
    A. After the person has recovered.
    B. When the person first seeks health care.
    C. When the person asks for help.
    D. When a discharge date has been set.
14. Which goal can be met through use of adaptive (assistive) devices?
    A. Recovering all former abilities
    B. Achieving independence in self-care
    C. Living alone in own home
    D. Using services provided by others
15. What is the nursing assistant's role when accompanying the occupational therapist who is teaching a person about assistive devices for cooking?
    A. Give the person emotional support while learning these new skills
    B. Listen to the therapist; similar words and phrases help the person to remember
    C. Help the therapist control the person physically and emotionally as needed
    D. Do whatever the therapist needs help with during the teaching session

16. Which information does the nursing assistant need to get from the nurse and the care plan when caring for a person who has dysphagia?
    A. Limitations of mobility
    B. Type of assistive device
    C. Type of diet
    D. Method of communication
17. Which type of program would a person who has had a joint replacement need?
    A. Spinal cord rehabilitation
    B. Amputee rehabilitation
    C. Orthopedic rehabilitation
    D. Stroke rehabilitation
18. What would the nursing assistant do when following the care plan and using a picture board to communicate with a person who has a speech disorder, but the person gets angry and yells?
    A. Try a different method of communicating that does not include the board
    B. Recognize that the person is frustrated, remain calm, talk to the nurse as needed
    C. Do not let the person take control; gently advise that anger is not necessary
    D. Be polite, ignore the angry outburst, and continue attempts to use the board
19. Which action could the home health nursing assistant perform to contribute to the safety of a person who needs rehabilitation?
    A. Help the person to install an automatic garage door opener
    B. Teach the person how to use the grab bars in the bathroom
    C. Determine where handrails are needed indoors and outdoors
    D. Make sure that there is a flashlight on the bedside table
20. Which rehabilitation program would help a person with a mental health disorder that is interfering with work, relationships, and activities of daily living?
    A. Drug and alcohol treatment
    B. Rehabilitation for complex medical and surgical conditions
    C. Brain injury rehabilitation
    D. Behavioral health treatment
21. Which task would the nursing assistant be assigned to assist a person who needs restorative nursing care?
    A. Taking and reporting frequent vital signs until the person is stable
    B. Performing total care for hygiene, nutrition, and elimination for a person
    C. Feeding a person who is unable to manipulate utensils and drinkware
    D. Helping the person to ambulate according to physical therapy plan
22. Which patient has the most factors that will affect recovery and rehabilitation?
    A. Patient A, aged 86 years, is highly motivated, has social support, and needs orthopedic rehabilitation for a hip fracture.
    B. Patient B, aged 26 years, has financial and social support and needs brain injury rehabilitation related to traumatic brain injury.
    C. Patient C, aged 71 years, suffered a stroke and has diabetes, heart, and respiratory disease, is low income, and needs stroke rehabilitation.
    D. Patient D, aged 35 years, is depressed after sustaining severe burns and needs rehabilitation for complex medical and surgical conditions.
23. Which rehabilitation program would help a person who is having difficulty managing diabetes and high blood pressure?
    A. Rehabilitation for complex medical and surgical conditions
    B. Cardiac rehabilitation
    C. Behavioral health treatment
    D. Hearing, speech, and vision rehabilitation
24. In which age-group does rehabilitation take longer?
    A. Infants
    B. Young children
    C. Middle-aged adults
    D. Older adults
25. Which goal would be appropriate for a resident in long-term care who has a progressive illness?
    A. Maintain the highest level of functioning
    B. Improve and return to own home as soon as possible
    C. Restore previous level of functioning
    D. Reverse declines in functioning and daily performance
26. Which rehabilitation program would help a person who cannot walk, or use the arms, and has lost bowel and bladder control after a serious car accident?
    A. Amputee rehabilitation
    B. Orthopedic rehabilitation
    C. Spinal cord rehabilitation
    D. Rehabilitation for complex medical and surgical conditions
27. What is the goal for a person who has a prosthesis?
    A. To have the device function and appear like the missing part
    B. To allow person to resume previous level of function
    C. To prevent deterioration of the affected extremity
    D. To improve the person's appearance
28. Why would the nursing assistant practice the task that the person must perform to achieve success in a rehabilitation program?
    A. To better assist the person
    B. To act as a role model for the person
    C. To experience difficulties of being disabled
    D. To decrease embarrassment for the person

29. Which rehabilitation program would help a person with leg fracture?
   A. Amputee rehabilitation
   B. Orthopedic rehabilitation
   C. Spinal cord rehabilitation
   D. Rehabilitation for complex medical and surgical conditions

Fill in the Blanks

30. The three goals of rehabilitation are to
   A. ______________________
   B. ______________________
   C. ______________________
31. A person with health problems or a disability needs to adjust in these four areas.
   A. ______________________
   B. ______________________
   C. ______________________
   D. ______________________
32. What are some adaptive (assistive) devices that will assist in self-feeding?
   A. ______________________
   B. ______________________
   C. ______________________
33. When assisting with rehabilitation and restorative care, what complications can be prevented if you report early signs and symptoms?
   A. ______________________
   B. ______________________
   C. ______________________
   D. ______________________
34. Who are the team members of the rehabilitation team?
   A. ______________________
   B. ______________________
   C. ______________________
   D. ______________________
   E. ______________________
35. Name seven things that you can do to promote the person's quality of life when a person is receiving rehabilitation and restorative care.
   A. ______________________
   B. ______________________
   C. ______________________
   D. ______________________
   E. ______________________
   F. ______________________
   G. ______________________

Optional Learning Exercises

Mrs. Mercer is 82 years old. She is a resident in a rehabilitation unit because she had a stroke that has caused weakness on her left side. Although she is right-handed, she needs to learn to use several adaptive (assistive) devices as she relearns ways to carry out activities of daily living (ADLs). She often becomes angry or depressed. Answer the following questions about Mrs. Mercer and her care

NOTE: Some of these questions will require information contained in other chapters.

36. Mrs. Mercer is having difficulty with controlling urinary and bowel elimination. What would be the goal of her care for these problems? ______________________ Her plan of care would include programs for ______________.
37. What should you do to prepare Mrs. Mercer's food at mealtime so she can feed herself? (see Chapter 31)
   ____
   ____
38. Mrs. Mercer can brush her teeth but needs help getting prepared. What should you do to get her ready to brush her teeth? (see Chapter 23)
   ____
39. Why does she need help at mealtime and to brush her teeth? (see Chapters 23 and 31) ______________________
   ____
40. Mrs. Mercer needs help to get in and out of bed. When helping her to transfer, you remember to position the chair on her ______________ side. (see Chapter 21)
41. When Mrs. Mercer becomes discouraged because progress is slow, how can you help her? You can stress ______________ and focus on ______________.

Use the FOCUS ON PRIDE section to complete these statements and then use the critical thinking and discussion question to develop your ideas

42. If a nursing assistant is being considered for promotion to a restorative aide position, list three qualities that are considered.
   A. ______________________
   B. ______________________
   C. ______________________
43. List seven things you can do to promote independence when a person is receiving rehabilitation and restorative care.
   A. ______________________
   B. ______________________
   C. ______________________
   D. ______________________
   E. ______________________
   F. ______________________
   G. ______________________

Critical Thinking and Discussion Question

44. You are working on a busy long-term care unit. You see another nursing assistant pushing one of the residents to the dining room in a wheelchair. You know that part of the rehabilitation goal for that resident is to encourage ambulation. Discuss reasons that may have caused the nursing assistant to use the wheelchair.

47 Hearing, Speech, and Vision Problems

Fill in the Blanks: Key Terms

Aphasia	Expressive aphasia (Broca's aphasia)	Low vision	Tinnitus
Blindness	Global aphasia (mixed aphasia)	Presbycusis	Vertigo
Braille	Hearing loss	Presbyopia	
Cerumen		Receptive aphasia (Wernicke's aphasia)	
Deafness			

1. ________________ is a touch reading and writing system that uses raised dots for each letter of the alphabet.
2. Decreased hearing ability due to aging; age-related hearing loss is ________________.
3. Another name for earwax is ________________.
4. ________________ is dizziness.
5. A ringing, roaring, hissing, or buzzing sound in the ears is ________________.
6. The total or partial loss of the ability to use or understand language is ________________.
7. ________________ is not being able to hear the normal range of sounds associated with normal hearing.
8. ________________ is difficulty expressing or sending out thoughts through speech or writing; motor aphasia.
9. Eyesight that cannot be corrected with eyeglasses, contact lenses, medicine, or surgery is ________________.
10. Difficulty understanding language is ________________.
11. A hearing loss in which it is impossible for the person to understand speech through hearing alone is ________________.
12. The gradual loss of the ability to focus on close-up objects that occurs with aging is ________________.
13. ________________ is difficulty expressing or sending out thoughts and difficulty understanding language.
14. The absence of sight is ________________.

Circle the Best Answer

15. Which person has occupational exposure that could cause hearing loss?
    A. Person A is a nursing assistant.
    B. Person B is a factory worker.
    C. Person C is a doctor.
    D. Person D is a plumber.
16. Which ear problem would be the easiest to resolve?
    A. Cerumen in the ear canal
    B. Tinnitus related to ear infection
    C. Risk for falling related to vertigo
    D. Loss of hearing related to aging
17. Which condition may develop if a person has chronic otitis media?
    A. Vertigo
    B. Permanent hearing loss
    C. Sore throat
    D. Nausea and vomiting
18. What would the nursing assistant expect to observe if an infant or young child has otitis media?
    A. Child pulls or tugs at the ear.
    B. Child sleeps more than usual.
    C. Child is frightened by normal sounds.
    D. Child turns the better ear toward sounds.
19. Which finding would the nursing assistant expect if a person with advanced dementia has otitis media?
    A. The person reports dizziness.
    B. Person's speech is barely audible.
    C. Person displays behavioral changes.
    D. The person reports tinnitus.
20. Which consideration is the most important when caring for a person who has Meniere disease?
    A. Risk for falls
    B. Difficulty with hearing
    C. Dietary restrictions
    D. Avoidance of flashing lights
21. Which of these is a preventable cause of hearing loss?
    A. Aging
    B. Heredity and genetics
    C. Exposure to loud sounds
    D. Birth defects
22. Which nursing assistant needs a reminder about communicating with a person who has hearing loss?
    A. Nursing assistant A lightly touches the person's arm.
    B. Nursing assistant B speaks very loudly and slowly.
    C. Nursing assistant C faces the person when speaking.
    D. Nursing assistant D uses gestures and facial expressions to give clues.
23. When does a child with normal hearing begin to babble in a speech-like way?
    A. Birth to 3 months
    B. 7 months to 1 year
    C. 4 to 6 months
    D. 1 to 2 years

24. What would the nursing assistant frequently observe when caring for person with a mild, but progressive hearing loss?
    A. Person can understand by reading lips.
    B. Person is usually very irritable.
    C. Drainage is often seeping from the ears.
    D. Person may deny a hearing loss.
25. Which information would the nursing assistant report to the nurse when caring for a person with a hearing aid?
    A. Time of turning the hearing aid off at night
    B. If a new battery is inserted
    C. If the hearing aid is lost or damaged
    D. When removing the battery at night
26. What would the nursing assistant expect to observe if a person has expressive aphasia?
    A. Person could not understand simple language.
    B. Person would give incorrect answers to questions.
    C. Person would have difficulty hearing what was said.
    D. Person might put words in the wrong order.
27. Which nursing measure is an effective way for the nursing assistant to develop communication with a speech-impaired person?
    A. Speak in a child-like way
    B. Ask the questions to which the answer is known
    C. Give complete and detailed instructions
    D. Make sure the TV and radio are turned on
28. What is the most common cause of cataracts?
    A. Aging
    B. Injury
    C. Poor diet
    D. Surgery
29. Which nursing measure is included for a person who had eye surgery for cataracts?
    A. Removing the eye shield or patch for naps and at night
    B. Having the person cover both eyes during a shower or shampoo
    C. Reminding the person not to rub or press on the affected eye
    D. Placing the overbed table on the operative side
30. Which behavior needs to be reported to the nurse at once for a patient who had cataract surgery?
    A. The person complains of eye pain.
    B. The person cannot see well enough to read.
    C. The person tries to wear their old glasses.
    D. The person asks for help with basic needs.
31. For which activity is a person with advanced age-related macular degeneration (AMD) most likely to need assistance?
    A. Standing up
    B. Brushing teeth
    C. Reading a menu
    D. Getting dressed
32. Which of these measures can reduce the risk for age-related macular degeneration (AMD)?
    A. Wearing sunglasses in bright light
    B. Eating a diet high in green leafy vegetables and fish
    C. Controlling diabetes as directed by doctor
    D. Having regular eye examinations
33. What causes diabetic retinopathy?
    A. Taking too much insulin
    B. Damage to tiny blood vessels in the retina
    C. Trauma that causes clouding of the lens
    D. Increased pressure in the eye
34. Which difficulty in seeing objects will occur for a person who has glaucoma?
    A. Objects that are far away will look enlarged.
    B. Objects in the peripheral vision will be blurred.
    C. Objects directly in front will be invisible.
    D. Objects that are brightly colored will look dark.
35. Which group has the greatest risk for glaucoma?
    A. Anyone older than 60 years
    B. Caucasians and Asians older than 40 years
    C. Younger persons with diabetic retinopathy
    D. Those who need corrective glasses or lens
36. Which parameters define vision for a person who is legally blind?
    A. Is totally unable to see anything including light
    B. Had normal vision at birth and became blind later in life
    C. Can see light at 200 feet, but cannot discern clear details
    D. Sees at 20 feet what a person with normal vision sees at 200 feet.
37. Which action would the nursing assistant take first upon entering the room of a blind person?
    A. Touch the person to let them know you are there
    B. Speak loudly to make sure the person knows you are there
    C. Make sure the lights are bright and the walkways are cleared
    D. Identify self and give name, title, and reason for being there
38. Which nursing measure would the nursing assistant use when caring for a person who is blind?
    A. Give extensive and detailed explanations for actions
    B. Avoid embarrassing words such as "see," "look," or "read"
    C. Offer an arm to assist the person to move about
    D. Perform most of the hygienic care for the person
39. Which action would the nursing assistant take when assisting a blind person to walk?
    A. Walk slightly behind the person and put an arm around the person's waist
    B. Walk slightly ahead with the person holding arm just above the elbow
    C. Grasp the person's arm firmly to guide the way
    D. Walk very slowly to allow the person to take small steps
40. Which nursing measure would the nursing assistant use to assist a blind person who uses a cane?
    A. Grasp the person by the arm holding the cane
    B. Come up behind the person and grasp the elbow
    C. Store the cane so it is out of the way
    D. Ask if assistance is required before trying to help

41. Which action is correct if a blind person uses a guide dog?
    A. Take the person by the arm on the side opposite from the dog
    B. Avoid distracting a guide dog by petting or feeding the dog
    C. Give the dog commands to avoid dangers
    D. Greet, praise, and pet the dog and compliment performance
42. What would the nursing assistant use to clean a person's eyeglasses?
    A. Warm water
    B. Hot water
    C. Detergent
    D. Paper towels
43. Which nursing measure would the nursing assistant take when cleaning an ocular prosthesis?
    A. Wash the artificial eye with mild soap and warm water
    B. Wash the eyelid and eyelashes with sterile water
    C. Dry the artificial eye before inserting it into the socket
    D. Use sterile technique throughout the entire procedure
44. Which type of infection often leads to otitis media?
    A. Urinary tract infection
    B. Brain infection
    C. Throat infection
    D. Eye infection
45. Why would the nursing assistant freely allow a person with visual impairment to move about the room when orienting the person to the room?
    A. To let the nurse know if the person seems confused
    B. To let the person touch and find the furniture and equipment
    C. To respect the person's privacy and individual space
    D. To observe for falls and dangerous obstacles
46. Which permanent condition can result from chronic otitis media?
    A. Hearing loss
    B. Meniere disease
    C. Cerumen impaction
    D. Acute otitis media
47. Which nursing assistant needs a reminder about safety practices when caring for a person who has Meniere disease?
    A. Nursing assistant A assists the person to lie down as needed.
    B. Nursing assistant B initiates fall prevention measures.
    C. Nursing assistant C reminds the person to avoid sudden movements.
    D. Nursing assistant D turns on a bright light for reading.
48. Which person is participating in a recreational activity that is less likely to cause hearing loss?
    A. Person A listens to loud music every day.
    B. Person B likes to watch old movies.
    C. Person C rides a motorcycle for fun and transportation.
    D. Person D regularly goes to shoot at a gun range.
49. Which resident behavior would the nursing assistant report to the nurse for a concern that the resident may have a hearing loss?
    A. Speaks very softly and quietly to others, especially small children
    B. Enjoys talking and frequently asks the nursing assistant to stay and chat
    C. Has trouble following a conservation when several people are speaking
    D. Wants to be invited and included in all activities at the nursing center
50. Which observation would the nursing assistant expect when communicating with a person who has apraxia?
    A. Person understands, but cannot speak.
    B. Person cannot hear so tries to read lips.
    C. Person can speak, but words are slurred.
    D. Person can hear, but does not understand.
51. Which member of the health-care team is likely to have the most trouble being heard when communicating with an elderly resident who has hearing loss?
    A. A 22-year-old male nursing student
    B. A 19-year-old female nursing assistant
    C. A 40-year-old male social worker
    D. A 68-year-old male doctor
52. Which communication problem would the nursing assistant anticipate when caring for a patient who has expressive aphasia?
    A. Person would have problems with speaking, gesturing, or writing.
    B. Person would have problems hearing soft tones or high-pitched voices.
    C. Person would have difficulties understanding directions.
    D. Person would immediately forget what was said or asked.
53. Which person has several risk factors for cataracts?
    A. Person A, aged 6 years, was treated for contagious pink eye infection.
    B. Person B, aged 67 years, had a heart attack last year, but has recovered.
    C. Person C, aged 23 years, has type 1 diabetes that is controlled with insulin.
    D. Person D, aged 72 years, is a smoker, drinks alcohol, and has high blood pressure.
54. At which distance does a legally blind person see an object that a person with normal vision sees at 200 feet?
    A. 2 feet
    B. 20 feet
    C. 100 feet
    D. 200 feet
55. Which reminder would the nursing assistant give to a person about wearing an eye shield after cataract surgery?
    A. Put it on before going to sleep
    B. Take it off when showering
    C. Secure it tightly over the eye
    D. Put it on if the eye starts hurting

56. Which nursing assistant is using the best body language to communicate with a person who has a hearing loss?
   A. Nursing assistant A chats with person while making the bed and cleaning up.
   B. Nursing assistant B faces and looks directly at person while speaking.
   C. Nursing assistant C stands beside the person's bed while conversing.
   D. Nursing assistant D looks in from the doorway and waves to the person.

Fill in the Blanks

57. Write out the abbreviations
   A. AMD ______
   B. ASL ______
   C. ADA ______
58. List four problems that could occur with a hearing loss.
   A. ______
   B. ______
   C. ______
   D. ______
59. Identify nine symptoms of hearing loss.
   A. ______
   B. ______
   C. ______
   D. ______
   E. ______
   F. ______
   G. ______
   H. ______
   I. ______
60. What are three common causes of speech disorders?
   A. ______
   B. ______
   C. ______
61. When communicating with a speech-impaired person, the nursing assistant would watch the person's ______ movements, ______ expressions, gestures, and body language.
62. When a person has receptive aphasia, the person has trouble ______.
63. The person with glaucoma sees through a ______, has blurred vision, and sees a ______ around lights.
64. Drugs and surgery are used with glaucoma to prevent further damage to the ______ nerve.
65. When assisting a blind or visually impaired person, list seven things that can be done to provide a consistent mealtime setting.
   A. ______
   B. ______
   C. ______
   D. ______
   E. ______
   F. ______
   G. ______
66. A person with age-related macular degeneration (AMD) would develop a blind spot ______.
67. For people who have diabetes, there is an increased risk for which eye disorder? ______.
68. How can a person with low vision use a computer as an adaptive device?
   A. ______
   B. ______

Optional Learning Exercises

Mr. Herman is an 85-year-old man with hearing loss that developed with aging. Answer these questions about his care.

69. Two nursing assistants, a male and a female, are caring for Mr. Herman. They notice that he answers questions asked by the male nursing assistant more quickly. What is the likely reason for this?
   ______
   ______
70. The nursing assistants have found that Mr. Herman is alert and oriented. They are surprised when Joan, another nursing assistant, tells them he is "senile." Why would Joan make this statement?
   ______
71. Mr. Herman says he is too tired to go to the game room for a party. He says no one likes him. What are some reasons for his actions and statements?
   A. Tired because
   ______
   B. No one likes him
   ______
72. When giving care, the nursing assistant turns off the TV and radio in Mr. Herman's room. Why is this done? ______

You are caring for Mrs. Sanchez, who is legally blind because of glaucoma. Answer these questions about her care.

73. When you enter the room, you notice that Mrs. Sanchez is looking at her mail with a magnifying glass. How is this possible since you thought she was blind? ______
   ______
74. When you enter the room, Mrs. Sanchez asks you to adjust the blinds. Why? ______
75. When you are helping Mrs. Sanchez to move about the room, you are careful to tell her where furniture is located. Why? ______
   ______

Use the FOCUS ON PRIDE section to complete these statements and then use the critical thinking and discussion questions to develop your ideas

76. When you are referring to a person who has speech, hearing, or vision problems, the person should be referred to by ______, not by the ______.
77. Braille signs for areas with public access are required by the ______.

Critical Thinking and Discussion Questions

78. A resident in a long-term care center has a hearing aid that she cannot independently use or maintain. She is pleasant and cooperative, but mildly confused. Sometimes she removes the hearing aid and then misplaces it. On other days, she wears it all day long without problems. Today, she has removed the hearing aid several times and you found it among the bed linens, on the bathroom sink, and on her roommate's bedside table. You tell the nurse, who instructs you to store it in the case for today. Later, the daughter visits and she is upset because the resident is not wearing the hearing aid.

    Discuss this situation:

    A. What are the issues for the staff?
    B. Why is the daughter upset?
    C. What could the staff do?

79. For the four American sign examples, identify the meaning of each sign.

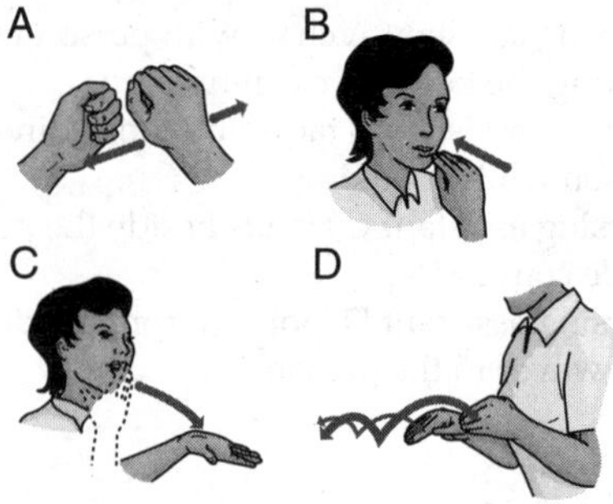

A. ______________________________
B. ______________________________
C. ______________________________
D. ______________________________

48 Cancer, Immune System, and Skin Disorders

Fill in the Blanks: Key Terms

Benign tumor
Biopsy
Cancer (malignant tumor)
Metastasis
Mole
Stomatitis
Tumor

1. A ______________________ is a tumor that invades and destroys nearby tissue and can spread to other body parts.
2. Inflammation of the mouth is ____________________.
3. A tumor that does not spread to other body parts is a ____.
4. A new growth of abnormal cells that may be benign or malignant is a ______________________________.
5. The spread of cancer to other body parts is ____.
6. A ____ is a procedure in which a piece of tissue is removed for testing.
7. A ____________________________________ is a brown, tan, or black spot on the skin that is flat or raised and round or oval.

Circle the Best Answer

8. Which goal for cancer treatment allows the nursing assistant to participate by taking responsibility for vigilant observing and reporting?
   A. Curing the cancer
   B. Controlling the disease
   C. Eliminating the signs and symptoms of the disease
   D. Reducing the signs and symptoms of the treatments
9. What would be an early sign or symptom of leukemia, which is the most common cancer that occurs in children?
   A. Seizures
   B. Fatigue
   C. Weight loss
   D. Black-colored mole
10. Which person is performing an action that represents a risk factor for cancer?
    A. Applying sunscreen
    B. Smoking a cigarette
    C. Eating an apple
    D. Drinking a soda
11. What is the primary purpose of doing surgery for patients who have cancer?
    A. Cure or control the cancer
    B. Kill the cancer cells
    C. Shrink the tumor
    D. Block hormone production
12. Which patient behavior would the nursing assistant expect to observe when caring for a person who is receiving radiation therapy?
    A. Wants more attention after therapy
    B. Needs extra rest related to fatigue
    C. Is at risk for bleeding and infections
    D. Has flu-like symptoms
13. What does chemotherapy involve?
    A. X-ray beams aimed at the tumor
    B. Local radiation to kill the tumor
    C. Therapies that spare normal cells
    D. Giving drugs that kill cells
14. Which action would the nursing assistant take when a person who is receiving chemotherapy is upset because her hair is falling out?
    A. Reassure that hair will regrow normally
    B. Tell her this is a symptom of her disease
    C. Report this to the nurse at once
    D. Change the subject so she will not be so upset
15. Which side effects may a woman experience when hormone therapy is used to treat cancer?
    A. Stomatitis and alopecia
    B. Flu-like symptoms
    C. Hot flashes, and loss of sexual desire
    D. Burns and skin breakdown
16. What is included in complementary and alternative medicine (CAM) treatment for cancer patients?
    A. Drugs or surgeries to remove hormone sources in the body
    B. Massage therapy, herbal products, and spiritual healing
    C. Implanting of radiation implants
    D. Giving blood-forming stem cells
17. Which nursing assistant needs a reminder about safety measures to protect self when caring for a patient with a radiation implant?
    A. Nursing assistant A checks on the person from the doorway.
    B. Nursing assistant B limits time spent in close proximity to the person.
    C. Nursing assistant C minimizes time in the room as much as possible.
    D. Nursing assistant D forgets to wear a radiation exposure badge.
18. Which nursing measure would the nursing assistant use when a person who has cancer expresses anger, fear, and depression?
    A. Tell the person not to worry or get upset
    B. Give the person privacy and time alone
    C. Be there when needed and listen to the person
    D. Change the subject to distract the person

19. For which activity of daily living, is a person with celiac disease most likely to require assistance?
    A. Toileting
    B. Ambulating
    C. Bathing
    D. Dressing
20. Which action would the nursing assistant perform when caring for a person who has acquired immunodeficiency syndrome (AIDS)?
    A. Assist the nurse to isolate the person using respiratory precautions
    B. Encourage self-care and avoid touching the person
    C. Assist with daily hygiene; avoid irritating soaps
    D. Double bag all linen and mark with a biohazard label
21. Which action would the nursing assistant take to protect self from human immunodeficiency virus (HIV) and acquired immunodeficiency syndrome (AIDS)?
    A. Avoid body fluids, such as urine, sputum, and saliva when giving care
    B. Wear filter mask, gloves, gown, and shoe covers for routine care
    C. Follow Standard Precautions and the Blood-borne Pathogen Standard
    D. Always use the sterile technique when giving any care
22. Which infectious disorder is caused by the same virus that causes shingles?
    A. Human immunodeficiency virus (HIV)
    B. Measles
    C. Chicken pox
    D. Mumps
23. Which person has a risk factor for cancer that can be avoided?
    A. Person A is 42 years old and is more than 70 pounds overweight.
    B. Person B had a liver transplant and takes medication to prevent rejection.
    C. Person C is 73 years old and has a history of dental problems.
    D. Person D has a significant family history for several types of cancer.
24. Which nursing assistant should notify the nurse for reassignment if the patient has radiation seed implants?
    A. Nursing assistant A has high blood pressure.
    B. Nursing assistant B is 4 months pregnant.
    C. Nursing assistant C just graduated and is newly hired.
    D. Nursing assistant D is older and has family history for cancer.
25. What is the cause of acquired immunodeficiency syndrome (AIDS)?
    A. Virus
    B. Bacteria
    C. Sexual intercourse
    D. Autoimmune response
26. Which finding would the nursing assistant expect to observe for a patient who is undergoing radiation therapy which destroys cancer cells and normal cells?
    A. Skin at the treatment site appears red and blistered.
    B. Large pieces of tissue slough off at the treatment site.
    C. Patient is unable to move or use body part that was treated.
    D. Patient has deep, disfiguring, and permanent burn scars.
27. Which nursing assistant needs a reminder about maintaining personal safety when caring for a person who is receiving chemotherapy?
    A. Nursing assistant A wears gloves for any contact with the person's body fluids.
    B. Nursing assistant B double bags incontinence products and waterproof underpads.
    C. Nursing assistant C forgets to put the lid down and flushes toilet once because of pets.
    D. Nursing assistant D empties and rinses bedpans, urinals, and kidney basins after use.
28. What is the main threat to personal health and risk for infection for nursing assistants when caring for a person with human immunodeficiency virus (HIV)?
    A. Needlesticks
    B. Cleaning perineal area
    C. Touching bloody linens
    D. Being close to the person
29. Which nursing assistant should notify the nurse for reassignment if the patient has shingles?
    A. Nursing assistant A had second dose of shingles vaccine last month.
    B. Nursing assistant B has a child who had chicken pox several years ago.
    C. Nursing assistant C received the vaccine to prevent chicken pox.
    D. Nursing assistant D is older and has a weakened immune system.

Fill in the Blanks

30. Write out the abbreviations
    A. AIDS ______________________________
    B. HIV ______________________________
    C. STD ______________________________
31. Cancer is the ____________________ leading cause of death in the United States.
32. A person with cancer may complain of constipation because of ________________.
33. The signs and symptoms of colon cancer are
    A. ______________________________
    B. ______________________________
    C. ______________________________
    D. ______________________________
    E. ______________________________
    F. ______________________________
    G. ______________________________
    H. ______________________________

34. List seven skin changes that are side effects of radiation therapy.
    A. ____________________
    B. ____________________
    C. ____________________
    D. ____________________
    E. ____________________
    F. ____________________
    G. ____________________
35. For a person who is receiving chemotherapy, list six side effects that might occur.
    A. ____________________
    B. ____________________
    C. ____________________
    D. ____________________
    E. ____________________
    F. ____________________
36. Complementary and Alternative Medicine (CAM) is sometimes used with standard cancer treatment. List seven treatments.
    A. ____________________
    B. ____________________
    C. ____________________
    D. ____________________
    E. ____________________
    F. ____________________
    G. ____________________
37. When a person has an autoimmune disorder, it means the ____________________ system attacks the ____________________.
38. List three treatment goals for autoimmune disorders.
    A. ____________________
    B. ____________________
    C. ____________________
39. How is human immunodeficiency virus (HIV) mainly transmitted?
    A. ____________________
    B. ____________________
40. Identify three groups of people who are at risk for developing shingles.
    A. ____________________
    B. ____________________
    C. ____________________

Optional Learning Exercises

Mrs. Myers is 62 years old who is having chemotherapy to treat cancer. She has not been eating well and complains of feeling very tired. When you assist her with personal care, you notice a large amount of hair on her pillow. Answer these questions about Mrs. Myers and her care.

41. Mrs. Myers may not be eating well because the chemotherapy ____________________ the gastrointestinal tract and causes ____________________, ____________________, ____________________, and ____________________.
42. She may also have inflammation of the mouth, which is called ____________________. You can help to relieve the discomfort from this side effect when you provide ____________________.
43. What is causing Mrs. Myers to lose her hair? ____________________. This condition is called ____________________.

Use the FOCUS ON PRIDE section to complete these statements and then use the critical thinking and discussion question to develop your ideas

44. If you work on an oncology unit, staff and patients value a person who is ____________________, ____________________, ____________________, and ____________________.
45. When you work closely with oncology patients and families, you must protect the person's privacy and rights and avoid crossing ____________________.

Critical Thinking and Discussion Question

46. You are caring for an older woman who was recently diagnosed with breast cancer. The nurse tells you that the woman is also human immunodeficiency virus (HIV) positive. You don gloves, before picking up soiled items and then discard the gloves and wash your hands after you are finished. The woman seems upset and remarks, "I have cancer. It's not contagious you know that don't you? Why are you wearing gloves and why do you keep washing your hands?" What should you say and do?

49 Nervous System and Musculoskeletal Disorders

Fill in the Blanks: Key Terms

Amputation
Arthritis
Arthroplasty
Closed fracture (simple fracture)
Fracture
Gangrene
Hemiparesis
Hemiplegia
Open fracture (compound fracture)
Paralysis
Paraplegia
Paresis
Quadriplegia (tetraplegia)

1. Weak or impaired muscle function without complete paralysis; partial paralysis is ______________________________.
2. ______________________________ is loss of muscle function.
3. The removal of all or part of an extremity is ______________________________.
4. A ______________________ is when the bone is broken, but the skin is intact.
5. ______________________________ is paralysis in the arms, legs, and trunk.
6. Paralysis on one side of the body is ______________________________.
7. Joint inflammation is ______________________________.
8. Partial paralysis on one side of the body is ______________________________.
9. A ______________________________ is a broken bone.
10. An ______________________________ occurs when the broken bone has come through the skin.
11. An ______________________________ is the surgical replacement of a joint.
12. Paralysis in the legs and lower trunk is ______________________________.
13. A condition in which there is death of tissue is ______________________________.

Circle the Best Answer

14. Which safety measure would the nursing assistant perform to help protect a person who has Parkinson disease?
    A. Suggest that the person should adhere to the exercise program
    B. Anticipate impaired balance and assist with standing and walking
    C. Follow the speech therapist's plan for speech improvement
    D. Administer drugs that are ordered to control the disease
15. Which nursing measure would the nursing assistant perform when a young woman has a flare-up of multiple sclerosis (MS) symptoms?
    A. Feed the woman small spoonfuls of soft food
    B. Encourage rest and naps for fatigue
    C. Perform passive range of motion for the patient
    D. Speak clearly and repeat as needed
16. Which action would the home health nursing assistant take when the patient's family reports that the patient had an episode of confusion and trouble speaking that lasted a few minutes and then resolved?
    A. Call the nurse at once and report situation and observations
    B. Advise the family that temporary signs and symptoms are not dangerous
    C. Assist the patient to lie down and rest for at least 24 hours
    D. Tell the family to make an appointment with the doctor
17. Which risk factor for stroke could be modified or controlled?
    A. Male gender
    B. Age older than 55 years
    C. Family history for heart disease
    D. High cholesterol
18. Which action would the nursing assistant perform when caring for a person who has right-sided "neglect" after a stroke?
    A. Assist the person to wash the left side of the face
    B. Approach the person on the right side
    C. Perform range-of-motion exercises on the right side
    D. Point out food items on the left side of the plate
19. Where would the nursing assistant place the call light for a person who has had a stroke?
    A. Positioned near the person's head
    B. Placed on the weak side of the body
    C. Placed on the strong side of the body
    D. Given to a family member to use for the person
20. What is a safety concern for a person with Parkinson disease?
    A. Changes in speech
    B. Swallowing problems
    C. A masklike expression
    D. Emotional changes

21. What is the main safety concern for a person with multiple sclerosis (MS)?
    A. Risk for falls
    B. Prone to infections
    C. Risk for aspiration
    D. Problems with breathing
22. What is expected when amyotrophic lateral sclerosis (ALS) progresses?
    A. Person becomes confused and disoriented.
    B. Person is able to walk with some assistance.
    C. Person is incontinent of bladder and bowel functions.
    D. Person is unable to move the arms, legs, and body.
23. Which nursing measure would the nursing assistant use if a person is in a vegetative state after traumatic brain injury?
    A. Assist with meals by spoon feeding small portions
    B. Gently wake the person up and explain care
    C. Encourage the person to participate in self-care
    D. Perform total hygienic care for the person
24. Which action would the nursing assistant most likely perform in caring for a person who has paraplegia from a spinal cord injury?
    A. Comb the person's hair
    B. Cut food into bite-size pieces
    C. Lock the wheelchair prior to transfer
    D. Assist the person to button the shirt
25. Which person is most likely to require the application of elastic stockings to prevent thrombi?
    A. Person A who had a stroke.
    B. Person B who has osteoarthritis.
    C. Person C who has an open wrist fracture.
    D. Person D who has multiple sclerosis (MS).
26. Which condition creates a risk for autonomic hyperreflexia?
    A. Recent traumatic brain injury
    B. Paralysis above the mid-thoracic level
    C. Stroke caused by cerebral hemorrhage
    D. Advanced amyotrophic lateral sclerosis (ALS)
27. Which observation needs to be reported to the nurse at once when caring for a person who has risk for autonomic hyperreflexia?
    A. The person reports a throbbing headache.
    B. The blood pressure is low.
    C. The person has pain below the level of the injury.
    D. The person has the urge to urinate.
28. Which nursing assistant needs a reminder about caring for a person who has risk for autonomic hyperreflexia?
    A. Nursing assistant A gives basic hygienic and daily care.
    B. Nursing assistant B removes wrinkles from clothing and linen.
    C. Nursing assistant C assists the person to zip up tight pants.
    D. Nursing assistant D repositions the person at least every 2 hours.
29. Which task would be part of the nursing assistant's responsibility when caring for a person who has rheumatoid arthritis?
    A. Identifying exercise activities that have low risk for joint stress
    B. Applying heat or cold applications according to the care plan
    C. Teaching the person how to use a cane or a walker
    D. Telling the person to eat low calorie foods
30. Which nursing measure would be most helpful to the person who has arthritis?
    A. Encouraging the person to stay in bed and to take frequent naps
    B. Keeping the room cool and well ventilated at all times
    C. Helping the person to use good body mechanics and good posture
    D. Telling the person to talk to the doctor about joint replacement surgery
31. Which action would the nursing assistant perform when caring for a person who has had a total hip replacement?
    A. Have a soft plush chair for the person to sit on
    B. Perform full range of motion on the affected side
    C. Remind the person not to cross legs while seated
    D. Place a low commode chair close to the bed
32. Which person requires gentle handling because of an increased risk for fractures?
    A. Person A has an amputated limb.
    B. Person B had traumatic brain injury.
    C. Person C has osteoporosis.
    D. Person D had a stroke.
33. Which person is displaying a sign or symptom of a fracture?
    A. Person A has full range of motion in the affected limb.
    B. Person B has bruising and color change in the affected area.
    C. Person C displays tremors and pill-rolling movements.
    D. Person D has sudden weakness and numbness in the affected limb.
34. What is the advantage of a closed reduction for treatment of a fracture?
    A. Infection is less likely to occur.
    B. Pain is significantly decreased.
    C. Dysfunction will not happen.
    D. Swelling is minimal.
35. How long does it take for a newly applied plaster cast to dry?
    A. 2 to 4 hours
    B. 3 to 4 days
    C. 24 to 48 hours
    D. 12 to 24 hours
36. Which action would the nursing assistant use to prevent flat spots on a cast?
    A. Position the cast on a hard, stable surface
    B. Support the entire cast with pillows
    C. Grasp the edge of the cast with your fingertips
    D. Cover the cast with a blanket

37. Which action would the nursing assistant take if a person complains of numbness in a limb that has a cast?
   A. Move the limb to relieve the numbness
   B. Reposition the limb to decrease pressure
   C. Gently rub the exposed toes or fingers
   D. Tell the nurse at once
38. Which nursing measure would the nursing assistant use when giving care to a person in traction?
   A. Put bottom linens on the bed from the top down
   B. Remove the weights while giving care
   C. Roll the person from side to side to give care
   D. Assist the person to use the commode chair when needed
39. Which nursing measure would the nursing assistant apply to the operated leg after surgery to repair a hip fracture?
   A. Keep it abducted at all times
   B. Maintain adduction at all times
   C. Massage the leg every 4 hours
   D. Position leg to maintain external rotation
40. Which nursing measure would the nursing assistant use when assisting a person to get up in a chair after hip surgery?
   A. Place the chair at the foot of the bed
   B. Place the chair on the unaffected side
   C. Have a low, soft comfortable chair for the person to use
   D. Encourage the person to briefly stand on the affected leg
41. Which action would the nursing assistant take if a person reported phantom pain in the amputated part?
   A. Report this to the nurse at once
   B. Be calm; the person is probably confused
   C. Reassure the person that this is a normal reaction
   D. Remind the person that body part is gone
42. Which nursing measure would the nursing assistant expect to perform in caring for a person who has amyotrophic lateral sclerosis (ALS)?
   A. Repeating instructions because of short-term memory loss
   B. Communicating with a white board for hearing loss
   C. Helping with hygiene related to bowel incontinence
   D. Assisting with transfers from bed to wheelchair
43. Which person will need range-of-motion exercises to prevent contractures?
   A. Person A had a transient ischemic attack.
   B. Person B had a stroke and the left arm is paralyzed.
   C. Person C experienced autonomic dysreflexia yesterday.
   D. Person D had a traumatic brain injury and needs supervision for ADLs.
44. Which nursing measure would the nursing assistant use to help relieve pain for a person who has arthritis?
   A. Tell the nurse to give the pain medication, right away
   B. Tell the person about personal successful strategies for weight loss
   C. Assist the person to take a warm bath or shower in the morning
   D. Suggest that the person talk to the doctor about joint replacement surgery
45. Which person is most likely to benefit from having a cane or walker to provide support when ambulating?
   A. Person A had a traumatic brain injury and is frequently frustrated.
   B. Person B is having frequent episodes of autonomic dysreflexia.
   C. Person C has arthritis and is awaiting knee replacement surgery.
   D. Person D was recently diagnosed with osteoporosis.
46. Which nursing assistant needs a reminder in caring for a person who had a hip replacement?
   A. Nursing assistant A avoids crossing the operated leg past the midline of the body.
   B. Nursing assistant B assists person to sit in a high chair with armrests.
   C. Nursing assistant C assists person to sit on an elevated toilet seat.
   D. Nursing assistant D flexes the hips past 90 degrees during hygienic care.
47. Which nutrients are emphasized in the prevention and treatment of osteoporosis?
   A. High-quality proteins
   B. Calcium and vitamin D
   C. Iron and vitamin C
   D. Low fat and low carbohydrate
48. Which nursing assistant needs a reminder about caring for a person in traction?
   A. Nursing assistant A changes a rope when noticing that it is frayed.
   B. Nursing assistant B performs range-of-motion exercises on uninvolved joints.
   C. Nursing assistant C reports redness and drainage at the pin site at once to the nurse.
   D. Nursing assistant D does not add or remove weights while giving care.
49. Which device would the nursing assistant use to prevent external rotation for a person who has a fractured hip?
   A. Splint
   B. Trochanter roll
   C. External fixation pin
   D. Hip abduction wedge
50. Which position is avoided when turning and positioning a person after hip surgery?
   A. Laying on the unaffected side
   B. Low Fowler's position
   C. Laying on the operative side
   D. Laying in the dorsal recumbent position

Fill in the Blanks

51. Write out the abbreviations
    A. AD ______
    B. ADL ______
    C. ALS ______
    D. CVA ______
    E. JA ______
    F. MS ______
    G. RA ______
    H. ROM ______
    I. TBI ______
    J. TIA ______
52. List five warning signs of stroke.
    A. ______
    B. ______
    C. ______
    D. ______
    E. ______
53. If a person has stroke-like symptoms that last a few minutes, it means that the person had a ______.
54. Name four signs and symptoms of Parkinson disease.
    A. ______
    B. ______
    C. ______
    D. ______
55. When symptoms of multiple sclerosis (MS) disappear, the person is in ______.
56. What are the five common causes of traumatic brain injury?
    A. ______
    B. ______
    C. ______
    D. ______
    E. ______
57. ______ are the major cause of head injuries in newborns.
58. When caring for a person with paralysis, you must check the person often if they are unable to use the ______.
59. A person with a spinal cord injury, reports blurred vision and a headache. You notice that the urinary catheter tube is kinked. You immediately notify the nurse because the person is having signs or symptoms of ______.
60. List six risk factors for developing osteoporosis.
    A. ______
    B. ______
    C. ______
    D. ______
    E. ______
    F. ______
61. What types of exercise are used to help prevent osteoporosis for weight-bearing joints?
    ______
62. When a person with a fracture has a cast, what do these symptoms mean?
    A. Pain ______
    B. Odor ______
    C. Numbness ______
    D. Cool skin ______
    E. Hot skin ______
63. If the person has an internal fixation device, the operative leg is not elevated when sitting in a chair because ______.
64. What disease is a common cause of vascular changes that can lead to an amputation?
    ______
65. Phantom pain after an amputation is considered a ______ reaction.

Optional Learning Exercises

You are caring for Mrs. Huber, who has had a stroke. The next five questions relate to Mrs. Huber and her care. The care plan gives the following instructions; explain the reason for these instructions.

66. Position Mrs. Huber in a side-lying position.
    ______
67. Approach Mrs. Huber from the unaffected side.
    ______
68. Mrs. Huber is given a dysphagia diet.
    ______
69. Elastic stockings are applied as part of her care.
    ______
70. Range-of-motion exercises are given.
    ______

You are caring for two persons who have arthritis. Read the information about each of them and answer the two questions about these persons.

- *Mr. Miller is 78 years old. He worked in construction for many years, where he did heavy physical work. He complains about pain in his hips and right knee. His fingers are deformed by arthritis and interfere with good range of motion.*
- *Mrs. Haxton is 40 years old. She has swelling, warmth, and tenderness in her wrists, several finger joints on both hands, and both knees. She tells you that she has had arthritis for about 10 years and it "comes and goes." At present, Mrs. Haxton has a temperature of 100.2°F and she states that she is tired and does not feel well.*

71. Which type of arthritis does Mr. Miller have? ________________ His ________ may have contributed to the joint pain. ________________.

72. Mrs. Haxton probably has ________________ arthritis. She complains of not feeling well because the arthritis affects ________________ as well as the joints.

Use the FOCUS ON PRIDE section to complete this statement and then use the critical thinking and discussion questions to develop your ideas

73. List four ways to promote independence when caring for persons with neurologic or musculoskeletal disorders.
    A. ________________
    B. ________________
    C. ________________
    D. ________________

Critical Thinking and Discussion Questions

74. You are assigned to care for a person who had a stroke. The nurse tells you that he has hemiplegia on the right side and will need assistance with most activities of daily living (ADLs) during the day. He is alert and he appears to understand your explanations and instructions. After you finish helping him with morning hygiene, you ensure that the call bell is within reach and the side rails are in place according to the care plan. You complete a safety check of the room before leaving. Thirty minutes later, you come back to check on him and he is attempting to climb over the side rails. You successfully help him get repositioned in the bed.
    A. What do you think caused the person to try and climb over the side rails?
    B. Why would you report this incident to the nurse?

50 Cardiovascular, Respiratory, and Lymphatic Disorders

Fill in the Blanks: Key Terms

Anemia	Congenital	Hypertension	Pneumonia
Apnea	Dysrhythmia (arrhythmia)	Lymphedema	Sleep apnea

1. An inflammation and infection of lung tissue is ______________________________.
2. An abnormal heart rhythm is ________________.
3. Pauses in breathing that occur during sleep is ______________________________.
4. The lack or absence of breathing is ________________.
5. ________________________ means to be born with a condition.
6. A decrease in the amount of healthy red blood cells is ______________________________
7. A buildup of lymph in the tissues causing edema is ______________________________.
8. The medical term for high blood pressure is ______________________________.

Circle the Best Answer

9. Which personal behavior should be discontinued if a person has bronchitis or emphysema?
   A. Drinking alcohol
   B. Eating red meat
   C. Smoking cigarettes
   D. Drinking caffeinated drinks
10. Which person needs assistance with a lifestyle change for the management of coronary artery disease?
    A. Person A walks at least 1 mile three to four times per week.
    B. Person B has reduced smoking cigarettes to one or two per day.
    C. Person C does stress reduction techniques one to two times per day.
    D. Person D eats fried foods at least five times per week.
11. What might the nursing assistant observe about the skin of an infant who has a congenital heart defect?
    A. Face and upper body are red.
    B. Skin is dry and flaky.
    C. Skin has a yellowish tint.
    D. Lips and skin have a bluish tint.
12. Which breakfast item could potentially contribute to plaque formation and atherosclerosis?
    A. Coffee
    B. Orange juice
    C. Oatmeal
    D. Bacon
13. Which blood pressure reading would the nursing assistant report because it is a warning signal for hypertension for a person who has risk factors, such as being overweight or having diabetes?
    A. 100/60
    B. 120/70
    C. 125/75
    D. 130/88
14. Which risk factor for hypertension cannot be modified?
    A. Stress
    B. Being overweight
    C. Age
    D. Lack of exercise
15. What is the most common cause of coronary artery disease?
    A. Lack of exercise
    B. Atherosclerosis
    C. Family history
    D. Stress
16. Which action is part of the nursing assistant's responsibilities for a person who needs cardiac rehabilitation?
    A. Develop an exercise training program for the person
    B. Teach the person about the heart condition
    C. Ensure that the person maintains strict bed rest
    D. Help the person select foods from a heart healthy menu
17. Which action usually relieves angina pain?
    A. Resting for several minutes
    B. Taking an aspirin or pain reliever
    C. Using oxygen therapy
    D. Getting up and walking for exercise
18. Which nursing measure would the nursing assistant use if a person takes a nitroglycerin tablet for angina?
    A. Give them a large glass of water to swallow the pill
    B. Take the pills back to the nurses' station
    C. Make sure the nurse knows that a pill was taken
    D. Encourage the person to walk around the room
19. Which equipment is the nurse most likely to ask the nursing assistant to obtain when a person is admitted to the long-term care facility and has a high risk for myocardial infarction?
    A. Oxygen tank and nasal cannula
    B. Continuous positive airway pressure (CPAP) device
    C. Cart with items for airborne precautions
    D. Elastic compression stockings
20. Which condition may be occurring and be must immediately assessed by the nurse when a person reports pain or numbness in the back, neck, jaw, or stomach?
    A. Person is having an angina attack.
    B. Person could be having early symptoms of a stroke.
    C. Person may be having a myocardial infarction.
    D. Person has worsening of chronic obstructive pulmonary disease (COPD).

21. Which signs and symptoms are observed when a patient has pulmonary edema secondary to heart failure?
    A. Dyspnea, cough, pink sputum, and gurgling sounds
    B. Irregular pulse and a low blood pressure
    C. Hot, red, dry skin with chills and fever
    D. Sneezing, coughing, and stuffy or runny nose
22. Which complication is a risk for an older person with heart failure?
    A. Contractures
    B. Skin breakdown
    C. Fractures
    D. Urinary tract infections
23. Which task will the home health nursing assistant perform related to the pacemaker?
    A. Test the battery function and change it as needed
    B. Check the lead wires to make sure that they are intact and not frayed or kinked
    C. Assist the person to check the function of the pacemaker via phone or internet
    D. Clean the pacemaker according to the manufacturer's instructions
24. What is the greatest risk factor for chronic obstructive pulmonary disease (COPD)?
    A. Family history
    B. Respiratory infections
    C. Cigarette smoking
    D. Exercise
25. Which physiologic function is adversely affected when a person has chronic obstructive pulmonary disease (COPD)?
    A. Oxygen (O_2) and carbon dioxide (CO_2) exchange in the lungs
    B. Blood flow to the heart and other organs
    C. The function of the kidneys and bladder
    D. Heart rhythm and the strength of the contractions
26. What is a common symptom of chronic bronchitis?
    A. Wheezing and tightening in the chest
    B. Shortness of breath on exertion
    C. A smoker's cough that produces a lot of mucus
    D. A high temperature for several days
27. Which information does the nursing assistant need to get from the nurse and the care plan when caring for a person with asthma?
    A. The allergens that trigger reactions
    B. The setting for the oxygen level
    C. The amount of fluid allowed
    D. How often to reposition the person?
28. Which nursing measure will the nursing assistant perform for a person who has sleep apnea?
    A. Wake the person every time there is loud snoring or gasping
    B. Position the person in a high Fowler's position for sleep and rest
    C. Alert nurse if the continuous positive airway pressure (CPAP) device is not working
    D. Encourage the person to take several naps during the day
29. Which finding can be observed when an older person has influenza?
    A. Body temperature below normal
    B. Chest pain and a hacking cough
    C. Thirst and hunger
    D. No symptoms of illness
30. Which signs and symptoms should the home health nursing assistant report to the nurse as a possible sign of anemia?
    A. Rapid pulse and dizziness
    B. Cough and stuffy nose
    C. Low-grade fever and body aches
    D. Thickening of the skin with itching
31. Which person needs Standard Precautions and airborne precautions?
    A. Person has emphysema and is unwilling to stop smoking.
    B. Person is admitted for asthma, probably allergy induced.
    C. Person was recently diagnosed with tuberculosis.
    D. Person has chronic bronchitis.
32. What is the purpose of increasing the fluid intake for a person who has pneumonia?
    A. Decrease the amount of bacteria in the lungs
    B. Dilute medication given to treat the disease
    C. Thin secretions and help reduce fever
    D. Decrease inflammation of the breathing passages
33. Which position eases the work of breathing for a person with pneumonia?
    A. Semi-Fowler's position
    B. Side-lying position
    C. Supine position
    D. Dorsal recumbent position
34. Which nursing measure must the nursing assistant remember when caring for a person who has lymphedema?
    A. Never use an affected arm to take a blood pressure
    B. Keep the affected arm or leg elevated at all times
    C. Keep the person on strict bed rest
    D. Restrict fluid intake
35. Which person has the greatest number of nonmodifiable risk factors for hypertension?
    A. A 65-year-old man with a family history of high blood pressure.
    B. A 25-year-old man who is overweight and has diabetes.
    C. A 55-year-old woman who is physically fit, but has stressful family situation.
    D. A 32-year-old woman who eats a diet that is high in fat, salt, and cholesterol.
36. Which person needs help to review activities that may bring on angina?
    A. Person A has a demanding and stressful job.
    B. Person B does regular moderate stretching exercises.
    C. Person C plans a vacation in an area with a temperate climate.
    D. Person D eats a light meal and then relaxes with friends.

37. Where are nitroglycerin tablets kept?
   A. In the bathroom medication cabinet
   B. In the person's bedside table
   C. At the nurses' station
   D. Within the person's reach at all times
38. Which factors in an older person who has heart failure increase the risk for skin breakdown?
   A. Urinary and bowel incontinence
   B. Poor circulation and tissue swelling
   C. Mental confusion and anxiety
   D. Increased appetite and weight gain
39. What is a common complication of influenza?
   A. Pneumonia
   B. Sleep apnea
   C. Myocardial infarction
   D. Human immunodeficiency virus
40. Which body system is involved when cancer invades and lymphoma occurs?
   A. Respiratory system
   B. Immune system
   C. Circulatory system
   D. Nervous system
41. Which patient would have a compression sleeve as part of the treatment?
   A. Patient A has right-sided heart failure.
   B. Patient B is weakened after myocardial infarction.
   C. Patient C sustained a fracture in the left wrist.
   D. Patient D has lymphedema of the right arm.
42. Which task would be assigned to the nursing assistant to help the person who is in a cardiac rehabilitation program?
   A. Help the person with yardwork and heavy lifting as needed
   B. Take and report vital signs before, during, and after exercise
   C. Suggest ways to cope with and manage depression and anxiety
   D. Help the person select foods to reduce weight and control cholesterol
43. Which tasks would be assigned to the nursing assistant to help to prevent skin breakdown in an older person with heart failure?
   A. Massage extremities and areas of fluid collection
   B. Assess peripheral pulses and circulation
   C. Monitor changes in tissue swelling
   D. Give skin care and frequently change position

Fill in the Blanks

44. Write out the abbreviations
   A. CAD ______________________
   B. CO_2 ______________________
   C. COPD ______________________
   D. MI ______________________
   E. O_2 ______________________
   F. RBC ______________________
   G. TB ______________________
   H. WBC ______________________
45. White blood cells (WBCs) are called *leukocytes*. They protect the body against ______________________.
46. Which component of the blood picks up oxygen and releases carbon dioxide? ______________________
47. Identify six activities or other factors that can cause angina.
   A. ______________________
   B. ______________________
   C. ______________________
   D. ______________________
   E. ______________________
   F. ______________________
48. List five descriptions of chest pain that indicate myocardial infarction.
   A. ______________________
   B. ______________________
   C. ______________________
   D. ______________________
   E. ______________________
49. List three goals of cardiac rehabilitation after a myocardial infarction.
   A. ______________________
   B. ______________________
   C. ______________________
50. Name four changes that occur in the lungs when a person has chronic obstructive pulmonary disease (COPD).
   A. ______________________
   B. ______________________
   C. ______________________
   D. ______________________
51. List nine signs and symptoms of sleep apnea.
   A. ______________________
   B. ______________________
   C. ______________________
   D. ______________________
   E. ______________________
   F. ______________________
   G. ______________________
   H. ______________________
   I. ______________________
52. List nine signs and symptoms that may be present if a person has active tuberculosis (TB).
   A. ______________________
   B. ______________________
   C. ______________________
   D. ______________________
   E. ______________________
   F. ______________________
   G. ______________________
   H. ______________________
   I. ______________________
53. List four treatment goals for lymphedema.
   A. ______________________
   B. ______________________
   C. ______________________
   D. ______________________

Matching

Match the symptom listed with disorders of coronary artery disease

A. Angina

B. Myocardial infarction

C. Heart failure

54. ________ Chest pain occurs with exertion.
55. ________ Blood flow to the heart is suddenly blocked.
56. ________ Blood backs up into the venous system.
57. ________ Fluid in the lungs.
58. ________ Rest and nitroglycerin often relieves the symptoms.
59. ________ Breaks out in a sweat for no reason.

Match the respiratory disorder with the related symptom

A. Chronic bronchitis

B. Emphysema

C. Asthma

60. ________ Person develops a barrel chest.
61. ________ Mucus and inflamed breathing passages obstruct airflow.
62. ________ Alveoli become less elastic.
63. ________ Sudden attacks can be mild or severe.
64. ________ The most common symptom is often a smoker's cough
65. ________ Normal O_2 and CO_2 exchange cannot occur in affected alveoli.
66. ________ Allergies and air pollutants are common causes.

Optional Learning Exercises

67. A parent with a congenital heart defect is at risk for having a child with one. What are other risk factors that may cause a congenital heart defect?
    A. ____________________
    B. ____________________
    C. ____________________
    D. ____________________
    E. ____________________
68. Older persons may not have typical symptoms of flu. List five symptoms that signal flu in an older person.
    A. ____________________
    B. ____________________
    C. ____________________
    D. ____________________
    E. ____________________

Use the FOCUS ON PRIDE section to complete these statements and then use the critical thinking and discussion questions to develop your ideas

69. When a person makes unhealthy choices, such as smoking, the health team
    A. Teaches the person the ____________ and encourages ____________
    B. Cannot force ____________
    C. Must be sure the person understands the ____________
70. Color-coded wristbands communicate ____________ or ____________.
71. If a color-coded bracelet says "limb alert" or "forbidden extremity," it means that an arm must not be used for
    A. ____________________
    B. ____________________
    C. ____________________

Critical Thinking and Discussion Questions

72. In the table below, check all the factors that apply to you. In the section of "factors you can change," select two or three that apply to you and answer the following questions.
    A. I'd like to change factor ____________, because ____________
    B. Three things that I could do to begin to change factor ____________ include
       a. ____________
       b. ____________
       c. ____________
    C. Three things that I could do to begin to change factor ____________ include
       a. ____________
       b. ____________
       c. ____________
    D. Three things that I could do to begin to change factor ____________ include
       a. ____________
       b. ____________
       c. ____________

	Cardiovascular Disorders—Risk Factors
	Factors You *Cannot* Control
	• Age—45 years or older for men; 55 years or older for women
	• Biological sex—risk increases for women after menopause
	• Family history—tends to run in families
	Factors You *Can* Control
	• Being overweight
	• Stress
	• Smoking and tobacco use
	• Poor diet—high in fat, salt, sugar, and cholesterol
	• Excessive alcohol
	• Lack of exercise
	• Not getting enough sleep
	• High blood pressure
	• Unhealthy blood cholesterol levels
	• Diabetes

51 Digestive and Endocrine Disorders

Fill in the Blanks: Key Terms

Heartburn (acid reflux)
Hyperglycemia
Hypoglycemia
Jaundice
Vomitus (emesis)

1. A high level of sugar in the blood is ______________________________.
2. ______________________________ is food and/or fluids that are expelled from the stomach through the mouth.
3. A low level of sugar in the blood is ______________________________.
4. A burning sensation in the chest and sometimes the throat is ______________________________.
5. ______________________________ is yellowish color of the skin or whites of the eyes.

Circle the Best Answer

6. Which nursing measure would the nursing assistant use to prevent aspiration when a person is vomiting?
   A. Turn the person's head well to one side
   B. Place a kidney basin under the person's chin
   C. Move the emesis away from the person
   D. Eliminate or reduce foul odors
7. Which observation needs to be reported to the nurse at once when caring for person with a peptic ulcer?
   A. Declines to eat anymore after eating a very small snack
   B. Vomits pink-tinged emesis with coffee ground–like particles
   C. Feels like stomach is full and bloated after eating
   D. Reports feeling nauseated and repeatedly belches after eating
8. Which request from the resident should be reported to the nurse for a resident who has gastroesophageal reflux disease (GERD)?
   A. Resident wants to frequently eat a small snack.
   B. Resident wants to sit in the dayroom after lunch.
   C. Resident wants to wear loose elastic-waist pants.
   D. Resident wants fried chicken and french fries for dinner.
9. Which complication is associated with aspirated vomitus?
   A. Hypovolemic shock
   B. Obstruction of airway
   C. Bleeding of esophagus
   D. Hiatal hernia
10. Why would the nursing assistant immediately report vomitus that looks like coffee grounds to the nurse?
    A. There could be bleeding in the gastrointestinal tract.
    B. The person may need a change in diet.
    C. This indicates an infection in the stomach.
    D. The person may have swallowed a foreign object.
11. Which procedure is the nursing assistant most likely to perform when caring for a person with diverticular disease who had surgery for the diseased portion of the bowel?
    A. Checking for and removing a fecal impaction
    B. Giving a small volume enema
    C. Assisting the person to empty an ostomy pouch
    D. Emptying a urinary drainage bag
12. Which task will the nursing assistant plan for extra time when caring for a person with ulcerative colitis?
    A. Frequently measuring emesis and cleaning the kidney basin
    B. Helping the person to clean up after frequent diarrheal episodes
    C. Reminding the person not to lie down after eating or drinking
    D. Donning and doffing personal protective equipment for isolation precautions
13. Which activity is most likely to precede a "gallbladder attack"?
    A. Eating a meal
    B. Overexertion
    C. Lying down
    D. Smoking
14. Which lifestyle modification is part of the treatment for hepatitis?
    A. Increasing exercise
    B. Smoking cessation
    C. Abstaining from alcohol
    D. Eating a high-protein diet
15. Which care measure will the nursing assistant use for a person with cirrhosis who needs good skin care because of symptoms caused by the disease process?
    A. Cleanse with cold water
    B. Apply lotion
    C. Report sweating
    D. Check for incontinence
16. Which person needs to be assisted to ambulate for exercise as part of the treatment for diabetes?
    A. A 17-year-old adolescent has just taken insulin for type 1 diabetes.
    B. An obese 50-year-old woman with hypertension has type 2 diabetes.
    C. A 26-year-old woman is pregnant and has gestational diabetes.
    D. An underweight 45-year-old woman with dizziness has type 2 diabetes.

17. Which action is the most important in caring for a person with diabetes who has thirst, frequent urination, a flushed face and rapid, deep, and labored respirations?
   A. Provide plenty of clear fluids
   B. Assist the person to the bathroom
   C. Count the respiratory rate
   D. Report your observations to the nurse
18. Which person has a risk factor related to diverticular disease?
   A. Person A fails to maintain regular exercise routine.
   B. Person B is slightly underweight for height.
   C. Person C eats low-fiber diet that is high in animal fat.
   D. Person D has poor personal hygiene after bowel movements.
19. Which person needs a reminder about lifestyle changes that help to reduce problems associated gastroesophageal reflux disease (GERD)?
   A. Person A eats small meals with portion control.
   B. Person B avoids drinking alcohol and stops smoking.
   C. Person C lies down to rest shortly after eating lunch.
   D. Person D is on a medically supervised weight loss diet.
20. Which infection prevention measure in the Bloodborne Pathogen Standard would help the nursing assistant to protect self against hepatitis?
   A. Avoiding items covered with blood
   B. Getting the hepatitis B vaccine
   C. Knowing which patients have hepatitis
   D. Using masks when caring for patients
21. Which nursing action would be assigned to the nursing assistant when caring for a patient who has cirrhosis of the liver with ascites of the abdomen and edema in the lower extremities?
   A. Telling family that mental status changes are expected
   B. Assessing for complications such as pneumonia
   C. Explaining diet and fluid restriction to the family
   D. Measuring daily weights and intake and output

Fill in the Blanks

22. Write out the meaning of the abbreviations
   A. BMs ____________________
   B. *C. diff* ____________________
   C. GERD ____________________
   D. GI ____________________
   E. IBD ____________________
   F. I&O ____________________
   G. TH ____________________
23. Peristalsis decreases with aging and can cause flatulence (gas) and ____________________.
24. List seven signs and symptoms of gastroesophageal reflux disease (GERD).
   A. ____________________
   B. ____________________
   C. ____________________
   D. ____________________
   E. ____________________
   F. ____________________
   G. ____________________
25. List the characteristics of the types of hepatitis.
   A. Hepatitis A is spread by the ____________________ route.
   B. Hepatitis B is present in the ____________________ of infected persons.
   C. Hepatitis C can be transmitted in ways similar to hepatitis ____________________.
   D. Hepatitis D is spread by having sex with someone who has ____________________.
   E. Hepatitis E can occur by eating undercooked ____________________.
26. A person with ____________________ diabetes can be treated with healthy eating, exercise, and sometimes oral drugs.

Matching

Match the type of hepatitis with the cause

A. Hepatitis A
B. Hepatitis B
C. Hepatitis C
D. Hepatitis D
E. Hepatitis E

27. ________ Born to a mother who has hepatitis B
28. ________ Received blood clotting factor before 1987
29. ________ Had unprotected sex with someone who has hepatitis D
30. ________ Oral contact with infected person's feces
31. ________ Drinking contaminated water; more common in Africa, Asia, or Central America

Match the symptom with either hypoglycemia or hyperglycemia

A. Hypoglycemia
B. Hyperglycemia

32. ________ Trembling, shakiness
33. ________ Sweet breath odor
34. ________ Tingling around the mouth
35. ________ Cold, clammy skin
36. ________ Rapid, deep, and labored respirations
37. ________ Leg cramps
38. ________ Flushed face
39. ________ Frequent urination

Optional Learning Exercises

You are caring for several persons with diabetes. Answer these questions about these persons.

Mr. Jones, a 75-year-old African American man

Ms. Miller, a 45-year-old White, overweight woman

Mrs. Thorpe, a 32-year-old pregnant woman

Ms. Hernandez, a 60-year-old Hispanic woman with hypertension

Emily F., a 12-year-old girl who has lost 15 pounds recently without dieting

40. Three of these persons are most likely to have type 2 diabetes. They are
    A. ______________________________
    B. ______________________________
    C. ______________________________
41. The 32-year-old probably has ______________ diabetes. She is at risk for developing ______________________ later in life.
42. The 12-year-old probably has ______________________ diabetes.
43. Which type of diabetes develops rapidly? ______________________________
44. Mrs. Hernandez has an open wound on her ankle. Why is this wound a concern? ______________________________
45. Why is Ms. Miller instructed to decrease her food intake? ______________________________
46. Mr. Jones tells you he feels shaky, dizzy, and has a headache when he misses a meal. He probably is experiencing ______________________.
47. Why does Emily F. take a snack with her when she goes to school? ______________________________.

Use the FOCUS ON PRIDE section to complete these statements and then use the critical thinking and discussion question to develop your ideas

48. Healthcare workers are at risk for exposure to the hepatitis B virus through ______________, ______________________, and ______________________.
49. Careful observation, prompt reporting, and nursing interventions are needed. Otherwise, the healthcare team could be liable for ______________, ______________, and other legal problems.

Critical Thinking and Discussion Question

50. Healthcare workers are at risk for hepatitis. In addition to getting the vaccine for hepatitis B, what can you do to protect yourself and others from getting hepatitis?

52 Urinary and Reproductive Disorders

Fill in the Blanks: Key Terms

Dialysis	Hematuria	Pyuria	Urostomy
Dysuria	Oliguria	Urinary diversion	

1. Scant urine is ______________________________.
2. Difficult or painful urination is ________________.
3. ____________ is a surgically created opening that connects to the urinary tract.
4. The process of removing waste products from the blood is ______________________________.
5. A surgically created pathway for urine to leave the body is a ______________________________.
6. Blood in the urine is ______________________.
7. ____________ is pus in the urine.

Circle the Best Answer

8. Which task is a nursing assistant's responsibility in the prevention of urinary tract infections (UTIs) among elderly residents in a long-term care center?
   A. Administer antibiotics as prescribed for UTIs
   B. Use sterile technique to insert indwelling catheters
   C. Give drinking water to those who are not on fluid restrictions
   D. Ensure that equipment for urologic examinations is sterile
9. Which anatomical or physiological characteristic places women at a higher risk for urinary tract infections (UTIs)?
   A. Female hormones affect immunity.
   B. The urethra is shorter in the female.
   C. The vagina harbors bacteria.
   D. Menstrual blood is contaminated.
10. Which nursing measure would be included in the care plan if a person has a urinary tract infection (UTI)?
    A. Restricting fluid intake
    B. Assisting with frequent ambulation
    C. Straining the urine
    D. Assisting with proper perineal care
11. Which condition is anticipated if a man has prostate enlargement?
    A. Will need urinary diversion
    B. Will have frequent voiding at night
    C. Frequently experiences severe back pain
    D. Eventually develops chronic renal failure
12. Which nursing measure will be included in the care plan after a person has surgery to correct benign prostatic hyperplasia (BPH)?
    A. A balanced diet to prevent constipation
    B. Increased activity with an exercise plan
    C. Restricted fluid intake
    D. Care of the surgical incision
13. How often is a urinary diversion pouch changed?
    A. Every shift
    B. Every 3 to 4 hours
    C. After showers or bathing
    D. One to two times per week or if it leaks
14. Which nursing measure will the nursing assistant use when caring for a person with kidney stones?
    A. Restricting fluids
    B. Maintaining strict bed rest
    C. Straining all urine
    D. Maintaining a strict diet
15. Which nursing measure will the care plan will include for a person with chronic renal failure?
    A. Increasing fluid intake to 2000 to 3000 mL/day
    B. Measuring and recording urine output
    C. Encouraging person to eat high-protein foods
    D. Assisting the person to ambulate in hallways
16. Which food item prompts the nursing assistant to check with the nurse before giving the meal tray to a person with chronic renal failure?
    A. Beef steak
    B. Green beans
    C. Whole wheat roll
    D. Tomato slices
17. Which nursing measure would be included in the care plan for a person who has chronic renal failure?
    A. Frequently check the linens for moisture
    B. Daily routine of moderate aerobic exercise
    C. Skin care to prevent itching
    D. Frequent bathing with soap
18. Which care measure is the most important for a woman who reports itching and painful urination and has a gray vaginal discharge with an odor?
    A. Make sure she has clean underwear
    B. Assist her with a sitz bath
    C. Obtain clean perineal pads for her
    D. Inform the nurse about the observations
19. Which nursing measure would the nursing assistant use when caring for a person after transurethral resection of the prostate (TURP)?
    A. Assist the person to empty the urinary pouch
    B. Help person select items from the renal diet menu
    C. Encourage person to drink at least eight cups of water every day
    D. Support person's efforts to cough and deep breathe

20. How much fluid per day should a person with kidney stones be encouraged to drink?
    A. 800 to 1200 mL
    B. 1000 to 1500 mL
    C. 2000 to 3000 mL
    D. 3000 to 5000 mL
21. Which snack item if selected by a person who is on a renal diet for chronic renal failure would prompt the nursing assistant to notify the nurse?
    A. Apple and pear slices
    B. Potato chips with ranch dip
    C. Yogurt with blueberries
    D. Hummus with celery sticks
22. Which safety measure would the nursing assistant use to protect self when caring for a person with a sexually transmitted disease (STD)?
    A. Assist the nurse to gather equipment for Transmission-Based precautions
    B. Practice Standard Precautions and follow Bloodborne Pathogen Standard
    C. Politely inquire if the person routinely uses condoms
    D. Ask the person to perform own perineal care and hygiene
23. Which person may need the nursing assistant's help to clean a pessary?
    A. Person A is being treated for a gonorrhea infection.
    B. Person B has pain related to pelvic inflammatory disease.
    C. Person C has benign prostatic hyperplasia (BPH).
    D. Person D has a uterine prolapse and may need surgery.
24. Which sign or symptom would the nursing assistant expect to observe when caring for a person who has kidney stones?
    A. Dry skin with itching
    B. Sharp severe pain in the lower back
    C. Edema in the feet, ankles, and legs
    D. Single, small, painless sore on genitals
25. Which task would be the most important for the nursing assistant to complete if the person is known to have oliguria?
    A. Measure intake and output
    B. Report and record temperature
    C. Assist with perineal hygiene
    D. Practice fall precautions

Fill in the Blanks

26. Write out the meaning of the abbreviations
    A. BPH ______________________________
    B. CKD ______________________________
    C. mL ______________________________
    D. STD ______________________________
    E. STI ______________________________
    F. TURP ______________________________
    G. UTI ______________________________
    H. AIDS ______________________________
    I. HIV ______________________________
    J. HPV ______________________________
27. Using ______________ prevents the spread of sexually transmitied diseases (STDs).

Matching

Match the sexually transmitted disease (STD) with the disease characteristics. Use Box 52.3 (p. 789) to complete the matching.

A. Herpes
B. Human papilloma viruses (HPV)
C. Gonorrhea
D. Chlamydia
E. Syphilis
F. Trichomoniasis
G. Human immunodeficiency virus (HIV)/acquired immunodeficiency syndrome (AIDS)

28. ____________ Virus stays in the body for life; repeated outbreaks are common
29. ____________ Causes genital warts
30. ____________ Yellow-green or gray vaginal discharge
31. ____________ Vaccines available for several types of virus
32. ____________ Men have pain on urination and a penile discharge
33. ____________ The immune system is harmed.
34. ____________ Painless sores develop first on genitals.
35. ____________ Common cause of pelvic inflammatory disease (PID), in addition to gonorrhea

Optional Learning Exercises

You give home care to Mrs. Eunice Weber twice a week. She is 92 years old and lives alone. She has severe osteoporosis and uses a walker to move about in her home. She receives Meals on Wheels and spends most of the day sitting on the sofa. She has periods of incontinence or dribbling because of poor bladder control. When you arrive to care for her today, she tells you she is not feeling well. She tells you it burns when she urinates. When she needs to urinate, the urge comes on suddenly and she often does not get to the toilet in time. Answer these questions about Mrs. Weber.

36. You should tell the ______________ because these symptoms may mean Mrs. Weber has ______________.
37. When the feeling to urinate comes on suddenly, it is called ______________________________.
38. How does Mrs. Weber's immobility affect the following?
    A. Fluid intake ______________ ______________
    B. Perineal care ______________ ______________
39. Why does gender increase Mrs. Weber's risk for urinary tract infections (UTIs)?
    ____
40. The doctor will probably order ______________ to treat the condition.
41. The care plan will probably include "Encourage fluids to ______________ per day."

Two weeks later you notice that Mrs. Weber has chills. When you take her temperature, it is 102°F (38.9°C). She tells you that she has been vomiting since yesterday. You observe her urine and see that it is very cloudy

42. You report these symptoms to the nurse, because it can indicate Mrs. Weber now has ________________. This means the infection has moved from the ____________________ to the _____________________.

Use the FOCUS ON PRIDE section to complete these statements

43. Proper ______________ care can prevent urinary tract infections (UTIs).
44. When a person has a urinary or reproductive disorder, you protect the person's rights and give respect when you give information only to ______________________.

Critical Thinking and Discussion Question

45. Poor fluid intake, healthcare–associated infections related to urinary catheters, and poor hygiene are mentioned as causes of urinary tract infections (UTIs). Based on previous chapters that you have studied, what skills and knowledge can you use in the prevention of UTIs?

53 Mental Health Disorders

Fill in the Blanks: Key Terms

Addiction
Alcoholism
Anxiety
Compulsion
Coping
Defense mechanism
Delusion
Delusion of persecution
Detoxification
Drug addiction
Flashback
Hallucination
Mental health
Mental health disorder (psychiatric disorder)
Obsession
Panic
Personality
Phobia
Psychosis
Stress
Stressor
Suicidal ideation
Suicide
Suicide contagion
Tolerance
Withdrawal syndrome

1. A feeling of worry, nervousness, or fear about an event or situation is ______________________________.
2. Alcohol dependence that involves craving, loss of control, physical dependence, and tolerance is ______________________________.
3. ______________ is using strategies to manage stress and reduce negative emotions caused by stress.
4. A ___________________________ is a serious illness that can affect a person's thinking, mood, behavior, function, and ability to relate to others.
5. A ______________________ is an event or factor that causes stress.
6. ________________ is the strong urge or craving to use the substance and cannot stop using; tolerance develops.
7. A frequent, upsetting and unwanted thought, idea, or an image is an ______________________________.
8. The response or change in the body caused by any emotional, psychological, physical, social, or economic factor is ______________________________.
9. A ___________________________ is an intense fear of something that has little or no real danger.
10. A false belief is a ______________________________.
11. When a person thinks about, considers, or plans suicide, the person is demonstrating ______________________________.
12. ______________________ is a condition that affects the mind and causes a loss of contact with reality.
13. A ___________________________ is seeing, hearing, feeling, or tasting things that are not real.
14. An overwhelming urge to repeat certain rituals, acts, or behaviors is a ______________________________.
15. _________________ involves a person's emotional, psychological, and social well-being.
16. The set of attitudes, values, behaviors, and traits of a person is ______________________________.
17. ____________________ is a false belief that one is being mistreated, abused, or harassed.
18. An intense and sudden feeling of fear, anxiety, or dread is ______________________________.
19. _________________ is needing more and more of a drug for the same effect.
20. A ____________ is an unconscious reaction that blocks unpleasant or threatening feelings.
21. ______________________ occurs with exposure to suicide or suicidal behaviors within one's family, or peer group, or media reports of suicide.
22. Reliving the trauma in thoughts during the day and in nightmares during sleep is ______________________.
23. The physical and mental response after stopping or severely reducing the use of a substance that was used regularly is ______________________________.
24. The process of removing a toxic substance from the body is ______________________________.
25. To end one's life on purpose is called ______________________________.
26. ______________________ is a chronic disease involving substance-seeking behaviors and use that is compulsive and hard to control despite the harmful effects

Circle the Best Answer

27. Which person is displaying an early warning sign of a mental health disorder?
    - A. Teenager likes to sleep in late on the weekends.
    - B. College student feels anxious about finding a job.
    - C. Middle-aged adult likes to have a drink with friends after work.
    - D. Older adult pulls away from friends and usual activities.
28. Which person has a risk factor for mental health disorders that is modifiable?
    - A. Person A's father and grandfather had bipolar disorder.
    - B. Person B sustained a traumatic brain injury during childhood.
    - C. Person C drinks alcohol and smokes marijuana.
    - D. Person D has cancer that is not responding to chemotherapy.

29. For which circumstance would anxiety be considered a normal and helpful reaction to stress?
    A. Person cannot sleep because work deadlines are looming.
    B. Student needs to study for a final examination.
    C. Building is on fire and the person cannot find the exit.
    D. Child refuses to go to school because of bullying.
30. What is an example of an unhealthy coping mechanism?
    A. Talking about the problem
    B. Playing music
    C. Overeating
    D. Exercising
31. Which defense mechanism is the student using after failing a test and blaming a friend for not being a better study partner?
    A. Conversion
    B. Projection
    C. Repression
    D. Displacement
32. Which nursing measure would the nursing assistant use when a person has a panic attack?
    A. Use short, simple sentences and give reassurance
    B. Ask the person what kind of help is required
    C. Tell the person that the voices are not real
    D. Call for help and restrain the person as needed
33. Which disorder is characterized by a person's repetitive action such as washing the hands over and over again?
    A. Schizophrenia
    B. Borderline personality disorder
    C. Anorexia nervosa
    D. Obsessive-compulsive disorder
34. Which sign or symptom is a young child likely to display when the medical diagnosis is posttraumatic stress disorder associated with abuse?
    A. Does many tasks at once without getting tired
    B. Sits for hours without moving or responding
    C. Hears the abuser's voice and answers
    D. Acts out the traumatic event during play
35. Which psychotic feature is manifesting when a person claims to be the president of the United States?
    A. Disorganized speech
    B. Delusion of persecution
    C. Hallucination
    D. Delusion of grandeur
36. What is the risk for a person who is in the manic phase of bipolar disorder?
    A. Immobility
    B. Constipation
    C. Pressure injuries
    D. Exhaustion
37. What is a safety risk for a person who has depression?
    A. May be very sad
    B. Has thoughts of suicide and death
    C. Has depressed body functions
    D. Cannot concentrate
38. Which nursing assistant needs a reminder about how to communicate with a patient who is having a severe panic attack?
    A. Nursing assistant A says, "You are safe. I am with you."
    B. Nursing assistant B says, "The nurse is coming. Focus on my voice."
    C. Nursing assistant C says, "Breathe slowly in through your mouth. Good job."
    D. Nursing assistant D says, "Calm down. There's nothing wrong with you."
39. Which behavior is characteristic of a person with an antisocial personality?
    A. Is suspicious and distrust others
    B. Displays emotional highs and lows
    C. Sees, hears, or feels things that are not real
    D. Has no regard for the safety of others
40. Which substance is most commonly abused among teenagers?
    A. Alcohol
    B. Hallucinogens
    C. Marijuana
    D. Stimulants
41. What occurs when alcohol is ingested?
    A. Stimulates alertness and agitation
    B. Causes drowsiness and reduces anxiety
    C. Causes hallucinations and delusions
    D. Stimulates hyperactivity and anger
42. Which change related to aging increases the risk for injury when an older person drinks alcohol?
    A. Slower reaction times
    B. Tolerance for alcohol
    C. Long-term memory loss
    D. Lapses in judgment
43. What is a sign of addiction when a person uses drugs over a period of time?
    A. Using two or three substances once or twice a month
    B. Taking larger amounts of the substance to get the same effect
    C. Using the substance occasionally in a social setting
    D. Taking the substance if a friend says the experience is safe
44. Which condition is characterized by eating large amounts of food and then forced vomiting?
    A. Anorexia nervosa
    B. Binge-eating disorder
    C. Substance abuse disorder
    D. Bulimia nervosa
45. Which action would the nursing assistant take if a person mentions suicide?
    A. Watch for psychosis
    B. Take the person seriously
    C. Change the topic of conversation
    D. Disregard the attention-seeking behavior

46. What occurs when a person who has posttraumatic stress disorder believes that trauma is happening all over again?
    A. A flashback
    B. A compulsion
    C. An obsession
    D. A hallucination
47. Which person has the most risk factors for a mental health disorder?
    A. Person A has history of abuse and helps other abuse victims.
    B. Person B has a chronic health condition, and it is well controlled.
    C. Person C feels lonely, but reaches out to friends and family.
    D. Person D suffered a traumatic brain injury and uses drugs and alcohol.
48. Which action will the nursing assistant take upon finding a patient with slow weak breathing, who has cold clammy skin and is limp and hard to arouse?
    A. Stimulate by shaking and speaking loudly
    B. Call the nurse for help and stay with the patient
    C. Help the patient to sit up to improve breathing
    D. Take vital signs and cover with a warm blanket
49. Which nursing assistant needs a reminder about nonverbal communication when interacting with patients who have mental health disorders?
    A. Nursing assistant A speaks calmly when patients get upset.
    B. Nursing assistant B hugs all new patients when they arrive.
    C. Nursing assistant C maintains eye contact with patients.
    D. Nursing assistant D faces the patients when interacting.
50. Which action would the nursing assistant use to protect self when a patient who has borderline personality disorder becomes inappropriately angry?
    A. Firmly instruct the patient to calm down
    B. Keep a safe distance between self and patient
    C. Distract the person by changing the subject
    D. Redirect by offering a snack or something to drink

Fill in the Blanks

51. Write out the meaning of the abbreviations
    A. BPD ________________
    B. CBT ________________
    C. GAD ________________
    D. OCD ________________
    E. PTSD ________________
52. When a person has an exaggerated belief about one's own importance, wealth, power, or talents, it is called ________________.
53. Depression may be overlooked in older persons because it may be mistaken for a __________ disorder.
54. Name the defense mechanism being used in these situations.
    A. After a heart attack a man continues to smoke. ________________
    B. A man does not like his boss. He buys the boss an expensive Christmas present. ________________
    C. A girl complains of a headache so she will not have to read aloud at school. ________________
    D. A child is angry with his teacher. He hits his brother. ________________
    E. A woman misses work frequently and is often late. She gets a bad evaluation. She says that the boss does not like her. ________________
55. Identify the phobia in each example.
    A. ________________ Being afraid of strangers
    B. ________________ Fear of pain or seeing others in pain
    C. ________________ Being trapped in an enclosed area
    D. ________________ Fear of darkness
56. Below are examples of problems that occur with schizophrenia. Identify each one.
    A. A woman says that voices told her to set fire to her apartment. ________________
    B. A man believes that others can hear his thoughts on the radio. ________________
    C. A woman tells you that she owns three mansions and is the governor of California. ________________

Optional Learning Exercises

57. Mr. Johnson is very worried about his surgery tomorrow. You notice that he is talking very fast and sweating. You give him directions to collect a urine specimen. Five minutes later, he turns on his call light to ask you to repeat the directions. He tells you that he is using the toilet "all the time" because he has diarrhea and frequent urination. The nurse tells you all of these things are signs and symptoms of ________________.
58. You are assigned to care for Mrs. Grand, a new resident. She is getting ready to go to the dining room. You assist her to get dressed and she tells you that she wants to wash her hands before going to the dining room. She goes to the bathroom and washes her hands for several minutes. As she leaves the room, she stops to turn off the light. Then she tells you she must wash her hands again. She repeats washing her hands and turning the lights on and off four or five times. You report this to the nurse, who tells you Mrs. Grand has ________________.

Use the FOCUS ON PRIDE section to complete these statements and then use the critical thinking and discussion question to develop your ideas

59. When caring for a person with mental illness, the team must react quickly to ____________________.
60. When caring for a person with a mental illness, you can take pride in working as a team when you ____________ when a team member calls for help.

Critical Thinking and Discussion Question

61. When you first begin to care for persons who have mental health disorders, you may feel a little anxious. How can you use this "normal" feeling of anxiety to improve your abilities and skills to care for people with mental health disorders?

54 Confusion and Dementia

Fill in the Blanks: Key Terms

Cognitive function
Confusion
Delirium
Delusion
Dementia
Elopement
Hallucination
Paranoia
Sundowning

1. ________________ occurs when a person leaves the agency without staff knowledge.
2. A false belief is a ________________________________.
3. Seeing, hearing, smelling, or feeling something that is not real is a ________________________________.
4. Increased signs, symptoms, and behavior of dementia during hours of darkness is ____________________.
5. ________________ is a state of sudden, severe confusion and rapid changes in brain function.
6. The loss of cognitive function that interferes with daily life and activities is ________________________.
7. ________________ is a mental state of being disoriented to person, place, situation, or identity.
8. ________________ involves memory, thinking, reasoning, ability to understand, judgment, and behavior.
9. ________________ is a disorder of the mind; the person has false beliefs and suspicions about a person or situation.

Circle the Best Answer

10. Which activity has safety implications related to changes in the nervous system that occur with aging?
    A. Driving a car
    B. Talking with friends
    C. Attending a party
    D. Petting a dog
11. Which sign or symptom would be considered a normal nervous system change related to aging?
    A. Inability to walk
    B. Depression
    C. Loss of appetite
    D. Change of sleep pattern
12. What is the primary difference between dementia and delirium?
    A. Rapidity of onset
    B. Level of confusion
    C. Ability to make judgments
    D. Degree of memory loss
13. Which nursing measure would the nursing assistant use when caring for a person who is confused?
    A. Repeat the date and time as often as necessary
    B. Change the routine each day to stimulate the person
    C. Keep the drapes pulled during the day
    D. Avoid talking too much to the person
14. Which communication technique would the nursing assistant use to compensate for changes in vision and hearing for a person who is confused?
    A. Speak in a loud voice
    B. Write out directions
    C. Face the person and speak clearly
    D. Stand by a window, so the person can see you
15. Which causative factor for dementia can be treated?
    A. Abnormal protein deposits
    B. Vitamin deficiency
    C. Stroke
    D. Alzheimer disease (AD)
16. Which reminder is the nursing assistant most likely to give to a person who has a mild cognitive disorder?
    A. To put on underpants before putting on trousers
    B. To put toothpaste on the toothbrush before brushing
    C. To call daughter about a scheduled appointment
    D. To ask for a snack if hungry in between meals
17. Which type of permanent dementia is most common among older persons?
    A. Alzheimer disease (AD)
    B. Vascular dementia
    C. Frontal-temporal disorder
    D. Lewy body dementia
18. Which disorder can mimic the signs and symptoms of dementia?
    A. Depression
    B. Schizophrenia
    C. Heart disease
    D. Diabetes
19. Which behavior is an example of the most common early symptom of Alzheimer disease (AD)?
    A. Person gets very upset and yells when the shoes are stored in the closet.
    B. Person cannot remember the instructions that were just given about the call bell.
    C. Person is lethargic, difficult to arouse, and speech is garbled.
    D. Person becomes confused and agitated in the early evening just before sunset.
20. Which action will the nursing assistant use when caring for a person with mild Alzheimer disease (AD)?
    A. Coach step-by-step for donning and buttoning shirt
    B. Perform perineal care for incontinence of bowel and bladder
    C. Allow more time to complete daily tasks, such as showering
    D. Introduce friends and family by name every time they visit

21. Which action will the nursing assistant use when caring for a person with moderate Alzheimer disease (AD)?
    A. Teach person to how to locate a personal item that is misplaced
    B. Consistently use the same routine for morning hygiene
    C. Ask the person if the family is handling the finances
    D. Monitor for seizure activity and report findings to the nurse
22. Which action will you use when caring for a person with severe Alzheimer disease (AD)?
    A. Wait patiently if he has trouble organizing his thoughts
    B. Tell him to focus on your voice when he has auditory hallucinations
    C. Be kind and matter of fact, say "It is time for a bath now."
    D. Ask him to explain what he wants you to do
23. Which safety issue is addressed by using a sign on the inside of the front door of the home that says, "STOP" for a person with Alzheimer disease (AD) who needs home care?
    A. Catastrophic reactions
    B. Wandering
    C. Paranoia
    D. Sundowning
24. Which care measure could the nursing assistant use to reduce the agitation for a person with Alzheimer disease (AD) who has symptoms of sundowning?
    A. Offer fluids and a snack
    B. Tell the person to calm down
    C. Have the person join a social group
    D. Put the person in quiet dark room
25. Which sign or symptom can be reduced or prevented by assisting a person with Alzheimer disease (AD) to wear prescribed glasses or hearing aids?
    A. Wandering
    B. Sundowning
    C. Hallucinations
    D. Paranoia
26. Which action would the nursing assistant take if a person with Alzheimer disease (AD) seems afraid or is worried about money?
    A. Change the conversation to a pleasant topic
    B. Tell the person that everything is okay
    C. Report the concern to the nurse
    D. Assume the person has paranoia
27. Which outcome is most likely to occur when a person who has dementia is overwhelmed by continuous talking, loud music, and noisy laughter in the background?
    A. Depression
    B. Catastrophic reactions
    C. Feelings of abandonment
    D. Wandering
28. Which caregiver behavior may cause agitation and aggression for a person with cognition dysfunction?
    A. Talking very slowly and using simple language
    B. Selecting activities that are interesting to the person
    C. Encouraging activity early in the day
    D. Expecting the person to complete care quickly
29. Which communication technique would the nursing assistant use to communicate with the person who has dementia?
    A. Make eye contact to get the person's attention
    B. List options for activities of interest
    C. Ask several open-ended questions
    D. Play soft music in the background
30. Which action would be included in the care plan if a person with Alzheimer disease (AD) frequently rubs the genitals?
    A. Inform the person that the behavior is not acceptable
    B. Make sure the person has good hygiene to prevent itching
    C. Isolate the person in a private room with the door closed
    D. Ignore the behavior because the disease causes it
31. Which nursing measure would the nursing assistant use when a person repeats the same motions or repeats the same words over and over?
    A. Remind the person to stop the repeating
    B. Report to the nurse; the behavior may have meaning
    C. Tell the nurse that the person is being tiresome
    D. Ask the person what is gained by repeating over and over again
32. What is the main purpose for encouraging a person with Alzheimer disease (AD) to take part in therapies and activities?
    A. To achieve a previous level of function and cognition
    B. To help the person to feel useful, worthwhile, and active
    C. To give family caregivers a respite from repetitive behaviors
    D. To improve physical problems such as incontinence and contractures
33. Which principle guides the placement, documentation, and ongoing review and revision of the care plan when a person is admitted to a memory care unit?
    A. Confidentiality
    B. Professionalism
    C. Least restrictive approach
    D. Standard precautions
34. Which criteria indicates that a person with Alzheimer disease (AD) no longer needs to stay in a secured unit?
    A. AD improves
    B. Person wants to return to own home.
    C. Person cannot sit or walk.
    D. Aggressive behaviors disrupt the unit.
35. What is a common reaction for family members who care for a person with dementia at home?
    A. They want to be with the person at all times.
    B. They have conflicted feelings of guilt and anger.
    C. They generally do not need any help from others.
    D. They will never consider a long-term care facility

36. Which person needs a reminder about lifestyle choices recommended by the National Institute on Aging (NIA) that help to maintain cognitive health?
   A. Person A gets regular exercise.
   B. Person B is seeing a counselor for depression.
   C. Person C has uncontrolled type 2 diabetes.
   D. Person D spends quality time with family and friends.
37. Which person is showing an early warning sign of dementia?
   A. Person A goes to the store and forgets to buy milk.
   B. Person B likes to wear bright colored clothes.
   C. Person C forgets where she placed her car keys.
   D. Person D goes outdoors in the snow without shoes.
38. Which mental health disorder is most likely to be mistaken for dementia?
   A. Schizophrenia
   B. Major depressive disorder
   C. Bipolar disorder
   D. Antisocial personality disorder
39. Which person is showing signs of delirium?
   A. A 73-year-old person with a urinary infection suddenly becomes confused.
   B. A 65-year-old person gets agitated, restless, and fearful every evening.
   C. A 59-year-old person displays low energy and difficulty concentrating.
   D. An 82-year-old person needs daily assistance with dressing and hygiene.
40. Which substance can cause treatable dementia?
   A. Cholesterol
   B. Tobacco
   C. Alcohol
   D. Artificial sweetener
41. Which nursing assistant needs a reminder about assisting a patient who has dementia with oral hygiene?
   A. Nursing assistant A coaches the patient step-by-step to prepare toothbrush.
   B. Nursing assistant B encourages the patient to do as much as possible.
   C. Nursing assistant C says to brush teeth and returns later to check on the patient.
   D. Nursing assistant D helps the patient to clean and store the dentures.
42. Which safety measure would the nursing assistant use to protect a person who has dementia?
   A. Play music that was popular in the person's past
   B. Remove harmful objects, such as knives or tools
   C. Perform activities that use more energy early in the day
   D. Treat the person with kindness and dignity
43. Which family caregiver needs to be reassessed by the nurse because of neglecting self-care measures?
   A. Youngest daughter asks for help when needed.
   B. Adult son keeps health, legal, and financial information current.
   C. Spouse tends to the patient every day and never leaves the house.
   D. Eldest adult daughter joins a support group and spends time with friends.

Fill in the Blanks

44. Write out the meaning of the abbreviations
   A. AD ______________________
   B. ADL ______________________
   C. CMS ______________________
   D. NIA ______________________
45. Cognitive functioning involves
   A. ______________________
   B. ______________________
   C. ______________________
   D. ______________________
   E. ______________________
   F. ______________________
46. Which senses decrease because of age-related changes in the nervous system?
   A. ______________________
   B. ______________________
   C. ______________________
   D. ______________________
   E. ______________________
47. In Alzheimer disease (AD) there is a slow, steady decline in mental functions, including
   A. ______________________
   B. ______________________
   C. ______________________
48. Certain behaviors are common with Alzheimer disease (AD). Name the behavior for each of these examples.
   A. The person becomes more anxious, confused, or restless during the night. ______________
   B. The person sits in a chair and folds the same napkin over and over. ______________
   C. The person begins to scream and cry when a visitor asks many questions. ______________
   D. The person walks away from home and cannot find the way back home. ______________
   E. The person becomes upset when the routine for activities of daily living (ADLs) is changed. ______________
   F. The person tells you he sees his dog sitting in the room but you do not see anything. ______________
   G. You frequently find the person looking for lost items in a wastebasket. ______________
   H. The person tries to hug and kiss other residents of the facility. ______________

Optional Learning Exercises

You are caring for Mr. Harris, a 78-year-old who is confused. You know that there are ways to help a person to be more oriented. Answer these questions about ways to help a confused person.

49. How can you help to orient Mr. Harris every time you are in contact with him? ______________
50. What are ways you can help to orient Mr. Harris to time?
   A. ______________________
   B. ______________________

51. What are ways you can maintain the day-night cycle?
   A. ______________________
   B. ______________________
   C. ______________________

You are caring for Mrs. Matthews, an 82-year-old resident. The nurse tells you that she lived with her daughter for the last 2 years, but the family is now concerned for her safety. She left the home when the temperature was 35°F (1.66°C) and was found 2 miles away, wearing a light sweater. On another occasion, she turned on the gas stove and could not remember how to turn it off. Sometimes, she does not recognize her daughter and resists getting a bath or changing clothes. Since admission to the care facility, she repeatedly tells everyone she must leave to go to her birthday party. She brushes her arms and legs and tells you "bugs" are crawling on her. Answer these questions about Mrs. Matthews and her care.

52. What is the most important reason that Mrs. Matthews is living in a special care unit in the nursing facility? ______________________
53. Mrs. Matthews is diagnosed with ______________ stage Alzheimer disease (AD). What activities or behaviors would indicate she is in this stage?
   A. ______________________
   B. ______________________
   C. ______________________
   D. ______________________
   E. ______________________
54. The nurse may encourage Mrs. Matthews's daughter to join an Alzheimer disease (AD) support group. How can this be helpful to the daughter?
   A. ______________________
   B. ______________________
   C. ______________________

Use the FOCUS ON PRIDE section to complete these statements and then use the critical thinking and discussion questions to develop your ideas

55. You demonstrate personal and professional responsibility when you treat each person as unique, with their own ______________________.
56. You show that you respect the rights of a person when you keep personal items ______________. It is important to protect the person's belongings from ______________ or damage.
57. You help to maintain independence for a person with Alzheimer disease (AD) by maintaining the person's ______________ when giving activities of daily living (ADLs).

Critical Thinking and Discussion Questions

58. Review Focus on Pride: Ethics and Laws (P. 819). There is an example of a licensed nursing assistant (LNA) reacting to a person who threw a food tray on the floor. The LNA was reprimanded by the Board of Nursing.
   A. Speculate about the circumstances that may have caused the LNA to react in such an unprofessional manner.
   B. What could the LNA have done to prevent the reaction?

55 Intellectual and Developmental Disabilities

Fill in the Blanks: Key Terms

Birth defect	Disability	Intellectual disability
Developmental disability	Inherited	Spastic

1. ______________________ is a lifelong condition that begins during the developmental period and limits intellectual function and adaptive behavior.
2. A ______________ is a problem that may develop during the first 3 months of pregnancy; it can affect a body structure or function.
3. ____________ means the uncontrolled contractions of skeletal muscles.
4. That which is passed down from parents to children is ______________________________________.
5. __________________is a lifelong condition that begins during the developmental period and impairs physical or intellectual function or both.
6. Any lost, absent, or impaired physical or mental function is a ______________________________.

Circle the Best Answer

7. Which observation would the nursing assistant report to the nurse because it could be a warning sign of intellectual or developmental disability in an infant?
   A. Likes to suck the thumb
   B. Cries when hungry
   C. Has delayed crawling
   D. Needs frequent diaper change
8. Which comment by a pregnant teenager would the nursing assistant report to nurse for follow-up to decrease the risk of intellectual disability for the unborn child?
   A. "I'm hungry; I'm going to eat pizza."
   B. "I am so tired I sleep all of the time."
   C. "Do I look fat? I think I am getting fat."
   D. "I am going to get so drunk this weekend."
9. Which action would the nursing assistant use when nurse says that the person has an IQ score of about 70?
   A. Use a spoon to feed the person
   B. Perform all hygienic care for person
   C. Assist the person to walk to the bathroom
   D. Repeat instructions using simple language
10. Which action would the nursing assistant use when caring for a person with an intellectual disability and significant limitations with social skills?
    A. Patiently remind about the rules
    B. Assist with the person to bath
    C. Assist the person to get dressed
    D. Help the person to read the menu
11. Which nursing measure would the nursing assistant most likely use when assisting a person with Down syndrome with morning hygiene?
    A. Explain tasks using step-by-step instructions
    B. Tell the person to take a shower
    C. Offer the person assistance as needed
    D. Perform perineal care for the person
12. Which signs or symptoms would the nursing assistant watch for and report when caring for a child with Down syndrome?
    A. Confusion and wandering behaviors
    B. Bruising or bleeding when brushing the teeth
    C. Evidence of ear or respiratory infections
    D. Seizure activity with urinary incontinence
13. Which care measure is specific to Fragile X syndrome?
    A. Skin is fragile; use mild soap and wash gently
    B. Joints are loose; avoid overextending joints
    C. Fats are not well digested; check frequently for diarrheal stools
    D. Hearing loss is common; face the person when speaking
14. Which information would the nursing assistant obtain from the nurse before starting the care of a person with autism?
    A. How the person reacts to being touched?
    B. How to enter the person's room?
    C. If talking to the person is acceptable?
    D. What to expect when smiling at the person?
15. Which approach will the healthcare team use in the care of a person with autism?
    A. Coach the person through every task
    B. Offer opportunities to explore new activities
    C. Allow the person to do whatever they want to do
    D. Maintain daily routines and schedules
16. Which category most accurately describes the disabilities and challenges for patients with cerebral palsy?
    A. Communication disorder
    B. Movement disorder
    C. Cognition disorder
    D. Sensory disorder
17. When a person has spastic cerebral palsy, what would the nursing assistant expect to observe?
    A. Constant slow weaving or writhing motions
    B. Intense muscles with jerking motions
    C. Muscle flaccidity with weak movements
    D. Stiff muscles and awkward movements

18. Which care measure will the nursing assistant plan to perform for a person has spina bifida; myelomeningocele type?
   A. Spoon feed during meals and give fluids in between meals
   B. Frequently check for bowel and bladder incontinence
   C. Assist with frequent oral hygiene and encourage fluids
   D. Assist with ambulation in the hallway three times per shift
19. Which area of the body needs special attention and good skin care when a child has hydrocephalus?
   A. The perineal area
   B. On the back of the head
   C. On the back of the heels
   D. Under the arms
20. Which behavior would the nursing assistant expect to see in a child who has fetal alcohol syndrome?
   A. Hyperactivity
   B. Lethargy
   C. Unresponsiveness
   D. Hypoactivity
21. Which care measure would be included in the care plan for a child who has autism spectrum disorder (ASD)?
   A. Providing stimulating group play times with other children
   B. Maintaining a daily routine without variation
   C. Teaching new games and ways to play with toys
   D. Limiting parental visitations during certain activity times
22. Which safety issue is a concern for a child with spastic cerebral palsy?
   A. Falls
   B. Wandering
   C. Aggression
   D. Suicide
23. Which nursing measure would the nursing assistant use when caring for a child who has attention deficit hyperactivity disorder (ADHD)?
   A. Give the child several attractive options as snack choices
   B. Keep to a schedule and insist that tasks are quickly completed
   C. Allow the child to discover and create own play opportunities
   D. Get child's attention and then give clear step-by-step directions
24. Which infection is associated with intellectual or developmental disabilities for the child if the mother has the infection during pregnancy?
   A. Influenza
   B. German measles
   C. Urinary tract infection
   D. Gastroenteritis
25. What is the general goal for persons with intellectual and developmental disabilities (IDDs)?
   A. Independence to the greatest extent possible
   B. To live at home with the family in the community
   C. To regain physical, intellectual, and social abilities
   D. To work and be a productive member of society
26. Which nutrient would be recommended during pregnancy to prevent neural tube defects, such as spina bifida?
   A. Iron
   B. Protein
   C. Folic acid
   D. Calcium

Fill in the Blanks

27. Write out the abbreviations
   A. ADA ______________________
   B. CP ______________________
   C. DS ______________________
   D. FAS ______________________
   E. FASDs ______________________
   F. Fragile X ______________________
   G. IDD ______________________
   H. IQ ______________________
   I. ASD ______________________
28. List two ways in which genetics can cause or contribute to intellectual disabilities.
   A. ______________________
   B. ______________________
29. According to the Arc of the United States, intellectual disabilities involve the condition being present before ______________ years of age.
30. The Arc supports opportunities such as living in a __________ home, learning, and __________ with children without disabilities.
31. If a child has Down syndrome (DS), what features are present in these areas?
   A. Head, ears, mouth ______________________
   B. Eyes ______________________
   C. Tongue ______________________
   D. Nose ______________________
   E. Hands and fingers ______________________
32. List the areas of therapy that are provided for persons with Down syndrome and other developmental disabilities.
   A. ______________________
   B. ______________________
   C. ______________________
   D. ______________________
   E. ______________________
33. The most common type of cerebral palsy is ______________________.
34. Symptoms of autism usually appear before the age of __________. A child with autism does not respond to own name by _____ months of age.

35. Which type of spina bifida would cause the problems in each of the examples given?
    A. The person has leg paralysis and a lack of bowel and bladder control. ____________________
    B. The person may have no symptoms. ____________
    C. Nerve damage usually does not occur and surgery corrects the defect. ____________________
36. If a hydrocephalus is not treated, pressure increases in the head and causes ____________ and ____________.

Optional Learning Exercises

Mr. Murphy is one of the residents you care for. He has Down syndrome. Answer the two questions that relate to this person.

37. Mr. Murphy is 40 years old. As an adult with Down syndrome, he has a risk for which disorder?

    ____

38. Mr. Murphy is encouraged to eat a well-balanced diet and to attend regular exercise classes. Including these in the care plan will help to prevent the problems of ____________________ and ____________________.

You care for Mary Reynolds, who has cerebral palsy. Answer the question about Ms. Reynolds.

39. Because Ms. Reynolds remains in bed or a special chair all the time, she is at special risk for __________ because of immobility and incontinence. She needs to be repositioned at least every ____________________.

Use the FOCUS ON PRIDE section to complete these statements and then use the critical thinking and discussion question to develop your ideas

40. Persons with developmental disabilities have a right to enjoy and maintain a good quality of life. Such a life involves
    A. ____
    B. ____
    C. ____
41. What signs or symptoms may alert the healthcare team that a developmentally disabled person is experiencing abuse?
    A. ____
    B. ____
    C. ____
    D. ____
    E. ____

Critical Thinking and Discussion Question

42. You are caring for a person who has Down syndrome. The person is around your age and you have a good working relationship with this person. The person asks you out on a date.
    A. Discuss how this would make you feel.
    B. What would you say to the person?

56 Caring for Mothers and Babies

Fill in the Blanks: Key Terms

Breastfeeding (nursing)	Episiotomy	Meconium	Prenatal care
Circumcision	Lochia	Postpartum	Umbilical cord

1. An ______________________________ is an incision into the perineum.
2. ______________________________ is the care a woman receives while pregnant.
3. The time period after childbirth is called __________.
4. ________________________ is the surgical removal of foreskin from the penis.
5. The vaginal discharge that occurs after childbirth is ______________________________.
6. The structure that carries blood, oxygen, and nutrients from the mother to the fetus is the ______________________________.
7. A dark green to black, tarry bowel movement is ______________________________.
8. Feeding a baby milk from the mother's breast is ______________________________.

Circle the Best Answer

9. Which position would the nursing assistant place the baby in for sleeping?
   A. Lay the baby on the stomach with head turned to the side
   B. Put the baby on the side with a pillow supporting the back
   C. Place the baby on the back remove soft pillows or plush toys
   D. Lay the baby in a bassinet with a small pillow under the head
10. Which action would the nursing assistant use to lift a newborn?
   A. Grasp the newborn's forearms and pull upward
   B. Scoop dominant hand under the newborn's back and buttocks
   C. Place hands under newborn's armpits and lifting upward
   D. Use both hands to support the head, back, and legs
11. Which action would the nursing assistant take if a baby is lying on a scale, bed, table, or other surface?
   A. Place pillows around the baby
   B. Tuck a blanket firmly around the baby
   C. Always keep one hand on the baby
   D. Keep an eye on the baby at all times
12. Which observation would the nursing assistant report to the nurse for follow-up assessment of possible postpartum depression?
   A. Mother seems sad and expresses feelings of inadequacy.
   B. Mother says she wants to take the baby home as soon as possible.
   C. Mother is irritated when a relative criticizes her breastfeeding method.
   D. Mother talks a lot about introducing the newborn to the older child.
13. Which of these crib features would the home health nursing assistant report to the nurse for follow-up investigation?
   A. The mattress is flush to the crib, without spaces or gaps.
   B. Side rails are fixed and drop-side latches are absent.
   C. Crib slats are closely spaced; about 2 inches apart.
   D. Headboard is decorated with a cute cut out design.
14. Which finding should the nursing assistant report to the nurse for follow-up assessment?
   A. Baby has a rectal temperature of 99.6°F.
   B. Baby has a soft, unformed stool after being breastfed.
   C. Baby turns head to one side or puts a hand to one ear.
   D. Baby cries when the diaper is wet or when hungry.
15. Which feeding schedule is typical for a breastfed newborn during the first month?
   A. Every 2 to 3 hours
   B. Every 8 to 12 hours
   C. Once an hour for a brief time
   D. On a very strict schedule
16. What will the nursing assistant place on the bedside table for a mother who will breastfeed the infant?
   A. Bottle with formula, in case the baby will not take the nipple
   B. Soap for cleaning the breast after feeding is complete
   C. Crackers and cheese; mother may experience hypoglycemia
   D. Milk, water, or juice; mother may get thirsty when breastfeeding

17. Which instruction would the mother be given about breastfeeding?
    A. Position the baby by using a pillow to prop up the baby
    B. Begin by stroking the baby's cheek with her nipple
    C. Nurse from one breast at each feeding
    D. Lay the baby on the stomach after feeding
18. Which action would the nursing assistant use when preparing bottles for feeding babies?
    A. Prepare and then refrigerate bottles for use within 24 hours
    B. Sterilize the bottles by boiling them for 20 minutes
    C. Rinse used bottles and nipples in boiling hot water
    D. Avoid using soap; it can cause gastrointestinal irritation
19. Which method would the nursing assistant use when preparing to give a bottle feeding to a baby?
    A. It may be used from the refrigerator without heating
    B. Place the bottle under warm running tap water
    C. Take the bottle out of the refrigerator and allow it to warm
    D. Heat the bottle in a microwave oven
20. How often should the nursing assistant burp an older baby during bottle feeding?
    A. Every 5 minutes
    B. After every 1/2 to 1 ounce of formula
    C. After every 2 to 3 ounces of formula
    D. When the newborn stops sucking
21. Which observation would the nursing assistant report to the nurse when diapering a baby?
    A. The stool is soft and unformed.
    B. The stool is hard and formed.
    C. The diaper is wet six to eight times a day.
    D. The baby has three stools in 1 day.
22. How often is the baby's diaper changed?
    A. When stool is present, usually 1 to 3 times a day
    B. When the diaper is wet or soiled, usually 6 to 8 times a day
    C. Before and after feeding and before and after sleep
    D. Before handing the baby to the mother for cuddling
23. Which action will the nursing assistant use for cord care?
    A. Apply petroleum jelly to the cord to keep it moist
    B. Wash with mild soap and pour warm water over the stump
    C. Keep the diaper below the cord to prevent irritation
    D. Gently pull off the cord if it looks ready to fall off
24. Which care measure would the nursing assistant perform for circumcision care?
    A. Clean the penis at each diaper change
    B. Clean the area with a sterile solution
    C. Apply a snug dressing to the area
    D. Avoid getting the penis wet
25. What should the water temperature be when giving a bath to a baby?
    A. Room temperature
    B. 80°F (26.6°C)
    C. 100°F (37.8°C)
    D. 110°F (43.3°C)
26. How often would the nursing assistant weigh a baby who is being breastfed?
    A. Once a day
    B. Before and after each feeding
    C. After every diaper change
    D. Once a week
27. Which observation for a postpartum patient would the nursing assistant report to the nurse at once?
    A. Small amount of bright red blood on sanitary napkin
    B. Saturating a sanitary napkin within 1 hour of application
    C. Saturating a sanitary napkin within 3 hours of application
    D. Dark red staining on sanitary napkin upon waking
28. Which finding would the nursing assistant report to the nurse when caring for the mother who is in postpartum period?
    A. Has occasional emotional reactions
    B. Has a whitish vaginal discharge 12 days after delivery
    C. Reports leg, abdominal, or perineal pain
    D. Has a menstrual period about 4 weeks after the baby is born
29. Which finding would the nursing assistant report to the nurse at once as a possible sign of postpartum infection for the mother?
    A. Pinkish brown lochia vaginal discharge
    B. Temperature of 99°F (37.2°C)
    C. Small gush of red fluid upon standing up in the morning
    D. Redness and foul-smelling drainage from episiotomy
30. Which action would the nursing assistant take when a postpartum patient reports pain in the left calf and area is swollen and tender to the touch?
    A. Assist the patient to get up and ambulate
    B. Help the patient to soak in a warm tub bath
    C. Report the observation and findings to the nurse
    D. Gently rub and massage the leg to stimulate circulation
31. Which site would the nursing assistant use to take a pulse on a baby?
    A. Brachial
    B. Radial
    C. Carotid
    D. Apical
32. Which rationale supports thoroughly rinsing of baby bottles, caps, and nipples to remove all soap?
    A. Soap can cause stomach and intestinal irritation.
    B. Soap scum is toxic and may cause genetic damage.
    C. Soap residue is unpleasant and indicates poor care.
    D. Soap taste will cause the baby to reject the bottle.

33. What is the purpose of applying petrolatum gauze dressing or jelly to an unhealed circumcision?
    A. Decreases the pain when newborn urinates
    B. Protects the penis from urine and feces
    C. Speeds healing and reduces scarring
    D. Prevents bleeding and purulent drainage
34. Which nursing assistant needs a reminder about safety measures that are followed to protect an infant during a bath?
    A. Nursing assistant A sets the room temperature at 80°F (26.7°C).
    B. Nursing assistant B keeps the bath water temperature at 110°F (43.3°C).
    C. Nursing assistant C never leaves the baby alone on a table top.
    D. Nursing assistant D never leaves the baby alone in the bathtub.
35. Which action should the nursing assistant take when changing the diaper and observes that the baby has an unhealed circumcision?
    A. Apply the diaper loosely so it will not irritate the penis
    B. Report this abnormal finding immediately to the nurse
    C. Leave the diaper off and place a waterproof pad under the hips
    D. Gently clean the incision using sterile technique
36. When would the nursing assistant expect to observe meconium stool during a diaper change?
    A. In the first 1 or 2 days after birth
    B. After the baby has the first breastfeeding
    C. When formula feeding is given
    D. When the baby is constipated
37. Which nursing measure would the nursing assistant use to enable the cord stump to heal faster?
    A. Cover the stump with a dry sterile dressing
    B. Expose the stump to let it air-dry
    C. Apply antibiotic ointment to the stump
    D. Gently wash the stump using clean technique

Fill in the Blanks

38. Write out the meaning of the abbreviations
    A. BM ______________________
    B. C ______________________
    C. CPSC ______________________
    D. C-section ______________________
    E. F ______________________
    F. SIDS ______________________
    G. SUID ______________________
39. What signs or symptoms related to each of these may indicate that the baby is ill?
    A. Skin color ______________________
    B. Respirations ______________________
    C. Eyes ______________________
    D. Stools ______________________
40. When a mother is breastfeeding, if the baby finished the last feeding at the right breast, the baby starts the next feeding at the ______________________ breast.
41. The baby is burped at least twice when breastfeeding. Burping is done
    A. ______________________
    B. ______________________
42. Sudden unexpected infant death may occur because of accidental suffocation or ______________________ in the bed.
43. You can prevent having air in the neck of the bottle or in the nipple by ______________________
    ______________________.
44. When changing a baby's diaper, what observations should be reported and recorded?
    A. ______________________
    B. ______________________
    C. ______________________
    D. ______________________
45. When caring for the umbilical cord, you should report the following to the nurse.
    A. ______________________
    B. ______________________
    C. ______________________
    D. ______________________
46. What steps are used to wash a baby's head?
    A. ______________________
    B. ______________________
    C. ______________________
    D. ______________________
    E. ______________________
47. A mother who had a baby 2 weeks ago has a whitish vaginal drainage. You document this finding and know that this is ______________ at this time, after having a baby.

Optional Learning Exercises

You are caring for Marilyn Hansen and her newborn son, Samuel, at home. Answer these questions about their care.

48. Ms. Hansen is breastfeeding. What would Ms. Hansen do to encourage Samuel to turn his head and start to suck? ______________________
49. Ms. Hansen is having difficulty in removing Samuel from her breast. How does she break the suction? ___
    ____
    ______________________.
50. What can Ms. Hansen do to prevent drying and cracking of the nipples?
    A. ______________________
    B. ______________________
    C. ______________________
    D. ______________________
51. When you are changing Samuel's diaper, clean the genital area from ______________________.
52. Ms. Hansen asks you when the cord stump will fall off. What will you tell her?
    ______________________.

53. Samuel has been circumcised and Ms. Hansen is concerned because the penis looks red, swollen, and sore. You know that this is normal. However, you should observe the circumcision for ________________, ________________, ________________, and ________________.

54. Ms. Hansen asks whether she should bathe Samuel in the morning or in the evening when they get home. You tell her an evening bath might work well because it
    A. ____
    ____
    B. ____
    ____

Use the FOCUS ON PRIDE section to complete these statements and then use the critical thinking and discussion question to develop your ideas

55. When you return a newborn to the mother, it is your professional responsibility to follow the agency policy for ____.

56. Newborns wear a security bracelet that will signal the agency when the baby is carried ____.

Critical Thinking and Discussion Question

57. You are assisting a new mother with care of the newborn, but she seems hesitant to try and wants you to do most of the care. What should you do?

57 Assisted Living

Fill in the Blanks: Key Terms

Assisted living
Service plan
Medication reminder

1. A ______________________ is reminding the person to take drugs, observing them being taken as prescribed, and recording that they were taken.
2. A written plan that lists the services needed by the person and who provides them is a ______________________.
3. ______________________ is a housing option for older persons who need help with activities of daily living (ADLs) but do not need 24-hour nursing care and supervision.

Circle the Best Answer

4. Which person would be the most likely candidate for assisted living?
   A. A person who needs help taking medications.
   B. A person who has a feeding tube and tracheostomy.
   C. A person who needs total help with all ADLs.
   D. A person who has advanced Alzheimer disease.
5. Which feature would be common to all assisted living residences?
   A. A private patio or balcony.
   B. 24-hour room service.
   C. Grab bars in the bathroom.
   D. A queen-sized bed.
6. Which housekeeping measure would help to prevent infection?
   A. Use air fresheners as needed.
   B. Clean bathroom surfaces with a disinfectant.
   C. Make beds and straighten up the living room.
   D. Open bathroom windows for a short time.
7. Which of these is included in the Assisted Living Residents' Rights?
   A. May take part in religious, social, community, and other activities.
   B. Receive personal care from preferred nursing assistants and nurses.
   C. Has a doctor or pharmacist assigned by the facility.
   D. Cannot be evicted or asked to vacate if unable to pay for service plan.
8. In which area will the nursing assistant need additional training if seeking employment in an assisted living residence?
   A. Using proper body mechanics.
   B. Assisting with daily hygiene.
   C. Using service plans.
   D. Measuring medications.
9. Which criteria must be met in order for the assisted living resident to meet safety needs in the event of an emergency?
   A. Residents are obliged to independently ambulate and help others as needed.
   B. Residents must be able to recognize and react appropriately to dangerous situations.
   C. Residents must give clear directions to others and follow instructions from the staff.
   D. Residents must leave the building with minimal assistance if helped into a wheelchair.
10. Which of these services, offered in an assisted living residence, would increase a resident's feeling of safety and security?
    A. A barber and a beauty service.
    B. A daily schedule of activities offered at the residence.
    C. A 24-hour emergency communication system.
    D. A common dining room and day area.
11. Which care measure would be the nursing assistant's responsibility related to meals in an assisted living residence?
    A. Give residents any foods they desire to eat.
    B. Take residents out to the restaurants of their choice.
    C. Assist residents, as needed, to go to the dining area.
    D. Ask residents about their special dietary needs.
12. Which task would the nursing assistant be expected to do when assisting with housekeeping?
    A. Clean the tub or shower after each use.
    B. Put out clean towels every week.
    C. Clean the carpet once a month.
    D. Dust furniture every day.
13. Which care measure should the nursing assistant follow when handling, preparing, or storing foods?
    A. Empty garbage at least once a week.
    B. Wash all pots and pans in a dishwasher.
    C. Save or discard leftovers.
    D. Use disinfectant to clean appliances, counters, and tables.
14. Which guideline would the nursing assistant follow when helping with the laundry?
    A. Sort and wash items using own laundry methods.
    B. Wear gloves when handling soiled laundry.
    C. Use hot water to wash all items.
    D. Use the highest dryer setting to sanitize the items.
15. Which task would be assigned to the nursing assistant for a person who needs help with medication in an assisted living situation?
    A. Opening containers if person is unable.
    B. Measuring the medications.
    C. Explaining the action of the medication.
    D. Preparing a pill organizer for each week.

16. Which action would the nursing assistant take if a drug error occurs?
    A. Tell the person not to do it again.
    B. Give the person the correct medication.
    C. Report the error to the nurse.
    D. Take all medications away from the person.
17. Which event represents a drug error?
    A. Taking a tablet from the pill organizer.
    B. Taking a drug after getting a medication reminder.
    C. Taking a pill from a presorted dose packet.
    D. Taking an extra dose of the medication.
18. What is the best recourse for the staff and administrators of an assisted living facility if a resident is a threat to the health and safety of self or others?
    A. Assign extra staff to monitor the resident's behavior.
    B. Have the resident transferred to a facility that can meet safety needs.
    C. Have the resident evicted to prevent injury and accidents.
    D. Ask the resident to leave voluntarily within a given time frame.
19. How would the nursing assistant respond when a resident who uses self-directed medication management says, "This pill looks different"?
    A. "Let's read the label; then you will know what you are taking."
    B. "Let me contact the nurse before you take the pill."
    C. "I'm sure the pharmacist knows to send the right medication."
    D. "Things can look and seem different when you are not at home."
20. What would be included in the service plan?
    A. Payment schedule and contact information for responsible party.
    B. Advance directives and power of attorney information.
    C. Individual social service and special service needs.
    D. Care measures for behavioral issues, such as agitation or confusion.
21. Why would a resident who had been in an assisted living facility for 2 years be moved to a nursing facility after having a stroke that caused left-sided paralysis?
    A. Assisted living facility can no longer meet the person's needs.
    B. Stroke always causes serious life-threatening consequences.
    C. Family typically prefers a facility that offers poststroke care.
    D. A rehabilitation facility is more cost-effective than assisted living.
22. Which nursing assistant needs remediation about responsibilities in caring for a person who needs a medication reminder?
    A. Nursing assistant A gives the injection as directed by the care plan.
    B. Nursing assistant B reminds the person to take the medications.
    C. Nursing assistant C observes that the drugs were taken as prescribed.
    D. Nursing assistant D records that the drugs were taken.

Fill in the Blanks

23. When working in an assisted living setting, the nursing assistant should follow ________________ when contact with blood, body fluids, secretions, excretions, or potentially contaminated items is likely.
24. Most persons living in assisted living residences need help with one or more activities of daily living (ADLs), such as
    A. ________________
    B. ________________
    C. ________________
    D. ________________
    E. ________________
    F. ________________
25. Assisted living residences cannot employ a person with a ________________.
26. The service plan is a written plan listing
    A. ________________
    B. ________________
    C. ________________
27. What 24-hour services are usually provided by the assisted living residences?
    A. ________________
    B. ________________
28. In which order would the nursing assistant wash cooking equipment, dishes, glassware, and utensils?
    ____
29. When assisting the person with taking medications, the six rights of drug administration include:
    A. ________________
    B. ________________
    C. ________________
    D. ________________
    E. ________________
    F. ________________
30. Some agencies use "10 rights of medication assistance." What are the 4 additional rights?
    A. ________________
    B. ________________
    C. ________________
    D. ________________
31. If you are assisting in drug administration, you should report any drug error to the RN. Errors would include:
    A. ________________
    B. ________________
    C. ________________
    D. ________________
    E. ________________
    F. ________________
    G. ________________
    H. ________________
    I. ________________
32. Residents have the right to not be photographed without consent, except for the purpose of resident ________________.

Optional Learning Exercises

You are working in an assisting living facility. What would you do in these situations?

33. Mrs. Jenkins tells you that she is expecting an important phone call and wants to eat her lunch in her room. What should you do? ____________________
____

34. Mr. Shante asks you to get his medicines ready for him to take. What assistance are you allowed to give after you have received the proper training?
A. ____________________
B. ____________________
C. ____________________
D. ____________________
E. ____________________
F. ____________________
G. ____________________
H. ____________________

35. When you are assisting Mrs. Clyde with her medicines, you notice two of the labels have an expired date. What should you do? ____________________
____

36. Mrs. Johnson asks you when the next meeting of the quilting group will be held. She also asks what days the community crafts fair is planned. Where would you direct her to find this information? ____________________
____

Use the FOCUS ON PRIDE section to complete these statements and then use the critical thinking and discussion question to develop your ideas

37. When you are caring for residents in assisted living, your interactions should assure the person and family that you will provide ____________________.

38. It is important to know your state's laws when you assist with drugs because if you act beyond those limits, you can lose ____________________ and your ability to work as a ____________________.

Critical Thinking and Discussion Question

39. Discuss some of the advantages and disadvantages of working in an assisted living residence.

58 Emergency Care

Fill in the Blanks: Key Terms

Anaphylaxis
Cardiopulmonary resuscitation (CPR)
Fainting
First aid
Frostbite
Hemorrhage
Hypothermia
Respiratory arrest
Resuscitate
Seizure (convulsion)
Shock
Sudden cardiac arrest (cardiac arrest)

1. ______________________ is an emergency procedure performed when the heart and breathing stop.
2. In ______________________, breathing stops but the heart action continues for several minutes.
3. The sudden loss of consciousness from an inadequate blood supply to the brain is ______________________.
4. When the heart stops suddenly and without warning, it is ______________________.
5. ______________________ results when there is not enough blood supply to organs and tissues.
6. Emergency care given to an ill or injured person before medical help arrives is ______________________.
7. Violent and sudden contractions or tremors of muscle groups, caused by abnormal electrical activity in the brain, is a ______________________.
8. ______________________ is the excessive loss of blood in a short period of time.
9. A life-threatening sensitivity to an antigen is ______________________.
10. ______________________ is an injury to the body caused by freezing of the skin and underlying tissues.
11. An abnormally low body temperature is ______________________.
12. ______________________ is to revive from apparent death or unconsciousness by using emergency measures.

Circle the Best Answer

13. What is the best way to stop bleeding from a wound?
    A. Use a tourniquet.
    B. Apply direct pressure.
    C. Cover with a thick dry dressing.
    D. Elevate the area that is bleeding.
14. Which nursing assistant needs additional practice during a cardiopulmonary training session?
    A. Nursing assistant A opens the airway using the head tilt-chin lift method.
    B. Nursing assistant B gives one breath every 2 to 3 seconds for an infant or child.
    C. Nursing assistant C checks for breathing; then gives one breath over 1 second every 2 seconds for an adult.
    D. Nursing assistant D checks pulse every 2 minutes; if no pulse starts cardiopulmonary resuscitation.
15. Which action should the nursing assistant take if the nurse instructs to activate the Emergency Medical Services (EMS) system?
    A. Tell the EMS operator the victim's name and the family's phone number.
    B. State name and employee identification number when calling EMS.
    C. Give the location, include street address and city to the EMS dispatcher.
    D. Tell EMS to hurry and send someone; then return to help the nurse.
16. Why is it important to quickly restore breathing and circulation during cardiac arrest?
    A. The person will have a seizure.
    B. The person will lose consciousness.
    C. Organ damage occurs within minutes.
    D. Life-threatening hemorrhage will occur.
17. Which set of signs and symptoms causes the nursing assistant to suspect that the person has had sudden cardiac arrest (SCA)?
    A. Chest pain, jaw pain, and nausea.
    B. No pulse, no breathing, and no response.
    C. Perspiration, dizziness, and pale skin.
    D. Trouble breathing, choking, and wheezing.
18. What is the purpose of chest compressions?
    A. To deflate the lungs.
    B. To increase oxygen in the blood.
    C. To force blood through the circulatory system.
    D. To help the heart work more effectively.
19. Which position must the person be in for chest compressions to be effective?
    A. In the prone position on any surface.
    B. Upright on a soft surface.
    C. Supine on a hard, flat surface.
    D. In bed in the semi-Fowler's position.
20. What is the depth of chest compression on the sternum when performing cardiopulmonary resuscitation on an adult?
    A. About 1 to 1½ inches.
    B. No more than 1 inch.
    C. At least 2 inches.
    D. About 3 inches.
21. What is the purpose of the head tilt-chin lift maneuver?
    A. Make the person more comfortable.
    B. Open the airway.
    C. Keep the head in alignment.
    D. Protect the jaw and teeth.

22. In which circumstance, would a barrier device be used for rescue breathing?
    A. Whenever possible to avoid contact with body fluids.
    B. In order to make a better seal for breathing.
    C. When ventilation through the mouth is not possible.
    D. Only when other methods will not work.
23. In which circumstance would mouth-to-mouth-and-nose breathing be used?
    A. When the person is semi-conscious.
    B. Rescuer wants to avoid contact with body fluids.
    C. In giving rescue breaths to an infant.
    D. When chest compressions are not needed.
24. At which point would an automated external defibrillator (AED) be used for a person who suffered a cardiac arrest?
    A. Use it after other methods have failed.
    B. Use when an RN or doctor are present.
    C. Use it as soon as possible.
    D. Use it once the person is responsive.
25. Which action occurs when an automated external defibrillator (AED) is used for a person who has cardiac arrest?
    A. Makes the heartbeat faster, stronger, and more efficiently.
    B. Slows down the heartbeat; then reestablishes a faster rhythm.
    C. Stops ventricular fibrillation and restores a regular heartbeat.
    D. Replaces chest compressions and rescue breathing.
26. When can cardiopulmonary resuscitation be stopped once it is initiated by bystanders at the scene of an automobile accident?
    A. Stop when the Emergency Medical Services (EMS) arrives.
    B. Pause when a bystander says to stop.
    C. Discontinue when the person seems dead.
    D. Cease when a family member says to stop.
27. Which action would the nursing assistant take before starting chest compressions?
    A. Make sure the person is breathing.
    B. Check carotid pulse for 10 seconds or less.
    C. Wait 30 seconds to see if the person responds.
    D. Turn the person to the side.
28. Which action would the nursing assistant do first when starting cardiopulmonary resuscitation?
    A. Give 30 chest compressions.
    B. Give two breaths.
    C. Look for the defibrillator.
    D. Report to the nurse.
29. Which action would the nursing assistant take to initiate rescue breathing if an adult is not breathing or not breathing adequately?
    A. Give one breath every 6 seconds.
    B. Give one breath every 2 seconds.
    C. Give two breaths that last about 5 seconds each.
    D. Give two breaths that last 10 seconds each.
30. What is the rate of chest compressions for an adult when performing cardiopulmonary resuscitation?
    A. 12 to 20 compressions per minute.
    B. 15 to 30 compressions per minute.
    C. 60 to 80 compressions per minute.
    D. 100 to 120 compressions per minute.
31. How long would the nursing assistant continue cycles of compressions and breathing when performing cardiopulmonary resuscitation?
    A. For 5 minutes.
    B. For 30 minutes.
    C. Until death is confirmed by the nurse.
    D. Until an automated external defibrillator (AED) arrives.
32. When is the recovery position used?
    A. During chest compressions.
    B. When mouth-to-mouth breathing is needed.
    C. After the person is breathing and has a pulse.
    D. When the automated external defibrillator (AED) is needed.
33. What is the depth of chest compressions when a 5-year-old child needs cardiopulmonary resuscitation?
    A. Move the sternum about $^1/_3$ of an inch.
    B. At least $^1/_3$ the depth of the chest.
    C. Push with fingers to cause blanching.
    D. Compress the sternum about 1 inch.
34. Which action would the nursing assistant use when giving breaths to an infant?
    A. Tip the head back as far as possible to open the airway.
    B. Pinch the nose closed and breathe through the mouth.
    C. Cover the infant's mouth and nose with own mouth.
    D. Always use a mouth barrier.
35. Which action would the nursing assistant take if a person has swallowed poison?
    A. Try to help the person to vomit.
    B. Give the person something to drink or eat.
    C. Contact the Poison Control Center as soon as possible.
    D. Ask the person why poison was swallowed.
36. Which of these is a sign of internal hemorrhage?
    A. Steady flow of blood from a wound.
    B. Pain, shock, vomiting blood, or coughing up blood.
    C. Bleeding occurs in bright red spurts.
    D. Dried blood at the site of an injury.
37. In which circumstance would the nursing assistant intervene when a child gets injured at a playground park and is bleeding?
    A. Bystander attempts to remove a stick embedded in the skin.
    B. Mother places a clean dry towel directly over the wound.
    C. Bystander applies direct pressure over the bleeding site.
    D. Father talks calmly and quietly to the child.

38. Which position is the best for a person who is experiencing the signs and symptoms of shock?
    A. Sitting position in a firm chair with head between legs.
    B. Recovery position with a small pillow under the head.
    C. High Fowler's position with legs slightly elevated.
    D. Supine position with legs elevated 6 to 12 inches.
39. Which factor causes anaphylactic shock?
    A. Hemorrhage.
    B. Allergies.
    C. Sudden cardiac arrest.
    D. Seizures.
40. Which action would the nursing assistant take if the person is having signs or symptoms of stroke?
    A. Make the person comfortable.
    B. Begin cardiopulmonary resuscitation immediately.
    C. Call Emergency Medical Services (EMS) at once.
    D. Ask the person to describe sensations and symptoms.
41. Which action is most important if a person has a seizure?
    A. Turn the person to one side.
    B. Note the time the seizure started.
    C. Put the person into the bed.
    D. Put something soft between the teeth.
42. Which action will the staff take first when a group of elderly residents are outside for a picnic and the nurse says some of people are showing signs or symptoms of heat-related illness?
    A. Move everyone to a cooler place.
    B. Loosen everyone's tight clothing.
    C. Give everyone a cold drink.
    D. Spray everyone with a cool mist.
43. Which action will the nursing assistant take when a person sustains a burn on the forearm?
    A. Apply direct pressure to the burned area.
    B. Remove jewelry that is not stuck to the skin.
    C. Give the person plenty of fluids.
    D. Apply oils or ointments to the burns.
44. Which nursing assistant needs remediation for giving emergency care for a burn?
    A. Nursing assistant A applies cool water for 10 to 15 minutes.
    B. Nursing assistant B places ice directly on the burn.
    C. Nursing assistant C covers burn area with a clean sheet.
    D. Nursing assistant D removes hot clothing that is not sticking to the skin.
45. Which action would the nursing assistant use to find the carotid pulse?
    A. Place index finger at jaw line, just below earlobe.
    B. Place thumb or index finger on the anterior wrist (thumb side).
    C. Place three fingers on the anterior upper arm above the elbow crease.
    D. Place two fingers on the trachea and slide fingers into the groove of the neck.
46. What is the time limit if compressions must be interrupted to apply the automated external defibrillator (AED)?
    A. Less than 5 seconds.
    B. Less than 10 seconds.
    C. About 30 seconds.
    D. Approximately 1 minute.
47. When would the health-care team start cardiopulmonary resuscitation for a young child?
    A. Child is sleeping very soundly; pulse is 80 beats/minute.
    B. Child will not arouse to stimuli that usually results in waking.
    C. Child is pale and lips are bluish; pulse is 45 beats/minute.
    D. Child is breathing 30 times per minute and is crying loudly.
48. Which action would the nursing assistant use to check for a response in an infant?
    A. Shake the infant gently.
    B. Tap the foot and shout.
    C. Call the infant by first name.
    D. Ask parent how infant usually responds.
49. What is the cycle of compressions and rescue breaths if a home health nursing assistant is the single rescuer performing cardiopulmonary resuscitation?
    A. 15 compressions followed by 1 breath.
    B. 15 compressions followed by 2 breaths.
    C. 30 compressions followed by 2 breaths.
    D. 100 compressions followed by 2 breaths.
50. Which nursing measure would the nursing assistant use if a person with a suspected concussion started vomiting?
    A. Quickly obtain oral suction equipment.
    B. Stay with the person and call the nurse for help.
    C. Logroll the person as a unit to a side-lying position.
    D. Sit the person upright and instruct to bend slightly forward.
51. Which step is correct when performing the head tilt-chin lift maneuver?
    A. Rescuer puts person in a prone position on a flat firm surface.
    B. Rescuer places one hand on the person's forehead.
    C. Rescuer applies pressure to the front of the person's neck.
    D. Rescuer pushes the chin downward with the fingers of both hands.
52. Which action would the nursing assistant take to protect the person's head during a seizure?
    A. Help the person to get back into bed.
    B. Help the person to sit upright.
    C. Cradle the person's body in arms or lap.
    D. Place something soft under the person's head.

Fill in the Blanks

53. Write out the abbreviations
    A. AED ____________________
    B. CPR ____________________
    C. EMS ____________________
    D. RRS ____________________
    E. SCA ____________________
    F. VF; V-fib ____________________
54. If you activate the Emergency Medical Services (EMS) system, what information should you give to the operator?
    A. ____________________
    B. ____________________
    C. ____________________
    D. ____________________
    E. ____________________
    F. ____________________
55. The three major signs of sudden cardiac arrest are
    A. ____________________
    B. ____________________
    C. ____________________
56. Rescue breaths are given when there is a ______________ but no ______________.
57. When doing chest compressions, you push ______________ and ______________ in the center of the chest.
58. When you perform mouth-to-mouth breathing, it is likely you will have contact with the person's ____________________ ____________________.
59. A bag valve mask is a ______________ device. It should be connected to an ______________ ______________.
60. The automated external defibrillator (AED) advises a "shock." What does the nurse say in a loud voice before pushing the SHOCK button? ____________________
61. What are the signs and symptoms of a heart attack?
    A. ____________________
    B. ____________________
    C. ____________________
    D. ____________________
    E. ____________________
    F. ____________________
62. Signs and symptoms of shock include
    A. ____________________
    B. ____________________
    C. ____________________
    D. ____________________
    E. ____________________
    F. ____________________
    G. ____________________
    H. ____________________
63. Anaphylaxis is an emergency because the reaction occurs within ____________________.
64. What are the signs and symptoms of an anaphylactic reaction?
    A. ____________________
    B. ____________________
    C. ____________________
    D. ____________________
    E. ____________________
    F. ____________________
    G. ____________________
    H. ____________________
    I. ____________________
    J. ____________________
    K. ____________________
65. Signs of a stroke include sudden
    A. ____________________
    B. ____________________
    C. ____________________
    D. ____________________
    E. ____________________
66. For people with suspected hypothermia or frostbite, you would move them into a ______________ ______________ as soon as possible.
67. What are the signs and symptoms of hypothermia?
    A. ____________________
    B. ____________________
    C. ____________________
    D. ____________________
    E. ____________________
    F. ____________________
    G. ____________________
    H. ____________________
    I. ____________________

Optional Learning Exercises

You are visiting a neighbor and she is washing dishes. As she washes a glass, it shatters and she sustains a deep cut on her wrist. Answer the following questions about how you would respond.

68. Clean rubber gloves are lying on the counter. How can they be useful to you? ____________________ ____________________
69. What materials in the home could be used to place over the wound? ____________________ ____________________
70. Your neighbor is restless and has a rapid and weak pulse. You notice her skin is cold, moist, and pale. These signs indicate she may be in ______________.
71. Her wound is still bleeding, and she loses consciousness. What should you do before you continue to give first aid? ____________________

Use the FOCUS ON PRIDE section to complete these statements and then use the critical thinking and discussion questions to develop your ideas

72. If a person has an emergency in a public place, you protect the person's right to privacy when you do what you can to ______________________________.

Critical Thinking and Discussion Questions

73. There is an emergency situation with a patient on the unit and you run to help. The charge nurse tells you to continue to care for the other patients, rather than assist with the emergency situation.
    A. Discuss how this would make you feel.
    B. Why would the nurse ask you to continue the care of the other patients?

59 End-of-Life Care

Fill in the Blanks: Key Terms

Advance directive
Autopsy
End-of-life care
Palliative care
Postmortem care
Rigor mortis
Terminal illness

1. The support and care given during the time surrounding death is ____________________.
2. The stiffness or rigidity of skeletal muscles that occurs after death is ____________________.
3. An ____________________ is a legal document stating a person's wishes about healthcare when that person is unable to make their own decisions.
4. Care of the body after death is ____________________.
5. An illness or injury from which a person will not likely recover and death is expected is a ____________________.
6. ____________________ is care that relieves or reduces the intensity of uncomfortable symptoms without producing a cure.
7. The examination of the body after death is an ____________________.

Circle the Best Answer

8. Which nursing assistant needs a reminder about communication when caring for a dying person?
   A. Nursing assistant A explains the care measures and actions.
   B. Nursing assistant B asks questions that need long answers.
   C. Nursing assistant C talks to a person who is in a coma.
   D. Nursing assistant D assumes that the dying person hears what is said.
9. Which care measure would be part of the nursing assistant's responsibility in caring for a person who has a terminal illness?
   A. Assisting a person to gather belongings for transfer to a rehabilitation unit.
   B. Helping a person to interpret and complete the advanced directive form.
   C. Helping a person with hygienic care for comfort and the quality of life.
   D. Assisting a person with range-of-motion exercises to increase strength.
10. What is the main difference between palliative care and hospice care?
    A. In hospice care, the focus of support is the family.
    B. In palliative care, treatment of the disease may continue.
    C. In palliative care, the person always remains at home.
    D. In hospice care, lifesaving measures are taken to prolong life.
11. Which criteria best describes hospice care?
    A. Is given when death is immediately imminent.
    B. Usually begins when terminal illness is diagnosed.
    C. May occur when a person has less than 6 months to live.
    D. Is given until the person recovers from the illness.
12. Which response is a barrier to communication when talking to a dying person?
    A. "Would you like to talk? I have time to listen."
    B. "You seem sad. Can I help?"
    C. "Is it okay if I quietly sit with you for a while?"
    D. "I understand what you are going through."
13. Which comment represents a 4-year-old child's understanding of death?
    A. "If grandma dies, she will be gone forever."
    B. "When grandma finishes dying, she's going to play with me."
    C. "If I get sick I might die, but I never get sick, so I won't die."
    D. "I don't think I will die; only old people die and I'm not old."
14. Which age-group is most likely to view death as freedom from pain, suffering, and disability?
    A. School-aged children.
    B. Young adults.
    C. Middle-aged adults.
    D. Older adults.
15. In which stage of dying does the person make promises and make "just one more" request?
    A. Acceptance.
    B. Anger.
    C. Depression.
    D. Bargaining.
16. Which care measure would the nursing assistant use if a dying person begins to talk about worries and concerns late at night?
    A. Call a spiritual leader.
    B. Tell the nurse.
    C. Listen quietly and use touch.
    D. Call the family.
17. What is the primary goal for care that is given when a person is dying?
    A. To meet the family's expectations.
    B. To promote comfort.
    C. To keep the person active.
    D. To prevent worsening.

18. Which care measure would the nursing assistant use to compensate for failing vision as death approaches?
    A. Explain actions and care.
    B. Have the room lit very brightly.
    C. Turn off all lights.
    D. Speak loudly and clearly.
19. Which care measure would the nursing assistant use, based on the knowledge that hearing is one of the last functions to be lost?
    A. Ask the person questions while giving care.
    B. Talk in a loud voice so the person can hear you.
    C. Provide reassurance and explanations about care.
    D. Ask the family to be quiet so they do not disturb the person.
20. How is oral hygiene handled as death nears?
    A. Given in the morning and in the evening.
    B. Done frequently when taking oral fluids is difficult.
    C. Offered occasionally to avoid disturbing the person.
    D. Never given because the person cannot swallow.
21. Which sign or symptom would prompt the nursing assistant to immediately notify the nurse because death is imminent for a person who has been in hospice for several weeks?
    A. Skin becomes red and warm to the touch.
    B. Person reports that pain is getting worse.
    C. Person seems more depressed than usual.
    D. Respirations become slow and shallow.
22. Which position is generally more comfortable for the dying person because of breathing difficulties?
    A. Supine position.
    B. Trendelenburg's position.
    C. Prone position.
    D. Semi-Fowler's position.
23. Which care measure for the family is likely to be included on the care plan when a person is dying?
    A. Allowing family members to stay as long as they wish.
    B. Ensuring privacy for the family and delaying care measures.
    C. Asking family members to leave so that care can be completed.
    D. Reassuring family members that the person is not in pain.
24. Which information would the healthcare team be able to obtain from a person's living will?
    A. Any religious or cultural considerations for postmortem care.
    B. Name and location of the hospital facility that the person prefers.
    C. Which interventions are allowed, such as tube feeding or resuscitation.
    D. Name and contact information for person who will make health-care decisions.
25. What is the implication of a "Do Not Resuscitate" (DNR) order?
    A. Chest compressions and rescue breathing are not initiated.
    B. The person will not be given food or fluid if death is inevitable.
    C. Doctor must be available to decide whether or not to resuscitate.
    D. The RN decides in some situations that resuscitation is needed.
26. Which sign indicates that death is near?
    A. Deep, rapid respirations.
    B. Body temperature changes.
    C. Muscles tense and contract in spasms.
    D. Peristalsis increases.
27. How is the body prepared when the family wishes to see the body after death?
    A. Body remains exactly as the person was at death.
    B. Body is positioned to appear comfortable and natural.
    C. Body is moved to a cheerful and well-lit room for viewing.
    D. Body is placed and supported in a semi-Fowler's position.
28. Which assumption would the nursing assistant make when air is expelled from the mouth when the body is turned during postmortem care?
    A. The person is still breathing. You must quickly get the nurse.
    B. Decaying tissues are causing bloating of intestinal organs.
    C. Cardiopulmonary resuscitation should be initiated.
    D. Moving the body has caused trapped air to be expelled.
29. Which action would the nursing assistant use when assisting with postmortem care?
    A. Place the body in a side-lying position.
    B. Tape all jewelry in place.
    C. Gently pull eyelids over the eyes.
    D. Dress the person in regular clothing.
30. Where is the second ID tag attached when the first ID tag from the postmortem kit is attached to the body, usually the right big toe or ankle?
    A. Person's dentures.
    B. Shroud, body bag, or sheet.
    C. Opposite toe or ankle.
    D. Bag of jewelry and other belongings.
31. Which nursing measure would the nursing assistant use when caring for a person who is dying because crusting and irritation of the nostrils can occur?
    A. Administer saline nasal spray or drops, as needed.
    B. Gently wash the wash and nose during tub bath or when showering.
    C. Assist the person to sit upright to facilitate breathing and nasal drainage.
    D. Clean the nose carefully. Apply lubricant as directed by the nurse and care plan.

32. Which fear is an adult person expressing when she says, "I wonder if my family will come to see me before I die?"
    A. Fear of dying alone.
    B. Fear of invasion of privacy.
    C. Fear of pain or suffering.
    D. Fear of the unknown.
33. Which elimination problem would prompt the nursing assistant to plan additional time for hygienic care when caring for a dying person?
    A. Constipation.
    B. Urinary infection.
    C. Urinary retention.
    D. Urinary and fecal incontinence.
34. Which task would be a nursing assistant's responsibility in the care of a person who is receiving palliative care?
    A. Offer the family tissues and express empathy and sympathy.
    B. Ensure that bed linens are clean, dry, and wrinkle-free.
    C. Coach and supervise person to do as much self-care as possible.
    D. Assist with postmortem care, according to the care plan.
35. Which documentation guides immediate actions if the nursing assistant is the first member of the healthcare team to discover a person who is in hospice to be in full cardiac arrest?
    A. Patient Self-Determination Act.
    B. Do Not Resuscitate Order.
    C. Omnibus Budget Reconciliation Act of 1987.
    D. Durable Power of Attorney for HealthCare.

Fill in the Blanks

36. Write out the abbreviations
    A. CPR ____________________
    B. DNR ____________________
    C. OBRA ____________________
    D. POLST ____________________
37. Hospice care focuses on these needs of the dying person and families.
    A. ____________________
    B. ____________________
    C. ____________________
    D. ____________________
38. Name the five stages of dying.
    A. ____________________
    B. ____________________
    C. ____________________
    D. ____________________
    E. ____________________
39. What are the end-of-life care comfort goals?
    A. ____________________
    B. ____________________
40. The Patient Self-Determination Act and *Omnibus Budget Reconciliation Act of 1987* (OBRA) give persons the right to ____________ or ____________ treatment.
41. When a person cannot make healthcare decisions, the authority to do so is given to the person with ____________________.
42. What are the signs that death is near?
    A. ____________________
    B. ____________________
    C. ____________________
    D. ____________________
    E. ____________________
    F. ____________________
43. As one of the signs of death, the pupils are ____________ and ____________.
44. When assisting with postmortem care, what information do you need from the nurse?
    A. ____________________
    B. ____________________
    C. ____________________
    D. ____________________
    E. ____________________

Optional Learning Exercises

You are assigned to care for Mrs. Adams, who is dying. Answer the questions regarding this situation.

45. You find Mrs. Adams crying in her room. When you ask her what is wrong, she tells you no one gave her fresh water this morning or helped her with a bath. She says, "Just to go away!" What stage of dying is she displaying? ____________________
46. Later in the day, Mrs. Adams tells you that she cannot wait until she is better to go home and plant her garden. She states that she knows the tests done last week were wrong and she will recover quickly from her illness. Now what stage is she displaying? ____________
    Why is she displaying two different stages so rapidly? ____________________
47. A minister comes to visit Mrs. Adams while you are giving care. What should you do? ____________________
48. You are working one night and find Mrs. Adams awake during the night. She asks you to sit with her. She begins to talk about her fears, worries, and anxieties. What are two things you can do to convey caring to her? ____________________
    ____
49. Mrs. Adams dies while you are working and the nurse asks you to assist with postmortem care. As you clean soiled areas, you assist the nurse to turn the body and air is expelled. This occurs because ____________________
    ____________________.
50. You wear gloves during postmortem care to protect yourself from ____________________.

Use the FOCUS ON PRIDE section to complete these statements and then use the critical thinking and discussion questions to develop your ideas

51. You are giving quality care to a dying person when you
    A. ______________________________
    B. ______________________________
    C. ______________________________
52. What are the dying person rights according to Omnibus Budget Reconciliation Act of 1987 (OBRA).
    A. ______________________________
    B. ______________________________
    C. ______________________________
    D. ______________________________
    E. ______________________________
    F. ______________________________
    G. ______________________________
    H. ______________________________

Critical Thinking and Discussion Questions

53. You are assisting in the care of a person who is dying. Initially, the person and the family were grateful for the care, but over the past week, the daughter has become increasingly unhappy and dissatisfied with everything that the staff tries to do. Today as you are doing helping with morning hygiene, the daughter says, "You are being too rough with her!"
    A. What would you do?
    B. What could contribute to the daughter's feelings of dissatisfaction and unhappiness in the past week?
54. Another nursing assistant was with a favorite resident and her family when the woman died. The nursing assistant posted a moving commentary about the last moments of the woman's life and the family's reaction on social media. Several staff members agreed that the woman will be missed and that the posted tribute reflected the staff's affection for the woman. However, the facility administration and the nursing supervisor decide to put the nursing assistant on suspension pending investigation of the incident. Why did the nursing assistant receive this reprimand?

60 Getting a Job

Fill in the Blanks: Key Terms

Discrimination
Job application
Job interview
Reasonable accommodation

1. During a ________________________________, a prospective employer asks questions about the applicant's education and career.
2. An agency's official form listing questions that require factual answers from the person seeking employment is a ____________________________.
3. Unjust treatment based on personal qualities is ____.
4. To assist or change a position or workplace to allow an employee to do a job despite having a disability is ____.

Circle the Best Answer

5. Which rationale supports displaying good work ethics as a student during clinical experiences because it may help you find a job?
   A. Improves the learning experience.
   B. Ethical behavior is mandatory.
   C. Grades will improve.
   D. Students are recruited as future employees.
6. Which nursing assistant has made the best choice for grooming and dressing for a job interview?
   A. Nursing assistant A wears her best black special occasion dress with matching heels.
   B. Nursing assistant B comes directly from a clinical rotation wearing school uniform.
   C. Nursing assistant C wears a bright-colored shirt that always gets compliments.
   D. Nursing assistant D wears a light blue long-sleeved shirt and tan-colored pants.
7. How does an employer know that you can perform the required job skills?
   A. Facility requires the National Assistant Training and Competency Evaluation Program (NATCEP).
   B. Agency requires a demonstration of selected skills.
   C. Employer asks a series of questions about performing certain skills.
   D. All prospective hires will be required to take and pass a written test.
8. Which question is allowed by the Equal Employment Opportunity Commission during an interview?
   A. Which religious holidays would do you observe?
   B. Have you ever had a substance abuse problem?
   C. Who will take care of your children while you are at work?
   D. Tell me about your last job; why did you leave?
9. What information do you need to give about each of your references when you are filling out a job application?
   A. Name, title, address, and phone number.
   B. Age, birth date, state of residence.
   C. Nature and duration of your relationship.
   D. Their qualifications to be your reference.
10. What would be the benefit of taking a practice run to a job interview?
    A. Shows you follow directions well.
    B. Shows that you are eager to work there.
    C. Provides information about time, distance, and parking.
    D. Allows you to look at the center to see if you want to work there.
11. Which action would be best to use when you are interviewing?
    A. Compliment the interviewer's appearance.
    B. Look directly at the interviewer.
    C. Ask for water if you feel very nervous.
    D. Convey animation and energy in your gestures.
12. What is a good way to share your list of skills with the interviewer?
    A. Tell the person verbally what you can do.
    B. Ask for a list of skills and check the ones you know.
    C. Prepare a list of your skills and give it to the interviewer.
    D. Tell the interviewer you will send a list as soon as possible.
13. What is the most important reason for you to ask questions at the end of the interview?
    A. Demonstrates your interests in taking the job.
    B. Helps you to decide if the job is right for you.
    C. Shows you have good communication skills.
    D. Helps you to anticipate problems related to the job.
14. What should you do after an interview?
    A. Send a thank you note within 24 hours of the interview.
    B. Call the interviewer every day to see if you are being hired.
    C. Wait for the employer to contact you.
    D. Call 1 week after the interview to thank the person for the interview.

Fill in the Blanks

15. Write out the abbreviations
    A. EEOC ________________________________
    B. NATCEP ______________________________
    C. OBRA ________________________________

16. List eight places you can find out about jobs.
 A. ______
 B. ______
 C. ______
 D. ______
 E. ______
 F. ______
 G. ______
 H. ______
 I. ______
17. When an employer requests proof of successful National Assistant Training and Competency Evaluation Program (NATCEP) completion, which items do you need?
 A. ______
 B. ______
 C. ______
18. When a section on a job application does not apply to you, you should ______.
19. List four reasons that could explain employment gaps.
 A. ______
 B. ______
 C. ______
 D. ______
20. If you lie on a job application, it is ______. If you do this, what can happen? ______
21. Which items do you need to provide when completing a job application?
 A. ______
 B. ______
 C. ______
 D. ______
22. You will soon be filling out job applications. Which documents and information will you collect in a file to make the process easier for yourself?
 A. ______
 B. ______
 C. ______
 D. ______
 E. ______
 F. ______
 G. ______
 H. ______
 I. ______
 J. ______

Optional Learning Experiences

Applying for a Job in Home Care

23. When the RN is not at the bedside to help you if problems occur, you are expected to be able to ______.
24. When you arrive at a person's home on time, you are using ______.
 What temptations should be avoided when you are giving home care? ______
25. When you shop for a person, what should you accurately report to the person or family? ______.
26. What questions should you ask if you are interviewing for a job in home care?
 A. ______
 B. ______
 C. ______
 D. ______
 E. ______
 F. ______

Use the FOCUS ON PRIDE section to complete these statements and then use the critical thinking and discussion questions to develop your ideas

27. Application and interview questions must relate to your ______ to do the job.
28. ______, ______, and interview questions help agencies decide if an applicant will meet safety and ethical standards.

Critical Thinking and Discussion Questions

29. A. What type of job setting would be your first preference?
 B. Why is that setting your first choice?
 C. What can you do to seek out that type of job?

Procedure Checklists

Relieving Choking—Adult or Child (Older Than 1 Year)

Name: ______________________ Date: ______________________

Procedure	S	U	Comments
1. Asked the person if they were choking.			
a. *If the person was coughing or talking,* proceeded for mild airway obstruction.	____	____	____________
b. *If the person was unresponsive,* and the cause unknown. Called for help and began cardiopulmonary resuscitation (CPR).	____	____	____________
c. *If the person nodded "yes" and could not talk,* continued to step 2.	____	____	____________
2. Had someone call for help.			
a. *In a public area,* had someone call 911 to activate the Emergency Medical Services (EMS) system. Sent someone to get an automated external defibrillator (AED).	____	____	____________
b. *In an agency,* had someone call the agency's Rapid Response System (RRS) and sent someone to get the defibrillator (AED).	____	____	____________
3. Gave abdominal thrusts.			
a. Stood or knelt behind the person.	____	____	____________
b. Wrapped your arms around the person's waist.	____	____	____________
c. Made fist with one hand.	____	____	____________
d. Placed the thumb side of the fist against the abdomen. The fist was slightly above the navel in the middle of the abdomen and well below the end of the sternum (breastbone).	____	____	____________
e. Grasped your fist with your other hand.	____	____	____________
f. Pressed your fist into the abdomen with a quick, upward thrust.			
g. Repeated thrusts until the object was expelled or the person became unresponsive.	____	____	____________
4. *If the object was dislodged,* encouraged hospital care. Injuries could occur from abdominal thrusts.	____	____	____________
5. *If the person became unresponsive,*			
a. Lowered the person to the floor. Positioned the person supine (lying flat on the back).	____	____	____________
b. Made sure the EMS or RRS was called.	____	____	____________
1) *If alone with a phone,* called while giving care.			
2) *If alone without a phone,* gave about 2 minutes of CPR first. Then called the EMS or RRS and got an AED.	____	____	____________
c. Started CPR. Did not check for a pulse.			
1) Gave 30 chest compressions.	____	____	____________
2) Opened the airway with the head tilt-chin lift method. Opened the person's mouth wide open. Looked for an object. Removed the object if you saw it and removed it easily.	____	____	____________
3) Gave two breaths.	____	____	____________
4) Continued cycles of 30 compressions, followed by 2 breaths. Looked for an object every time you opened the airway.	____	____	____________

Procedure—cont'd	S	U	Comments
d. *If choking was relieved*, checked for a response, breathing, and a pulse. (NOTE: Choking was relieved when you felt air move and saw the chest rise and fall when giving breaths.)			
1) *If no response, no normal breathing, and no pulse*—continued CPR. Used the AED as soon as possible.	______	______	______
2) *If no response and no normal breathing, but there was a pulse*—gave rescue breaths. For an adult, gave one breath every 6 seconds. For a child, gave one breath every 2 to 3 seconds. Checked for a pulse every 2 minutes. If no pulse, began CPR.	______	______	______
3) *If the person had normal breathing and a pulse*—placed the person in the recovery position if there was no response. Continued to check the person until help arrived. Encouraged hospital care.	______	______	______

Relieving Choking—In the Infant (Younger Than 1 Year)

Name: ______________________ Date: ______________________

Procedure	S	U	Comments
1. Had someone call for help.			
a. *In a public area,* had someone activate the Emergency Medical Services (EMS) by calling 911. Sent someone to get an automated external defibrillator (AED).	____	____	____________
b. *In an agency,* had someone call the agency's Rapid Response System (RRS) and obtain an AED.	____	____	____________
2. Knelt next to the infant. Or sat with the infant in your lap.	____	____	____________
3. Held the infant face down over your forearm. (Supported your arm on your thigh or lap.) The infant's head was lower than the chest. Supported the head and jaw with your hand.	____	____	____________
4. Gave up to five forceful back slaps (back blows). Used the heel of your hand. Gave the back slaps between the shoulder blades. (Stopped the back slaps if the object was expelled.)	____	____	____________
5. Turned the infant as a unit.			
a. Continued to support the infant's face, jaw, head, neck, and chest with one hand.	____	____	____________
b. Supported the back and the back of the infant's head with your other hand. Your palm supported the back of the head.	____	____	____________
c. Turned the infant as a unit. The infant was face up on your forearm. Your forearm rested on your thigh. The infant's head was lower than the chest.	____	____	____________
6. Gave up to five chest thrusts.			
a. Placed two fingers in the center of the chest just below the nipple line.	____	____	____________
b. Gave chest thrusts at a rate of about 1 every second. The thrusts are quick and downward.	____	____	____________
c. Stopped chest thrusts if the object was expelled.	____	____	____________
7. Continued giving five back slaps followed by five chest thrusts until the object was expelled or the infant became unresponsive.	____	____	____________
8. *If the infant became unresponsive*:			
a. Made sure the EMS system or RRS was called.	____	____	____________
1) *If alone with a phone,* called while giving care.	____	____	____________
2) If alone without a phone, gave about 2 minutes of CPR first. Then called the EMS or RRS and got an AED.	____	____	____________
b. Placed the infant on a firm, flat surface.	____	____	____________
c. Started CPR. Did not check for a pulse. Gave 30 compressions.	____	____	____________
d. Opened the airway. Used the head tilt-chin lift method. Opened the infant's mouth. Looked for an object. Removed the object if you saw it and could remove it easily. Used your fingers.	____	____	____________
e. Gave two breaths.	____	____	____________
f. Continued cycles of 30 compressions and 2 breaths. Looked for an object. Removed the object if you saw it and could remove it easily. Used your fingers.	____	____	____________
g. Continued CPR until help arrived or until choking was relieved.	____	____	____________

Using a Fire Extinguisher

Name: ______________________________ Date: ______________________________

Procedure	S	U	Comments
1. Pulled the fire alarm.	______	______	____________________
2. Got the nearest fire extinguisher.	______	______	____________________
3. Took it to the fire. Carried it upright.	______	______	____________________
4. Positioned self so you could exit safely. Did not allow the fire, smoke, or heat to block your exit path.	______	______	____________________
5. Followed the word *PASS*.			
a. *P*—for *pull the safety pin*. This unlocked the handle.	______	______	____________________
b. *A*—for *aim low*. Directed the hose or nozzle at the base of the fire. Did not try to spray the tops of the flames.	______	______	____________________
c. *S*—for *squeeze the lever*. Squeezed or pushed down on the lever, handle, or button to start the stream. Released the lever, handle, or button to stop the stream.	______	______	____________________
d. *S*—for *sweep back and forth*. Swept the stream back and forth (side to side) at the base of the fire.	______	______	____________________
6. Evacuated immediately if the fire was spreading or could not be extinguished.	______	______	____________________

Using a Transfer/Gait Belt

VIDEO CLIP VIDEO

Name: ______________________ Date: ______________________

Procedure	S	U	Comments
Quality of Life			
• Knocked before entering the person's room.			
• Addressed the person by name.			
• Introduced yourself by name and title.			
• Explained the procedure before starting and during the procedure.			
• Protected the person's rights during the procedure.			
• Handled the person gently during the procedure.			
Preprocedure			
1. Saw *Promoting Safety and Comfort: Transfer/Gait Belts.*			
2. Practiced hand hygiene.			
3. Obtained a transfer/gait belt of the correct type and size.			
4. Identified the person. Checked the identification (ID) bracelet against the assignment sheet. Used two identifiers. Also called the person by name.			
5. Provided for privacy.			
Procedure			
6. Assisted the person to sitting position. Applied slip-resistant footwear if not already on.			
7. Applied the belt. Held the belt by the buckle. Wrapped the belt around the person's waist over clothing. Did not apply it over the bare skin.			
a. *For a belt with a metal buckle*:			
1) Inserted the belt's metal tip into the buckle. Passed the belt through the side with the teeth first.			
2) Brought the belt tip across the front of the buckle. Inserted the tip through the buckle's smooth side.			
b. *For a belt with a quick-release buckle,* pushed the belt ends together to secure the buckle.			
8. Tightened the belt so it was snug. It did not cause discomfort or impair breathing. You were able to slide your open, flat hand under the belt. Asked about the person's comfort. If the belt was too loose or too tight, adjusted the belt as needed.			
9. Made sure that the person's breasts were not caught under the belt.			
10. Placed the buckle off-center in the front or off-center in the back for the person's comfort. A quick-release buckle was turned around to the back out of the person's reach. The buckle was not over the spine.			
11. Tucked any excess strap into the belt.			
12. Completed the transfer or ambulation procedure. Grasped the belt from underneath with two hands. Used an upward grasp. Or grasped the belt by the handles.			

Postprocedure	S	U	Comments
13. Removed the belt after completing the transfer or ambulation. The person was not left alone wearing the belt.	______	______	______
a. *For a belt with a metal buckle*:			
1) Brought the belt strap back through the buckle's smooth side.	______	______	______
2) Pulled the belt through the side with the teeth.	______	______	______
b. *For a belt with a quick-release buckle*, pushed inward on the quick-release buttons.	______	______	______
c. Removed the belt from the person's waist. Did not drag the belt across the waist.	______	______	______
14. Provided for comfort.	______	______	______
15. Placed the call light and other needed items within reach.	______	______	______
16. Followed the care plan and the person's preferences for privacy measures. Left the privacy curtain, window coverings, and door open or closed as person preferred.	______	______	______
17. Completed a safety check of the room.	______	______	______
18. Returned the transfer/gait belt to its proper place.	______	______	______
19. Practiced hand hygiene.	______	______	______
20. Reported and recorded your care and observations.	______	______	______

Helping the Falling Person

Name: ______________________ Date: ______________________

Procedure	S	U	Comments
1. Stood behind the person with your feet apart. Kept your back straight.	_____	_____	__________
2. Brought the person close to your body as fast as possible. Used the transfer/gait belt. Or wrapped your arms around the person's waist. If necessary, you held the person under the arms.	_____	_____	__________
3. Moved your leg so the person's buttocks rested on it.	_____	_____	__________
4. Lowered the person to the floor. The person slid down your leg to the floor. Bent at your hips and knees as you lowered the person.	_____	_____	__________
5. Called a nurse to check the person. Stayed with the person.	_____	_____	__________
6. Followed the nurse's directions to return the person to bed. Asked other staff to help, if needed.	_____	_____	__________
Postprocedure			
7. Provided for comfort.	_____	_____	__________
8. Placed the call light and other needed items within reach.	_____	_____	__________
9. Raised or lowered bed rails. Followed the care plan.	_____	_____	__________
10. Completed a safety check of the room.	_____	_____	__________
11. Practiced hand hygiene.	_____	_____	__________
12. Reported and recorded the following:			
• How the fall occurred	_____	_____	__________
• If the person was standing or walking	_____	_____	__________
• How activity was tolerated before the fall	_____	_____	__________
• Complaints before the fall	_____	_____	__________
• How much help the person needed while walking	_____	_____	__________
13. Completed an incident report.	_____	_____	__________

Applying Restraints

Name: ______________________ Date: ______________________

Procedure	S	U	Comments
Quality of Life			
• Knocked before entering the person's room.			
• Addressed the person by name.			
• Introduced yourself by name and title.			
• Explained the procedure before starting and during the procedure.			
• Protected the person's rights during the procedure.			
• Handled the person gently during the procedure.			
Preprocedure			
1. Followed *Delegation Guidelines: Applying Restraints*. Saw *Promoting Safety and Comfort: Applying Restraints*.			
2. Practiced hand hygiene and got the following supplies as instructed by the nurse.			
• Correct type and size of restraint			
• Padding for the skin and bony areas			
• Bed rail pads or gap protectors (if needed)			
3. Arranged items in the person's room. 4. Practiced hand hygiene.			
5. Identified the person. Checked the ID (identification) bracelet against the assignment sheet. Used two identifiers. Also called the person by name.			
6. Provided for privacy.			
Procedure			
7. Positioned the person for comfort and good alignment.			
8. Placed the bed rail pads or gap protectors (if needed) on the bed if the person was in bed. Followed the manufacturer's instructions.			
9. Padded bony areas. Followed the nurse's instructions and the care plan.			
10. Read and followed the manufacturer's instructions. Noted the front and back of the restraint.			
11. *For limb holders to the wrist*:			
a. Placed the soft or foam part toward the skin.			
b. Secured the holder so it was snug but not tight. Made sure you could slide one finger under the holder. Adjusted the straps if the holder was too loose or too tight. Checked for snugness again.			
c. Secured the straps to the movable part of the bed frame out of the person's reach. Used the buckle or quick-release knot.			
d. Repeated the following for the other wrist.			
1) Placed the soft or foam part toward the skin.			
2) Secured the restraint so it was snug but not tight. Made sure you could slide one finger under the restraint. Adjusted the straps if the restraint was too loose or too tight. Checked for snugness again.			
3) Secured the straps to the movable part of the bed frame out of the person's reach. Used the buckle or quick-release knot.			
12. *For mitt restraints*:			
a. Cleaned and dried the person's hands.			

Procedure—cont'd	S	U	Comments
b. Inserted the person's hand into the restraint with the palm down.			
c. Wrapped the wrist strap around the smallest part of the wrist. Secured the strap with the hook-and-loop or other closure.			
d. Secured the restraint to the bed if directed to do so. Secured the straps to the movable part of the bed frame out of the person's reach. Used the buckle or a quick-release tie.			
e. Checked for snugness. Slid one finger between the restraint and the wrist. Adjusted the straps if the restraint was too loose or too tight. Checked for snugness again.			
f. Repeated the following for the other hand.			
1) Inserted the person's hand into the restraint with the palm down.			
2) Wrapped the wrist strap around the smallest part of the wrist. Secured the strap with the hook-and-loop or other closure.			
3) Secured the restraint to the bed if directed to do so. Secured the straps to the movable part of the bed frame out of the person's reach. Used the buckle or a quick-release tie.			
4) Checked for snugness. Slid one finger between the restraint and the wrist. Adjusted the straps if the restraint was too loose or too tight. Checked for snugness again.			
13. *For elbow splints*:			
a. Released the adjustment straps (hook-and-loop).			
b. Placed buckles toward the person.			
c. Wrapped a splint over one arm. Or slid the splint up the arm. The splint was centered over the elbow. Opening was toward the inside of the arm. Followed the manufacturer's instructions.			
d. Secured the splint by following the manufacturer's instructions. Used the clips provided by the manufacturer to secure the splint to a sleeve.			
e. Checked for snugness. Followed the manufacturer's instructions. Adjusted the splint if it was too loose or too tight. Checked for snugness again.			
f. Repeated for the other arm:			
1) Released the adjustment straps (hook-and-loop).			
2) Placed buckles toward the person.			
3) Wrapped a splint over one arm. Or slid the splint up the arm. The splint was centered over the elbow. Opening was toward the inside of the arm. Followed the manufacturer's instructions.			
4) Secured the splint by following the manufacturer's instructions. Used the clips provided by the manufacturer to secure the splint to the sleeve.			
5) Checked for snugness. Followed the manufacturer's instructions. Adjusted the splint if it was too loose or too tight. Checked for snugness again.			
14. *For a belt restraint*:			
a. Assisted the person to a sitting position.			
b. Applied the restraint.			
c. Removed wrinkles or creases from the front and back.			
d. Brought the ties through the slots in the back.			

Procedure—cont'd	S	U	Comments
e. Positioned the straps at a 45-degree angle between the wheelchair seat and sides. If in bed, helped the person lie down.	______	______	______
f. Made sure the person was comfortable and in good alignment.	______	______	______
g. Secured the straps to the movable part of the bed frame. Used the buckle or a quick-release knot. The buckle or knot was out of the person's reach. For a wheelchair, crisscrossed and secured the straps.	______	______	______
h. Checked for snugness. Slid an open hand between the restraint and the person. Adjusted the restraint if it was too loose or too tight. Checked for snugness again.	______	______	______
15. *For a vest restraint; assisted the nurse as directed.*			
a. Assisted the person to a sitting position. If in a wheelchair:			
1) Person was as far back in the wheelchair as possible.	______	______	______
2) Buttocks were against the chair back.	______	______	______
b. Applied the restraint. The "V" neck was in front.	______	______	______
c. Brought the straps through the slots if the vest crisscrossed.	______	______	______
d. Ensured that side seams were under the arms. Removed wrinkles in the front and back. Closed the zipper or fastened with other closures.	______	______	______
e. Positioned the straps at a 45-degree angle between the wheelchair seat and sides. If in bed, helped the person lie down.	______	______	______
f. Made sure the person was comfortable and in good alignment.	______	______	______
g. Secured the straps to the movable part of the bed frame at waist level. Used the buckle or a quick-release knot. The buckle or knot was out of the person's reach. For a wheelchair, crisscrossed and secured the straps.	______	______	______
h. Checked for snugness. Slid an open hand between the restraint and the person. Adjusted the restraint if it was too loose or too tight. Checked for snugness again.	______	______	______
16. *For a jacket restraint; assisted the nurse as directed.*			
a. Assisted the person to a sitting position. If in a wheelchair:			
1) Person was as far back in the wheelchair as possible.	______	______	______
2) Buttocks were against the chair back.	______	______	______
b. Applied the restraint. The jacket opening went in the back.	______	______	______
c. Made sure the side seams were under the arms. Removed wrinkles in the front and back.__________			
d. Closed the back with the zipper or other closures.	______	______	______
e. Positioned the straps at a 45-degree angle between the wheelchair seat and sides. If in bed, helped the person lie down.	______	______	______
f. Made sure the person was comfortable and in good alignment.	______	______	______
g. Secured the straps to the movable part of the bed frame at waist level. Used the buckle or quick-release knot. The buckle or knot was out of the person's reach. For a wheelchair, crisscrossed and secured the straps.	______	______	______
h. Checked for snugness. Slid an open hand between the restraint and the person. Adjusted the restraint if it was too loose or too tight. Checked for snugness again.	______	______	______

Postprocedure	S	U	Comments
17. Positioned the person as the nurse directed.			
18. Provided for comfort.			
19. Placed the call light and other need items within the person's reach.			
20. Raised or lowered bed rails. Followed the care plan and the manufacturer's instructions for restraints.			
21. Followed the care plan and the nurse's instructions for privacy measures.			
22. Completed a safety check of the room.			
23. Practiced hand hygiene.			
24. Checked the person and the restraint at least every 15 minutes or as often as directed by the nurse and the care plan. Reported and recorded your care and observations.			
a. *For limb holders, mitt restraints, or elbow splints*: checked the pulse, color, and temperature of restrained parts.			
b. *For vest, jacket, or belt restraint*: checked the person's breathing. Made sure the restraint was properly positioned in the front and back. *Released the restraint and called for the nurse at once if the person was not breathing or was having problems breathing.*			
25. Did the following at least every 2 hours for at least 10 minutes.			
a. Removed or released the restraint.			
b. Measured vital signs.			
c. Repositioned the person.			
d. Met food, fluid, hygiene, and elimination needs.			
e. Gave skin care.			
f. Performed ROM exercises or helped the person walk. Followed the care plan.			
g. Provided for physical and emotional support.			
h. Reapplied the restraint.			
26. Completed a safety check of the room.			
27. Practiced hand hygiene.			
28. Reported and recorded your observations and the care given.			

NATCEP™ VIDEO

Handwashing

Name: ______________________ Date: ______________________

Procedure	S	U	Comments
1. Saw *Promoting Safety and Comfort: Hand Hygiene.*			
2. Made sure you had soap, paper towels, an orangewood stick or nail file, and a wastebasket. Collected missing items.			
3. Pushed your watch up your arm 4 to 5 inches. Pushed long uniform sleeves up too.			
4. Stood away from the sink so your clothes did not touch the sink. Stood so the soap and faucet were easy to reach. Did not touch the inside of the sink at any time.			
5. Turned on and adjusted the water until it felt warm.			
6. Wet your wrists and hands. Kept your hands lower than your elbows. Was sure to wet the area 3 to 4 inches above your wrists.			
7. Applied about one teaspoon of soap to your hands. Followed the manufacturer's instructions for the amount to use.			
8. Rubbed your palms together and interlaced your fingers to work up a good lather. Lathered your wrists, hands, and fingers. Kept your hands lower than your elbows. Steps 8 through 10 should have lasted at least 20 seconds.			
9. Washed each hand and wrist thoroughly. Cleaned the back of your fingers and between your fingers.			
10. Cleaned under the fingernails. Rubbed your fingernails against your palms.			
11. Cleaned under the fingernails with a nail file or orangewood stick. Did this for the first hand hygiene of the day and when your hands were highly soiled.			
12. Rinsed your wrists, hands, and fingers well. Water flowed from above the wrists to your fingertips.			
13. Repeated steps 7 through 12, if needed. a. Applied about one teaspoon of soap to your hands.			
b. Rubbed your palms together and interlaced your fingers to work up a good lather. Lathered your wrists, hands, and fingers. Kept your hands lower than your elbows. This step should have lasted at least 20 seconds.			
c. Washed each hand and wrist thoroughly. Cleaned the back of your fingers and between your fingers.			
d. Cleaned under the fingernails. Rubbed your fingertips against your palms.			
e. Cleaned under the fingernails with a nail file or orangewood stick. Did this for the first handwashing of the day and when your hands were highly soiled.			

Procedure	S	U	Comments
f. Rinsed your wrists, hands, and fingers well. Water flowed from above the wrists to your fingertips.	______	______	______
14. Dried your fingers, hands, and wrists with clean, dry paper towels. Patted dry starting at your fingertips.	______	______	______
15. Discarded used paper towels into the wastebasket.	______	______	______
16. Used clean, dry paper towels to turn off faucets. This prevented you from contaminating your clean hands. Or used knee or foot controls to turn off the faucet.	______	______	______
17. Discarded the paper towels into the wastebasket.	______	______	______

NATCEP™ VIDEO VIDEO CLIP

Using an Alcohol-Based Hand Sanitizer

Name: ______________________ Date: ______________________

Procedure	S	U	Comments
1. Saw *Promoting Safety and Comfort: Hand Hygiene.*	______	______	______________________
2. Applied a palmful of an alcohol-based hand sanitizer into a cupped hand. Followed the manufacturer's instructions for the amount to use.	______	______	______________________
3. Rubbed your palms together. Covered all surfaces of the hands and fingers.	______	______	______________________
a. Rubbed your palms together.	______	______	
b. Rubbed the palm of one hand over the back of the other. Did the same for the other hand.	______	______	______________________
c. Rubbed your palms together with your fingers interlaced.	______		
d. Interlocked your fingers. Rubbed your fingers back and forth.	______	______	______________________
e. Rubbed the thumb of one hand into the palm of the other. Did the same for the other thumb.	______	______	______________________
f. Rubbed the fingers of one hand into the palm of the other hand. Used a circular motion. Did the same for the fingers of the other hand.	______	______	______________________
4. Continued rubbing your hands until they were dry.	______	______	______________________

Sterile Gloving

Name: ______________________ Date: ______________________

Procedure	S	U	Comments
1. Followed *Delegation Guidelines: Assisting With Sterile Procedures*. Saw *Promoting Safety and Comfort: Sterile Gloving*.			
2. Practiced hand hygiene.			
3. Inspected the package of sterile gloves for sterility.			
a. Checked the expiration date.			
b. Checked if the package was dry.			
c. Checked for tears, holes, punctures, and watermarks.			
4. Created a work surface with enough room.			
a. Arranged the work surface at waist level and within your vision.			
b. Cleaned and dried the work surface.			
c. Did not reach over or turn your back on the work surface.			
5. Opened the package. Grasped the flaps. Gently peeled them back.			
6. Removed the inner package. Placed it on your work surface.			
7. Noted the labels on the inner package—*left, right, up*, and *down*.			
8. Arranged the inner package for left, right, up, and down. Left glove was on your left. Right glove was on your right. Glove openings were near you, the fingers pointed away from you.			
9. Grasped the folded edges of the inner package. Used the thumb and index finger of each hand.			
10. Folded back the inner package to expose the gloves. Did not touch or otherwise contaminate the inside package or the gloves. The inside of the inner package was a sterile field.			
11. Noted that about 2 to 3 inches of each glove is folded so the inside of the glove is to the outside. This is called the cuff. The insides of the gloves were *not sterile*. These were the only parts that you can touch with bare hands.			
12. Put on the right glove if you were right handed. Put on the left glove if you were left handed.			
a. Picked up the glove with your other hand. Used your thumb and index and middle fingers. Touched only the cuff and the inside of the glove.			
b. Turned the hand to be gloved palm side up.			
c. Slid your fingers and hand into the glove.			
d. Pulled the glove up over your hand. If some fingers got stuck, left them that way until the other glove was on. *Did not use your ungloved hand to straighten the glove. Did not let the outside of the glove touch any nonsterile surface.*			
e. Left the cuff folded at the wrist.			
13. Put on the other glove. Used your gloved hand.			
a. Reached under the cuff of the second glove. Used the four fingers of your gloved hand.			
b. Put on the second glove. Your gloved hand did not touch the cuff or any surface. Held the thumb of your first gloved hand away from the other hand.			

Procedure—cont'd	S	U	Comments
14. Adjusted each glove with the other hand. The gloves were smooth and comfortable.	______	______	______
15. Slid the fingers of one hand under the cuff of the glove on the other hand. Touched only the outer surface of the glove. Pulled upward to unfold the cuff. Repeated for the other hand.	______	______	______
16. Touched only sterile items.	______	______	______
17. Removed and discarded the gloves.	______	______	______
18. Practiced hand hygiene.	______	______	______

NATCEP™ VIDEO VIDEO CLIP

Donning and Removing Personal Protective Equipment (PPE)

Name: ______________________ Date: ______________________

Procedure	S	U	Comments
1. Followed *Delegation Guidelines: Transmission-Based Precautions*. Saw *Promoting Safety and Comfort:*			
a. *Transmission-Based Precautions*	____	____	____________
b. *Goggles and Face Shields*	____	____	____________
c. *Gloves*	____	____	____________
d. *Donning and Removing PPE*	____	____	____________
2. Removed your watch and all jewelry.	____	____	____________
3. Rolled up uniform sleeves.	____	____	____________
4. Practiced hand hygiene.	____	____	____________
5. Put on a gown.			
a. Held a clean gown out in front of you.	____	____	____________
b. Unfolded the gown. Faced the back of the gown. Did not shake it.	____	____	____________
c. Put your hands and arms through the sleeves.	____	____	____________
d. Made sure the gown covered you from your neck to your knees. It covered your arms to the end of your wrists.	____	____	____________
e. Tied the strings at the back of the neck.	____	____	____________
f. Overlapped the back of the gown. Made sure it covered your uniform. The gown was snug, not loose.	____	____	____________
g. Tied the waist strings. Tied them at the back or the side. Did not tie them in front.	____	____	____________
6. Put on a mask or respirator.			
a. Picked up a mask by its upper ties. Did not touch the part that covered your face.	____	____	____________
b. Placed the mask over your nose and mouth.	____	____	____________
c. Placed the upper strings above your ears. Tied them at the back in the middle of your head.	____	____	____________
d. Tied the lower strings at the back of your neck. The lower part of the mask was under your chin.	____	____	____________
e. Pinched the metal band around your nose. The top of the mask was snug over your nose. If you wore eyeglasses, the mask was snug under the bottom of the eyeglasses.	____	____	____________
f. Made sure the mask was snug over your face and under your chin.	____	____	____________
7. Put on goggles or a face shield (if needed and was not part of the mask).			
a. Placed the device over your face and eyes.	____	____	____________
b. Adjusted the device to fit.	____	____	____________
8. Put on gloves. Made sure the gloves covered the wrists of the gown.	____	____	____________
9. Provided care.	____	____	____________
10. Removed and discarded the PPE. Practiced hand hygiene between each step if your hands became contaminated.			
a. *Method 1: Gloves, goggles, or face shield, gown, mask, or respirator.*			
1) Removed and discarded the gloves.			
a) Made sure that glove touched only glove.	____	____	____________
b) Grasped a glove at the palm. Grasped it on the outside.	____	____	____________
c) Pulled the glove down over your hand so it was inside out.	____	____	____________

Procedure—cont'd	S	U	Comments
d) Held the removed glove with your other gloved hand.	______	______	______
e) Reached inside the other glove. Used the first two fingers of the ungloved hand.	______	______	______
f) Pulled the glove down (inside out) over your hand and the other glove.	______	______	______
g) Discarded the gloves.	______	______	______
2) Removed and discarded the goggles or face shield if worn.			
a) Lifted the headband or earpieces from the back. Did not touch the front of the device.	______	______	______
b) Discarded the device. If reusable, followed agency policy.	______	______	______
3) Removed and discarded the gown. Did not touch the outside of the gown.			
a) Untied the neck and then the waist strings.	______	______	______
b) Pulled the gown down and away from your neck and shoulders. Only touched the inside of the gown.	______	______	______
c) Turned the gown inside out as it was removed. Held it at the inside shoulder seams and brought your hands together.	______	______	______
d) Folded or rolled up the gown away from you. Kept it inside out. Did not let the gown touch the floor.	______	______	______
e) Discarded the gown.	______	______	______
4) Removed and discarded the mask if worn. (Note: Removed a respirator after leaving the room and closing the door.)			
a) Untied the lower strings of the mask.	______	______	______
b) Untied the top strings.	______	______	______
c) Held the top strings. Removed the mask.	______	______	______
d) Discarded the mask.	______	______	______
b. *Method 2: Gown and gloves, goggles or face shield, mask or respirator.*			
1) Removed and discarded the gown and gloves.			
a) Grasped the gown in front with your gloved hands. Pulled away from your body so the ties broke. Only touched the outside of the gown.	______	______	______
b) Folded or rolled the gown inside out into a bundle while removing the gown. Kept it inside-out. Did not let the gown touch the floor.	______	______	______
c) Peeled off your gloves as you removed the gown. Only touched the inside of the gloves and the gown with your bare hands.	______	______	______
d) Discarded the gown and gloves.	______	______	______
2) Removed and discarded the goggles or face shield.			
a) Lifted the headband or earpieces from the back. Did not touch the front of the device.	______	______	______
b) Discarded the device. If reusable, followed agency policy.	______	______	______

Procedure—cont'd	S	U	Comments
3) Removed and discarded the mask if worn. (Note: Removed a respirator after leaving the room and closing the door.)			
a) Untied the lower strings of the mask.	______	______	______
b) Untied the top strings.	______	______	______
c) Held the top strings. Removed the mask without touching the front of the mask.	______	______	______
d) Discarded the mask.	______	______	______
11. Practiced hand hygiene after removing all PPE.	______	______	______

Double-Bagging

Name: ______________________ Date: ______________________

Procedure	S	U	Comments
1. Asked a coworker to help you. Coworker stood outside the doorway. You were in the room.	____	____	____
2. Sealed the *dirty* bags securely.	____	____	____
3. Asked your coworker to make a wide cuff on a *clean* bag. It was held wide open. The cuff protected the hands from contamination.	____	____	____
4. Placed the *dirty* bag into the *clean* bag. Did not touch the outside of the *clean* bag.	____	____	____
5. Asked your coworker to seal the *clean* bag. Followed agency procedures for use of color-coded or *BIOHAZARD* bags.	____	____	____
6. Repeated the following steps for other *dirty* bags.	____	____	____
a. Sealed the *dirty* bags securely.	____	____	____
b. Asked your coworker to make a wide cuff on a *clean* bag. It was held wide open. The cuff protected the hands from contamination.	____	____	____
c. Placed the *dirty* bag into the *clean* bag. Did not touch the outside of the *clean* bag.	____	____	____
d. Asked your coworker to seal the *clean* bag. Followed agency procedures for use of color-coded or *BIOHAZARD* bags	____	____	____
7. Asked your coworker to take or send the bags to the appropriate department for for laundering, disinfection, sterilization, or disposal.	____	____	____

Raising the Person's Head and Shoulders

Name: ______________________ Date: ______________________

Quality of Life

	S	U	Comments
• Knocked before entering the person's room.			
• Addressed the person by name.			
• Introduced yourself by name and title.			
• Explained the procedure before starting and during the procedure.			
• Protected the person's rights during the procedure.			
• Handled the person gently during the procedure.			

Preprocedure

1. Followed *Delegation Guidelines*:
   a. *Moving the Person*
   b. *Moving Persons in Bed*

   Saw *Promoting Safety and Comfort*:
   a. *Moving the Person*
   b. *Planning a Safe Move*
2. Asked a coworker to help you if needed.
3. Practiced hand hygiene.
4. Identified the person. Checked the ID (identification) bracelet against the assignment sheet. Used two identifiers. Also called the person by name.
5. Provided for privacy.
6. Locked the brakes on bed wheels.
7. Raised the bed for body mechanics. Bed rails were up if used.

Procedure

8. If you were working alone and the person had a weaker side, stood on the weak side. Had your coworker stand on the other side of the bed (if needed).
9. Lowered one or both bed rails if up. Raised the head of the bed.
10. Locked arms and supported the person's neck and shoulders.
    a. Placed your near arm behind the person's near arm and shoulder. Had the person do the same to your arm. The person's hand rested on your shoulder. If you were working with a coworker, your coworker did the same on the other side.
    b. Brought your other arm around the person's back. Grasped the person's far shoulder. Your arm supported the neck and shoulder. If you were working with a coworker, your coworker also placed a hand behind the back and supported the person.
11. Helped the person rise to a sitting or semi-sitting position on the "count of 3."
12. Continued to support the person with your near arm if needed. Gave care with your far arm. If you were working with a coworker, one of you supported the person. The other gave care.
13. Helped the person lie down. Provided support with your locked arm. Supported the person's neck and shoulders with your other arm. Your coworker did the same.

Postprocedure

14. Positioned the person in good alignment. Lowered the head of the bed to a position of comfort.	______	______	______
15. Provided for comfort.	______	______	______
16. Placed the call light and other needed items within reach.	______	______	______
17. Lowered the bed to a safe and comfortable level. Followed the care plan.	______	______	______
18. Raised or lowered bed rails. Followed the care plan.	______	______	______
19. Followed the care plan and the person's preferences for privacy measures to maintain. Leaving the privacy curtain, window coverings, and door open or closed were examples.	______	______	______
20. Completed a safety check of the room.	______	______	______
21. Practiced hand hygiene.	______	______	______
22. Reported and recorded your care and observations.	______	______	______

Moving the Person Up in Bed With a Friction-Reducing Device

Name: ____________________ Date: ____________________

Quality of Life	S	U	Comments
• Knocked before entering the person's room.			
• Addressed the person by name.			
• Introduced yourself by name and title.			
• Explained the procedure before starting and during the procedure.			
• Protected the person's rights during the procedure.			
• Handled the person gently during the procedure.			

Preprocedure

	S	U	Comments
1. Followed *Delegation Guidelines*:			
a. *Moving the Person*			
b. *Moving Persons in Bed*			
Saw *Promoting Safety and Comfort*:			
a. *Moving the Person*			
b. *Planning a Safe Move*			
c. *Friction-Reducing Devices*			
d. *Moving the Person Up in Bed*			
2. Asked at least one coworker to help you.			
3. Practiced hand hygiene and obtained the needed friction-reducing device.			
4. Identified the person. Checked the ID (identification) bracelet against the assignment sheet. Used two identifiers. Also called the person by name.			
5. Provided for privacy.			
6. Locked brakes on the bed wheels.			
7. Raised the bed for body mechanics. Bed rails were up if used.			

Procedure

	S	U	Comments
8. Stood on one side of the bed. Your coworker stood on the other side.			
9. Lowered the head of the bed to a level appropriate for the person. It was as flat as possible.			
10. Lowered the bed rails if up.			
11. Removed pillows as directed by the nurse. Placed a pillow upright against the headboard if the person could be without it.			
12. If a trapeze was used.			
a. Had the person grasp the trapeze and flex both knees.			
b. Placed one arm under the person's shoulder and one arm under the thighs. Your coworker did the same. Grasped each other's forearms. Or used a friction-reducing device under the person.			
13. If using a friction-reducing device under the person:			
a. Positioned the device.			
b. Had the person cross the arms over the chest, unless the person used the arms to assist with the move.			
c. Rolled the sides of the device up close to the person or omitted this step if the device had handles.			
d. Grasped the device firmly near the person's shoulders and hips. Or grasped it by the handles. Ensured that the person's head was supported. ________			

Procedure—cont'd	S	U	Comments
14. Explained that:			
a. You would count "1, 2, 3."	____	____	____
b. The move would be on "3."	____	____	____
c. On "3," the person pushed against the bed with the feet if able. If a trapeze was used, the person pulled up with the trapeze.	____	____	____
15. Stood with a wide base of support and good posture. Bent your hips and knees, not your back. Positioned the leg near the head of the bed slightly forward in the direction of the move.	____	____	____
16. Moved the person up in bed on the "count of 3." Shifted your weight from your rear leg to your front leg. Used the strong muscles in your legs.	____	____	____
17. Repeated steps 15 and 16 if necessary.	____	____	____
18. Unrolled the sides of the friction-reducing device if used or omitted this step if the device had handles. Removed the slide sheet if used. Had the person release the trapeze.	____	____	____

Postprocedure

19. Placed the pillow under the person's head and neck. Straightened linens.	____	____	____
20. Positioned the person in good alignment. Raised the head of the bed to a level appropriate for the person.	____	____	____
21. Provided for comfort.	____	____	____
22. Placed the call light and other needed items within reach.	____	____	____
23. Lowered the bed to a safe and comfortable level. Followed the care plan.	____	____	____
24. Raised or lowered bed rails. Followed the care plan.	____	____	
25. Followed the care plan and the person's preferences for privacy measures to maintain. Leaving the privacy curtain, window coverings, and door open or closed were examples.	____	____	____
26. Completed a safety check of the room.	____	____	____
27. Practiced hand hygiene.	____	____	____
28. Reported and recorded your care and observations.	____	____	____

Moving the Person to the Side of the Bed

Name: ________________________ Date: ________________________

Quality of Life	**S**	**U**	**Comments**
• Knocked before entering the person's room.	______	______	______
• Addressed the person by name.	______	______	______
• Introduced yourself by name and title.	______	______	______
• Explained the procedure before starting and during the procedure.	______	______	______
• Protected the person's rights during the procedure.	______	______	______
• Handled the person gently during the procedure.	______	______	______
Preprocedure			
1. Followed *Delegation Guidelines*:			
a. *Moving the Person*	______	______	______
b. *Moving Persons in Bed*	______	______	______
Saw *Promoting Safety and Comfort*:			
a. *Moving the Person*	______	______	______
b. *Planning a Safe Move*	______	______	______
c. Friction-Reducing Devices	______	______	______
d. *Moving the Person to the Side of the Bed*	______	______	______
2. Asked one or two coworkers to help you if you used a friction-reducing device.	______	______	______
3. Practiced hand hygiene and got the needed friction-reducing device if it was not already in place. (This procedure used a drawsheet.)	______	______	______
4. Identified the person. Checked the ID (identification) bracelet against the assignment sheet. Used two identifiers. Also called the person by name.	______	______	______
5. Provided for privacy.	______	______	______
6. Locked brakes on the bed wheels.	______	______	______
7. Raised the bed for body mechanics. Bed rails were up if used.	______	______	______
Procedure			
8. Stood on the side of the bed to which you were moving the person.	______	______	______
9. Lowered the head of the bed to a level appropriate for the person. It was as flat as possible.	______	______	______
10. Lowered the bed rail near you if bed rails were used. (Both bed rails were lowered for Method 2.)	______	______	______
11. Removed pillows as directed by the nurse.	______	______	______
12. Crossed the person's arms over the chest.			
13. Stood with a wide base of support and good posture. Bent your hips and knees, not your back. One foot was in front of the other.	______	______	______
14. *Method 1—moving the person in segments*:			
a. Placed your arm under the person's neck and shoulders. Grasped the far shoulder.	______	______	______
b. Placed your other arm under the midback.	______	______	______
c. Moved the upper part of the person's body toward you. Rocked backward and shifted your weight to your rear leg.	______	______	______
d. Placed one arm under the person's waist and one under the thighs.	______	______	______
e. Rocked backward to move the lower part of the person toward you.	______	______	______
f. Placed your arms under the person's thighs and calves. Repeated the procedure for the legs and feet.	______	______	______

Procedure—cont'd	S	U	Comments
15. *Method 2—moving the person with a drawsheet*:			
a. Positioned the drawsheet if it was not already in place under the person.			
b. Rolled up the drawsheet close to the person.	______	______	______
c. Grasped the rolled-up drawsheet near the person's shoulders and hips. Your coworker did the same. Ensured that the person's head was supported.	______	______	______
d. Rocked backward on the "count of 3," moving the person toward you. Your coworker rocked backward slightly and then forward toward you while keeping the arms straight.	______	______	______
e. Unrolled the drawsheet. Removed any wrinkles.	______	______	______

Postprocedure

16. Placed the pillow under the person's head and neck. Straightened linens.	______	______	______
17. Turned and positioned the person on the side. Or returned the person to the center of the bed after completing care at the side of the bed.	______	______	______
18. Position the person in good alignment.	______	______	______
19. Provided for comfort.	______	______	______
20. Placed the call light and other needed items within reach.	______	______	______
21. Lowered the bed to a safe and comfortable level. Followed the care plan.	______	______	______
22. Raised or lowered bed rails. Followed the care plan.	______	______	______
23. Followed the care plan and the person's preferences for privacy measures to maintain. Leaving the privacy curtain, window coverings, and door open or closed were examples.	______	______	______
24. Completed a safety check of the room.	______	______	______
25. Practiced hand hygiene.	______	______	______
26. Reported and recorded your care and observations.	______	______	______

NATCEP™ VIDEO VIDEO CLIP

Turning and Positioning the Person on the Side

Name: ______________________ Date: ______________________

Quality of Life	S	U	Comments
• Knocked before entering the person's room.			
• Addressed the person by name.			
• Introduced yourself by name and title.			
• Explained the procedure before starting and during the procedure.			
• Protected the person's rights during the procedure.			
• Handled the person gently during the procedure.			
Preprocedure			
1. Followed *Delegation Guidelines*:			
a. *Moving the Person*			
b. *Moving Persons in Bed*			
c. *Turning Persons*			
Saw *Promoting Safety and Comfort*:			
a. *Moving the Person*			
b. *Planning a Safe Move*			
c. *Moving the Person to the Side of the Bed*			
d. *Turning Persons*			
2. Practiced hand hygiene.			
3. Identified the person. Checked the ID (identification) bracelet against the assignment sheet. Used two identifiers. Also called the person by name.			
4. Provided for privacy.			
5. Locked brakes on the bed wheels.			
6. Raised the bed for body mechanics. Bed rails were up if used.			
Procedure			
7. Stood on the side of the bed opposite to where you will turn the person.			
8. Lowered the head of the bed to a level appropriate for the person. It was as flat as possible.			
9. Lowered the bed rail.			
10. Moved the person to the side near you.			
11. Crossed the person's arms over the chest. Crossed the leg near you over the far leg.			
12. *Turning the person away from you*:			
a. Stood with a wide base of support and good posture. Bent your hips and knees, not your back. One foot was in front of the other.			
b. Placed one hand on the person's shoulder. Placed the other on the hip near you.			
c. Rolled the person gently away from you toward the raised bed rail.			
d. Shifted your weight from your rear leg to your front leg. If the person could assist with the turn, the person grasped the far bed rail when able.			
13. *Turning the person toward you*:			
a. Raised the bed rail.			
b. Went to the other side of the bed. Lowered the bed rail.			
c. Stood with a wide base of support and good posture. Bent your hips and knees, not your back. One foot was in front of the other.			

d. Placed one hand on the person's shoulder. Placed the other on the far hip.	_____	_____	_____
e. Rolled the person gently toward you. Shifted your weight from your front leg to your rear leg.	_____	_____	_____
14. Positioned the person. Followed the nurse's directions and the care plan. For a lateral (side-lying) position:			
a. Placed a pillow under the head and neck.	_____	_____	_____
b. Adjusted the shoulder. The person was not on an arm.	_____	_____	_____
c. Positioned a pillow against the back.	_____	_____	_____
d. Placed a small pillow under the top hand and arm.	_____	_____	_____
e. Flexed the top hip and knee. Supported the top leg and ankle on a pillow. The top leg did not rest on the bottom leg.	_____	_____	_____

Postprocedure

15. Provided for comfort.	_____	_____	_____
16. Placed the call light and other needed items within reach.	_____	_____	_____
17. Lowered the bed to a safe and comfortable level appropriate. Followed the care plan.	_____	_____	_____
18. Raised or lowered bed rails. Followed the care plan.	_____	_____	_____
19. Followed the care plan and the person's preferences for privacy measures to maintain. Leaving the privacy curtain, window coverings, and door open or closed were examples.	_____	_____	_____
20. Completed a safety check of the room.	_____	_____	_____
21. Practiced hand hygiene.	_____	_____	_____
22. Reported and recorded your care and observations.	_____	_____	_____

NATCEP™ VIDEO

Logrolling the Person

Name: ______________________ Date: ______________________

Quality of Life	S	U	Comments
• Knocked before entering the person's room.			
• Addressed the person by name.			
• Introduced yourself by name and title.			
• Explained the procedure before starting and during the procedure.			
• Protected the person's rights during the procedure.			
• Handled the person gently during the procedure.			

Preprocedure	S	U	Comments
1. Followed *Delegation Guidelines*:			
a. *Moving the Person*			
b. *Moving Persons in Bed*			
c. *Turning Persons*			
Saw *Promoting Safety and Comfort*:			
a. *Moving the Person*			
b. Planning a Safe Move			
c. Friction-Reducing Devices			
d. *Turning Persons*			
e. *Logrolling*			
2. Asked a coworker to help you.			
3. Practiced hand hygiene and got the needed friction-reducing device if it was not already in place. (This procedure used a turning pad.)			
4. Identified the person. Checked the identification (ID) bracelet against the assignment sheet. Used two identifiers. Also called the person by name.			
5. Provided for privacy.			
6. Locked brakes on the bed wheels.			
7. Raised the bed for body mechanics. Bed rails were up if used.			

Procedure	S	U	Comments
8. Stood on the side opposite to which you turned the person. Your coworker stood on the other side.			
9. Made sure the bed was flat.			
10. Lowered the bed rails if used.			
11. Positioned the turning pad or other friction-reducing device if needed.			
12. Moved the person as a unit to the side of the bed near you. Used the turning pad. (If the person had a spinal cord injury or had spinal cord surgery, assisted the nurse as directed.)			
13. Placed the person's arms across the chest. Placed a pillow between the knees.			
14. Raised the bed rail if used.			
15. Went to the other side.			
16. Stood near the shoulders and chest. Your coworker stood near the hips and thighs.			
17. Stood with a wide base of support and good posture. Bent your hips and knees, not your back. One foot was in front of the other.			
18. Asked the person to hold the body rigid.			
19. Grasped the turning pad. Rolled the person toward you. Turned the person as a unit.			
20. Positioned the person in good alignment. Use pillows as directed by the nurse and care plan.			

Postprocedure

21. Provided for comfort.	_______	_______	_______________
22. Placed the call light and other needed items within reach.	_______	_______	_______________
23. Lowered the bed to a safe and comfortable level. Followed the care plan.	_______	_______	_______________
24. Raised or lowered bed rails. Followed the care plan.	_______	_______	_______________
25. Followed the care plan and the person's preferences for privacy measures to maintain. Leaving the privacy curtain, window coverings, and door open or closed were examples.	_______	_______	_______________
26. Completed a safety check of the room.	_______	_______	_______________
27. Practiced hand hygiene.	_______	_______	_______________
28. Reported and recorded your care and observations.	_______	_______	_______________

Sitting on the Side of the Bed (Dangling)

Name: ______________________ Date: ______________________

Quality of Life	S	U	Comments
• Knocked before entering the person's room.			
• Addressed the person by name.			
• Introduced yourself by name and title.			
• Explained the procedure before starting and during the procedure.			
• Protected the person's rights during the procedure.			
• Handled the person gently during the procedure.			

Preprocedure	S	U	Comments
1. Followed *Delegation Guidelines*:			
a. *Moving the Person*			
b. *Dangling*			
Saw *Promoting Safety and Comfort*:			
a. *Moving the Person*			
b. *Planning a Safe Move*			
c. *Dangling*			
2. Asked a coworker to help you.			
3. Practiced hand hygiene.			
4. Identified the person. Checked the identification (ID) bracelet against the assignment sheet. Used two identifiers. Also called the person by name.			
5. Provided for privacy.			
6. Locked brakes on the bed wheels.			
7. Raised the bed for body mechanics. Bed rails were up if used.			

Procedure	S	U	Comments
8. Decided which side of the bed to use. Stood on that side.			
9. Lowered the bed rail if up.			
10. Positioned the person in a side-lying position facing you. The person laid on the strong side. The bottom arm was flat on the bed. The top arm was crossed over the chest. The hips and knees were flexed (bent).			
11. Raised the head of the bed, if possible, raised it to a semi-sitting position.			
12. Stood by the person's hips.			
13. Slid one arm under the person's shoulders. Placed your other hand over the thighs near the knees.			
14. Stood with a wide base of support. Bent your hips and knees, not your back.			
15. Moved the person's legs over the side of the bed. Assist the person to an upright position.			
a. *If the person could assist,* had the person push off of the mattress to help move from the lying to the sitting position.			
b. *If the person could not assist,* the procedure was done with a coworker. You moved the upper body. Your coworker moved the lower body.			
16. Had the person hold on to the edge of the mattress. This supported the person in the sitting position. If possible, raised a half-length bed rail (on the person's strong side) for the person to grasp. Had your coworker support the person at all times.			

Procedure—cont'd	S	U	Comments
17. Checked the person's condition.			
a. Asked how the person felt. Asked if the person felt dizzy or light headed.			
b. Checked the pulse and respirations.			
c. Checked for difficulty breathing.			
d. Noted if the skin was pale or bluish in color.			
18. Reversed the procedure to return the person to bed. (Or prepared the person to walk or for a transfer to a chair or wheelchair. Lowered the bed to a safe and comfortable level. The person's feet were flat on the floor.)			
19. Lowered the head of the bed after the person returned to bed. Helped the person move to the center of the bed.			
20. Positioned the person in good alignment.			

Postprocedure

21. Provided for comfort.			
22. Placed the call light and other needed items within reach.			
23. Lowered the bed to a safe and comfortable level appropriate. Followed the care plan.			
24. Raised or lowered bed rails. Followed the care plan.			
25. Followed the care plan and the person's preferences for privacy measures to maintain. Leaving the privacy curtain, window coverings, and door open or closed were examples.			
26. Completed a safety check of the room.			
27. Practiced hand hygiene.			
28. Reported and recorded your care and observations.			

NATCEP™ VIDEO VIDEO CLIP

Transferring the Person to a Chair or Wheelchair

Name: ______________________ Date: ______________________

Quality of Life	S	U	Comments
• Knocked before entering the person's room.			
• Addressed the person by name.			
• Introduced yourself by name and title.			
• Explained the procedure before starting and during the procedure.			
• Protected the person's rights during the procedure.			
• Handled the person gently during the procedure.			

Preprocedure

	S	U	Comments
1. Followed *Delegation Guidelines: Transferring the Person*, Saw *Promoting Safety and Comfort*:			
a. *Transfer/Gait Belts*			
b. *Transferring the Person*			
c. *Stand and Pivot Transfers*			
d. *Bed to Chair or Wheelchair Transfers*			
2. Practiced hand hygiene and got the following supplies:			
• Wheelchair or armchair			
• Bath blanket or cushion (if needed)			
• Lap blanket (if used)			
• Robe (if needed) and slip-resistant footwear			
• Paper towel or towel (if needed)			
• Transfer belt (if needed)			
3. Arranged items in the person's room.			
4. Practiced hand hygiene.			
5. Identified the person. Checked the identification (ID) bracelet against the assignment sheet. Used two identifiers. Also called the person by name.			
6. Provided for privacy.			
7. Decided which side of the bed to use. Moved furniture (as needed) for a safe transfer.			

Procedure

	S	U	Comments
8. Raised the wheelchair footplates. Removed or swung front rigging out of the way if possible. Positioned the chair or wheelchair near the bed on the person's strong side.			
a. If at the head of the bed, it faced the foot of the bed.			
b. If at the foot of the bed, it faced the head of the bed.			
c. The armrest almost touched the bed.			
9. Placed a folded bath blanket or cushion on the seat (if needed).			
10. Locked (braked) the wheelchair wheels. Made sure that bed wheels were locked.			
11. Fanfolded top linens to the foot of the bed.			
12. Placed the paper towel or towel under the person's feet. (This protected linens from footwear.) Put footwear on the person or applied footwear when the person was seated on the side of the bed.			
13. Lowered the bed to a safe and comfortable level. Followed the care plan.			

Procedure—cont'd	S	U	Comments
14. Helped the person sit on the side of the bed. Feet were flat on the floor.			
15. Ensured that the person's clothing would properly cover the person during the transfer. Helped the person put on a robe (if needed).			
16. Applied the transfer belt if needed. It was applied at the waist over clothing.			
17. *Method 1: Using a transfer belt*:			
a. Stood in front of the person.			
b. Had the person hold on to the mattress.			
c. Made sure the person's feet were flat on the floor.			
d. Had the person lean slightly forward.			
e. Grasped the transfer belt at each side. Grasped the handles or grasped the belt from underneath. Hands were in an upward position (upward grasp).			
f. Prevented the person from sliding or falling. Did one of the following:			
1) Braced your knees against the person's knees. Blocked their feet with your feet.			
2) Used the knee and foot of one leg to block the person's weak leg or foot. Placed your other foot slightly behind you for balance.			
3) Straddled your legs around the person's weak leg.			
g. Explained the following:			
1) You will count "1, 2, 3."			
2) The move will be on "3."			
3) On "3," the person pushes down on the mattress and stands.			
h. Asked the person to push down on the mattress and to stand on the "count of 3." Assisted the person to a standing position as you straightened your knees.			
18. *Method 2: No transfer belt*. (Note: Used this method only if directed by the nurse and the care plan and you are comfortable doing so.)			
a. Followed steps 17, a–c.			
1) Stood in front of the person.			
2) Had the person hold on to the mattress.			
3) Made sure the person's feet were flat on the floor.			
b. Placed your hands under the person's arms. Your hands were around the person's shoulder blades.			
c. Had the person lean slightly forward.			
d. Prevented the person from sliding or falling. Did one of the following:			
1) Braced your knees against the person's knees. Blocked the person's feet with your feet.			
2) Used the knee and foot of one leg to block the person's weak leg or foot. Placed your other foot slightly behind you for balance.			
3) Straddled your legs around the person's weak leg.			
e. Explained the "count of 3."			
1) You will count "1, 2, 3."			
2) The move will be on "3."			
3) On "3," the person pushes down on the mattress and stands.			

Procedure—cont'd	S	U	Comments
f. Asked the person to push down on the mattress and to stand on the "count of 3." Assisted the person up into a standing position as you straightened your knees.			
19. Supported the person in the standing position. Held the transfer belt or kept your hands around the person's shoulder blades. Steadied the person to prevent sliding or falling.			
20. Helped the person pivot (turn) so they could grasp the far arm of the chair or wheelchair. The legs touched the edge of the seat.			
21. Continued to help the person pivot (turn) until the other armrest was grasped.			
22. Lowered the person into the chair or wheelchair as you bent your hips and knees. The person leaned slightly forward and bent the elbows and knees.			
23. Made sure the hips were to the back of the seat. Positioned the person in good alignment.			
24. Removed the transfer belt if used.			
25. Attached wheelchair front rigging for a wheelchair transfer. Positioned the person's feet on the footplates.			
26. Covered the person's lap and legs with a lap blanket (if used). Kept the blanket off the floor and the wheels.			
27. Positioned the chair as the person preferred. Locked (braked) the wheelchair wheels according to the care plan.			

Postprocedure

	S	U	Comments
28. Provided for comfort.			
29. Placed the call light and other needed items within reach.			
30. Followed the care plan and the person's preferences for privacy measures to maintain. Leaving the privacy curtain, window coverings, and door open or closed were examples.			
31. Completed a safety check of the room.			
32. Practiced hand hygiene.			
33. Reported and recorded your care and observations.			
34. Saw procedure: *Transferring the Person From a Chair or Wheelchair to Bed* to return the person to bed.			

NATCEP™

Transferring the Person From a Chair or Wheelchair to Bed

Name: ______________________ Date: ______________________

Quality of Life	S	U	Comments
• Knocked before entering the person's room.	____	____	____
• Addressed the person by name.	____	____	____
• Introduced yourself by name and title.	____	____	____
• Explained the procedure before starting and during the procedure.	____	____	____
• Protected the person's rights during the procedure.	____	____	____
• Handled the person gently during the procedure.	____	____	____

Preprocedure

	S	U	Comments
1. Followed *Delegation Guidelines*:			
a. *Transferring the Person*	____	____	____
Saw *Promoting Safety and Comfort*:			
a. *Transfer/Gaits Belts*	____	____	____
b. *Transferring the Person*	____	____	____
c. *Stand and Pivot Transfer*	____	____	____
d. *Bed to Chair or Wheelchair Transfers*	____	____	____
2. Practiced hand hygiene and got a transfer belt if needed.	____	____	
3. Identified the person. Checked the identification (ID) bracelet against the assignment sheet. Used two identifiers. Called the person by name.	____	____	____
4. Provided privacy.	____	____	____
5. Moved furniture as needed for safe transfer.	____	____	____

Procedure

	S	U	Comments
6. Raised the head of the bed to a sitting position. Ensured that the bed was at a safe and comfortable level for the person. Followed the care plan. When the person transferred to the bed, the feet were flat on the floor while sitting on the side of the bed.	____	____	____
7. Moved the call light so it was on the person's strong side when in bed.	____	____	____
8. Positioned the chair or wheelchair so the person's strong side was next to the bed. Had a coworker help you if necessary.	____	____	____
9. Locked (braked) the wheelchair and bed wheels.	____	____	____
10. Removed and folded the lap blanket.	____	____	____
11. Lifted the person's feet from the footplates. Raised the footplates. Removed or swung front rigging out of the way. Put slip-resistant footwear on the person if not already done.	____	____	____
12. Applied the transfer belt if needed.	____	____	____
13. Made sure the person's feet were flat on the floor.	____	____	____
14. Stood in front of the person.	____	____	____
15. Had the person hold on to the armrests. (If the nurse directed you to do so, placed your arms under the person's arms. Your hands were around the shoulder blades.)	____	____	____
16. Had the person lean slightly forward.	____	____	____
17. Grasped the transfer belt on each side if using it. Grasped underneath the belt. Hands were in an upward position (upward grasp).	____	____	____
18. Prevented the person from sliding or falling. Did one of the following:			

Procedure—cont'd	S	U	Comments
a. Braced your knees against the person's knees. Blocked the feet with your feet.	_____	_____	_____
b. Used the knee and foot of one leg to block the person's weak leg or foot. Placed your other foot slightly behind you for balance.	_____	_____	_____
c. Straddled your legs around the person's weak leg.	_____	_____	_____
19. Explained the count of "3."			
a. You will count "1, 2, 3."	_____	_____	_____
b. The move will be on "3."	_____	_____	_____
20. Asked the person to push down on the armrest on the "count of 3." Assisted the person into a standing position as you straightened your knees.	_____	_____	_____
21. Supported the person in the standing position. Held the transfer belt or kept your hands around the person's shoulder blades. Steadied the person to prevent sliding or falling.	_____	_____	
22. Helped the person pivot (turn) to reach the edge of the mattress. The legs touched the mattress. The person could reach the mattress with both hands.	_____	_____	_____
23. Lowered the person onto the bed as you bent your hips and knees. The person leaned slightly forward and bent the elbows and knees.	_____	_____	_____
24. Removed the transfer belt.	_____	_____	_____
25. Removed the robe (if worn) and footwear.	_____	_____	_____
26. Helped the person lie down.	_____	_____	_____

Postprocedure

27. Provided for comfort.	_____	_____	_____
28. Placed the call light and other needed items within reach.	_____	_____	_____
29. Raised or lowered bed rails. Followed the care plan.	_____	_____	_____
30. Arranged furniture to meet the person's needs.	_____	_____	_____
31. Followed the care plan and the person's preferences for privacy measures to maintain. Leaving the privacy curtain, window coverings, and door open or closed were examples.	_____	_____	_____
32. Completed a safety check of the room.	_____	_____	_____
33. Practiced hand hygiene.	_____	_____	_____
34. Reported and recorded your care observations.	_____	_____	_____

Transferring the Person To and From the Toilet

Name: ______________________ Date: ______________________

Quality of Life	S	U	Comments
• Knocked before entering the person's room.			
• Addressed the person by name.			
• Introduced yourself by name and title.			
• Explained the procedure before starting and during the procedure.			
• Protected the person's rights during the procedure.			
• Handled the person gently during the procedure.			

Preprocedure

	S	U	Comments
1. Followed *Delegation Guidelines: Transferring the Person,* Saw Promoting Safety and Comfort:			
a. *Transfer/Gait Belts*			
b. *Transferring the Person*			
c. *Stand and Pivot Transfer*			
d. *Bed to Chair or Wheelchair Transfers*			
e. *Transferring the Person To and From the Toilet*			
2. Practiced hand hygiene and got the following supplies: • Transfer belt • Slip-resistant footwear (if not already on)			
3. Provided for privacy.			

Procedure

	S	U	Comments
4. Placed slip-resistant footwear on the person (if no already on).			
5. Wheeled the wheelchair into the bathroom near the toilet. Closed the bathroom door for privacy.			
6. Lifted the person's feet from the footplates. Raised the footplates. Removed or swung front rigging out of the way.			
7. Positioned the wheelchair close to the toilet with the person's strong side near the toilet. Grab bars were within reach.			
a. Method 1—at the front of the toilet			
b. Method 2—next to the toilet			
8. Locked (brake) the wheelchair wheels.			
9. Applied the transfer belt.			
10. Helped the person unfasten clothing.			
11. Used the transfer belt to help the person stand and to pivot (turn) to the toilet. The person used the grab bars for support.			
12. Supported the person with the transfer belt while they lowered clothing. Or had the person hold on to the grab bars for support while you lowered the person's clothing.			
13. Used the transfer belt to lower the person onto the toilet seat. Checked for proper positioning on the toilet.			
14. Removed the transfer belt.			
15. Told the person you would stay nearby. Reminded the person to use the call light or call for you when help was needed. Stayed with the person if required by the care plan.			
16. Closed the bathroom door for privacy.			

Procedure—cont'd	S	U	Comments
17. Stayed near the bathroom. Completed other tasks in the person's room. Checked on the person every 5 minutes.	______	______	______
18. Knocked on the bathroom door when the person called for you.	______	______	______
19. Helped with wiping, perineal care, flushing, and hand hygiene as needed. Wore gloves and practiced hand hygiene after removing the gloves.	______	______	______
20. Applied the transfer belt.	______	______	______
21. Used the transfer belt to help the person stand.	______	______	______
22. Helped the person raise and secure clothing as needed.	______	______	______
23. Used the transfer belt to transfer the person to the wheelchair.	______	______	______
24. Made sure the person's buttocks were to the back of the seat. Positioned the person in good alignment.	______	______	______
25. Removed the transfer belt.	______	______	______
26. Rolled the wheelchair back away from the toilet. Reattached front rigging. Lowered the footplates. Positioned the feet on the footplates.	______	______	______
27. Covered the lap and legs with a lap blanket. Kept the blanket off the floor and wheels.	______	______	______
28. Positioned the chair as the person preferred. Locked (braked) the wheelchair wheels according to the care plan.	______	______	______

Postprocedure

29. Provided for comfort.	______	______	______
30. Placed the call light and other needed items within reach.	______	______	______
31. Followed the care plan and the person's preferences for privacy measures to maintain. Leaving the privacy curtain, window coverings, and door open or closed were examples.	______	______	______
32. Completed a safety check of the room.	______	______	______
33. Practiced hand hygiene.	______	______	______
34. Reported and recorded your care and observations.	______	______	______

NATCEP™ VIDEO

Moving the Person to a Stretcher

Name: ______________________ Date: ______________________

Quality of Life	S	U	Comments
• Knocked before entering the person's room.	____	____	____
• Addressed the person by name.	____	____	____
• Introduced yourself by name and title.	____	____	____
• Explained the procedure before starting and during the procedure.	____	____	____
• Protected the person's rights during the procedure.	____	____	____
• Handled the person gently during the procedure.	____	____	____
Preprocedure			
1. Followed *Delegation Guidelines: Transferring the Person*, Saw *Promoting Safety and Comfort*:	____	____	____
a. *Transferring the Person*	____	____	____
b. *Moving the Person to a Stretcher*	____	____	____
2. Asked one or two staff members to help you.	____	____	____
3. Practiced hand hygiene and got the following supplies:			
• Stretcher covered with a sheet or bath blanket	____	____	____
• Bath blanket or sheet	____	____	____
• Pillow(s) if needed	____	____	____
• Lateral transfer device (this procedure uses a slide board)	____	____	____
4. Arranged items in the person's room.	____	____	
5. Practiced hand hygiene.	____	____	____
6. Identified the person. Checked the identification (ID) bracelet against the assignment sheet. Used two identifiers. Also called the person by name.	____	____	____
7. Provided for privacy.	____	____	____
8. Moved furniture as needed for space.	____	____	____
Procedure			
9. Raised the bed for body mechanics. Lowered the head of the bed. It was as flat as possible. Lowered the bed rails if used. Bed wheels were locked (braked).	____	____	____
10. Fanfolded top linens to the foot of the bed.	____	____	____
11. Positioned the lateral transfer device. Followed the manufacturer's instructions and the nurse's directions. To position a slide board:			
a. Loosened the drawsheet if it was tucked in. Used the drawsheet to assist with turning.	____	____	____
b. Turned the person to the side. Turned the person toward you.	____	____	____
c. Had a coworker place the slide board on the bed.	____	____	____
d. Turned the person onto the back. The person was lying on the board. The drawsheet was between the board and the person.	____	____	____
12. Had a coworker position the stretcher next to the bed. Held the far side of the drawsheet to protect the person from falling.	____	____	____
13. Raised the stretcher as directed by the nurse. It was either at the same level as the bed or slightly lower (about ½ inch).	____	____	____
14. Locked (brake) the stretcher wheels.	____	____	____
15. Positioned yourself and coworkers.	____	____	____
a. One or two workers stood at the side of the stretcher.	____	____	____
b. One worker remained at the side of the bed.	____	____	____

Procedure—cont'd	S	U	Comments
16. Grasped the handles on the slide board.	_____	_____	_____
17. Slid the person to the stretcher on the "count of 3." Ensured that the person was fully on the stretcher.	_____	_____	_____
18. Had the worker(s) on the stretcher side hold the far side of the drawsheet to protect the person from falling. Unlocked the stretcher wheels (released the brakes). Moved the stretcher away from the side of the bed.	_____	_____	_____
19. Removed the slide board.			
a. Locked (brake) the stretcher wheels.	_____	_____	_____
b. Had the worker(s) use the drawsheet to turn the person. Turned toward the worker(s).	_____	_____	_____
c. Removed the slide board.	_____	_____	_____
d. Turned the person onto the back. The person was centered on the stretcher.	_____	_____	_____
20. Placed a pillow or pillows under the person's head and shoulder if allowed. Raised the head of the stretcher if allowed.	_____	_____	_____
21. Covered the person. Provided for comfort.	_____	_____	_____
22. Fastened the safety straps. Raised the side rails.	_____	_____	_____
23. Unlocked the stretcher wheels (released the brakes). Transported the person.	_____	_____	_____
Postprocedure			
24. Practiced hand hygiene.	_____	_____	_____
25. Reported and recorded:			
• The time of the transport	_____	_____	_____
• Where the person was transported to	_____	_____	_____
• Who went with him or her	_____	_____	_____
• How the transfer was tolerated	_____	_____	_____
26. Reversed the procedure to return the person to bed.	_____	_____	_____

Transferring the Person Using a Stand-Assist Mechanical Lift

Name: ______________________ Date: ______________________

Quality of Life	S	U	Comments
• Knocked before entering the person's room.			
• Addressed the person by name.			
• Introduced yourself by name and title.			
• Explained the procedure before starting and during the procedure.			
• Protected the person's rights during the procedure.			
• Handled the person gently during the procedure.			

Preprocedure

	S	U	Comments
1. Followed *Delegation Guidelines*:			
a. *Transferring the Person,*			
b. *Using a Mechanical Lift*			
Saw *Promoting Safety and Comfort*:			
a. *Transferring the Person*			
b. *Using a Mechanical Lift*			
2. Asked a coworker to help you (if needed).			
3. Practiced hand hygiene and got the following supplies:			
• Stand-assist mechanical lift and sling			
• Armchair or wheelchair			
• Slip-resistant footwear			
• Bath blanket or cushion (if needed)			
• Lap blanket (if used)			
4. Arranged items in the person's room.			
5. Practiced hand hygiene.			
6. Identified the person. Checked the identification (ID) bracelet against the assignment sheet. Used two identifiers. Also called the person by name.			
7. Provided for privacy.			

Procedure

	S	U	Comments
8. Placed the chair (wheelchair) at the head of the bed. It was even with the headboard and about one foot away from the bed. Locked (braked) the wheelchair wheels. Placed a folded bath blanket or cushion in the seat if needed.			
9. Assisted the person to a seated position on the side of the bed. The person's feet were flat on the floor. Bed wheels were locked.			
10. Put footwear on the person.			
11. Applied the sling.			
a. Positioned the sling at the lower back.			
b. Brought the straps around to the front of the chest. The straps were positioned under the arms.			
c. Secured the waist belt around the person's waist. Adjusted the belt so it was snug but not tight.			
12. Positioned the lift in front of the person.			
13. Widened the lift's base.			
14. Locked (braked) the lift's wheels.			
15. Had the person place the feet on the footplate and the knees against the knee pad. Assisted as needed. If the lift had a knee strap, secured the strap around the legs. Adjusted the strap so it was snug but not tight.			
16. Attached the sling to the sling hooks.			
17. Had the person grasp the lift's hand grips.			

Procedure—cont'd	S	U	Comments
18. Unlocked the lift's wheels (released the brakes) following the manufacturer's instructions.			
19. Raised the person slightly off the bed. Checked that the sling was secure, the feet were on the footplate, and the knees were against the knee pad. If not, lowered the person and corrected the problem.			
20. Raised the lift until the person was clear of the bed. Or raised the person to a standing position. Followed the care plan.			
21. Adjusted the base's width to move from the bed to the chair (wheelchair) if needed. Kept the base in the wide or open position as much as possible.			
22. Moved the lift to the chair (wheelchair). The person's back was toward the seat.			
23. Lowered the person into the chair (wheelchair). Guided the person into the seat.			
24. Locked (braked) the lift's wheels following the manufacturer's instructions.			
25. Unhooked the sling from the sling hooks.			
26. Unbuckled the waist belt. Removed the sling.			
27. Unlocked the lift's wheels (released the brakes).			
28. Had the person lift the feet off of the footplate. Assisted as needed. Moved the lift. Positioned the person's feet flat on the floor or on the wheelchair footplates.			
29. Covered the lap and legs with a lap blanket (if used). Kept it off the floor.			

Postprocedure

30. Provided for comfort.			
31. Placed the call light and other needed items within reach.			
32. Followed the care plan and the person's preferences for privacy measures to maintain. Leaving the privacy curtain, window coverings, and door open or closed were examples.			
33. Completed a safety check of the room.			
34. Practiced hand hygiene.			
35. Reported and recorded your care and observations.			
36. Reversed the procedure to return the person to bed.			

NATCEP™ VIDEO

Transferring the Person Using a Full-Sling Mechanical Lift

Name: ______________________ Date: ______________________

Quality of Life	S	U	Comments
• Knocked before entering the person's room.			
• Addressed the person by name.			
• Introduced yourself by name and title.			
• Explained the procedure before starting and during the procedure.			
• Protected the person's rights during the procedure.			
• Handled the person gently during the procedure.			

Preprocedure	S	U	Comments
1. Followed *Delegation Guidelines*:			
a. *Transferring the Person,*			
b. *Using a Mechanical Lift*			
Saw *Promoting Safety and Comfort*:			
a. *Transferring the Person*			
b. *Using a Mechanical Lift*			
2. Asked a coworker to help you.			
3. Practiced hand hygiene and got the following supplies:			
• Full-sling mechanical lift and sling			
• Armchair or wheelchair			
• Slip-resistant footwear			
• Bath blanket or cushion (if needed)			
• Lap blanket (if used)			
4. Arranged items in the person's room.			
5. Practice hand hygiene.			
6. Identified the person. Checked the identification (ID) bracelet against the assignment sheet. Used two identifiers. Also called the person by name.			
7. Provided for privacy.			
8. Raised the bed for body mechanics. Bed rails were up if used.			

Procedure	S	U	Comments
9. Lowered the head of the bed to a level appropriate for the person. It is as flat as possible.			
10. Stood on one side of the bed. Your coworker stood on the other side.			
11. Lowered the bed rails if up. Locked (braked) the bed wheels.			
12. Centered the sling under the person. To position the sling, turned the person from side to side. Followed the manufacturer's instructions to position the sling.			
13. Positioned the person in the semi-Fowler's position.			
14. Placed the chair (wheelchair) at the head of the bed. It was even with the headboard and about one foot away from the bed. Placed a folded bath blanket or cushion in the seat if needed. Locked (brake) the wheelchair wheels.			
15. Lowered the bed so it was level with the chair.			
16. Raised the lift to position it over the person.			
17. Positioned the lift over the person.			
18. Widened the lift's base. Locked (braked) the lift wheels.			
19. Attached the sling to the sling hooks.			

Procedure—cont'd	S	U	Comments
20. Raised the head of the bed to a comfortable level for the person.			
21. Crossed the person's arms over the chest. The arms were inside the sling.			
22. Unlocked the lift wheels (released the brakes). Followed the manufacturer's instructions.			
23. Raised the person slightly from the bed. Checked that the sling was secure. If not, lowered the person and corrected the problem.			
24. Raised the lift until the person and sling were free of the bed.			
25. Had your coworker support the person's legs as you moved the lift and the person away from the bed.			
26. Adjusted the base's width to move from the bed to the chair (wheelchair) if needed. Kept the base in the wide or open position as much as possible.			
27. Positioned the lift so the person's back was toward the chair (wheelchair).			
28. Adjusted the position of the chair (wheelchair) as needed to lower the person into it. Locked (braked) the wheelchair wheels.			
29. Lowered the person into the chair (wheelchair). Guided the person into the seat.			
30. Locked (braked) the lift wheels. Followed the manufacturer's instructions.			
31. Unhooked the sling. Unlocked the lift's wheels (released the brakes). Moved the lift away from the person. Removed the sling from under the person unless otherwise indicated.			
32. Put footwear on the person. Positioned the feet flat on the floor or on the wheelchair footplates.			
33. Covered the lap and legs with a lap blanket (if used). Kept it off the floor and wheels.			
34. Positioned the chair (wheelchair) as the person preferred. Locked (braked) the wheelchair wheels according to the care plan.			

Postprocedure	S	U	Comments
35. Provided for comfort.			
36. Placed the call light and other needed items within reach.			
37. Followed the care plan and the person's preferences for privacy measures to maintain. Leaving the privacy curtain, window coverings, and door open or closed were examples.			
38. Completed a safety check of the room.			
39. Practiced hand hygiene.			
40. Reported and recorded your care and observations.			
41. Reversed the procedure to return the person to bed. Followed the manufacturer's instructions to position a sling on a person seated in a chair or wheelchair.			
a. Had the person lean forward. Had your coworker help the person if needed.			
b. Slid the sling behind the person's back. Tucked the sling down along the back to the seat of the chair or wheelchair.			
c. Brought the leg straps around the sides of the person. The straps were at the sides of the legs.			
d. Passed the leg straps under the legs.			

NATCEP™ VIDEO

Making a Closed Bed

Name: ______________________ Date: ______________________

Quality of Life	S	U	Comments
• Knocked before entering the person's room.	___	___	___
• Addressed the person by name.	___	___	___
• Introduced yourself by name and title.	___	___	___
• Explained the procedure before starting and during the procedure.	___	___	___
• Protected the person's rights during the procedure.	___	___	___
• Handled the person gently during the procedure.	___	___	___

Preprocedure

	S	U	Comments
1. Followed *Delegation Guidelines: Making Beds.* Saw *Promoting Safety and Comfort: Making Beds.*	___	___	___
2. Practiced hand hygiene and got the following clean linens and supplies:	___	___	___
• Mattress pad (if needed)	___	___	___
• Bottom sheet (flat sheet or fitted sheet)	___	___	___
• Drawsheet (if needed)	___	___	___
• Waterproof underpad (if needed)	___	___	___
• Top sheet	___	___	___
• Blanket (if needed)	___	___	___
• Bedspread	___	___	___
• A pillowcase for each pillow	___	___	___
• Personal hygiene lines (as needed)—bath towel, hand towel, washcloth, gown or pajamas, bath blanket	___	___	___
• Gloves	___	___	___
• Laundry bag	___	___	___
• Towel, paper towels, or disposable bed protector (as a barrier for clean linens)	___	___	___
3. Arranged items in the person's room. Placed linens on a clean surface. First placed the barrier between the clean surface and the clean linens if required by agency policy.	___	___	___
4. Raised the bed for body mechanics. Bed rails are down.	___	___	___

Procedure

	S	U	Comments
5. Put on gloves if contact with blood or body fluids might occur.	___	___	___
6. Removed linens. Rolled each piece away from you. Placed each piece in a laundry bag. (Note: Discarded the incontinence product, disposable bed protector, and disposable drawsheet in the trash. Did not put them in the laundry bag.)	___	___	___
7. Cleaned the bed frame and mattress (if this was your job).	___	___	___
8. Removed and discarded the gloves. Practiced hand hygiene.	___	___	___
9. Moved the mattress to the head of the bed.	___	___	___
10. Put the mattress pad on the mattress. It was even with the top of the mattress.	___	___	___
11. Applied the bottom sheet to one side of the bed. Unfolded the sheet lengthwise. Placed the center crease in the middle of the bed.			
a. For a flat sheet:			

Procedure—cont'd	S	U	Comments
1) Placed the lower edge even with the foot of the mattress.			
i) If there was a large and small hem, placed the large hem at the head and the small hem at the foot.			
ii) Placed the stitched side of the hem downward, away from the person. The smooth side is up, against the skin.			
2) Opened the sheet. Fanfolded it to the other side of the bed.			
3) Tucked the top of the sheet under the mattress. Smoothed the sheet from the head to the foot.			
4) Made a mitered corner at the top. Tucked in the sheet along the side of the mattress.			
b. For a fitted sheet:			
1) Open and fanfold the sheet to the other side of the bed.			
2) Tuck the corners over the mattress at the head and the foot of the bed on one side.			
12. Placed the drawsheet (if used) on the bed. It was in the middle of the mattress.			
a. Opened and fanfolded the drawsheet to the other side of the bed.			
b. Tucked the drawsheet under the mattress.			
13. Went to the other side of the bed.			
14. Tucked in the bottom sheet on the other side of the bed. Made sure the sheet is smooth and tight without wrinkles.			
a. *For a flat sheet*, mitered the top corner. Tucked in the sheet along the side of the mattress.			
b. *For a fitted sheet*, tucked the corners over the mattress at the head and the foot of the bed.			
15. Pulled the drawsheets tight so there were no wrinkles.			
16. *If using a waterproof underpad*, placed the waterproof underpad on the bed. It was in the middle of the mattress.			
17. Put the top sheet on the bed.			
a. Unfolded it lengthwise with the center crease in the middle.			
b. Placed the large hem even with the top of the mattress.			
1) If there was a large hem and small hem, the large hem was at the head. The small hem was at the foot.			
2) Placed the stitched side of the hem outward, away from the person. The smooth side was down, against the skin.			
c. Opened and fanfolded the sheet to the other side. Did not tuck the sheet in yet. Never tucked top linens in on the sides.			
18. Placed the blanket on the bed (if used).			
a. Unfolded it with the center crease in the middle.			
b. Put the upper hem about 6 to 8 inches from the top of the mattress.			
c. Opened and fanfolded the blanket to the other side.			
19. Placed the bedspread on the bed.			
a. Unfolded it with the center crease in the middle.			

Procedure—cont'd	S	U	Comments
b. Placed the top edge even with the head of the mattress.	______	______	______
c. Opened and fanfolded the bedspread to the other side.	______	______	______
20. Went to the other side.	______	______	______
21. Brought the top linens down over the side of the bed. Straightened all top linens. Made sure the bedspread facing the door was even. It covered all top linens.	______	______	______
22. Tucked in top linens together at the foot of the bed so they were smooth and tight. Made mitered corners at the foot of the bed. Left the side of the top linens untucked.	______	______	______
23. Put the pillowcase on the pillow. The zipper, tag, or seam end of the pillow was inserted into the pillowcase first. Kept the pillow and pillowcase away from your body and uniform. Folded extra material under the pillow at the open end of the pillowcase.	______	______	______
24. Followed the person's preference and agency practices for finishing the bed. The bed looked neat and wrinkle free. Linens were not touching the floor. The open end of the pillowcase did not face the door.			
a. Method 1—Turned the top hem of the bedspread under the blanket to form a cuff. Turned the top sheet over the bedspread. Hemstitching was down. The smooth side was up. Placed the pillow on the bed.			
b. Method 2—Folded the top of the bedspread back (enough to fit the pillow in the area). Placed the pillow on the bed. Brought the bedspread up over the pillow. Tucked the bedspread under the pillow.			
c. Method 3—Pulled the bedspread up to the head of the mattress. Placed the pillow on top.			

Postprocedure

	S	U	Comments
25. Provided for comfort. Note: Omitted this step if the bed was prepared for a new patient or resident.	______	______	______
26. Attached the call light to the bed. Or placed it within the person's reach.	______	______	______
27. Lowered the bed to a safe and comfortable level. Followed the care plan. Locked (braked) the bed wheels.	______	______	______
28. Raised or lowered bed rails. Followed the care plan or the nurse's directions.			
29. Put the towels, washcloth, gown or pajamas, and bath blanket in the bedside stand.	______	______	______
30. Completed a safety check of the room.	______	______	______
31. Followed agency policy for used linens.	______	______	______
32. Practiced hand hygiene.	______	______	______

NATCEP™ VIDEO

Making an Occupied Bed

Name: ______________________ Date: ______________________

Quality of Life	S	U	Comments
• Knocked before entering the person's room.	______	______	______
• Addressed the person by name.	______	______	______
• Introduced yourself by name and title.	______	______	______
• Explained the procedure before starting and during the procedure.	______	______	______
• Protected the person's rights during the procedure.	______	______	______
• Handled the person gently during the procedure.	______	______	______

Preprocedure

	S	U	Comments
1. Followed *Delegation Guidelines: Making Beds.* Saw *Promoting Safety and Comfort*:			
a. *Making Beds*	______	______	______
b. *The Occupied Bed*	______	______	______
2. Asked a coworker to help you if needed.	______	______	______
3. Practiced hand hygiene and got the following supplies:	______	______	______
• Clean linens (same as closed bed)	______	______	______
• Bath blanket	______	______	______
• Gloves	______	______	______
• Laundry bag	______	______	______
• Towel, paper towels, or disposable bed protector (as a barrier for clean linens)	______	______	______
4. Arranged items in the person's room. Placed linens on a clean surface. First place the barrier between the clean surface and clean linens if required by agency policy.	______	______	______
5. Practiced hand hygiene.	______	______	______
6. Identified the person. Checked the identification (ID) bracelet against the assignment sheet. Used two identifiers. Also called the person by name.	______	______	______
7. Provided for privacy.	______	______	______
8. Moved the call light off of the bed.	______	______	______
9. Raised the bed for body mechanics. Bed rails were up if used. Bed wheels were locked (braked).	______	______	______
10. Lowered the head of the bed. It was as flat as possible.	______	______	______

Procedure

	S	U	Comments
11. Put on gloves if contact with blood or body fluids might have occurred.	______	______	______
12. Loosened top linens at the foot of the bed.	______	______	______
13. Lowered the bed rail near you if up.	______	______	______
14. Folded and removed the bedspread. Did the same for the blanket (if used). Placed each over the chair or on a clean surface.	______	______	______
15. Covered the person with a bath blanket from the bedside stand.			
a. Unfolded the bath blanket over the top sheet.	______	______	______
b. Had the person hold the bath blanket. If the person was unable, tucked the top part under the person's shoulders.	______	______	______
c. Grasped the top sheet under the bath blanket at the shoulders. Brought the sheet down toward the foot of the bed. Removed the sheet from under the blanket.	______	______	______

Procedure—cont'd	S	U	Comments
16. Explained the safety measures you used to prevent falling from the bed. Helped the person turn onto the side facing away from you. Adjusted the pillow for comfort.			
17. Loosened bottom linens on the side of the bed near you.			
18. Fanfolded bottom linens one at a time toward the person. If reusing a mattress pad, did not fanfold it.			
19. Removed and discarded the gloves. Practiced hand hygiene. Put on clean gloves if you had to handle soiled linens again on the other side of the bed.			
20. Placed a clean mattress pad on the bed if needed. Unfolded it lengthwise with the center crease in the middle. Fanfolded the top part toward the person. If reusing a mattress pad, straightened and smoothed any wrinkles.			
21. Placed the bottom sheet on the side of the bed near you.			
a. For a flat sheet,			
1) Placed the lower edge even with the foot of the mattress.			
i) If there was a large and small hem, placed the large hem at the head and the small hem at the foot.			
ii) Placed the stitched side of the hem downward, away from the person. The smooth side is up, against the skin.			
b. For a fitted sheet,			
1) Tucked the corners over the mattress at the head and the foot of the bed on the side near you. Fanfolded the sheet toward the person.			
22. *If using a drawsheet*:			
a. Placed the drawsheet on the bed. It was in the middle of the mattress.			
b. Opened the drawsheet.			
c. Fanfolded it toward the person.			
d. Tucked in excess fabric at the side of the bed.			
23. *If using a waterproof underpad*:			
a. Placed the waterproof underpad on the bed. It was in the middle of the mattress.			
b. Fanfolded it toward the person.			
24. Explained to the person that there was a "bump" to roll back over. Helped the person turn to the other side. Adjusted the pillow for comfort.			
25. Raised the bed rail. Went to the other side and lowered the bed rail. (NOTE: Omitted this step if you were working with a coworker. Your coworker removed used linens and placed clean linens on the other side of the bed.)			
26. Loosened bottom linens. Removed one piece at a time. Placed each piece in the laundry bag. (Note: Discarded the disposable bed protector, incontinence product, and disposable drawsheet in the trash. Did not put them in the laundry bag.)			
27. Removed and discarded the gloves. Practiced hand hygiene.			
28. Straightened and smoothed the mattress pad if used.			

Procedure—cont'd	S	U	Comments
29. Pulled the clean bottom sheet toward you and tucked it in. For a flat sheet, made a mitered corner at the top. Tucked the sheet under the mattress from the head to the foot of the bed. For a fitted sheet, tucked the corners over the mattress at the head and the foot of the bed.			
30. Pulled the drawsheets tightly toward you and tucked it in.			
31. Positioned the person supine in the center of the bed. Adjusted the pillow for comfort.			
32. Put the top sheet on the bed. Unfolded it lengthwise with the crease in the middle. The large hem was even with the head of the mattress. Hemstitching was on the outside.			
33. Had the person hold the top sheet so you could remove the bath blanket. Or tucked the top sheet under the person's shoulders. Removed the bath blanket. Placed it in the laundry bag.			
34. Unfolded the blanket on the bed (if used). The crease was in the middle and it covered the person. The upper hem was 6 to 8 inches from the head of the mattress.			
35. Unfolded the bedspread on the bed. The center crease was in the middle and it covered the person. The top hem was even with the head of the mattress.			
36. Straightened and smooth top linens.			
37. Raised the bed rail. Went to foot of the bed.			
38. Made a 2-inch toe pleat across the foot of the bed. The pleat (fold) was about 6 to 8 inches from the foot of the bed. The pleat prevented pressure on the toes from top linens.			
39. Tucked in all top linens together at the foot of the bed. Avoided removing the toe pleat. Mitered the corners at the foot of the bed. Left the top linens untucked at the sides.			
40. Followed the person's preference and agency practices for finishing the bed. If a blanket was used, turned the top hem of the bedspread under the blanket to make a cuff. Brought the top sheet down over the bedspread to form a cuff.			
41. Changed the pillowcase(s).			

Postprocedure

42. Provided for comfort.			
43. Placed the call light and other needed items within reach.			
44. Lowered the bed to a safe and comfortable level. Followed the care plan. The bed wheels were locked (braked).			
45. Raised or lowered bed rails. Followed the care plan.			
46. Put the clean towels, washcloth, gown or pajamas, and bath blanket in the bedside stand.			
47. Followed the care plan and the person's preferences for privacy measures to maintain. Leaving the privacy curtain, window coverings, and door open or closed were examples.			
48. Completed a safety check of the room.			
49. Followed agency policy for used linens.			
50. Practiced hand hygiene.			
51. Reported and recorded your care and observations.			

Making a Surgical Bed

VIDEO

Name: ______________________ Date: ______________________

Preprocedure	S	U	Comments
1. Followed *Delegation Guidelines: Making Beds*. Saw *Promoting Safety and Comfort*:			
a. *Making Beds*	____	____	________
b. *The Surgical Bed*	____	____	________
2. Practiced hand hygiene and got the following supplies:			
• Clean linens (same as for closed bed)	____	____	________
• Gloves	____	____	________
• Laundry bag	____	____	________
• Equipment requested by the nurse	____	____	________
• Towel, paper towels, or disposable bed protector (as a barrier for clean linens)	____	____	________
3. Arranged items in the person's room. Placed linens on a clean surface. First placed the barrier between the clean surface and clean linens if required by agency policy.	____	____	________
4. Moved the call light off of the bed.	____	____	________
5. Raised the bed for body mechanics. Bed rails were down.	____	____	________

Procedure	S	U	Comments
6. Put on gloves if contact with blood or body fluids may have occurred them.	____	____	________
7. Removed and placed all linens in the laundry bag. Removed gloves. Practiced hand hygiene after removing and discarding gloves.	____	____	________
8. Made a closed bed. Did not tuck top linens under the mattress.	____	____	________
9. Folded all top linens at the foot of the bed back onto the bed. The fold was even with the edge of the mattress.	____	____	________
10. Knew on which side of the bed the stretcher would be placed. Fanfolded linens lengthwise to the other side of the bed.	____	____	________
11. Put a pillowcase on each pillow.	____	____	________
12. Placed the pillow(s) on a clean surface.	____	____	________

Postprocedure	S	U	Comments
13. Left the bed in its highest position.	____	____	________
14. Left both bed rails down.	____	____	________
15. Put the clean towels, washcloth, gown or pajamas, and bath blanket in the bedside stand.	____	____	________
16. Moved furniture away from the bed. Allowed room for the stretcher and the staff.	____	____	________
17. Did not attach the call light to the bed.	____	____	________
18. Completed a safety check of the room.	____	____	________
19. Followed agency policy for used linens.	____	____	________
20. Practiced hand hygiene.	____	____	________

Assisting the Person to Brush and Floss the Teeth

Name: ______________________ Date: ____________ ______________________

Quality of Life	S	U	Comments
• Knocked before entering the person's room.	____	____	____
• Addressed the person by name.	____	____	____
• Introduced yourself by name and title.	____	____	____
• Explained the procedure before starting and during the procedure.	____	____	____
• Protected the person's rights during the procedure.	____	____	____
• Handled the person gently during the procedure.	____	____	____

Preprocedure

1. Followed *Delegation Guidelines: Purpose of Oral Hygiene*. Saw *Promoting Safety and Comfort: Purpose of Oral Hygiene*.	____	____	____
2. Practiced hand hygiene and got the following supplies:	____	____	____
• Toothbrush with soft bristles	____	____	____
• Toothpaste	____	____	____
• Mouthwash (or solution noted on care plan)	____	____	____
• Floss or other interdental cleaner (if used)	____	____	____
• Water cup with cool water	____	____	____
• Straw	____	____	____
• Kidney basin (if needed)	____	____	____
• Hand towel	____	____	____
• Towel or paper towels (as a barrier for supplies)	____	____	____
• Gloves	____	____	____
• Laundry bag	____	____	____
3. Arranged items in the person's room or bathroom. Placed the barrier (towel, paper towels) on the over-bed table or bathroom counter. Arranged items on top.	____	____	____
4. Practiced hand hygiene.	____	____	____
5. Identified the person. Checked the ID (identification) bracelet against the assignment sheet. Used two identifiers. Also called the person by name.	____	____	____
6. Provided for privacy.	____	____	____

Procedure

7. Positioned the person for oral hygiene (sitting up in bed or at the bathroom sink).	____	____	____
8. Placed the towel over the person's chest. This protected garments from spills.	____	____	____
9. Ensured that the person could reach needed supplies. Adjusted the over-bed table in front of the person if used.	____	____	____
10. Had the person perform hand hygiene.	____	____	____
11. Had the person perform oral hygiene. This included brushing the teeth and tongue, rinsing the mouth, flossing, and using mouthwash or other solution. If in bed, the person spit into a kidney basin.	____	____	____
12. Removed the towel when the person was done. Placed the towel in the laundry bag.	____	____	____
13. Returned the person to a comfortable position. Assisted the person out of the bathroom if needed.	____	____	____

Postprocedure

14. Provided for comfort.
15. Made sure the bed was at a safe and comfortable level. Followed the care plan.
16. Raised or lowered bed rails. Followed the care plan.
17. Cleaned up and stored supplies and equipment. (Wore gloves.)
    a. Discarded disposable items.
    b. Rinsed the toothbrush and returned it to its proper place.
    c. Followed agency procedures to clean and disinfect reusable equipment. Returned supplies and equipment to their proper place.
    d. Followed agency policy for dirty linens.
    e. Cleaned and dried the over-bed table. Dried with paper towels. Discarded paper towels. Positioned the over-bed table as the person preferred.
    f. Removed and discarded gloves. Practiced hand hygiene.
18. Placed the call light and other needed items within reach.
19. Followed the care plan and the person's preferences for privacy measures to maintain. Leaving the privacy curtain, window coverings, and door open or closed were examples.
20. Completed a safety check of the room.
21. Practiced hand hygiene.
22. Reported and recorded your care and observations.

NATCEP™ VIDEO VIDEO CLIP

Brushing and Flossing the Person's Teeth

Name: ______________________ Date: ______________________

Quality of Life	S	U	Comments
• Knocked before entering the person's room.			
• Addressed the person by name.			
• Introduced yourself by name and title.			
• Explained the procedure before starting and during the procedure.			
• Protected the person's rights during the procedure.			
• Handled the person gently during the procedure.			

Preprocedure	S	U	Comments
1. Followed *Delegation Guidelines: Purpose of Oral Hygiene*. Saw *Promoting Safety and Comfort*: a. *Purpose of Oral Hygiene*.			
2. Practiced hand hygiene and got the following supplies:			
• Toothbrush with soft bristles			
• Toothpaste			
• Mouthwash (or solution noted on care plan)			
• Floss or other interdental cleaner (if used)			
• Water cup with cool water			
• Straw			
• Kidney basin (if needed)			
• Hand towel			
• Towel or paper towels (as a barrier for supplies)			
• Gloves			
• Laundry bag			
3. Arranged items in the person's room or bathroom. Placed the barrier (towel or paper towels) on the over-bed table or bathroom counter. Arranged items on top.			
4. Practiced hand hygiene.			
5. Identified the person. Checked the ID (identification) bracelet against the assignment sheet. Used 2 identifiers. Also called the person by name.			
6. Provided for privacy.			
7. Raised the bed for body mechanics. Bed rails were up if used.			

Procedure	S	U	Comments
8. Lowered the bed rail near you if up.			
9. Assisted the person to a sitting position or side-lying position near you. (Some state competency tests require that the person is at a 60- to 90-degree angle. Other states require a 75- to 90-degree angle.)			
10. Placed the towel across the person's chest.			
11. Adjusted the over-bed table so you could reach it with ease.			
12. Practiced hand hygiene. Put on the gloves.			
13. Held the toothbrush over the kidney basin. Poured some water over the brush.			
14. Applied toothpaste to the toothbrush.			
15. Brushed the teeth gently. Brushed the inner, outer, and chewing surfaces of upper and lower teeth.			
16. Brushed the tongue gently. Also gently brushed the roof of the mouth, inside of the cheeks, and gums.			

Procedure—cont'd	S	U	Comments
17. Allowed the person to rinse the mouth with water. Held the kidney basin under the person's chin. Repeated this step as needed.			
18. Flossed the person's teeth (optional).			
a. Broke off an 18-inch piece of dental floss from the dispenser.			
b. Wrapped most of the floss around one of your middle fingers. Wrapped a small amount around the middle finger on the other hand. (As floss was used, unwrapped clean floss from the first middle finger. Wrapped used floss around the middle finger on the other hand.)			
c. Stretched the floss with your thumbs. Held the floss between your thumbs and index fingers.			
d. Started at the back side of an upper back tooth. Worked around to the other side of the mouth.			
e. Gently inserted the floss between the teeth with a rubbing motion. Did not jerk or snap the floss.			
f. Gently slid the floss into the space between the gum and the tooth.			
g. Rubbed the floss gently against the side of the tooth. Moved away from the gum with slow back-and-forth and up-and-down motions.			
h. Used a new section of floss for each tooth. Remembered to floss the back side of the last tooth.			
i. Flossed the lower teeth. Started on the one side. Worked around to the other side. Remembered to floss the back side of the last tooth.			
j. Discarded the floss.			
19. Allowed the person to use mouthwash or other solution. Held the kidney basin under the chin.			
20. Wiped the person's mouth. Removed the towel. Placed the towel in the laundry bag.			
21. Removed and discarded the gloves. Practiced hand hygiene.			
22. Returned the person to a safe and comfortable position.			
Postprocedure			
23. Provided for comfort.			
24. Lowered the bed to a safe and comfortable level appropriate for the person.			
Raised or lowered bed rails. Followed the care plan.			
25. Cleaned up and stored supplies and equipment. (Wore gloves. Changed gloves as needed.)			
a. Discarded disposable items.			
b. Rinsed the toothbrush and returned it to its proper place.			
c. Followed agency procedures to clean and disinfect reusable equipment. Returned supplies and equipment to their proper place.			
d. Followed agency policy for used linens.			
e. Cleaned and dried the over-bed table. Dried with paper towels. Discarded paper towels. Positioned the over-bed table as the person preferred.			
f. Removed and discarded gloves. Practiced hand hygiene.			
26. Placed the call light and other needed items within reach.			

Postprocedure—cont'd	S	U	Comments
27. Followed the care plan and the person's preferences for privacy measures to maintain. Leaving the privacy curtain, window coverings, and door open or closed were examples.	______	______	______________________
28. Completed a safety check of the room.	______	______	______________________
29. Practiced hand hygiene.	______	______	______________________
30. Reported and recorded your care and observations.	______	______	______________________

Providing Mouth Care for the Unconscious Person

VIDEO

Name: ______________________ Date: ______________________

Quality of Life	S	U	Comments
• Knocked before entering the person's room.			
• Addressed the person by name.			
• Introduced yourself by name and title.			
• Explained the procedure before starting and during the procedure.			
• Protected the person's rights during the procedure.			
• Handled the person gently during the procedure.			

Preprocedure

	S	U	Comments
1. Followed *Delegation Guidelines: Purpose of Oral Hygiene*. Saw *Promoting Safety and Comfort*:			
a. *Purpose of Oral Hygiene*			
b. *Mouth Care for the Unconscious Person*			
2. Practiced hand hygiene and got the following supplies:			
• Cleaning agent (checked care plan)			
• Sponge swabs			
• Bite block or plastic tongue depressor			
• Water cup with cool water			
• Hand towel			
• Kidney basin			
• Lip lubricant (check the care plan)			
• Towels or paper towels (as a barrier for supplies)			
• Gloves			
• Laundry bag			
3. Arranged items in the person's room. Placed the barrier (towel, paper towels) on the over-bed table. Arranged items on top.			
4. Practiced hand hygiene.			
5. Identified the person. Checked the ID (identification) bracelet against the assignment sheet. Used two identifiers. Also called the person by name.			
6. Provided for privacy.			
7. Raised the bed for body mechanics. Bed rails were up if used.			

Procedure

	S	U	Comments
8. Lowered the bed rail near you.			
9. Positioned the person in a side-lying position near you. Turned the person's head well to the side.			
10. Placed the towel under the person's face and along the chest. This protected the person and the bed.			
11. Practiced hand hygiene. Put on gloves.			
12. Placed the kidney basin under the chin.			
13. Separated the upper and lower teeth. Used the bite block or plastic tongue depressor. Was gentle. Never used force. If you had problems, asked the nurse for help.			
14. Moistened the sponge swabs moistened with the cleaning agent. Squeezed out excess cleaning agent.			
15. Cleaned the mouth. (Use new swabs as needed. Discard used swabs.)			
a. Cleaned the inner, outer, and chewing surfaces of the upper and lower teeth.			

Procedure—cont'd	S	U	Comments
b. Cleaned the gums and tongue.	_____	_____	_____
c. Swabbed the roof of the mouth, inside of the cheek, and the lips.	_____	_____	_____
16. Moistened and squeezed out a clean swab. Swabbed the mouth to rinse. Discarded the swab.	_____	_____	_____
17. Removed the kidney basin.	_____	_____	_____
18. Wiped the person's mouth. Removed the towel. Placed the towel in the laundry bag.	_____	_____	_____
19. Applied lubricant to the lips.	_____	_____	_____
20. Removed and discarded the gloves. Practiced hand hygiene.	_____	_____	_____
21. Returned the person to a safe and comfortable position.			
Postprocedure			
22. Provided for comfort.	_____	_____	_____
23. Lowered the bed to a safe and comfortable level. Followed the care plan.	_____	_____	_____
24. Raised or lowered bed rails. Followed the care plan.	_____	_____	_____
25. Cleaned up and stored supplies and equipment.			
a. Discarded disposable items.	_____	_____	_____
b. Followed agency procedures to clean and disinfect reusable equipment. Returned supplies and equipment to their proper place.	_____	_____	_____
c. Followed agency policy for used linens.	_____	_____	_____
d. Cleaned and dried the over-bed table. Dried with paper towels. Discarded paper towels. Positioned the over-bed table near the bed for staff use.	_____	_____	_____
e. Removed and discarded the gloves. Practiced hand hygiene.	_____	_____	_____
26. Placed the call light and other needed items within reach for staff and visitor use.	_____	_____	_____
27. Followed the care plan and the person's preferences for privacy measures to maintain. Leaving the privacy curtain, window coverings, and door open or closed were examples.	_____	_____	_____
28. Completed a safety check of the room.	_____	_____	_____
29. Told the person that you were leaving the room. Said when you would return.	_____	_____	_____
30. Practiced hand hygiene.	_____	_____	_____
31. Reported and recorded your care and observations.	_____	_____	_____

Providing Denture Care

Name: ____________________ Date: ____________________

Quality of Life

Quality of Life	S	U	Comments
• Knocked before entering the person's room.			
• Addressed the person by name.			
• Introduced yourself by name and title.			
• Explained the procedure before starting and during the procedure.			
• Protected the person's rights during the procedure.			
• Handled the person gently during the procedure.			

Preprocedure

Preprocedure	S	U	Comments
1. Followed *Delegation Guidelines: Purpose of Oral Hygiene*. Saw *Promoting Safety and Comfort*:			
a. *Purpose of Oral Hygiene*			
b. *Denture Care*			
2. Practiced hand hygiene and got the following supplies:			
• Denture brush			
• Denture cup and lid labeled with the person's name and room and bed number			
• Denture cleaning agent			
• Denture adhesive as noted in the care plan (if needed)			
• Mouthwash (or other noted solution)			
• Kidney basin			
• Two hand towels			
• Gauze squares			
• Sponge swabs			
• Towel or paper towels (as a barrier for supplies)			
• Gloves			
• Laundry bag			
3. Arranged items in the person's room and near the sink.			
a. Placed a barrier (towel, paper towels) on the over-bed table. Arranged items needed at the bedside on top—gloves, hand towel, gauze squares, kidney basin, mouthwash (or other solution), denture adhesive (if needed).			
b. Placed a barrier (towel, paper towels) on the counter near the sink. Arranged needed items on top—denture cup and lid, hand towel, denture brush, denture cleaning agent.			
4. Practiced hand hygiene.			
5. Identified the person. Checked the ID (identification) bracelet against the assignment sheet. Used two identifiers. Also called the person by name.			
6. Provided for privacy.			

Procedure

Procedure	S	U	Comments
7. Positioned the person for oral hygiene (sitting up in bed or at the sink). (For this procedure, the person was in bed.) Placed the towel over the person's chest.			
8. Had the person practice hand hygiene if they were handling dentures. Practiced hand hygiene. Put on gloves.			
9. Had the person remove the dentures and placed them in the kidney basin (if able).			

Procedure—cont'd	S	U	Comments
10. Removed the dentures if the person could not do so. Used gauze squares to get a good grip on the slippery dentures.			
a. Grasped the upper denture with your thumb and index finger. Moved it up and down slightly to break the seal. Gently removed the denture. Placed it in the kidney basin.			
b. Grasped and removed the lower denture with your thumb and index finger. Turned it slightly and lifted it out of the person's mouth. Placed it in the kidney basin.			
11. Took the kidney basin with dentures to the sink.			
12. Rinsed the denture cup and lid.			
13. Lined the bottom of the sink with a towel. Did not use paper towels. Filled the sink halfway with water.			
14. Rinsed each denture under cool or warm running water. Followed center policy for water temperature.			
15. Returned dentures to the kidney basin.			
16. Applied denture cleaning agent to the brush.			
17. Brushed each denture. Brushed the inner, outer, and chewing surfaces and all surfaces that touched the gums.			
18. Rinsed the dentures under running water. Used warm or cool water as directed by the cleaning agent manufacturer.			
19. Placed dentures in the denture cup. Covered the dentures with cool or warm water. Followed center policy for water temperature. Closed the lid tightly.			
20. *If dentures were not worn*, stored them in a safe place. Followed agency policy and the person's preference for where to store dentures. Dentures were placed in water or in a denture soaking solution.			
21. Rinsed the kidney basin. Took the kidney basin to the over-bed table. Took the denture cup if dentures were worn.			
22. Used moistened gauze or sponge swabs to clean the gums, tongue, roof of the mouth, and inside the cheeks. Had the person use mouthwash (or noted solution). Held the kidney basin under the chin. Wiped the person's mouth.			
23. If dentures were worn:			
a. Applied denture adhesive if used. Some products were applied to wet dentures. Others were applied to dry dentures. Followed the manufacturer's instructions for how to apply and the amount to use.			
b. Had the person insert the dentures. Inserted them if the person could not.			
1) Held the upper denture firmly with your thumb and index finger. Raised the upper lip with the other hand. Inserted the denture. Gently pressed on the denture with your index finger to make sure it was in place.			
2) Held the lower denture with your thumb and index finger. Pulled the lower lip down slightly. Inserted the denture. Gently pressed down on it to make sure it was in place.			
24. Wiped the person's mouth if needed. Removed the towel. Placed it in the laundry bag.			
25. Removed and discarded the gloves. Practiced hand hygiene.			

Postprocedure

26. Provided for comfort. ______ ______ ______
27. Made sure the bed was at a safe and comfortable level. Followed the care plan. ______ ______ ______
28. Raised or lowered bed rails. Followed the care plan. ______ ______ ______
29. Drained the sink. ______ ______ ______
30. Cleaned up and stored supplies and equipment. (Wear gloves.)
    a. Discarded disposable items. ______ ______ ______
    b. Rinsed the brush. Emptied and rinsed the denture cup if dentures are worn. Returned them to their proper place. ______ ______ ______
    c. Followed agency procedures to clean and disinfect reusable equipment. Returned supplies and equipment to their proper place. ______ ______ ______
    d. Cleaned and dried the over-bed table. Dried with paper towels. Discarded paper towels. Positioned the over-bed table as the person preferred. ______ ______ ______
    e. Removed the towel from the sink. Squeezed to remove excess water. Placed the towel in the laundry bag.
    f. Followed center policy for used linens. ______ ______ ______
    g. Removed and discarded gloves. Practiced hand hygiene. ______ ______ ______
31. Placed the call light and other needed items within reach. ______ ______ ______
32. Followed the care plan and the person's preferences for privacy measures to maintain. Leaving the privacy curtain, window coverings, and door open or closed were examples. ______ ______ ______
33. Completed a safety check of the room. ______ ______ ______
34. Practiced hand hygiene. ______ ______ ______
35. Reported and recorded your care and observations. ______ ______ ______

Giving a Complete Bed Bath

NATCEP™ VIDEO VIDEO CLIP

Name: ______________________ Date: ______________________

Quality of Life	S	U	Comments
• Knocked before entering the person's room.			
• Addressed the person by name.			
• Introduced yourself by name and title.			
• Explained the procedure before starting and during the procedure.			
• Protected the person's rights during the procedure.			
• Handled the person gently during the procedure.			

Preprocedure	S	U	Comments
1. Followed *Delegation Guidelines*: *Bathing*.			
Saw *Promoting Safety and Comfort*:			
a. *Daily Hygiene and Bathing*			
b. *Bathing*			
2. Practiced hand hygiene.			
3. Identified the person. Checked the identification (ID) bracelet against the assignment sheet. Used two identifiers. Also called the person by name.			
4. Collected clean linens. Placed linens on a clean surface.			
5. Got the following supplies:			
• Wash basin (if available, a second basin could be used—one for washing and one for rinsing)			
• Soap or bodywash			
• Water thermometer			
• Orangewood stick or nail file			
• Washcloth one or more for washing and rinsing (some state competency tests specify a clean, "soap-free" washcloth for rinsing) and at least four washcloths for perineal care			
• Towels—at least one hand towel, two bath towels, a separate towel for perineal care			
• Bath blanket			
• Clothing or sleepwear			
• Skin care products (as needed)—lotion, powder, deodorant (antiperspirant)			
• Brush and comb			
• Other grooming items as requested			
• Towel or paper towels (as a barrier for supplies)			
• Gloves			
• Laundry bag			
6. Placed a barrier (towel, paper towels) on the over-bed table. Arranged items on the over-bed table. Adjusted the height as needed.			
7. Provided for privacy.			
8. Raised the bed for body mechanics. Bed rails were up if used. Lowered the bed rail near you if up.			

Procedure

9. Covered the person with a bath blanket. Removed top linens.
10. Removed the sleepwear. Did not expose the person. Followed agency policy for used clothing or sleepwear. (Wore gloves if clothing was wet or soiled. Practiced hand hygiene after removing and discarding gloves.)
11. Filled the wash basin ⅔ (two-thirds) full with water. (Followed the care plan for bed rail use. Raised the rail if used. Lowered the bed to a safe level.) Followed the care plan for water temperature. Water temperature is usually 110°F to 115°F (43.3°C–46.1°C) for adults. Measured water temperature. Used the water thermometer. Or dipped your elbow or inner wrist into the basin to test the water.
12. Asked the person to check the water temperature. Adjusted the water temperature as needed
13. Placed the basin on the over-bed table.
14. Raised the bed for body mechanics. Lowered the bed rail near you if up.
15. Lowered the head of the bed. It was as flat as possible. The person had at least one pillow.
16. Practiced hand hygiene. Put on gloves.
17. Placed a hand towel over the person's chest.
18. Made a mitt with the washcloth. Used a mitt for the entire bath. (NOTE: Some state competency tests require that the corners of the washcloth be contained during bathing. This was one method.)
19. Had the person close the eyes. Washed the eyelids and around the eyes with water. Did not use soap.
    a. Cleaned the far eye. Gently wiped from the inner to the outer aspect of the eye with a corner of the mitt.
    b. Cleaned around the eye near you. Used a clean part of the washcloth for each stroke.
20. Washed, rinsed, and dried the face, ears, and neck.
    a. Asked if the person wanted soap or bodywash used on the face. If so, applied soap or bodywash to the washcloth. If not, just used water. Washed the face and ears.
    b. Washed the neck using soap or bodywash.
    c. Rinsed all areas. Used a soap-free washcloth.
    d. Patted dry with the towel on the chest.
21. Help the person move to the side of the bed near you.
22. Washed, rinsed, and dried the far arm.
    a. Exposed the arm. Placed a bath towel lengthwise under the arm.
    b. Applied soap or bodywash to the washcloth.
    c. Supported the arm with your palm under the person's elbow. The person's forearm rested on your forearm.
    d. Washed the arm, shoulder, and underarm. Used long, firm strokes
    e. Rinsed all areas.
    f. Patted dry. Dried well under the underarm.
23. Washed, rinsed, and dried the far hand.
    a. Method 1—Placed the basin on the towel. Put the person's hand into the water. Had the person exercise the hand and fingers. Washed the hand well. Removed the basin.

Procedure—cont'd	S	U	Comments
b. Method 2—Applied soap or bodywash to the washcloth. Washed the hand well.			
c. Cleaned under the nails if nail care was done during the bath. Or performed nail care separately. Used an orangewood stick or nail file.			
d. Rinsed the hand. Used a soap-free washcloth.			
e. Patted dry.			
f. Removed the towel under the arm. Covered the arm with the bath blanket.			
24. Repeated steps for near arm and hand. Washed, rinsed, and dried the near arm.			
a. Exposed the arm. Placed a bath towel lengthwise under the arm.			
b. Applied soap or bodywash to the washcloth.			
c. Supported the arm with your palm under the person's elbow. The person's forearm rested on your forearm.			
d. Washed the arm, shoulder, and underarm. Used long, firm strokes.			
e. Rinsed all areas.			
f. Patted dry. Dried well under the underarm.			
25. Washed, rinsed, and dried the near hand.			
a. Method 1—Placed the basin on the towel. Put the person's hand into the water. Had the person exercise the hand and fingers. Washed the hand well. Removed the basin.			
b. Method 2—Applied soap or bodywash to the washcloth. Washed the hand well.			
c. Cleaned under the nails if nail care was done during the bath. Or performed nail care separately. Used an orangewood stick or nail file.			
d. Rinsed the hand. Used a soap-free washcloth.			
e. Patted dry.			
f. Removed the towel under the arm. Covered the arm with the bath blanket.			
26. Washed, rinsed, and dried the chest.			
a. Placed a bath towel over the chest crosswise. Held the towel in place. Pulled the bath blanket from under the towel to the waist.			
b. Applied soap or bodywash to the washcloth.			
c. Lifted the towel slightly and washed the chest. Did not expose the person.			
d. Rinsed the chest. Used a soap-free washcloth.			
e. Patted dry. Dried well under breasts.			
27. Washed, rinsed, and dried the abdomen.			
a. Moved the towel lengthwise over the chest and abdomen. Did not expose the person. Pulled the bath blanket down to the pubic area.			
b. Applied soap or bodywash to the washcloth.			
c. Lifted the towel slightly and wash the abdomen.			
d. Rinsed the abdomen. Used a soap-free washcloth.			
e. Patted dry. Dried well under abdominal skin folds.			
28. Pulled the bath blanket up to the shoulders. Covered both arms. Removed the towel.			
29. Changed soapy or cool water as needed. Followed these safety measures.			
a. Raised the bed rail if used. Lowered the bed to a safe level.			

Procedure—cont'd	S	U	Comments
b. Measured bath water temperature. Followed the care plan for water temperature. Water temperature is usually 110°F to 115°F (43.3°C–46.1°C) for adults. Measured water temperature. Used the water thermometer. Or dipped your elbow or inner wrist into the basin to test the water. Had the person check the water temperature.	______	______	______
c. Raised the bed for body mechanics and lower the bed rail if used when you return.	______	______	______
30. Washed, rinsed, and dried the far leg.	______	______	______
a. Uncovered the far leg. Did not expose the genital area. Placed a towel lengthwise under the foot and leg.	______	______	______
b. Applied soap or bodywash to a washcloth.	______	______	______
c. Bent the knee and supported the leg with your arm. Washed it with long, firm strokes. Washed the skin fold area of the groin.	______	______	______
d. Rinsed the leg. Used a soap-free washcloth.	______	______	______
e. Patted dry. Dried the groin area well.	______	______	______
31. Washed, rinsed, and dried the far foot.	______	______	
a. Method 1—Placed the basin on the towel near the foot. Bent the knee and lifted the leg slightly. Slid the basin under the foot. Placed the foot in the basin. Washed the foot well. Carefully separated the toes. Removed the basin.	______	______	______
b. Method 2—Applied soap or bodywash to the washcloth. Washed the foot well. Carefully separated the toes.	______	______	______
c. Cleaned under the nails if instructed to do so and if nail care was done during the bath. Or performed nail care separately. Used an orangewood stick or nail file.	______	______	______
d. Rinsed the foot. Used a soap-free washcloth.	______	______	______
e. Patted dry. Dried well between the toes.	______	______	______
f. Applied lotion to the foot if directed by the nurse and the care plan. Did not apply lotion between the toes.	______	______	______
g. Covered the leg with the bath blanket. Removed the towel.	______	______	______
32. Repeated steps for the near leg and foot. Washed, rinsed, and dried the far leg.	______	______	______
a. Uncovered the far leg. Did not expose the genital area. Placed a towel lengthwise under the foot and leg.	______	______	______
b. Applied soap or bodywash to a washcloth.	______	______	______
c. Bent the knee and supported the leg with your arm. Washed it with long, firm strokes. Washed the skin fold area of the groin.	______	______	______
d. Rinsed the leg. Used a soap-free washcloth.	______	______	______
e. Patted dry. Dried the groin area well.	______	______	______
33. Washed, rinsed, and dried the near foot.	______	______	______
a. Method 1—Placed the basin on the towel near the foot. Bent the knee and lifted the leg slightly. Slid the basin under the foot. Placed the foot in the basin. Washed the foot well. Carefully separated the toes. Removed the basin.	______	______	______
b. Method 2—Applied soap or bodywash to the washcloth. Washed the foot well. Carefully separated the toes.	______	______	______

Procedure—cont'd	S	U	Comments
c. Cleaned under the nails if instructed to do so and if nail care was done during the bath. Or performed nail care separately. Used an orangewood stick or nail file.	_____	_____	_____
d. Rinsed the foot. Used a soap-free washcloth.	_____	_____	_____
e. Patted dry. Dried well between the toes.	_____	_____	_____
f. Applied lotion to the foot if directed by the nurse and the care plan. Did not apply lotion between the toes.	_____	_____	_____
g. Covered the leg with the bath blanket. Removed the towel.	_____	_____	_____
34. Changed the water. Followed these safety measures.	_____	_____	_____
a. Raised the bed rail if used. Lowered the bed to a safe level.	_____	_____	_____
b. Measured bath water temperature. Followed the care plan for water temperature. Water temperature is usually 110°F to 115°F (43.3°C–46.1°C) for adults. Measured water temperature. Used the water thermometer. Or dipped your elbow or inner wrist into the basin to test the water. Had the person check the water temperature.	_____	_____	_____
c. Raised the bed for body mechanics and lower the bed rail if used when you return.	_____	_____	_____
35. Washed, rinsed, and dried the back and buttocks.	_____	_____	_____
a. Turned the person onto the side away from you. The person was covered with the bath blanket.	_____	_____	_____
b. Uncovered the back and buttocks. Did not expose the person. Placed a towel lengthwise on the bed along the back.	_____	_____	_____
c. Applied soap or bodywash to a washcloth.	_____	_____	_____
d. Washed the back. Worked from the back of the neck to the lower end of the buttocks. Used long, firm, continuous strokes.	_____	_____	_____
e. Rinsed the back and buttocks. Used a soap-free washcloth.	_____	_____	_____
f. Patted dry.	_____	_____	_____
36. Placed used washcloths and towels in the laundry bag.	_____	_____	_____
37. Turned the person onto the back.	_____	_____	_____
38. Washed, rinsed, and dried the genital and anal areas.	_____	_____	_____
a. Changed the water. Followed the safety measures and the care plan for water temperature. Raised the bed rail if used. Lowered the bed to a safe level. Water temperature for perineal care is lower [usually 105°F–109°F (40.5°C–42.7°C)]. Measured water temperature. Used the water thermometer. Or dipped your elbow or inner wrist into the basin to test the water. Had the person check the water temperature.	_____	_____	_____
b. Allowed the person to clean the genital and anal areas if able. If the person could not do so, performed perineal care with clean gloves. At least four washcloths and a clean towel were needed. Placed each washcloth in the laundry bag after one use. Washcloths were not reused for perineal care.	_____	_____	_____
39. Removed and discarded the gloves. Practiced hand hygiene.	_____	_____	_____
40. Gave a back massage.	_____	_____	_____

Procedure—cont'd	S	U	Comments
41. Applied lotion, powder, deodorant, or antiperspirant as requested. Safely applied powder.			
42. Put clean garments on the person.			
43. Combed and brushed the hair.			
44. Made the bed. Removed the bath blanket and placed it in the laundry bag.			

Postprocedure

	S	U	Comments
45. Provided for comfort.			
46. Lowered the bed to a safe and comfortable level.			
Raised or lowered bed rails. Followed the care plan.			
47. Cleaned up and stored supplies and equipment. (Wore gloves.)			
a. Discarded disposable items.			
b. Emptied the wash basin.			
c. Followed agency procedures to clean and disinfect reusable equipment. Returned supplies and equipment to their proper place.			
d. Followed center policy for used linens.			
e. Cleaned and dried the over-bed table. Dried with paper towels. Discarded paper towels. Positioned the over-bed table as the person preferred.			
f. Removed and discarded gloves. Practiced hand hygiene.			
48. Placed the call light and other needed items within reach.			
49. Followed the care plan and the person's preferences for privacy measures to maintain. Leaving the privacy curtain, window coverings, and door open or closed were examples.			
50. Completed a safety check of the room.			
51. Practiced hand hygiene.			
52. Reported and recorded your care and observations.			

NATCEP™ VIDEO

Assisting With the Partial Bath

Name: ______________________ Date: ______________________

Quality of Life	S	U	Comments
• Knocked before entering the person's room.	____	____	____
• Addressed the person by name.	____	____	____
• Introduced yourself by name and title.	____	____	____
• Explained the procedure before starting and during the procedure.	____	____	____
• Protected the person's rights during the procedure.	____	____	____
• Handled the person gently during the procedure.	____	____	____

Preprocedure

1. Followed *Delegation Guidelines: Bathing*. Saw *Promoting Safety and Comfort*:			
a. *Daily Hygiene and Bathing*	____	____	____
b. *Bathing*	____	____	____
2. Practiced hand hygiene.	____	____	____
3. Identified the person. Checked the identification (ID) bracelet against the assignment sheet. Used two identifiers. Also called the person by name.	____	____	____
4. Collected clean linens. Placed linens on a clean surface.	____	____	____
5. Got the following supplies:			
• Wash basin (if available, a second basin could be used—one for washing and one for rinsing)	____	____	____
• Soap or bodywash	____	____	____
• Water thermometer	____	____	____
• Orangewood stick or nail file	____	____	____
• Washcloth one or more for washing and rinsing (some state competency tests specify a clean, "soap-free" washcloth for rinsing) and at least four washcloths for perineal care	____	____	____
• Towels—at least one hand towel, two bath towels, a separate towel for perineal care	____	____	____
• Bath blanket	____	____	____
• Clothing or sleepwear	____	____	____
• Skin care products (as needed)—lotion, powder, deodorant (antiperspirant)	____	____	____
• Brush and comb	____	____	____
• Other grooming items as requested	____	____	____
• Towel or paper towels (as a barrier for supplies)	____	____	____
• Gloves	____	____	____
• Laundry bag	____	____	____
6. Placed a barrier (towel, paper towels) on the over-bed table. Arranged items on the over-bed table. Adjusted the height as needed.	____	____	____
7. Provided for privacy.	____	____	____

Procedure

8. Made sure the bed was in the lowest position.	____	____	____
9. Covered the person with a bath blanket. Removed top linens.	____	____	____
10. Filled the wash basin 2⁄3 (two-thirds) full with water. Water temperature was 110°F to 115°F (43.3°C–46.1°C) or as directed by the nurse. Measured water temperature with the water thermometer. Or tested bath water by dipping your elbow or inner wrist into the basin.	____	____	____

Procedure—cont'd	S	U	Comments
11. Asked the person to check the water temperature. Adjusted the water temperature as needed.			
12. Placed the basin on the over-bed table.			
13. Positioned the person in Fowler's position or seated at the bedside.			
14. Adjusted the over-bed table so the person could reach the basin and supplies.			
15. Helped the person undress. (Wore gloves if clothing was wet or soiled. Practiced hand hygiene after removing and discarding gloves.) Used the bath blanket for privacy and warmth.			
16. Had the person wash easy-to-reach body parts. Explained that you would wash the back and areas the person could not reach.			
17. Ensured that the call light was within reach. Asked the person to signal when help was needed or bathing was completed.			
18. Practiced hand hygiene. Then left the room.			
19. Returned when the call light was on. Knocked before entering. Practiced hand hygiene.			
20. Washed and dried areas the person could not reach.			
a. Changed the bath water. Measured bath water temperature. Water temperature is usually 110°F to 115°F (43.3°C–46.1°C) or as directed by the nurse. Measured water temperature with the water thermometer. Or tested bath water by dipping your elbow or inner wrist into the basin. Had the person check the water temperature.			
b. Raised the bed for body mechanics. The far bed rail was up if used.			
c. Put on gloves.			
d. Asked what was washed. Washed and dried areas the person could not reach. The face, hands, underarms, back, buttocks, and perineal area were washed for the partial bath.			
21. Placed used washcloths and towels in the laundry bag.			
22. Removed and discarded the gloves. Practiced hand hygiene.			
23. Gave a back massage.			
24. Applied lotion, powder, and deodorant or antiperspirant as requested.			
25. Helped the person put on clean garments			
26. Assisted with hair care and other grooming needs.			
27. Made the bed. Remove the bath blanket and placed it in the laundry bag.			

Postprocedure

	S	U	Comments
28. Provided for comfort.			
29. Lowered the bed to a safe and comfortable level.			
Raised or lowered bed rails. Followed the care plan.			
30. Cleaned up and stored supplies and equipment. (Wore gloves.)			
a. Discarded disposable items.			
b. Emptied the wash basin.			
c. Followed agency procedures to clean and disinfected reusable equipment. Returned supplies and equipment to their proper place.			
d. Followed center policy for used linens.			

Postprocedure—cont'd	S	U	Comments
e. Cleaned and dried the over-bed table. Dried with paper towels. Discarded paper towels. Positioned the over-bed table as the person preferred.			
f. Removed and discarded gloves. Practiced hand hygiene.			
32. Placed the call light and other needed items within reach.			
33. Followed the care plan and the person's preferences for privacy measures to maintain. Leaving the privacy curtain, window coverings, and door open or closed were examples.			
34. Completed a safety check of the room.			
35. Practiced hand hygiene.			
36. Reported and recorded your care and observations.			

NATCEP™ VIDEO VIDEO CLIP

Assisting With a Tub Bath or Shower

Name: ______________________ Date: ______________________

Quality of Life	S	U	Comments
• Knocked before entering the person's room.			
• Addressed the person by name.			
• Introduced yourself by name and title.			
• Explained the procedure before starting and during the procedure.			
• Protected the person's rights during the procedure.			
• Handled the person gently during the procedure.			

Preprocedure

	S	U	Comments
1. Followed *Delegation Guidelines*:			
a. *Bathing*			
b. *Tub Baths and Showers*			
Saw *Promoting Safety and Comfort*:			
a. *Daily Hygiene and Bathing*			
b. *Bathing*			
c. *Tub Baths and Showers*			
2. Reserved the tub or shower room.			
3. Practiced hand hygiene.			
4. Identified the person. Checked the identification (ID) bracelet against the assignment sheet. Used two identifiers. Also called the person by name.			
5. Got the following supplies:			
• Washcloth—at least one for bathing or showering and washcloths for perineal care			
• Bath towels—at least two			
• Bath blanket			
• Soap or bodywash			
• Water thermometer (for tub bath)			
• Clothing or sleepwear			
• Grooming items as requested			
• Robe and slip-resistant footwear			
• Rubber bath mat if needed			
• Disposable bath mat if needed			
• Gloves			
• Laundry bag			
• Wheelchair, shower chair, shower bench, and so on as needed			

Procedure

	S	U	Comments
6. Placed items in the tub or shower room. Used the space provided or a chair.			
7. Followed agency procedures to clean and disinfect the tub or shower and shared equipment (e.g., a shower chair). (Wore gloves for this step. Practiced hand hygiene after removing and discarding the gloves.)			
8. Placed a rubber bath mat in the tub or on the shower floor. Did not block the drain.			
9. Placed the disposable bath mat on the floor in front of the tub or shower.			
10. Placed the occupied sign on the door.			
11. Returned to the person's room. Provided for privacy. Practiced hand hygiene.			
12. Helped the person sit on the side of the bed.			

Procedure—cont'd	S	U	Comments
13. Helped the person put on a robe and slip-resistant footwear. Or the person left clothing on.			
14. Assisted or transported the person to the tub or shower room.			
15. Had the person sit on a chair if they walked to the tub or shower room.			
16. Provided for privacy.			
17. *For a tub bath*:			
a. Filled the tub halfway with warm water (usually 105°F; 40.5°C). Followed the care plan for water temperature.			
b. Measured water temperature. Used the water thermometer or checked the digital display.			
c. Asked the person to check the water temperature. Adjusted the water temperature as needed.			
18. *For a shower*:			
a. Turned on the shower.			
b. Adjusted water temperature and pressure. Checked the digital display. Water temperature is usually 105°F; 40.5°C.			
c. Asked the person to check the water temperature. Adjusted the water temperature as needed.			
19. Helped the person undress and remove footwear.			
20. Helped the person into the tub or shower. Positioned the shower chair and locked (braked) the wheels.			
21. Assisted with washing as necessary. Wore gloves.			
a. Washed the face, neck, arms, hands, chest, abdomen, legs, feet, back, and buttocks.			
b. Provided perineal care if the person was unable to do it. Wore clean gloves and used clean washcloths. Removed and discarded gloves. Practiced hand hygiene.			
c. Followed the care plan and the person's preferences for shampooing hair. Assisted with shampooing as needed.			
22. Had the person use the call light when done or when help was needed. Reminded the person that a tub bath lasts no longer than 20 minutes.			
23. Placed a towel across the chair.			
24. Stayed in the room or nearby if the person could be left alone. Checked on the person at least every 5 minutes.			
25. Responded when the person signaled for you.			
26. Turned off the shower or drained the tub. Covered the person with the bath blanket while the tub drained.			
27. Helped the person out of the shower or tub and onto a chair.			
28. Helped the person dry off. Patted gently. Dried well under the breasts, between skin folds, between the toes, and in the perineal area.			
29. Place used washcloths and towels in the laundry bag.			
30. Applied lotion, powder, and deodorant or antiperspirant as requested.			

Procedure—cont'd	S	U	Comments
31. Helped the person dress and put on footwear. Placed the bath blanket in the laundry bag.	______	______	______
32. Practiced hand hygiene.	______	______	______
33. Helped the person return to the room. Provided for privacy.	______	______	______
34. Assisted the person to a chair or into bed.	______	______	______
35. Provided a back massage if the person returned to bed.	______	______	______
36. Assisted with hair care and other grooming needs.	______	______	______

Postprocedure

37. Provided for comfort.	______	______	______
38. Make sure the bed is at a safe and comfortable level. Followed the care plan.	______	______	______
39. Raised or lowered bed rails. Followed the care plan.	______	______	______
40. Placed the call light and other needed items within reach.	______	______	______
41. Followed the care plan and the person's preferences for privacy measures to maintain. Leaving the privacy curtain, window coverings, and door open or closed were examples.	______	______	______
42. Completed a safety check of the room.	______	______	______
43. Practiced hand hygiene. Returned to the tub or shower room.	______	______	______
44. Cleaned up and stored supplies and equipment. (Wore gloves.)	______	______	______
a. Discarded disposable items.	______	______	______
b. Followed agency procedures to clean and disinfected the tub or shower and shared equipment. Returned supplies and equipment to their proper place.	______	______	______
c. Followed center policy for used linens.	______	______	______
d. Removed and discarded gloves. Practiced hand hygiene.	______	______	______
45. Put the unoccupied sign on the door.	______	______	______
46. Practiced hand hygiene.	______	______	______
47. Reported and recorded your care and observations.	______	______	______

Giving Female Perineal Care

Name: ______________________ Date: ______________________

Quality of Life	S	U	Comments
• Knocked before entering the person's room.			
• Addressed the person by name.			
• Introduced yourself by name and title.			
• Explained the procedure before starting and during the procedure.			
• Protected the person's rights during the procedure.			
• Handled the person gently during the procedure.			
Preprocedure			
1. Followed *Delegation Guidelines: Perineal Care.*			
Saw *Promoting Safety and Comfort:* a. *Daily Hygiene and Bathing*			
b. *Perineal Care*			
2. Practiced hand hygiene and got the following supplies:			
• Soap, bodywash, or other cleaning agent as directed			
• At least four washcloths			
• Bath towel			
• Bath blanket			
• Water thermometer			
• Wash basin			
• Waterproof underpad			
• Gloves			
• Laundry bag			
• Towel or paper towels (as a barrier for supplies)			
3. Placed the barrier (towel, paper towels) on the over-bed table. Arranged items on top.			
4. Practiced hand hygiene.			
5. Identified the person. Checked the identification (ID) bracelet against the assignment sheet. Used two identifiers. Also called the person by name.			
6. Provided for privacy.			
7. Raised the bed for body mechanics. Bed rails were up if used. Lowered the bed rail near you if up.			
Procedure			
8. Positioned the person on the back			
9. Covered the person with a bath blanket. Moved top linens to the foot of the bed.			
10. Draped the person.			
11. Raised the bed rail if used. Lowered the bed to a safe level.			
12. Filled the wash basin. Water temperature was 105°F to 109°F (40.5°C–42.7°C). Followed the care plan for water temperature. Measured water temperature according to agency policy. Had the person check the water temperature. Adjusted the water temperature as needed.			
13. Placed the basin on the over-bed table.			
14. Raised the bed for body mechanics. Lowered the bed rail if up.			
15. Practiced hand hygiene. Put on gloves.			

Procedure—cont'd	S	U	Comments
16. Placed a waterproof underpad under the buttocks. Had the person raise the hips or turn from side to side. Positioned the person on the back.			
17. Helped the person to bed the knees and spread the legs. Or helped the person to spread the legs as much as possible with the knees straight.			
18. Folded the corner of the bath blanket between the legs onto the abdomen.			
19. Wet the washcloths.			
20. Squeezed out water from a washcloth. Made a mitted washcloth. Applied soap, bodywash, or other cleansing agent. (Squeezed out excess water every time you changed washcloths. Put used washcloths in the laundry bag. *Did not place used washcloths back in the basin.*)			
21. Cleaned the perineum. Changed washcloths as needed.			
a. Separated the labia.			
b. Cleaned one side of the labia. Cleaned downward from front to back (top to bottom) with 1 stroke. Used one part of a washcloth.			
c. Cleaned the other side of the labia. Cleaned downward from front to back (top to bottom) with one stroke. Used a clean part of a washcloth.			
d. Cleaned the vaginal area. Cleaned downward from front to back (top to bottom) with one stroke. Used a clean part of a washcloth.			
22. Rinsed the perineum using a clean washcloth. Changed washcloths as needed.			
a. Separated the labia.			
b. Rinsed one side of the labia. Rinsed downward from front to back (top to bottom) with one stroke. Used one part of a washcloth.			
c. Rinsed the other side of the labia. Rinsed downward from front to back (top to bottom) with one stroke. Used a clean part of a washcloth.			
d. Rinsed the vaginal area. Rinsed downward front to back (top to bottom) with one stroke. Used a clean part of a washcloth.			
23. Patted the perineal area dry with the towel. Dried from front to back.			
24. Folded the blanket back between the legs.			
25. Helped the person lower the legs and turn onto the side away from you.			
26. Applied soap, bodywash, or other cleansing agent to a clean mitted washcloth.			
27. Cleaned and rinsed the rectal area.			
a. Cleaned from the vagina to the anus with one stroke. Used one part of the washcloth.			
b. Repeated and applied soap, bodywash, or other cleansing agent to a clean mitted washcloth. Cleaned the rectal area, until the area was clean. Used a clean part of the washcloth for each stroke. Changed washcloths as needed.			
c. Rinsed the rectal area with a clean washcloth. Rinsed from the vagina to the anus. Repeated as necessary. Used a clean part of the washcloth for each stroke. Changed washcloths as needed.			

Procedure—cont'd	S	U	Comments
28. Patted the rectal area dry with the towel. Dried from the vagina to the anus. Placed the towel in the laundry bag.			
29. Folded and tucked the waterproof underpad under the person. The wet side was inside. Had the person turn toward you or lay on the back and lift the buttocks. Removed the waterproof underpad. Placed it in the laundry bag. Positioned the person on the back. Person was covered with bath blanket.			
30. Removed and discarded the gloves. Practiced hand hygiene.			
31. Applied clean and dry garments and linens as needed. Removed the bath blanket. Placed it in the laundry bag.			
32. Positioned the person for comfort.			

Postprocedure

33. Provided for comfort.			
34. Lowered the bed to a safe and comfortable level.			
Raised or lowered bed rails. Followed the care plan.			
35. Cleaned up and stored supplies and equipment. (Wore gloves.)			
a. Discarded disposable items.			
b. Emptied the wash basin.			
c. Followed agency procedures to clean and disinfect reusable equipment. Returned supplies and equipment to their proper place.			
d. Followed agency policy for used linens.			
e. Cleaned and dried the over-bed table. Dried with paper towels. Discarded paper towels. Positioned the over-bed table as the person preferred.			
f. Removed and discarded gloves. Practiced hand hygiene.			
36. Placed the call light and other needed items within reach.			
37. Followed the care plan and the person's preferences for privacy measures to maintain. Leaving the privacy curtain, window coverings, and door open or closed were examples.			
38. Completed a safety check of the room.			
39. Practiced hand hygiene.			
40. Reported and recorded your care and observations.			

NATCEP™ VIDEO VIDEO CLIP

Giving Male Perineal Care

Name: ______________________ Date: ______________________

Quality of Life	S	U	Comments
• Knocked before entering the person's room.			
• Addressed the person by name.			
• Introduced yourself by name and title.			
• Explained the procedure before starting and during the procedure.			
• Protected the person's rights during the procedure.			
• Handled the person gently during the procedure.			
Preprocedure			
1. Followed *Delegation Guidelines: Perineal Care.*			
Saw *Promoting Safety and Comfort*: a. *Daily Hygiene and Bathing*			
b. *Perineal Care*			
2. Practiced hand hygiene and got the following supplies:			
• Soap, bodywash, or other cleaning agent as directed			
• At least four washcloths			
• Bath towel			
• Bath blanket			
• Water thermometer			
• Wash basin			
• Waterproof underpad			
• Gloves			
• Laundry bag			
• Towel or paper towels (as a barrier for supplies)			
3. Placed the barrier (towel, paper towels) on the over-bed table. Arranged items on top.			
4. Practiced hand hygiene.			
5. Identified the person. Checked the identification (ID) bracelet against the assignment sheet. Used two identifiers. Also called the person by name.			
6. Provided for privacy.			
7. Raised the bed for body mechanics. Bed rails were up if used. Lowered the bed rail near you if up.			
Procedure			
8. Positioned the person on the back.			
9. Covered the person with a bath blanket. Moved top linens to the foot of the bed.			
10. Draped the person.			
11. Raised the bed rail if used. Lowered the bed to a safe level.			
12. Filled the wash basin. Water temperature was 105°F to 109°F (40.5°C–42.7°C). Followed the care plan for water temperature. Measured water temperature according to agency policy. Had the person check the water temperature. Adjusted the water temperature as needed.			
13. Placed the basin on the over-bed table.			
14. Raised the bed for body mechanics. Lowered the bed rail if up.			
15. Practiced hand hygiene. Put on gloves.			

Procedure—cont'd	S	U	Comments
16. Placed a waterproof underpad under the buttocks. Had the person raise the hips or turn from side to side. Positioned the person on the back.			
17. Folded the corner of the bath blanket between the legs onto the person's abdomen.			
18. Wetted the washcloths.			
19. Squeezed out water from a washcloth. Made a mitted washcloth. Applied soap. (Squeezed out water every time you changed washcloths. Did not place used washcloths back in the basin. Put used washcloths in the laundry bag.)			
20. Grasped the penis.			
21. Retracted the foreskin if the person was uncircumcised.			
22. Cleaned the tip. Started at the meatus. Used a circular motion. Repeated as needed. Used a clean part of the washcloth each time.			
23. Rinsed the tip with another washcloth. Used the same circular motion.			
24. Dried the tip (uncircumcised). Returned the foreskin to its natural position.			
25. Cleaned the shaft of the penis. Used firm downward strokes. Used a clean part of a washcloth for each stoke.			
26. Rinsed the shaft. Used firm downward strokes. Used a clean part of a washcloth for each stoke.			
27. Helped the person bend the knees and spread the legs. Or helped him spread the legs as much as possible with the knees straight.			
28. Cleaned the scrotum. Used a clean part of a washcloth.			
29. Rinsed the scrotum. Used a clean part of a washcloth. Observed for redness and irritation of the skin folds.			
30. Patted dry the penis and the scrotum. Used the towel.			
31. Folded the bath blanket back over the legs.			
32. Helped the person lower the legs and turn onto the side away from you.			
33. Applied soap, bodywash, or other cleansing agent to a clean mitted washcloth. Cleaned the rectal area.			
34. Cleaned from the scrotum (front or top) to the anus (back or bottom). Used one part of the washcloth.			
35. Repeated until the area is clean. Used a clean part of the washcloth for each stroke. Changed washcloths as needed.			
36. Rinsed and dried well. Placed used washcloths and the towel in the laundry bag.			
37. Patted the rectal area dry with the towel. Place the towel in the laundry bag.			
38. Folded and tucked the waterproof underpad under the person. The wet side was inside. Had the person turn toward you or lay on the back and lift the buttocks. Removed the waterproof underpad. Placed it in the laundry bag. Positioned the person on the back.			
39. Removed and discarded the gloves. Practiced hand hygiene.			
40. Provided clean and dry garments and linens as needed. Removed the bath blanket. Placed it in the laundry bag.			
41. Positioned the person for comfort			

Postprocedure

38. Lowered the bed to a safe and comfortable level. Followed the care plan.
39. Raised or lowered bed rails. Followed the care plan.
40. Cleaned up and stored supplies and equipment. (Wore gloves.)
    a. Discarded disposable items.
    b. Emptied the wash basin.
    c. Followed agency procedures to clean and disinfect reusable equipment. Returned supplies and equipment to their proper place.
    d. Followed agency policy for used linens.
    e. Cleaned and dried the over-bed table. Dried with paper towels. Discarded paper towels. Positioned the over-bed table as the person preferred.
    f. Removed and discarded gloves. Practiced hand hygiene.
41. Placed the call light and other needed items within reach.
42. Followed the care plan and the person's preferences for privacy measures to maintain. Leaving the privacy curtain, window coverings, and door open or closed were examples.
43. Completed a safety check of the room.
44. Practiced hand hygiene.
45. Reported and recorded your care and observations.

NATCEP™ VIDEO VIDEO CLIP

Brushing and Combing Hair

Name: ______________________ Date: ______________________

Quality of Life	S	U	Comments
• Knocked before entering the person's room.			
• Addressed the person by name.			
• Introduced yourself by name and title.			
• Explained the procedure before starting and during the procedure.			
• Protected the person's rights during the procedure.			
• Handled the person gently during the procedure.			

Preprocedure

	S	U	Comments
1. Followed *Delegation Guidelines: Brushing and Combing Hair*. Saw *Promoting Safety and Comfort: Brushing and Combing Hair*.			
2. Practiced hand hygiene.			
3. Identified the person. Checked the ID (identification) bracelet against the assignment sheet. Used two identifiers. Also called the person by name.			
4. Asked the person how to style hair.			
5. Got the following supplies:			
• Comb and brush			
• Bath towel			
• Other hair care items as requested			
• Laundry bag			
6. Arranged items nearby.			
7. Provided for privacy.			

Procedure

	S	U	Comments
8. Positioned the person.			
a. *In a chair*—Helped the person to the chair. The person wore slip-resistant footwear for a transfer. Clothing properly covered the person. Or a robe was applied.			
b. *In bed*—Raised the bed for body mechanics. Bed rails were up if used. Lowered the bed rail near you. Assisted the person to a semi-Fowler's position if allowed.			
9. Placed a towel across the person's back and shoulders or across the pillow.			
10. Had the person remove eyeglasses. Put them in the eyeglass case. Put the case inside the bedside stand.			
11. *Hair that was not matted or tangled.*			
a. Used the comb to part the hair.			
1) Parted hair down the middle into two sides.			
2) Divided one side into two smaller sections.			
b. Brushed one of the small sections of hair. Started at the scalp and brushed toward the hair ends. Did the same for the other small section of hair. If the person preferred, brushed long hair starting at the hair ends.			
c. Repeated for the other side.			
1) Divided side into two smaller sections.			

Procedure—cont'd	S	U	Comments
2) Brushed one of the small sections of hair. Started at the scalp and brushed toward the hair ends. Did the same for the other small section of hair. If the person preferred, brushed long hair starting at the hair ends.	_____	_____	_____
12. *Matted or tangled hair.*			
a. Took a small section of hair near the ends. Held above the area to be combed or brushed.	_____	_____	_____
b. Combed or brushed through to the hair ends.	_____	_____	_____
c. Added small sections of hair as you worked up to the scalp.	_____	_____	_____
d. Combed or brushed through each longer section to the hair ends.	_____	_____	_____
13. Styled the hair as the person preferred.	_____	_____	_____
14. Removed the towel. Placed it in the laundry bag.	_____	_____	_____
15. Had the person put on eyeglasses, if worn.	_____	_____	_____

Postprocedure

	S	U	Comments
16. Provided for comfort.	_____	_____	_____
17. Lowered the bed to a safe and comfortable level.	_____	_____	_____
Raised or lowered bed rails. Followed the care plan.	_____	_____	_____
18. Cleaned up and stored supplies and equipment. (Wore gloves.)	_____	_____	_____
a. Removed hair from the brush or comb. Discarded hair.	_____	_____	_____
b. Followed agency procedures to clean equipment. Returned hair care items to their proper place.	_____	_____	_____
c. Followed agency policy for used linens.	_____	_____	_____
d. Cleaned and dried the over-bed table (if used). Dried with paper towels. Discarded paper towels. Positioned the over-bed table as the person preferred.	_____	_____	_____
e. Removed and discarded gloves. Practiced hand hygiene.	_____	_____	_____
19. Placed the call light and other needed items within reach.	_____	_____	_____
20. Followed the care plan and the person's preferences for privacy measures to maintain. Leaving the privacy curtain, window coverings, and door open or closed were examples.	_____	_____	_____
21. Completed a safety check of the room.	_____	_____	_____
22. Practiced hand hygiene.	_____	_____	_____
23. Report and record your care and observations.	_____	_____	_____

Shampooing the Person's Hair in Bed

Name: ______________________ Date: ______________________

Quality of Life

	S	U	Comments
• Knocked before entering the person's room.			
• Addressed the person by name.			
• Introduced yourself by name and title.			
• Explained the procedure before starting and during the procedure.			
• Protected the person's rights during the procedure.			
• Handled the person gently during the procedure.			

Preprocedure

	S	U	Comments
1. Followed *Delegation Guidelines: Shampooing*. Saw *Promoting Safety and Comfort: Shampooing*.			
2. Practiced hand hygiene and got the following supplies:			
• Two bath towels			
• Washcloth			
• Shampoo			
• Hair conditioner (if requested)			
• Water thermometer			
• Water Pitcher			
• Shampoo basin			
• Collecting basin			
• Waterproof underpad			
• Gloves (if needed)			
• Comb and brush			
• Hair dryer			
• Laundry bag			
3. Arranged items nearby. Placed the collecting basin on a chair by the bed.			
4. Practiced hand hygiene.			
5. Identified the person. Checked the ID (identification) bracelet against the assignment sheet. Used two identifiers. Also called the person by name.			
6. Provided for privacy.			
7. Raised the bed for body mechanics. Bed rails were up if used. Lowered the bed rail near you if up.			

Procedure

	S	U	Comments
8. Brushed and combed hair to remove tangles.			
9. Positioned the person for a shampoo in bed.			
a. Lowered the head of the bed and removed the pillow.			
b. Placed the waterproof underpad and shampoo basin under the head and shoulders.			
c. Supported the head and neck with a folded towel if necessary.			
10. Covered the person's chest with a bath towel.			
11. Filled the water pitcher. Followed these safety measures.			
a. Raised the bed rail if used. Lowered the bed to a safe level.			

Procedure—cont'd	S	U	Comments
b. Measured water temperature following agency policy. Water temperature is usually 105°F (40.5°C). Had the person check the water temperature. Adjusted water temperature as needed.			
c. Raised the bed for body mechanics. Lowered the bed rail if used when you return.			
12. Put on gloves (if needed).			
13. Had the person hold a washcloth over the eyes. It did not cover the nose and mouth. (Note: A damp washcloth is easier to hold. It does not slip. However, your agency may require a dry washcloth.)			
14. Used the water pitcher to wet the hair. Asked the person about the water temperature and adjusted as needed.			
15. Applied a small amount of shampoo.			
16. Worked up a lather with both hands. Started at the hairline. Worked toward the back of the head.			
17. Massaged the scalp with your fingertips. Did not scratch the scalp with your fingernails.			
18. Rinsed the hair until the water ran clear.			
19. Repeated the following steps: a. Applied a small amount of shampoo.			
b. Worked up a lather with both hands. Started at the hairline. Worked toward the back of the head.			
c. Massaged the scalp with your fingertips. Did not scratch the scalp with your fingernails.			
d. Rinsed the hair until the water ran clear.			
20. Applied conditioner if used. Followed directions on the container.			
21. Squeezed water from the hair.			
22. Covered the hair with a bath towel.			
23. Removed the shampoo basin, collecting basin, and waterproof underpad.			
24. Dried the person's face with the towel on the chest.			
25. Rubbed the hair and scalp with the towel. Rubbed gently. Used the second towel if the first one was wet.			
26. Placed towels in the laundry bag. Removed and discarded gloves (if worn). Practiced hand hygiene after removing and discarding gloves.			
27. Raise the head of the bed.			
28. Combed the hair to remove snarls and tangles. Dried and styled hair as the person preferred. [Wore gloves if needed. Removed and discarded the gloves (if used). Practiced hand hygiene after removing and discarding gloves.]			

Postprocedure

	S	U	Comments
29. Provided for comfort.			
30. Lowered the bed to a safe and comfortable level. Raised or lowered bed rails. Followed the care plan.			
31. Cleaned up and stored supplies and equipment. (Wore gloves.)			
a. Discarded disposable items.			

Postprocedure—cont'd	S	U	Comments
b. Removed hair from the brush or comb. Discarded hair.	_____	_____	_____
c. Followed agency procedures to clean and disinfect reusable equipment. Returned supplies and equipment to their proper place.	_____	_____	_____
d. Followed agency policy for used linens.	_____	_____	_____
e. Cleaned and dried the over-bed table (if used). Dried with paper towels. Discarded paper towels. Positioned the over-bed table as the person preferred.	_____	_____	_____
f. Removed and discarded gloves. Practiced hand hygiene.	_____	_____	_____
32. Placed the call light and other needed items within reach.	_____	_____	_____
33. Followed the care plan and the person's preferences for privacy measures to maintain. Leaving the privacy curtain, window coverings, and door open or closed were examples.	_____	_____	_____
34. Completed a safety check of the room.	_____	_____	_____
35. Practiced hand hygiene.	_____	_____	_____
36. Reported and recorded your care and observations.	_____	_____	_____

NATCEP™ VIDEO VIDEO CLIP

Shaving the Person's Face With a Safety Razor

Name: ______________________ Date: ______________________

Quality of Life	S	U	Comments
• Knocked before entering the person's room.			
• Addressed the person by name.			
• Introduced yourself by name and title.			
• Explained the procedure before starting and during the procedure.			
• Protected the person's rights during the procedure.			
• Handled the person gently during the procedure.			

Preprocedure	S	U	Comments
1. Followed *Delegation Guidelines: Shaving*. Saw *Promoting Safety and Comfort: Shaving*.			
2. Practiced hand hygiene and got the following supplies:			
• Wash basin			
• Bath towel			
• Washcloth or hand towel			
• Towels or paper towels (to wipe razor)			
• Safety razor			
• Mirror			
• Shaving cream or shaving gel			
• Shaving brush if used			
• Aftershave or lotion if used			
• Towel or paper towels (as a barrier for supplies)			
• Gloves			
• Laundry bag			
3. Placed the barrier (towel, paper towels) on the over-bed table. Arranged supplies on top.			
4. Practiced hand hygiene.			
5. Identified the person. Checked the ID (identification) bracelet against the assignment sheet. Used two identifiers. Also called the person by name.			
6. Provided for privacy.			

Procedure	S	U	Comments
7. Filled the wash basin with warm water. Placed the basin on the over-bed table.			
8. Raised the bed for body mechanics. Bed rails are up if used. Lowered the bed rail near you if up.			
9. Assisted the person to semi-Fowler's position if allowed or the supine position.			
10. Adjusted lighting to clearly see the person's face.			
11. Placed the towel over the person's chest and shoulders.			
12. Adjusted the over-bed table for easy reach.			
13. Put on gloves.			
14. Attached the razor blade to the shaver if necessary.			
15. Washed the person's face. Did not dry.			
16. Wet the washcloth or towel. Wrung it out.			
17. Applied the washcloth or towel to the face for a few minutes.			

Procedure—cont'd	S	U	Comments
18. Applied shaving cream with your hands. If using gel, lathered it before applying it. (If needed, changed your gloves or wiped excess shaving cream from your gloves using a towel or paper towel. Or used a shaving brush to apply lather.)			
19. Held the skin taut with one hand.			
20. Shaved in the direction of hair growth. Used shorter strokes around the chin and lips.			
21. Rinsed the razor often. Wiped it with tissues or paper towels.			
22. Applied direct pressure to any bleeding areas.			
23. Washed off any remaining shaving cream or soap. Patted dry with the towel on the person's chest.			
24. Applied aftershave or lotion if requested. (If there were nicks or cuts, did not apply aftershave or lotion.)			
25. Removed the towel. Placed the towel and washcloth (or hand towel) in the laundry bag. Removed and discarded gloves. Practiced hand hygiene.			

Postprocedure

26. Provided for comfort.			
27. Lowered the bed to a safe and comfortable level.			
Raised or lowered bed rails. Followed the care plan.			
28. Cleaned up and stored supplies and equipment. (Wore gloves.)			
a. Discarded disposable items. Discarded the razor blade or disposable razor into the sharps container.			
b. Emptied the wash basin.			
c. Followed agency procedures to clean and disinfect reusable equipment. Returned supplies and equipment to their proper place.			
d. Followed agency policy for used linens.			
e. Cleaned and dried the over-bed table. Dried with paper towels. Discarded paper towels. Positioned the over-bed table as the person preferred.			
f. Removed and discarded gloves. Practiced hand hygiene.			
29. Placed the call light and other needed items within reach.			
30. Followed the care plan and the person's preferences for privacy measures to maintain. Leaving the privacy curtain, window coverings, and door open or closed were examples.			
31. Completed a safety check of the room.			
32. Practiced hand hygiene.			
33. Reported and recorded your care and observations. Reported nicks, cuts, irritation, or bleeding to the nurse at once.			

NATCEP™ VIDEO VIDEO CLIP

Shaving the Person's Face With an Electric Shaver

Name: ______________________ Date: ______________________

	S	U	Comments

Quality of Life

- Knocked before entering the person's room.
- Addressed the person by name.
- Introduced yourself by name and title.
- Explained the procedure before starting and during the procedure.
- Protected the person's rights during the procedure.
- Handled the person gently during the procedure.

Preprocedure

1. Followed *Delegation Guidelines: Shaving*. See *Promoting Safety and Comfort: Shaving*.
2. Practiced hand hygiene and got the following supplies:
   - Wash basin
   - Bath towel
   - Washcloth or hand towel
   - Electric shaver
   - Mirror
   - Pre-electric shave product if used
   - Aftershave or lotion if used
   - Towel or paper towels (as a barrier for supplies)
   - Gloves
   - Laundry bag
3. Placed the barrier (towel, paper towels) on the over-bed table. Arranged supplies on top.
4. Practiced hand hygiene.
5. Identified the person. Checked the ID bracelet against the assignment sheet. Used two identifiers. Also called the person by name.
6. Provided for privacy.

Procedure

7. Ensured that the shaver was clean. Followed the manufacturer's instructions. The shaver was clean and dry before use.
8. Filled the wash basin with warm water. Placed the basin on the over-bed table.
9. Raised the bed for body mechanics. Bed rails were up if used. Lowered the bed rail near you if up.
10. Assisted the person to semi-Fowler's position if allowed or the supine position.
11. Adjusted lighting to clearly see the person's face.
12. Placed the towel over the person's chest and shoulders.
13. Adjusted the over-bed table for easy reach.
14. Put on gloves.
15. Washed and dried the person's face.
16. Applied a pre-electric shave product (if used). Followed the instructions on the product.
17. Held the skin taut with one hand.
18. Turned on the shaver. Shaved facial hair. Followed the manufacturer's instructions for the motion to use and the direction of the shave. Shaved any sensitive areas first. Pressed lightly. Avoided going over the same area many times.

Procedure—cont'd	S	U	Comments
a. *Rotary-type shaver*—Moved the shaver in small circles over the face.			
b. *Foil (oscillating blade) shaver*—Moved the shaver in straight lines up and down or across the face in the direction of hair growth. Followed the manufacturer's instructions. Used short strokes.			
19. Applied direct pressure to any bleeding areas. The risk of bleeding with electric shavers was low. However, irritation and breaks in the skin were possible.			
20. Applied aftershave or lotion if requested. (If there were irritated areas, did not apply aftershave or lotion.)			
21. Removed the towel. Placed the towel and washcloth (or hand towel) in the laundry bag. Removed and discarded gloves. Practiced hand hygiene.			

Postprocedure

	S	U	Comments
22. Provided for comfort.			
23. Lowered the bed to a safe and comfortable level.			
Raised or lowered bed rails. Followed the care plan.			
24. Cleaned up and stored supplies and equipment. (Wore gloves.)			
a. Discarded disposable items.			
b. Emptied the wash basin.			
c. Emptied hair from the shaver. Followed the manufacturer's instructions and agency procedures to clean and dry the device. Returned the shaver to its proper place.			
d. Followed agency procedures to clean and disinfect reusable equipment. Returned supplies and equipment to their proper place.			
e. Followed agency policy for used linens.			
f. Cleaned and dried the over-bed table. Dried with paper towels. Discarded paper towels. Positioned the over-bed table as the person preferred.			
g. Removed and discarded gloves. Practiced hand hygiene.			
25. Placed the call light and other needed items within reach.			
26. Followed the care plan and the person's preferences for privacy measures to maintain. Leaving the privacy curtain, window coverings, and door open or closed were examples.			
27. Completed a safety check of the room.			
28. Practiced hand hygiene.			
29. Reported and recorded your care and observations. Reported irritation or bleeding to the nurse at once.			

Giving Nail and Foot Care

Name: ______________________ Date: ______________________

Quality of Life	S	U	Comments
• Knocked before entering the person's room.			
• Addressed the person by name.			
• Introduced yourself by name and title.			
• Explained the procedure before starting and during the procedure.			
• Protected the person's rights during the procedure.			
• Handled the person gently during the procedure.			

Preprocedure	S	U	Comments
1. Followed *Delegation Guidelines: Nail and Foot Care.* Saw *Promoting Safety and Comfort: Nail and Foot Care.*			
2. Practiced hand hygiene and got the following supplies:			
a. Wash basin or whirlpool foot bath			
b. Kidney basin			
c. Soap			
d. Water thermometer			
e. Bath towel			
f. Washcloth and hand towel			
g. Nail clippers			
h. Orangewood stick			
i. Emery board or nail file			
j. Lotion for the hands			
k. Lotion or petroleum jelly for the feet			
l. Towel or paper towels (as a barrier for supplies)			
m. Disposable waterproof pad			
n. Gloves			
o. Laundry bag			
3. Placed the barrier (towel, paper towels) on the over-bed table. Arranged supplies on top.			
4. Practiced hand hygiene.			
5. Identified the person. Checked the ID (identification) bracelet against the assignment sheet. Used two identifiers. Also called the person by name.			
6. Provided for privacy.			

Procedure	S	U	Comments
7. Assisted the person to the bedside chair. Removed footwear and socks or stockings. Placed the call light and other needed items within reach.			
8. Placed the disposable waterproof pad under the feet.			
9. Filled the wash basin or whirlpool foot bath 2⁄3 (two-thirds) full with water. Water temperature is usually 105°F (40.5°C). Measured the temperature with a water thermometer. Had the person check the water temperature. Adjusted as needed.			
10. Placed the basin or foot bath on the disposable waterproof pad.			
11. Helped the person put the bare feet into the water. Both feet were completely covered by water.			
12. Adjusted the over-bed table in front of the person.			

Procedure—cont'd	S	U	Comments
13. Filled the kidney basin 2⁄3 (two-thirds) full with water. Water temperature is usually 105°F (40.5°C). Measured the temperature with a water thermometer. Had the person check the water temperature. Adjusted as needed.	______	______	
14. Placed the kidney basin on the over-bed table.	______	______	______
15. Placed the person's fingers into the basin. Positioned the arms for comfort.	______	______	______
16. Allowed the fingers to soak for 5 to 10 minutes. Allowed the feet to soak for 15 to 20 minutes. Rewarmed water as needed.	______	______	______
17. Put on gloves.	______	______	
18. Cleaned the hands with soap and water if needed or if required by your state's competency exam. Cleaned between the fingers. Rinsed the hands.	______	______	______
19. Removed the kidney basin.	______	______	______
20. Dried the hands and between the fingers thoroughly.	______	______	______
21. Cleaned under the fingernails with the flat edge of the orangewood stick. Wiped the orangewood stick with a towel after each nail.	______	______	______
22. Pushed cuticles back gently with the orangewood stick or a washcloth if requested by the person.	______	______	______
23. Trimmed fingernails straight across with nail clippers. You carefully rounded the corners slightly.	______	______	______
24. Filed and shaped nails with an emery board or nail file. Nails were smooth with no rough edges. Checked each nail for smoothness. Filed as needed. Filed in one direction.	______	______	______
25. Applied lotion to the hands. Warmed lotion first. To warm lotion, rubbed some between your hands or held the bottle under warm water.	______	______	______
26. Moved the over-bed table to the side. (NOTE: If your agency or state competency test requires clean gloves for foot care, removed and discarded gloves. Practiced hand hygiene. Put on clean gloves.)	______	______	______
27. Lifted a foot out of the water. Supported the foot and ankle with one hand. With your other hand, washed the foot and between the toes with soap and a washcloth. Returned the foot to the water to rinse the foot and between the toes.	______	______	______
28. Repeated for the other foot. Lifted foot out of the water. Supported the foot and ankle with one hand. With your other hand, washed the foot and between the toes with soap and a washcloth. Returned the foot to the water to rinse the foot and between the toes.	______	______	______
29. Removed the feet from the water. Dried thoroughly, especially between the toes. Supported the foot and ankle as needed.	______	______	______
30. Applied lotion or petroleum jelly to the tops, soles, and heels of the feet. Did not apply between the toes. Warmed lotion or petroleum jelly first, by rubbing some between your hands or held bottle under warm water. Removed excess lotion or petroleum jelly with a towel. Supported the foot and ankle as needed.	______	______	______
31. Place the used towels and washcloth in the laundry bag. Removed and discarded the gloves. Practiced hand hygiene.	______	______	______
32. Helped the person put on slip-resistant footwear.	______	______	______

Postprocedure

33. Provided for comfort. ______ ______ ______
34. Made sure the bed is at a safe and comfortable level. Followed the care plan. ______ ______ ______
35. Raised or lowered bed rails. Followed the care plan. ______ ______ ______
36. Cleaned up and stored supplies and equipment. (Wore gloves.) ______ ______ ______
    a. Discarded disposable items. ______ ______ ______
    b. Emptied the kidney basin and wash basin (whirlpool foot bath). ______ ______ ______
    c. Followed agency procedures to clean and disinfect reusable equipment. Returned supplies and equipment to their proper place. ______ ______ ______
    d. Followed agency policy for used linens. ______ ______ ______
    e. Cleaned and dried the over-bed table. Dried with paper towels. Discarded paper towels. Positioned the over-bed table as the person preferred. ______ ______ ______
    f. Removed and discarded gloves. Practiced hand hygiene. ______ ______ ______
37. Placed the call light and other needed items within reach. ______ ______ ______
38. Followed the care plan and the person's preferences for privacy measures to maintain. Leaving the privacy curtain, window coverings, and door open or closed were examples. ______ ______ ______
39. Completed a safety check of the room. ______ ______ ______
40. Practiced hand hygiene. ______ ______ ______
41. Reported and recorded your care and observations. ______ ______ ______

NATCEP™ VIDEO VIDEO CLIP

Undressing the Person

Name: ______________________ Date: ______________________

Quality of Life	S	U	Comments
• Knocked before entering the person's room.	___	___	___
• Addressed the person by name.	___	___	___
• Introduced yourself by name and title.	___	___	___
• Explained the procedure before starting and during the procedure.	___	___	___
• Protected the person's rights during the procedure.	___	___	___
• Handled the person gently during the procedure.	___	___	___

Preprocedure

1. Followed *Delegation Guidelines: Changing Garments.* Saw *Promoting Safety and Comfort: Changing Garments.*	___	___	___
2. Asked a coworker to help turn and position the person if needed.	___	___	___
3. Practiced hand hygiene.	___	___	___
4. Identified the person. Checked the ID (identification) bracelet against the assignment sheet. Used two identifiers. Also called the person by name.	___	___	___
5. Got the following supplies:			
• Bath blanket	___	___	___
• Laundry bag	___	___	___
• Clothing requested by the person	___	___	___
6. Provided for privacy.	___	___	___
7. Raised the bed for body mechanics. Bed rails were up if used.	___	___	___

Procedure

8. Stood on the person's affected (weak) side if the person had one. Lowered the bed rail near you if up.	___	___	___
9. Positioned the person for the procedure. The head of the bed was raised if the person could sit up and lean forward. The head of the bed was flat if the person could turn from side to side.	___	___	___
10. Covered the person with a bath blanket. Fanfolded linens to the foot of the bed. Kept the person covered as much as possible throughout the procedure.	___	___	___
11. Removed garments that opened in the back.	___	___	___
a. *If the person could sit up and lean forward*	___	___	___
1) Had the person lean forward.	___	___	___
2) Undid buttons, zippers, ties, snaps, or other closures.	___	___	___
3) Brough the sides of the garment to the sides of the person.	___	___	___
4) Had the person sit back.	___	___	___
b. *If the person could not sit up and lean forward*	___	___	___
1) Turned the person away from you.	___	___	___
2) Undid buttons, zippers, ties, snaps, or other closures.	___	___	___
3) Tucked the far side of the garment under the person. Folded the near side onto the chest.	___	___	___
4) Positioned the person supine.	___	___	___
c. Slid the garment off of the shoulder and arm on the unaffected (strong) side. Removed the garment from the affected (weak) side.	___	___	___

Procedure—cont'd | **S** | **U** | **Comments**

12. Removed pullover garments.
    a. Undid any buttons, zippers, ties, snaps, or other closures.
    b. Removed the garment from the arm and shoulder on the unaffected (strong) side.
    c. Had the person lean forward if able or turned the person toward you to bring the garment up to the neck. Had the person sit back. Or positioned the person supine.
    d. Brought the garment over the head.
    e. Removed the garment from the affected (weak) side.
13. Removed garments that opened in the front.
    a. Undid buttons, zippers, ties, or snaps or other closures.
    b. Slid the garment off the shoulder and arm on the unaffected (strong) side.
    c. *If the person could sit up and lean forward:*
        1) Had the person lean forward.
        2) Brought the garment around the back to the affected (weak) side.
        3) Had the person sit back.
    d. *If the person could not sit up and lean forward:*
        1) Turned the person toward you.
        2) Tucked the removed part of the garment under the person.
        3) Turned the person away from you.
        4) Pulled the side of the garment out from under the person. Made sure the person would not lie on it when supine.
        5) Positioned the person supine.
    e. Removed the garment from the affected (weak) side.
14. Removed pants or slacks.
    a. Removed footwear and socks.
    b. Positioned the person supine.
    c. Undid buttons, zippers, ties, snaps, or buckles. Removed the belt if worn.
    d. *If the person could raise the hips to lift the buttocks off of the bed:*
        1) Had the person lift the buttocks off the bed.
        2) Brought the pants down over the hips and buttocks.
        3) Had the person lower the hips and buttocks.
    e. *If the person could not raise the hips off the bed:*
        1) Turned the person toward you.
        2) Slid the pants off the hip and buttocks on the unaffected (strong) side.
        3) Turned the person away from you.
        4) Slid the pants off the hip and buttocks on the affected (weak) side.
        5) Positioned the person supine.
    f. Slid the pants down the legs and over the feet.
15. Dressed the person.

Postprocedure

16. Provided for comfort.	______	______	______
17. Lowered the bed to a safe and comfortable level. Raised or lowered bed rails. Followed the care plan.	______	______	______
18. Followed agency policy for soiled clothing.	______	______	______
19. Placed the call light and other needed items within reach.	______	______	______
20. Followed the care plan and the person's preferences for privacy measures to maintain. Leaving the privacy curtain, window coverings, and door open or closed were examples.	______	______	______
21. Completed a safety check of the room.	______	______	______
22. Practiced hand hygiene.	______	______	______
23. Reported and recorded your care and observations.	______	______	______

Dressing the Person

Name: ______________________ Date: ______________________

Quality of Life	S	U	Comments
• Knocked before entering the person's room.			
• Addressed the person by name.			
• Introduced yourself by name and title.			
• Explained the procedure before starting and during the procedure.			
• Protected the person's rights during the procedure.			
• Handled the person gently during the procedure.			

Preprocedure

	S	U	Comments
1. Followed *Delegation Guidelines: Changing Garments.* Saw *Promoting Safety and Comfort: Changing Garments.*			
2. Asked a coworker to help turn and position the person if needed.			
3. Practiced hand hygiene.			
4. Identified the person. Checked the ID (identification) bracelet against the assignment sheet. Used two identifiers. Also called the person by name.			
5. Got the following supplies:			
• Bath blanket			
• Laundry bag			
• Clothing requested by the person			
6. Provided for privacy.			
7. Raised the bed for body mechanics. Bed rails were up if used.			
8. Stood on the person's affected (weak) side if the person had one. Lowered the bed rail near you if up.			
9. Positioned the person for the procedure. The head of the bed was raised if the person could sit up and lean forward. The head of the bed was flat if the person could turn from side to side.			
10. Covered the person with a bath blanket. Fanfolded linens to the foot of the bed. Kept the person covered as much as possible throughout the procedure.			
11. Removed garments that opened in the back			
a. *If the person could sit up and lean forward*			
1) Had the person lean forward.			
2) Undid buttons, zippers, ties, snaps, or other closures.			
3) Brought the sides of the garment to the sides of the person.			
4) Had the person sit back.			
b. *If the person could not sit up and lean forward*			
1) Turned the person away from you.			
2) Undid buttons, zippers, ties, snaps, or other closures.			
3) Tucked the far side of the garment under the person. Folded the near side onto the chest.			
4) Positioned the person supine.			
c. Slid the garment off of the shoulder and arm on the unaffected (strong) side. Removed the garment from the affected (weak) side.			

Preprocedure—cont'd	S	U	Comments
12. Removed pullover garments			
a. Undid any buttons, zippers, ties, snaps, or other closures.			
b. Removed the garment from the arm and shoulder on the unaffected (strong) side.			
c. Had the person lean forward if able or turned the person toward you to bring the garment up to the neck. Had the person sit back. Or positioned the person supine.			
d. Brought the garment over the head.			
e. Removed the garment from the affected (weak) side.			
13. Removed garments that opened in the front.			
a. Undid buttons, zippers, ties, or snaps or other closures.			
b. Slid the garment off the shoulder and arm on the unaffected (strong) side.			
c. *If the person could sit up and lean forward:*			
1) Had the person lean forward.			
2) Brought the garment around the back to the affected (weak) side.			
3) Had the person sit back.			
d. *If the person could not sit up and lean forward:*			
1) Turned the person toward you.			
2) Tucked the removed part of the garment under the person.			
3) Turned the person away from you.			
4) Pulled the side of the garment out from under the person. Made sure the person would not lie on it when supine.			
5) Positioned the person supine.			
e. Removed the garment from the affected (weak) side.			
14. Removed pants or slacks.			
a. Removed footwear and socks.			
b. Positioned the person supine.			
c. Undid buttons, zippers, ties, snaps, or buckles. Removed the belt if worn.			
d. *If the person could raise the hips to lift the buttocks off of the bed:*			
1) Had the person lift the buttocks off the bed.			
2) Brought the pants down over the hips and buttocks.			
3) Had the person lower the hips and buttocks.			
e. *If the person could not raise the hips off the bed:*			
1) Turned the person toward you.			
2) Slid the pants off the hip and buttocks on the unaffected (strong) side.			
3) Turned the person away from you.			
4) Slid the pants off the hip and buttocks on the affected (weak) side.			
5) Positioned the person supine.			
f. Slid the pants down the legs and over the feet.			

Procedure

15. Dressed person. Put on garments that opened in the back.
    a. Slid the correct sleeve of the garment onto the arm and shoulder of the affected (weak) side.
    b. Slid the garment's other sleeve onto the arm and shoulder of the unaffected (strong) side.
    c. *If the person could sit up and lean forward:*
        1) Had the person lean forward.
        2) Brought the sides of the garment to the back.
        3) Fastened buttons, zippers, ties, snaps, or other closures.
        4) Had the person sit back.
    d. *If the person could not sit up and lean forward:*
        1) Turned the person toward you. Brought the side of the garment around the back.
        2) Turned the person away from you. Brought the side of the garment around the back on the other side.
        3) Brought the sides of the garment together. Fastened buttons, zippers, ties, snaps, or other closures.
        4) Positioned the person supine.
16. Put on pullover garments.
    a. Slid the correct sleeve of the garment onto the arm and shoulder on the affected (weak) side.
    b. Brought the garment over the head.
    c. Slid the garment's other sleeve onto the arm and shoulder of the unaffected (strong) side.
    d. Brought the garment down.
    e. *If the person could sit up and lean forward,* had the person lean forward. Pulled the garment down. Had the person sit back.
    f. *If the person could not sit up and lean forward:*
        1) Turned the person away from you.
        2) Pulled the garment down on the affected (weak) side.
        3) Turned the person toward you.
        4) Pulled the garment down on the unaffected (strong) side.
        5) Positioned the person supine.
17. Put on garments that opened in the front.
    a. Slid the correct sleeve of the garment onto the arm and shoulder on the affected (weak) side.
    b. *If the person can sit up and lean forward:*
        1) Had the person lean forward.
        2) Brought the garment around the back to the unaffected (strong) side.
        3) Slid the garment's other sleeve onto the arm and shoulder of the unaffected (strong) side.
        4) Had the person sit back.
    c. *If the person could not sit up and lean forward.*
        1) Turned the person away from you. Brought the garment around the person's back. Tucked the far side of the garment under the person.
        2) Turned the person toward you. Brought the garment around the person's unaffected (strong) side.
        3) Positioned the person supine.
        4) Slid the garment onto the arm and shoulder on the unaffected (strong) side.
    d. Fastened buttons, zippers, ties, snaps, or other closures.

Preprocedure—cont'd	S	U	Comments
18. Put on pants or slacks.	____	____	____
a. Positioned the person supine.	____	____	____
b. Slid the pants over the feet and up the legs.	____	____	____
c. *If the person could raise the hips to lift the buttocks off of the bed.*	____	____	____
1) Had the person raise the hips.	____	____	____
2) Brought the pants up over the hips and buttocks.	____	____	____
3) Had the person lower the hips.	____	____	____
d. *If the person could not raise the hips*	____	____	____
1) Turned the person away from you.	____	____	____
2) Slid the pants over the hip and buttocks on the affected (weak) side.	____	____	____
3) Turned the person toward you.	____	____	____
4) Slid the pants over the hip and buttocks on the unaffected (strong) side.	____	____	____
5) Positioned the person supine.	____	____	____
e. Fastened buttons, zippers, ties, snaps, a belt buckle, or other closures.	____	____	____
19. Put socks on the person. Socks were up all the way and smooth. Applied slip-resistant footwear if the person was getting out of bed.	____	____	____
20. Removed the bath blanket. Placed it in the laundry bag.	____	____	____
21. Covered the person or helped the person out of bed.	____	____	____

Postprocedure			
22. Provided for comfort.	____	____	____
23. Lowered the bed to a safe and comfortable level.	____	____	____
Raised or lowered bed rails. Followed the care plan.	____	____	____
24. Followed agency policy for soiled clothing.	____	____	____
25. Placed the call light and other needed items within reach.	____	____	____
26. Followed the care plan and the person's preferences for privacy measures to maintain. Leaving the privacy curtain, window coverings, and door open or closed were examples.	____	____	____
27. Completed a safety check of the room.	____	____	____
28. Practiced hand hygiene.	____	____	____
29. Reported and recorded your care and observations.	____	____	____

Changing a Standard Patient Gown on a Person With an IV

Name: ____________________ Date: ____________________

Quality of Life	S	U	Comments
• Knocked before entering the person's room.			
• Addressed the person by name.			
• Introduced yourself by name and title.			
• Explained the procedure before starting and during the procedure.			
• Protected the person's rights during the procedure.			
• Handled the person gently during the procedure.			

Preprocedure	S	U	Comments
1. Followed *Delegation Guidelines: Changing Garments, Changing Patient Gowns*. Saw *Promoting Safety and Comfort: Changing Garments, Changing Patient Gowns*.			
2. Practiced hand hygiene.			
3. Identified the person. Checked the ID (identification) bracelet against the assignment sheet. Used two identifiers. Also called the person by name.			
4. Got the following supplies:			
• Clean gown			
• Bath blanket			
• Laundry bag			
5. Provided for privacy.			
6. Raised the bed for body mechanics. Bed rails were up if used.			

Procedure	S	U	Comments
7. Lowered the bed rail near you (if up).			
8. Covered the person with a bath blanket. Fanfolded linens to the foot of the bed.			
9. Untied the gown. Freed parts that the person was lying on.			
10. Removed the gown from the arm with *no IV*.			
11. Gathered up the sleeve of the arm *with the IV*. Slid it over the IV site and tubing. Removed the arm and hand from the sleeve.			
12. Kept the sleeve gathered. Slid the gathered sleeve along the tubing to the bag.			
13. Removed the bag from the pole. Slid the bag and tubing through the sleeve. Did not pull on the tubing. Kept the bag above the person.			
14. Hung the IV bag on the pole.			
15. Placed the used gown in the laundry bag.			
16. Gathered the sleeve of the clean gown that went on the arm with the IV infusion.			
17. Removed the bag from the pole. Slipped the sleeve over the bag at the shoulder part of the gown. Hung the bag.			
18. Slid the gathered sleeve over the tubing, hand, arm, and IV site. Then slid it onto the shoulder.			
19. Put the other side of the gown on the person. Fastened the gown.			
20. Covered the person. Removed and stored the bath blanket. Or placed it in the laundry bag.			

Postprocedure

21. Provided for comfort.			
22. Lowered the bed to a safe and comfortable level. Raised or lowered bed rails. Followed the care plan.			
23. Followed agency policy for used linens.			
24. Placed the call light and other needed items within reach.			
25. Followed the care plan and the person's preferences for privacy measures to maintain. Leaving the privacy curtain, window coverings, and door open or closed were examples.			
26. Completed a safety check of the room.			
27. Practiced hand hygiene.			
28. Asked the nurse to check the flow rate.			
29. Reported and recorded your care and observations.			

NATCEP™ VIDEO VIDEO CLIP

Giving the Bedpan

Name: ____________________ Date: ____________________

Quality of Life	S	U	Comments
• Knocked before entering the person's room.			
• Addressed the person by name.			
• Introduced yourself by name and title.			
• Explained the procedure before starting and during the procedure.			
• Protected the person's rights during the procedure.			
• Handled the person gently during the procedure.			

Preprocedure	S	U	Comments
1. Followed *Delegation Guidelines:*			
a. *Bedpans*			
Saw *Promoting Safety and Comfort:*			
a. *Urinary Needs*			
b. Voiding Equipment			
c. *Bedpans*			
2. Practiced hand hygiene.			
3. Provided for privacy.			
4. Got the following supplies:			
• Bedpan			
• Bedpan cover			
• Toilet paper			
• Waterproof underpad			
• Disposable waterproof underpad (as a barrier for the bedpan)			
• Bath blanket			
• Gloves			
• Laundry bag			
5. Arranged equipment nearby. Placed the bedpan on the chair or bed. Used the disposable waterproof pad as a barrier between the bedpan and the surface.			
6. Raised the bed for body mechanics. Bed rails were up if used. Lowered the bed rail near you (if up).			

Procedure	S	U	Comments
7. Lowered the head of the bed. Positioned the person supine. Or raised the head of the bed slightly for comfort.			
8. Covered the person with a bath blanket. Folded the top linens and gown out of the way.			
9. Applied gloves.			
10. Folded back the person's gown and the bath blanket as needed. Kept the person covered as much as possible.			
11. Placed the bedpan.			
a. *If the person could raise the hips to lift the buttocks off of the bed:*			
1) Had the person flex (bend) the knees and raise the buttocks. The person pushed against the mattress with the feet.			
2) Slid your hand under the lower back. Helped raise the buttocks.			

Preprocedure—cont'd	S	U	Comments
3) Placed a waterproof underpad under the buttocks if not already in place.			
4) Slid the bedpan under the person.			
5) Had the person lower the buttocks onto the bedpan.			
b. *If the person could not raise the hips:*			
1) Turned the person to position a waterproof underpad if not already in place.			
2) Turned the person onto the side away from you.			
3) Placed the bedpan firmly against the buttocks. Pushed downward on the bedpan and toward the person.			
4) Held the bedpan securely. Turned the person onto the back.			
c. Made sure the bedpan was centered under the person. When the person sat up, the urethra and anus were over the opening.			
12. Covered the person with the bath blanket.			
13. Removed and discarded the gloves. Practiced hand hygiene.			
14. Raised the head of the bed so the person was in a sitting position (Fowler's position) for a standard bedpan. Or raised the head of the bed to a comfortable level for the person.			
15. Ensured that the person was correctly positioned on the bedpan.			
16. Raised the bed rail if used. Lowered the bed.			
17. Placed the toilet paper and call light within reach.			
18. Asked the person to signal when done or when help was needed. (NOTE: For some state competency tests, you ask the person to use hand-wipes for hand hygiene after wiping with toilet paper.)			
19. Stayed with the person if necessary. Or left the room and closed the door. (Practiced hand hygiene before leaving.) Was respectful. Provided as much privacy as possible.			
20. Returned when the person signaled. Or checked on the person every 5 minutes. Knocked before entering. Practiced hand hygiene.			
21. Raised the bed for body mechanics. Lowered the bed rail (if used) and lowered the head of the bed.			
22. Applied gloves.			
23. Had the person raise the buttocks. Removed the bedpan. Or held the bedpan and turned the person onto the side away from you. Placed the bedpan on the disposable waterproof pad or in the cover (if used).			
24. Cleaned the genital area if the person could not do so.			
a. Cleaned from the meatus (front or top) to the anus (back or bottom) with toilet paper. Used fresh toilet paper for each wipe. Placed used toilet paper in the bedpan.			
b. Provided perineal care if needed.			

Preprocedure—cont'd	S	U	Comments
c. Removed and discarded the waterproof underpad (if used). Placed it in the laundry bag.	_____	_____	_____
d. Covered the person with the bath blanket.	_____	_____	_____
e. Removed and discarded the gloves. Practiced hand hygiene. Applied clean gloves.	_____	_____	_____
f. Lowered the person's gown. Covered the person with the top linens. Removed the bath blanket. Placed it in the laundry bag.	_____	_____	_____
25. Raised the bed rail if used. Lowered the bed.	_____	_____	_____
26. Took the bedpan to the bathroom. Noted the color, amount (output), and character of urine or feces.	_____	_____	_____
27. Emptied the bedpan contents into the toilet. Rinsed the bedpan. Poured the rinse into the toilet and flushed.	_____	_____	_____
28. Followed agency procedures to clean and disinfect the bedpan. Returned the bedpan to its proper place.	_____	_____	_____
29. Removed and discarded the gloves. Practiced hand hygiene and put on clean gloves.	_____	_____	_____
30. Helped the person with hand hygiene.	_____	_____	_____
31. Removed and discarded the gloves. Practiced hand hygiene.			

Postprocedure	S	U	Comments
32. Provided for comfort.	_____	_____	_____
33. Lowered the bed to a safe and comfortable level. Raised or lowered bed rails. Followed the care plan.	_____	_____	_____
34. Cleaned up and stored supplies and equipment. (Wore gloves. Changed gloves as needed.)	_____	_____	_____
a. Discarded disposable items.	_____	_____	_____
b. Followed agency procedures to clean and disinfect reusable equipment. Returned supplies and equipment to their proper place.	_____	_____	_____
c. Followed agency policy for used linens.	_____	_____	_____
d. Cleaned and dried the over-bed table if used. Dried with paper towels. Discarded paper towels. Positioned the over-bed table as the person preferred.	_____	_____	_____
e. Removed and discarded gloves. Practiced hand hygiene.	_____	_____	_____
35. Placed the call light and other needed items within reach.	_____	_____	_____
36. Followed the care plan and the person's preferences for privacy measures to maintain. Leaving the privacy curtain, window coverings, and door open or closed were examples.	_____	_____	_____
37. Completed a safety check of the room.	_____	_____	_____
38. Practiced hand hygiene.	_____	_____	_____
39. Reported and recorded your care and observations.	_____	_____	_____

Giving the Male Urinal

Name: ______________________ Date: ______________________

Quality of Life

S U Comments

- Knocked before entering the person's room.
- Addressed the person by name.
- Introduced yourself by name and title.
- Explained the procedure before starting and during the procedure.
- Protected the person's rights during the procedure.
- Handled the person gently during the procedure.

Preprocedure

1. Followed *Delegation Guidelines:*
   a. *Urinals*
   Saw *Promoting Safety and Comfort:*
   a. *Urinary Needs*
   b. *Voiding Equipment*
   c. *Urinals*
2. Practiced hand hygiene.
3. Provided for privacy.
4. Determined if the man would stand, sit, or lie in bed.
5. Got the following supplies:
   - Urinal
   - Slip-resistant footwear if the man would stand to void
   - Transfer belt (if needed)
   - Gloves

Procedure

6. Put on gloves
7. *Standing to use the urinal:*
   a. Prepared the person to stand. Helped the person sit on the side of the bed. Applied slip-resistant footwear. Applied a transfer belt if needed.
   b. Helped the person to stand. Provided support if the person is unsteady.
   c. Gave the person the urinal.
8. *Using the urinal in bed:*
   a. Gave the person the urinal.
   b. Reminded the person to tilt the bottom down to prevent spills.
9. Positioned the urinal and placed the penis in the urinal if the person could not do so.
10. *If the person could be left alone:*
   a. Removed and discarded the gloves. Practiced hand hygiene.
   b. Placed the call light within reach. Asked the person to signal when done or when help is needed.
   c. Maintained privacy measures. Covered the person for privacy if in bed.
   d. Stayed in the room or left the room and closed the door. Followed the care plan. Was respectful. Provided as much privacy as possible. (Practiced hand hygiene before leaving the room.)
   e. Returned when the person signaled. Or checked on the person every 5 minutes. Knocked before entering the room.
   f. Practiced hand hygiene. Applied gloves.

Procedure—cont'd	S	U	Comments
11. Closed the urinal cap.			
12. Assisted with clothing and sitting as needed.			
13. Took the urinal to the bathroom.			
14. Noted the color, amount (output), and clarity of urine.			
15. Emptied the urinal into the toilet and flushed. Rinsed the urinal with cold water. Poured rinse into the toilet and flushed.			
16. Followed agency procedures to clean and disinfect the urinal. Returned the urinal to its proper place.			
17. Removed and discarded the soiled gloves. Practiced hand hygiene and put on clean gloves.			
18. Assisted with hand hygiene.			
19. Removed and discarded the gloves. Practiced hand hygiene.			
Postprocedure			
20. Provided for comfort.			
21. Ensured that the bed was at a safe and comfortable level. Raised or lowered bed rails. Followed the care plan.			
22. Returned supplies to their proper place.			
23. Followed agency policy for used linens.			
24. Placed the call light and other needed items within reach.			
25. Followed the care plan and the person's preferences for privacy measures to maintain. Leaving the privacy curtain, window coverings, and door open or closed were examples.			
26. Completed a safety check of the room.			
27. Practiced hand hygiene.			
28. Reported and recorded your care and observations.			

Helping the Person to the Commode

Name: ______________________ Date: ______________________

Quality of Life	S	U	Comments
• Knocked before entering the person's room.	____	____	________
• Addressed the person by name.	____	____	________
• Introduced yourself by name and title.	____	____	________
• Explained the procedure before starting and during the procedure.	____	____	________
• Protected the person's rights during the procedure.	____	____	________
• Handled the person gently during the procedure.	____	____	________

Preprocedure	S	U	Comments
1. Followed *Delegation Guidelines:*			
a. *Commodes*	____	____	________
Saw *Promoting Safety and Comfort:*			
a. *Urinary Needs*	____	____	________
b. Voiding Equipment	____	____	________
c. *Commodes*	____	____	________
2. Practiced hand hygiene.	____	____	________
3. Provided for privacy.	____	____	________
4. Got the following supplies:			
• Commode	____	____	________
• Toilet paper	____	____	________
• Bath blanket	____	____	________
• Transfer belt	____	____	________
• Slip-resistant footwear	____	____	________
• Gloves	____	____	________
• Laundry bag	____	____	________
5. Arranged equipment. The commode was next to the bed. Checked that the wheels were locked (braked) if present.	____	____	________

Procedure	S	U	Comments
6. Helped the person sit on the side of the bed. Followed the care plan for raising or lowering the bed rail.	____	____	________
7. Helped the person put on slip-resistant footwear.	____	____	________
8. Applied the transfer belt.	____	____	________
9. Applied gloves if contact with urine or feces (stools) was expected.	____	____	________
10. Assisted the person to the commode. Used the transfer belt. Helped the person lower clothing as needed.	____	____	________
11. Removed and discarded the gloves if worn and soiled. Practiced hand hygiene after removing and discarding gloves.	____	____	________
12. Covered the person's lap and legs with a bath blanket for warmth and privacy. Removed the transfer belt.	____	____	________
13. Placed the toilet paper within reach. (Provided hand-wipes if they were to be used for hand hygiene. Asked the person to use them after wiping with toilet paper.)	____	____	________
14. *If the person could be left alone:*			
a. Placed the call light within reach. Asked the person to signal when done or when help is needed.	____	____	________
b. Maintained privacy measures.	____	____	________

Procedure—cont'd	S	U	Comments
c. Stayed in the room or left the room and closed the door. Followed the care plan. Was respectful. Provided as much privacy as possible. (Practiced hand hygiene before leaving the room.)			
d. Returned when the person signaled. Or checked on the person every 5 minutes. Knocked before entering.			
e. Practiced hand hygiene.			
15. Applied gloves.			
16. Removed the bath blanket. Placed it in the laundry bag.			
17. Helped the person clean the genital area as needed. Removed and discarded the gloves. Practiced hand hygiene.			
18. Applied the transfer belt. Helped the person stand and fasten clothing as needed. Helped the person back to bed using the transfer belt. Removed the transfer belt and footwear. Raised the bed rail if used.			
19. Put on clean gloves. Removed and covered the commode container.			
20. Took the container to the bathroom.			
21. Observed urine and feces for color, amount (output), and character.			
22. Emptied the container contents into the toilet and flushed. Rinsed the container. Poured the rinse into the toilet and flushed.			
23. Followed agency procedures to clean and disinfect the container. Returned the container to the commode. Closed the lid.			
24. Disinfected other parts of the commode if necessary.			
25. Removed and discarded the gloves. Practiced hand hygiene. Applied clean gloves.			
26. Assisted with hand hygiene.			
27. Removed and discarded the gloves. Practiced hand hygiene.			

Postprocedure

28. Provided for comfort.			
29. Ensured that the bed was at a safe and comfortable level. Raised or lowered bed rails. Followed the care plan.			
30. Returned other supplies to their proper place.			
31. Followed agency policy for used linens.			
32. Placed the call light and other needed items within reach.			
33. Followed the care plan and the person's preferences for privacy measures to maintain. Leaving the privacy curtain, window coverings, and door open or closed were examples.			
34. Completed a safety check of the room.			
35. Practiced hand hygiene.			
36. Reported and recorded your care and observations.			

NATCEP™ VIDEO VIDEO CLIP

Applying Incontinence Products

Name: ____________________ Date: ____________________

Quality of Life	S	U	Comments
• Knocked before entering the person's room.			
• Addressed the person by name.			
• Introduced yourself by name and title.			
• Explained the procedure before starting and during the procedure.			
• Protected the person's rights during the procedure.			
• Handled the person gently during the procedure.			

Preprocedure	S	U	Comments
1. Followed *Delegation Guidelines: Applying Incontinence Products*. Saw *Promoting Safety and Comfort:*			
a. *Urinary Needs*			
b. Voiding Equipment			
c. *Applying Incontinence Products*			
2. Practiced hand hygiene.			
3. Provided for privacy.			
4. Got the following supplies:			
• Incontinence product as directed by the nurse			
• Barrier cream or moisturizer as directed by the nurse			
• Cleaning agent—soap, bodywash, or perineal cleanser			
• Items for perineal care			
• Waterproof underpad—one or two as needed			
• Bath blanket			
• Slip-resistant footwear if the person stands			
• Towel or paper towels (as barrier for supplies)			
• Plastic trash bag			
• Gloves			
• Laundry bag			
5. Placed the barrier (towel, paper towels) on the over-bed table. Arranged items on top.			
6. Practiced hand hygiene.			
7. Identified the person. Checked the ID (identification) bracelet against the assignment sheet. Used two identifiers. Also called the person by name.			
8. Marked the date, time, and your initials on the new product.			
9. Filled the wash basin and placed it on the over-bed table. Water temperature was 105°F to 109°F (40.5°C–42.7°C). Measured water temperature according to agency policy. Asked the person to check the water temperature. Adjusted water temperature as needed.			
10. Raised the bed for body mechanics (unless the person will stood). Bed rails were up if used. Lowered the bed rail near you if up.			

Procedure

11. Positioned the person for changing the product in bed. Person was on the back. Head of the bed was lowered as much as possible. _______ _______ _______________
12. Applied gloves. _______ _______ _______________
13. Covered the person with a bath blanket. Lowered top linens to the foot of the bed. If linens were wet, removed them and placed them in the laundry bag. _______ _______ _______________
14. Placed a waterproof underpad under the buttocks if not already in place. Asked the person to raise the buttocks off the bed. Or turned the person from side to side. Positioned the person supine. _______ _______ _______________
15. Moved or removed clothing as needed. Lowered or removed pants (slacks) if worn. Raised the person's gown if worn. Removed any wet garments. Followed agency policy for removed clothing. _______ _______ _______________
16. Folded back the bath blanket. Kept the person covered as much as possible. Had the person spread the legs. _______ _______ _______________
17. Removed the used product and applied a new product. _______________
    1) *For removal of a brief with the person in bed:*
        a. Loosened the tabs on each side of the used brief. _______ _______ _______________
        b. Turned the person onto the side away from you. Had the person spread the legs. Removed the used brief from front to back (top to bottom). Rolled the front of the product toward the back (bottom) with the soiled side inside. Removed the brief. _______ _______ _______________
        c. Observed the urine as you rolled the product up. Estimated the amount of urine: small, moderate, large. Observed for urine color and blood. _______ _______ _______________
        d. Placed the used brief in the trash bag. Tied and sealed the bag and set the bag aside. _______ _______ _______________
        e. Performed perineal care wearing clean gloves. Cleaned all areas that had contact with urine. Washed, rinsed, and dried the skin fold areas of the groin. Applied the barrier cream (ointment) as directed. _______ _______ _______________
        f. Removed soiled or wet waterproof underpad. Placed it in the laundry bag. _______ _______ _______________
        g. Removed and discarded the gloves. Practiced hand hygiene. Put on clean gloves. _______ _______ _______________
        h. Placed a clean waterproof underpad under the buttocks if needed. Followed the care plan. _______ _______ _______________
    2) *For application of a brief with the person in bed:*
        a. Opened the new brief. Folded it in half lengthwise along the center. _______ _______ _______________
        b. Inserted the brief lengthwise between the legs from front to back (top to bottom). _______ _______ _______________
        c. Unfolded and spread the back panel. _______ _______ _______________
        d. Centered the brief in the perineal area. _______ _______ _______________
        e. Turned the person onto their back. _______ _______
        f. Made sure the brief was positioned high in the groin folds and fit the shape of the body. _______ _______ _______________

Procedure—cont'd	S	U	Comments
g. Secured the brief. Pulled the lower tape tab forward on the side near you. Attached it at a slightly upward angle. Did the same for the other side.	______	______	______
h. Smoothed out all wrinkles and folds.	______	______	______
3) *For removal of a pad worn with an undergarment with the person in bed.*			
a. Placed a waterproof underpad under the buttocks if not already in place. Asked the person to raise the buttocks off the bed. Or turned the person from side to side.	______	______	______
b. Turned the person onto the side away from you.	______	______	______
c. Pulled the undergarment down. The waistband was over the knee.	______	______	______
d. Removed the used pad from the front to back (top to bottom). Observed the urine as you rolled the product up. Estimated the amount of urine in the used product: small, moderate, large. Observed for urine color and blood.	______	______	______
e. Placed the used pad in the trash bag. Tied and sealed the bag and set the bag aside.	______	______	______
f. Performed perineal care wearing clean gloves. Cleaned all areas that had contact with urine. Washed, rinsed, and dried the skin fold areas of the groin. Applied barrier cream (ointment) as directed.	______	______	______
g. Removed and discarded the gloves. Practiced hand hygiene. Put on clean gloves.	______	______	______
4) *To apply a pad worn with an undergarment with the person in bed:*			
a. Folded the new pad in half lengthwise along the center.	______	______	______
b. Inserted the pad between the legs from front to back (top to bottom).	______	______	______
c. Unfolded and spread the back panel. Centered the pad in the perineal area.	______	______	______
d. Pulled the garment up at the back.	______	______	______
e. Turned the person onto their back.	______	______	
f. Pulled the garment up in front. Adjusted the pad and undergarment for a good fit. Smoothed out all wrinkles and folds.	______	______	______
g. Placed a clean waterproof underpad under the buttocks if needed. Followed the care plan.	______	______	______
5) *To remove pull-on underwear with the person standing:*			
a. Helped the person stand. Removed the pants or slacks.	______	______	______
b. Tore the side seams to remove the used underwear.	______	______	______
c. Removed the underwear from front to back (top to bottom). Observed the urine as you rolled the underwear up. Estimated the amount of urine in the used product: small, moderate, large. Observed for urine color and blood.	______	______	______

Procedure—cont'd	S	U	Comments
d. Placed the used underwear in the trash bag. Tied and sealed the bag and set the bag aside.	______	______	______
e. Performed perineal care wearing clean gloves. Cleaned all areas that had contact with urine. Washed, rinsed, and dried the skin fold areas of the groin. Applied barrier cream (ointment) as directed.	______	______	______
f. Removed and discarded the gloves. Practiced hand hygiene. Put on clean gloves.	______	______	______
6) *To apply pull on underwear for a person who can stand:*			
a. Had the person sit on the side of the bed.	______	______	______
b. Slid the new underwear over the feet to past the knees.	______	______	______
c. Helped the person stand.	______	______	______
d. Pulled the underwear up. Adjusted as needed for a good fit. Smoothed out all wrinkles and folds.	______	______	______
18. Asked about comfort. Asked if the product felt too loose or too tight. Checked for wrinkles or creases. Made sure the product did not rub or irritate the groin. Adjusted the product as needed.	______	______	______
19. Raised or put on pants or slacks or lowered person's gown.	______	______	______
20. Positioned the person for comfort. Covered the person. Removed the bath blanket. Placed it in the laundry bag.	______	______	______
21. Removed and discarded gloves. Practiced hand hygiene.	______	______	______

Postprocedure

22. Provided for comfort.	______	______	______
23. Lowered the bed to a safe and comfortable level. Raised or lowered the bed rails. Followed the care plan.	______	______	______
24. Cleaned up and stored supplies and equipment. (Wore gloves. Changed gloves as needed.)	______	______	______
a. Discarded disposable items.	______	______	______
b. Emptied the wash basin.	______	______	______
c. Followed agency procedures to clean and disinfected reusable equipment. Returned supplies and equipment to their proper place.	______	______	______
d. Followed agency policy for used linens.	______	______	______
e. Cleaned and dried the over-bed table. Dried with paper towels. Discarded paper towels. Positioned the over-bed table as the person preferred.	______	______	______
f. Removed and discarded gloves. Practiced hand hygiene.	______	______	______
25. Placed the call light and other needed items within reach.	______	______	______
26. Followed the care plan and the person's preferences for privacy measures to maintain. Leaving the privacy curtain, window coverings, and door open or closed were examples.	______	______	______
27. Completed a safety check of the room.	______	______	______
28. Practiced hand hygiene.	______	______	______
29. Reported and recorded your care and observations.	______	______	______

NATCEP™ VIDEO VIDEO CLIP

Giving Catheter Care

Name: ______________________ Date: ______________________

Quality of Life	S	U	Comments
• Knocked before entering the person's room.			
• Addressed the person by name.			
• Introduced yourself by name and title.			
• Explained the procedure before starting and during the procedure.			
• Protected the person's rights during the procedure.			
• Handled the person gently during the procedure.			

Preprocedure

	S	U	Comments
1. Followed *Delegation Guidelines:*			
a. *Perineal Care*			
b. *Catheter Care*			
Saw *Promoting Safety and Comfort:*			
a. *Perineal Care*			
c. *Urinary Catheters*			
d. *Catheter Care*			
2. Practiced hand hygiene and got the following supplies:			
• Items for perineal care			
• At least two washcloths and one towel for catheter care			
• Bath blanket			
• Towels or paper towels (as a barrier for supplies)			
• Gloves			
• Laundry bag			
3. Placed the barrier (towel, paper towels) on the over-bed table. Arranged items on top of them.			
4. Practiced hand hygiene.			
5. Identified the person. Checked the ID (identification) bracelet against the assignment sheet. Used two identifiers. Also called the person by name.			
6. Filled the wash basin. Water temperature was 105°F to 109°F (40.5°C–42.7°C). Measured water temperature according to agency policy. Asked the person to check the water temperature. Adjusted water temperature as needed.			
7. Provided for privacy.			
8. Raised the bed for body mechanics. Bed rails were up if used. Lowered the bed rail near you if up.			

Procedure

	S	U	Comments
9. Covered the person with a bath blanket. Fanfolded top linens to the foot of the bed.			
10. Placed the waterproof underpad under the buttocks. Had the person raise the buttocks off the bed. Or turned the person from side to side.			
11. Positioned and draped the person for perineal care.			
12. Practiced hand hygiene. Put on the gloves.			
13. Folded back the bath blanket to expose the perineal area.			
14. Checked the drainage tubing. Made sure it was not kinked and that urine could flow freely.			

Procedure—cont'd	S	U	Comments
15. Separated the labia (female). In an uncircumcised male, retracted the foreskin. Checked for crusts, abnormal drainage, or secretions. Checked for signs of pressure at the meatus.			
16. Gave perineal care. Kept the foreskin of the uncircumcised male retracted through step 19.			
17. Cleaned, rinsed, and dried the catheter.			
a. Applied soap, bodywash, or other cleansing agent to a clean, wet washcloth.			
b. Held the catheter at the meatus. Do so for all of step 17.			
c. Cleaned the catheter from the meatus down the catheter at least 4 inches. Cleaned downward, away from the meatus with one stroke. Did not tug or pull on the catheter. Repeated as needed with a clean area of the washcloth. Used another clean washcloth if needed.			
d. Wet a clean, soap-free washcloth.			
e. Rinsed from the meatus down the catheter at least 4 inches. Rinsed downward, away from the meatus with one stroke. Did not tug or pull on the catheter. Repeated as needed with a clean area of the washcloth. Used another clean washcloth if needed.			
f. Dried from the meatus down the catheter at least 4 inches. Did not tug or pull on the catheter.			
18. Patted dry the perineal area. Dried from front to back (top to bottom).			
19. Returned the foreskin (uncircumcised male) to its natural position.			
20. Secured the catheter. Positioned the tubing in a straight line or coiled on the bed. Followed the nurse's directions. Secured the tubing to the bottom linens.			
21. Covered the person with the bath blanket. Removed the waterproof underpad.			
22. Removed and discarded the gloves. Practiced hand hygiene.			
23. Covered the person. Removed the bath blanket. Placed it in the laundry bag.			

Postprocedure	S	U	Comments
24. Provided for comfort.			
25. Lowered the bed to a safe and comfortable level. Raised or lowered bed rails. Followed the care plan.			
26. Cleaned up and stored supplies and equipment. (Wore gloves. Changed gloves as needed.)			
a. Discarded disposable items.			
b. Emptied the wash basin.			
c. Followed agency procedures to clean and disinfect reusable equipment. Returned supplies and equipment to their proper place.			
d. Followed center policy for used linens.			
e. Cleaned and dried the over-bed table. Dried with paper towels. Discarded paper towels. Positioned the over-bed table as the person preferred.			
f. Removed and discarded gloves. Practiced hand hygiene.			
27. Placed the call light and other needed items within reach.			

Postprocedure—cont'd	S	U	Comments
28. Followed the care plan and the person's preferences for privacy measures to maintain. Leaving the privacy curtain, window coverings, and door open or closed were examples.			
29. Completed a safety check of the room.			
30. Practiced hand hygiene.			
31. Reported and recorded your care and observations.			

Changing a Leg Bag to a Standard Drainage Bag

Name: ____________________ Date: ____________________

Quality of Life	S	U	Comments
• Knocked before entering the person's room.			
• Addressed the person by name.			
• Introduced yourself by name and title.			
• Explained the procedure before starting and during the procedure.			
• Protected the person's rights during the procedure.			
• Handled the person gently during the procedure.			

Preprocedure

	S	U	Comments
1. Followed *Delegation Guidelines: Urine Drainage Systems.*			
Saw *Promoting Safety and Comfort:*			
a. *Urinary Catheters*			
b. *Urine Drainage Systems*			
2. Practiced hand hygiene and got the following supplies:			
• Standard drainage bag and tubing			
• Antiseptic wipes			
• Sterile cap and plug			
• Catheter clamp			
• Items to empty the drainage bag			
• Waterproof underpad			
• Bath blanket			
• Bedpan and cover (if used)			
• Disposable waterproof pad (as a barrier for the bedpan)			
• Paper towels			
• Towel or paper towels (as a barrier for supplies			
• Gloves			
• Laundry bag			
3. Placed the barrier (towel, paper towels) on the over-bed table. Arranged items on top. Placed the bedpan on the chair or bed. Used the disposable waterproof pad as a barrier between the bedpan and the surface.			
4. Practiced hand hygiene.			
5. Identified the person. Checked the ID (identification) bracelet against the assignment sheet. Used two identifiers. Also called the person by name.			
6. Provided for privacy.			

Procedure

	S	U	Comments
7. Raised the bed to a safe height for dangling and for body mechanics. Had the person sit on the side of the bed. Followed the care plan for bed rail use.			
8. Practiced hand hygiene. Put on gloves.			
9. Exposed the catheter and leg bag.			
10. Emptied the drainage bag			
11. Clamped the catheter. This prevented urine from draining from the catheter into the drainage tubing.			
12. Allowed urine to drain from below the clamp into the drainage tubing. This emptied the lower end of the catheter.			

Procedure—cont'd	S	U	Comments
13. Helped the person to lie down.			
14. Covered the person with a bath blanket. Fanfolded top linens to the foot of the bed. Exposed the catheter and leg bag.			
15. Unfastened the straps on the leg bag. Placed the waterproof underpad under the catheter and leg bag.			
16. Opened the package with the standard drainage bag and tubing.			
17. Attached the standard drainage bag to the bed frame.			
18. Opened the package with the sterile cap and plug. Did not let anything touch the sterile cap or plug.			
19. Disconnected the catheter from the drainage tubing. Did not allow anything to touch the ends.			
20. Inserted the sterile plug into the catheter end. Touched only the end of the plug. Did not touch the part that went inside the catheter. (If you contaminated the end of the catheter, wiped the end with an antiseptic wipe. Did so before you inserted the sterile plug.)			
21. Placed the sterile cap on the end of the leg bag drainage tube. (If you contaminated the tubing end, wiped the end with an antiseptic wipe. Did so before you applied the sterile cap.) Placed the leg bag in the bedpan if the bag would be reused.			
22. Removed the cap from the new standard drainage tubing.			
23. Removed the sterile plug from the catheter.			
24. Inserted the end of the drainage tubing into the catheter.			
25. Removed the clamp from the catheter.			
26. Positioned drainage tubing in a straight line or coiled on the bed. Followed the nurse's directions. Secured the tubing to the bottom linens.			
27. Removed and discarded the waterproof underpad. Placed it in the laundry bag.			
28. Removed and discarded the gloves. Practice hand hygiene.			
29. Covered the person. Removed the bath blanket. Placed it in the laundry bag.			

Postprocedure

30. Provided for comfort.			
31. Lowered the bed to a safe and comfortable level. Raised or lowered bed rails. Followed the care plan.			
32. Cleaned up and stored supplies and equipment. (Wore gloves. Changed gloves as needed.)			
a. Discarded disposable items.			
b. Cleaned and disinfected reusable equipment. Returned supplies and equipment to their proper place.			
c. Followed the manufacturer's instructions and agency policy to discard or reuse the leg bag. Followed agency procedures to clean, disinfect, and store a reused leg bag. Or discarded following agency policy.			

Postprocedure—cont'd	S	U	Comments
d. Followed center policy for used linens.	_______	_______	_______
e. Cleaned and dried the over-bed table. Dried with paper towels. Discarded paper towels. Positioned the over-bed table as the person preferred.	_______	_______	_______
f. Removed and discarded gloves. Practiced hand hygiene.	_______	_______	_______
33. Placed the call light and other needed items within reach.	_______	_______	_______
34. Followed the care plan and the person's preferences for privacy measures to maintain. Leaving the privacy curtain, window coverings, and door open or closed were examples.	_______	_______	_______
35. Completed a safety check of the room.	_______	_______	_______
36. Practiced hand hygiene.	_______	_______	_______
37. Reported and recorded your care and observations.	_______	_______	_______

Emptying a Urine Drainage Bag

Name: ______________________ Date: ______________________

Quality of Life	S	U	Comments
• Knocked before entering the person's room.			
• Addressed the person by name.			
• Introduced yourself by name and title.			
• Explained the procedure before starting and during the procedure.			
• Protected the person's rights during the procedure.			
• Handled the person gently during the procedure.			

Preprocedure	S	U	Comments
1. Followed *Delegation Guidelines: Urine Drainage Systems.*			
Saw *Promoting Safety and Comfort:*			
a. *Urinary Catheters*			
b. *Urine Drainage Systems*			
2. Practiced hand hygiene and got the following supplies:			
• Graduate (measuring container)			
• Gloves			
• Towel or paper towels (as a barrier for supplies)			
• Antiseptic wipes			
3. Arranged items in the person's room.			
4. Practiced hand hygiene.			
5. Identified the person. Checked the ID (identification) bracelet against the assignment sheet. Used two identifiers. Also called the person by name.			
6. Provided for privacy.			

Procedure	S	U	Comments
7. Put on the gloves.			
8. Placed paper towel or disposable waterproof pad on the floor. Placed graduate on top of it.			
9. Positioned the graduate under the drainage bag.			
10. Opened the clamp on the drain.			
11. Allowed all urine to drain into the graduate. Did not let the drain touch the graduate.			
12. Cleaned the end of the drain with an antiseptic wipe. Discarded the wipe following agency policy.			
13. Clamped and positioned the drain in the holder.			
14. Measured the urine.			
15. Removed and discarded the paper towel or disposable waterproof pad.			
16. Emptied the contents of the graduate into the toilet Rinsed the graduate. Emptied the rinse into the toilet and flushed.			
17. Followed agency procedures to clean and disinfect the graduate. Returned the graduate to its proper place.			
18. Removed and discarded the gloves. Practiced hand hygiene.			
19. Recorded the time and amount of the urine on the intake and output (I&O) record.			

Postprocedure

20. Provided for comfort. _____ _____ _____
21. Placed the call light and other needed items within reach. _____ _____ _____
22. Followed the care plan and the person's preferences for privacy measures to maintain. Leaving the privacy curtain, window coverings, and door open or closed were examples. _____ _____ _____
23. Completed a safety check of the room. _____ _____ _____
24. Practiced hand hygiene. _____ _____ _____
25. Reported and recorded your care and observations. _____ _____ _____

Removing an Indwelling Catheter

Name: ______________________ Date: ______________________

Quality of Life	S	U	Comments
• Knocked before entering the person's room.			
• Addressed the person by name.			
• Introduced yourself by name and title.			
• Explained the procedure before starting and during the procedure.			
• Protected the person's rights during the procedure.			
• Handled the person gently during the procedure.			

Preprocedure

	S	U	Comments
1. Followed *Delegation Guidelines: Removing Indwelling Catheters.*			
Saw *Promoting Safety and Comfort:*			
a. *Urinary Catheters*			
b. *Removing Indwelling Catheters*			
2. Practiced hand hygiene and got the following supplies:			
• Disposable waterproof pad			
• Syringe in the size directed by the nurse			
• Towel			
• Bath blanket			
• Disposable bag			
• Items to empty the drainage bag			
• Gloves			
• Laundry bag			
3. Arranged items in the person's room.			
4. Practiced hand hygiene.			
5. Identified the person. Checked the ID (identification) bracelet against the assignment sheet. Used two identifiers. Also called the person by name.			
6. Provided for privacy.			
7. Raised the bed for body mechanics. Bed rails were up if used. Lowered the bed rail near you if up			

Procedure

	S	U	Comments
8. Positioned and draped the person as for perineal care.			
9. Checked the size of the syringe. Knew the amount of water in the balloon. Made sure the syringe was large enough to withdraw all the water from the balloon.			
10. Practiced hand hygiene. Applied gloves.			
11. Folded the bath blanket back to expose the catheter.			
12. Removed the tube holder, leg band, or tape securing the catheter to the person.			
13. Positioned the disposable waterproof pad.			
a. Female—between the legs			
b. Male—over the thighs			
14. Removed all the water from the balloon. (Knew how much water was in the balloon. If the balloon was filled with 10 mL of water, you removed 10 mL of water.)			
a. Slid the syringe plunger up and down several times. This loosened the plunger.			
b. Pulled the plunger back to the 0.5 (one-half) mL mark.			

Procedure—cont'd	S	U	Comments
c. Attached the syringe to the catheter's balloon port gently. Used only enough force to get the syringe to stay in the port.	_____	_____	_____
d. Allowed the water to drain into the syringe. Waited at least 30 seconds to allow the full amount to drain. Did not pull back on the plunger. Pressure in the balloon forced the plunger back and filled the syringe. If the water was draining slowly or not at all, called the nurse. Did not remove the catheter if there was water in the balloon. The nurse may have directed you to:			
1. Gently reposition the syringe in the port.	_____	_____	_____
2. Reposition the person.	_____	_____	_____
3. Pull back on the syringe gently and slowly. Forceful pulling would collapse the catheter.	_____	_____	_____
15. Pulled the catheter straight out once all the water was removed. Had the person breathe out slowly during removal. Removed the catheter gently.	_____	_____	_____
16. Wrapped the catheter in the disposable waterproof pad.	_____	_____	_____
17. Dried the perineal area with the towel. Placed the towel in the laundry bag.	_____	_____	_____
18. Covered the person with the bath blanket.	_____	_____	_____
19. Lifted the drainage tubing to ensure that all urine has drained from the drainage tubing into the drainage bag. Emptied the drainage bag. Noted the amount of urine. Unhooked the bag from the bed. Placed the used catheter, tubing, and drainage bag in the disposable bag.	_____	_____	_____
20. Removed and discarded the gloves. Practiced hand hygiene.	_____	_____	_____
21. Covered the person. Removed the bath blanket. Placed it in the laundry bag.	_____	_____	_____

Postprocedure

22. Provided for comfort.	_____	_____	_____
23. Lowered the bed to a safe and comfortable level. Raised or lowered bed rails. Followed the care plan.	_____	_____	_____
24. Cleaned up and stored supplies and equipment. (Wore gloves. Changed gloves as needed.)	_____	_____	_____
a. Discarded disposable items. Discarded the used catheter, tubing, and drainage bag following agency policy.	_____	_____	_____
b. Emptied the graduate into the toilet. Rinsed the graduate. Emptied the rinse into the toilet and flush. Followed agency procedures to clean and disinfect the graduate. Returned supplies and equipment to their proper place.	_____	_____	_____
c. Followed center policy for used linens.	_____	_____	_____
d. Cleaned and dried the over-bed table if used. Dried with paper towels. Discarded paper towels. Positioned the over-bed table as the person preferred.	_____	_____	_____
e. Removed and discarded gloves. Practiced hand hygiene.	_____	_____	_____
25. Placed the call light and other needed items within reach.	_____	_____	_____

Procedure—cont'd	S	U	Comments
26. Followed the care plan and the person's preferences for privacy measures to maintain. Leaving the privacy curtain, window coverings, and door open or closed were examples.	______	______	______
27. Completed a safety check of the room.	______	______	______
28. Practiced hand hygiene.	______	______	______
29. Reported and recorded your care and observations.	______	______	______

Applying a Condom Catheter

Name: ______________________ Date: ______________________

Quality of Life	S	U	Comments
• Knocked before entering the person's room.			
• Addressed the person by name.			
• Introduced yourself by name and title.			
• Explained the procedure before starting and during the procedure.			
• Protected the person's rights during the procedure.			
• Handled the person gently during the procedure.			

Preprocedure	S	U	Comments
1. Followed *Delegation Guidelines:*			
a. *Perineal Care*			
b. *Condom Catheters*			
Saw *Promoting Safety and Comfort:*			
a. *Perineal Care*			
c. *Urinary Catheters*			
d. *Condom Catheters*			
2. Practiced hand hygiene and got the following supplies:			
• Condom catheter (with adhesive strip if needed)			
• Standard drainage bag or leg bag			
• Cap for the drainage bag			
• Basin of warm water			
• Soap, bodywash, or other cleansing agent			
• Towel and washcloths			
• Bath blanket			
• Waterproof underpad			
• Items to empty the drainage bag			
• Towel or paper towels (as a barrier for supplies)			
• Gloves			
• Laundry bag			
3. Placed a barrier (towel, paper towels) on the over-bed table. Arranged items on top.			
4. Practiced hand hygiene.			
5. Identified the person. Checked the ID (identification) bracelet against the assignment sheet. Used two identifiers. Also called the person by name.			
6. Provided for privacy.			
7. Raised the bed for body mechanics. Bed rails were up if used. Lowered the bed rail near you if up.			

Procedure	S	U	Comments
8. Covered the person with a bath blanket. Lowered top linens.			
9. Positioned the waterproof underpad under the person. Had the person to raise the buttocks off the bed. Or turned the person from side to side.			
10. Positioned and draped the person for perineal care.			
11. Practiced hand hygiene. Put on the gloves.			
12. Secured the standard drainage bag to the bed frame. Or had a leg bag ready. Closed the drain.			
13. Folded back the bath blanket to expose the genital area. Kept the person covered as much as possible.			

Procedure—cont'd	S	U	Comments
14. Removed the condom catheter.			
a. For a catheter with a single-sided adhesive strip (outside)—removed the adhesive strip.			
b. For a self-adhesive catheter—if needed, wet a washcloth with warm water. Applied it to the penis for a few minutes. This helped release the adhesive.			
c. Rolled the sheath off of the penis.			
d. For a catheter with a double-sided adhesive strip (inside)—removed the adhesive strip after rolling the sheath off of the penis.			
15. Disconnected the used tubing form the condom catheter. Capped the drainage tube.			
16. Discarded the condom catheter and adhesive strip (if used).			
17. Provided perineal care. Ensured that the penis was dried well. For an uncircumcised male, the foreskin was returned to its natural position before the new condom catheter was applied.			
18. Observed the penis for reddened areas, skin breakdown, and irritations. If present, did not apply a new catheter. Called for the nurse.			
19. Removed and discarded the gloves. Practiced hand hygiene. Put on clean gloves.			
20. Applied the new condom catheter. Followed the manufacturer's instructions.			
a. Grasped the penis.			
b. *For a catheter with a double-sided adhesive strip (inside):*			
1) Removed the paper liner from one side of the adhesive strip.			
2) Applied the adhesive strip in a spiral on the penis. Began just behind the penis head. Did not apply the adhesive strip completely around the penis.			
3) Removed the paper liner from the other side of the adhesive strip.			
4) Rolled the condom onto the penis. Followed the manufacturer's instructions for the amount of space to leave between the catheter and the penis tip. A 1-inch space was common.			
5) Gently pressed the condom to the adhesive strip on the penis.			
c. *For a catheter with a single-sided adhesive strip (outside):*			
1) Rolled the condom onto the penis. Followed the manufacturer's instructions for the amount of space to leave between the catheter and the penis tip. A 1-inch space was common.			
2) Removed the paper liner from the adhesive strip.			
3) Applied the adhesive strip in a spiral over the condom catheter. Began at the penis head. Did not apply the adhesive strip completely around the penis.			

Procedure—cont'd	S	U	Comments
d. *For a self-adhesive catheter:* Rolled the condom onto the penis. Followed the manufacturer's instructions for the amount of time to hold. About 1 minute was common.			
21. Ensured that the penis tip did not touch the condom. Ensured that the condom was not twisted.			
22. Connected the condom to the drainage tubing. Secured excess tubing on the bed. Or attached a leg bag.			
23. Covered the person. Removed the bath blanket. Removed the waterproof underpad and gloves. Placed it in the laundry bag.			
24. Emptied the used drainage bag. Measured and record the urine amount.			
25. Removed and discarded the gloves. Practiced hand hygiene.			
26. Covered the person. Removed the bath blanket. Placed it in the laundry bag.			

Postprocedure

	S	U	Comments
27. Provided for comfort.			
28. Lowered the bed to a safe and comfortable level. Raised or lowered bed rails. Followed the care plan.			
29. Cleaned up and stored supplies and equipment. (Wore gloves. Changed gloves as needed.)			
a. Discarded disposable items.			
b. Followed the manufacturer's instructions and agency policy to discard or reuse the drainage bag. Followed agency procedures to clean, disinfect, and store a reused bag. Or discarded following agency policy.			
c. Empty washbasin.			
d. Followed agency procedures to clean and disinfect reusable equipment. Returned supplies and equipment to their proper place.			
e. Followed agency policy for used linens.			
f. Cleaned and dried the over-bed table. Dried with paper towels. Discarded paper towels. Positioned the over-bed table as the person preferred.			
g. Removed and discarded gloves. Practiced hand hygiene.			
30. Placed the call light and other needed items within reach.			
31. Followed the care plan and the person's preferences for privacy measures to maintain. Leaving the privacy curtain, window coverings, and door open or closed were examples.			
32. Completed a safety check of the room.			
33. Practiced hand hygiene.			
34. Reported and recorded your care and observations.			

Giving a Cleansing Enema to an Adult

Name: ____________________ Date: ____________________

Quality of Life	S	U	Comments
• Knocked before entering the person's room.			
• Addressed the person by name.			
• Introduced yourself by name and title.			
• Explained the procedure before starting and during the procedure.			
• Protected the person's rights during the procedure.			
• Handled the person gently during the procedure.			

Preprocedure

	S	U	Comments
1. Followed *Delegation Guidelines:*			
a. *Bowel Needs*			
b. *Enemas*			
c. Cleansing Enemas			
Saw *Promoting Safety and Comfort:*			
a. *Bowel Needs*			
d. *Enemas*			
2. Practiced hand hygiene and got the following supplies:			
• Disposable enema kit as directed by the nurse (enema bag, and tube with clamp)			
• Enema solution as directed by the nurse			
• Additive (if needed)—3 to 5 mL (1 teaspoon) castile soap for SSE			
• Graduate (measuring container)			
• Water thermometer or other means of measuring solution temperature as directed by agency procedure			
• Lubricant			
• IV (intravenous) pole			
• Commode or bedpan as needed (this procedure uses a commode)			
• Toilet paper			
• Bath blanket			
• Waterproof underpad			
• Slip-resistant footwear			
• Robe (if needed)			
• Transfer/gait belt (if needed)			
• Disposable bag			
• Gloves			
• Laundry bag			
3. Arranged items in the person's room and bathroom.			
4. Practiced hand hygiene.			
5. Identified the person. Checked the ID (identification) bracelet against the assignment sheet. Used two identifiers. Also called the person by name.			
6. Provided for privacy.			

Procedure

	S	U	Comments
7. Positioned the IV pole so the enema bag was 12 inches above the anus. Or it was at the height directed by the nurse.			
8. Prepared the enema.			
a. Closed the clamp on the tube.			

Procedure—cont'd	S	U	Comments
b. Filled the enema bag with the correct amount of solution. Followed agency procedures for warming and checking the temperature. (Added castile soap for an SSE as directed by the nurse. Added it to the bag after the water to reduce suds.)			
c. Sealed the bag.			
d. Hung the bag on the IV pole.			
e. Removed air from the tubing. Held the opening of the tube over a receptacle (graduate, sink, bedpan). Released the clamp. Allowed the solution flow to the end of the tubing. Clamped the tube.			
9. Positioned the person. Covered the person for warmth and privacy.			
a. Raised the bed for body mechanics. Bed rails were up if used. Lowered the bed rail near you if up.			
b. Covered the person with a bath blanket. Fanfolded top linens to the foot of the bed.			
c. Placed a waterproof underpad under the buttocks.			
d. Positioned the person in the left semi-prone or left side-lying position.			
10. Applied gloves.			
11. Gave the enema.			
a. Lubricated the tip of the tube. Lubricated 2 to 4 inches of the tube.			
b. Folded back the bath blanket to expose the anal area. Separated the buttocks to see the anus.			
c. Asked the person to take a deep breath and breathe out slowly through the mouth.			
d. Inserted the tube gently 2 to 4 inches into the adult's rectum. Did this when the person was exhaling. Stopped if the person reportedd pain, you felt resistance, or bleeding occurred.			
e. Checked the amount of solution in the bag.			
f. Unclamped the tube. Gave the solution slowly.			
g. Asked the person to take slow, deep breaths. This helped the person relax.			
h. Clamped the tube if the person needed to have a bowel movement (BM), had cramping, or started to expel solution. Also clamped the tube if the person was sweating or complained of nausea or weakness. Unclamped when symptoms subsided.			
i. Gave the amount of solution ordered. Stopped if the person did not tolerate the procedure.			
j. Clamped the tube before it emptied. This prevented air from entering the bowel.			
k. Held toilet paper around the tube and against the anus. Removed the tube. Placed the enema bag and tube in a bag for disposal.			
12. Covered the person with the bath blanket.			
13. Removed and discarded the gloves. Practiced hand hygiene.			
14. Encouraged retention of the enema for the time ordered. Maintained the left semi-prone or left side-lying position.			

Procedure—cont'd	S	U	Comments
15. Lowered the bed to a safe and comfortable level. Raised or lower bed rails. Followed the care plan. Provided for comfort.			
16. Discarded disposable items. Discarded the enema bag and tube following agency policy.			
17. Assisted the person to the commode when the person requested. Followed these privacy and safety measures.			
a. Ensured that the person's clothing properly covered the person or applied a robe when up.			
b. Applied slip-resistant footwear.			
c. Used a transfer/gait belt as needed.			
d. Ensured that the bed was at a level that was safe for a transfer.			
e. Raised or lowered bed rails according to the care plan.			
f. Wore gloves as needed. Practiced hand hygiene after removing and discarding gloves.			
g. Replaced the waterproof underpad on the bed if it was soiled.			
h. Stayed with the person as needed. Or left the room and closed the door. (Placed the call light and toilet paper in reach. Practiced hand hygiene before leaving.) Was respectful. Provided as much privacy as possible. Returned when the person signals. Or checked on the person every 5 minutes. Knocked before entering the room. Practiced hand hygiene after returning.			
18. Applied gloves.			
19. Assisted with wiping and perineal care as needed. Removed and discarded the gloves. Practiced hand hygiene.			
20. Assisted the person back to bed. Covered the person. Placed the bath blanket in the laundry bag.			
21. Observed enema results for amount, color, consistency, shape, and odor. Called the nurse to observe results.			
22. Assisted with hand hygiene. (Wore gloves for this step. Practiced hand hygiene after removing and discarding the gloves.)			

Postprocedure	S	U	Comments
23. Provided for comfort.			
24. Lowered the bed to a safe and comfortable level. Raised or lowered the bedrails. Followed the care plan.			
25. Cleaned up and stored supplies and equipment. (Wore gloves. Changed gloves as needed.)			
a. Discarded disposable items.			
b. Emptied the commode after the nurse observed the results.			
c. Followed agency procedures to clean and disinfect the commode and other reusable equipment. Returned supplies and equipment to their proper place.			
d. Followed center policy for used linens and used supplies.			
e. Cleaned and dried the over-bed table if used. Dried with paper towels. Discarded paper towels. Positioned the over-bed table as the person preferred.			

Procedure—cont'd	S	U	Comments
f. Removed and discarded gloves. Practiced hand hygiene.	______	______	______
26. Placed the call light and other needed items within reach.	______	______	______
27. Followed the care plan and the person's preferences for privacy measures to maintain. Leaving the privacy curtain, window coverings, and door open or closed were examples.	______	______	______
28. Completed a safety check of the room.	______	______	______
29. Practiced hand hygiene.	______	______	______
30. Reported and recorded your care and observations.	______	______	______

Giving a Small-Volume Enema

Name: ______________________ Date: ______________________

Quality of Life	S	U	Comments
• Knocked before entering the person's room.			
• Addressed the person by name.			
• Introduced yourself by name and title.			
• Explained the procedure before starting and during the procedure.			
• Protected the person's rights during the procedure.			
• Handled the person gently during the procedure.			
Preprocedure			
1. Followed *Delegation Guidelines:*			
a. *Bowel Needs*			
b. *Enemas*			
Saw *Promoting Safety and Comfort:*			
a. *Bowel Needs*			
b. *Enemas*			
2. Practiced hand hygiene and got the following supplies:			
• Small-volume enema			
• Commode or bedpan (this procedure uses a bedpan)			
• Bedpan cover (if used)			
• Disposable waterproof underpad			
• Toilet paper			
• Bath blanket			
• Waterproof underpad			
• Gloves			
• Laundry bag			
3. Arranged items in the person's room.			
4. Practiced hand hygiene.			
5. Identified the person. Checked the ID (identification) bracelet against the assignment sheet. Used two identifiers. Also called the person by name.			
6. Provided for privacy.			
7. Raised the bed for body mechanics. Bed rails are up if used. Lower the bed rail near you if up.			
Procedure			
8. Positioned the person. Covered the person for warmth and privacy.			
a. Covered the person with a bath blanket. Fanfolded top linens to the foot of the bed.			
b. Placed a waterproof underpad under the buttocks.			
c. Positioned the person in the left semi-prone or in the left side-lying position.			
9. Applied clean gloves.			
10. Positioned the bedpan nearby. Used the disposable waterproof pad as a barrier.			
11. Gave the enema.			
a. Folded the bath blanket back to expose the anal area.			
b. Removed the cap from the enema tip.			
c. Separated the buttocks to see the anus.			

Procedure—cont'd	S	U	Comments
d. Asked the person to take a deep breath and breathe out slowly through the mouth.			
e. Inserted the tube gently 2 inches into the adult's rectum. Did this as the person exhaled. Stopped if the person reported pain, you felt resistance, or bleeding occurred.			
f. Squeezed and rolled up the container gently. Released pressure on the bottle after you removed the tip from the rectum.			
g. Put the container into the box, tip first. Discarded the container and box.			
12. Covered the person with the bath blanket.			
13. Encouraged retention of the enema. Maintained the left semi-prone or left side-lying position. Provided for comfort.			
14. Assisted the person onto the bedpan when the person had the urge to have a bowel movement (BM).			
15. Removed and discarded the gloves. Practiced hand hygiene.			
16. Lowered the bed to a safe level. Raised or lowered bed rails according to the care plan.			
17. Stayed with the person as needed. Or left the room and close the door. (Placed the call light and toilet paper in reach. Practiced hand hygiene before leaving.) Was respectful. Provided as much privacy as possible. Returned when the person signals. Or checked on the person every 5 minutes. Knocked before entering the room. Practiced hand hygiene after returning.			
18. Raised the bed for body mechanics. Lowered the bed rail if up.			
19. Applied gloves.			
20. Removed the bedpan. Observed enema results for amount, color, consistency, shape, and odor. Called the nurse to observe the results.			
21. Assisted with wiping and perineal care as needed. Removed the waterproof underpad as needed. Covered the person with the bath blanket. Removed and discarded gloves. Practiced hand hygiene.			
22. Covered the person with the top linens. Removed the bath blanket. Placed it in the laundry bag.			
23. Raised the bed rail if used. Lowered the bed.			
24. Assisted with hand hygiene. (Wore gloves. Practiced hand hygiene after removing and discarding the gloves.)			
Postprocedure			
25. Provided for comfort.			
26. Ensured that the bed was at a safe and comfortable level. Raised or lowered bed rails. Followed the care plan.			
27. Cleaned up and stored supplies and equipment. (Wore gloves. Changed gloves as needed.)			
a. Discarded disposable items.			
b. Emptied the bedpan after the nurse observed the results.			

Procedure—cont'd	S	U	Comments
c. Followed agency procedures to clean and disinfect the bedpan and other reusable equipment. Returned supplies and equipment to their proper place.	_______	_______	_______________
d. Followed center policy for used linens.	_______	_______	_______________
e. Cleaned and dried the over-bed table if used. Dried with paper towels. Discarded paper towels. Positioned the over-bed table as the person preferred.	_______	_______	_______________
f. Removed and discarded the gloves. Practiced hand hygiene.	_______	_______	_______________
28. Placed the call light and other needed items within reach.	_______	_______	_______________
29. Followed the care plan and the person's preferences for privacy measures to maintain. Leaving the privacy curtain, window coverings, and door open or closed were examples.	_______	_______	_______________
30. Completed a safety check of the room.	_______	_______	_______________
31. Practiced hand hygiene.	_______	_______	_______________
32. Reported and recorded your care and observations.	_______	_______	_______________

Giving an Oil-Retention Enema

VIDEO

Name: ______________________ Date: ______________________

Quality of Life	S	U	Comments
• Knocked before entering the person's room.			
• Addressed the person by name.			
• Introduced yourself by name and title.			
• Explained the procedure before starting and during the procedure.			
• Protected the person's rights during the procedure.			
• Handled the person gently during the procedure.			
Preprocedure			
1. Followed *Delegation Guidelines:*			
a. *Bowel Needs*			
b. *Enemas*			
Saw *Promoting Safety and Comfort:*			
a. *Bowel Needs*			
b. *Enemas*			
c. *Oil-Retention Enemas*			
2. Practiced hand hygiene and got the following supplies:			
• Oil-retention enema			
• Commode or bedpan as needed (this procedure uses a toilet)			
• Slip-resistant footwear and transfer/gait belt (if needed)			
• Waterproof underpads			
• Gloves			
• Bath blanket			
• Laundry bag			
3. Arranged items in the person's room.			
4. Practiced hand hygiene.			
5. Identified the person. Checked the ID (identification) bracelet against the assignment sheet. Used two identifiers. Also called the person by name.			
6. Provided for privacy.			
7. Raised the bed for body mechanics. Bed rails were up if used. Lowered the bed rail near you if up.			
Procedure			
8. Positioned the person. Covered the person for warmth and privacy. (Eliminated use of a bedpan if not needed. Or kept a bedpan nearby for prompt use.)			
a. Covered the person with a bath blanket. Fanfolded top linens to the foot of the bed.			
b. Placed a waterproof underpad under the buttocks.			
c. Positioned the person in the left semi-prone or in left side-lying position.			
9. Applied clean gloves.			
10. Positioned the bedpan nearby. Used the disposable waterproof pad as a barrier.			
11. Gave the enema.			
a. Folded the bath blanket back to expose the anal area.			

Procedure—cont'd	S	U	Comments
b. Removed the cap from the enema tip.			
c. Separated the buttocks to see the anus.			
d. Asked the person to take a deep breath and breathe out slowly through the mouth.			
e. Inserted the tube gently 2 inches into the adult's rectum. Did this as the person exhaled. Stopped if the person reported pain, you felt resistance, or bleeding occurred.			
f. Squeezed and rolled up the container gently. Released pressure on the bottle after you removed the tip from the rectum.			
g. Put the container into the box, tip first. Discarded the container and box.			
12. Covered the person with the bath blanket.			
13. Encouraged retention of the enema. Maintained the left semi-prone or left side-lying position. Provided for comfort.			
14. Removed and discarded gloves. Practiced hand hygiene.			
15. Provided for comfort.			
16. Ensured that the bed was at a safe and comfortable level. Raised or lowered bed rails. Followed the care plan.			
17. Cleaned up and stored supplies and equipment. Followed center policy for used linens and used supplies.			
18. Placed the call light and other needed items within reach.			
19. Followed the care plan and the person's preferences for privacy measures to maintain. Leaving the privacy curtain, window coverings, and door open or closed were examples.			
20. Completed a safety check of the room.			
21. Practiced hand hygiene.			
22. Reported and recorded your care and observations.			
23. Checked the person often. Replaced the waterproof underpad on the bed as needed if there was leakage. (Wore gloves. Practiced hand hygiene after removing and discarding gloves.) Reminded the person to call before flushing if the person uses the bathroom without help.			
24. Returned when the person signaled.			
25. Practiced hand hygiene.			
26. Assisted the person to and from the bathroom if help was needed. Practiced safety measures for transfers and walking. Provided as much privacy as possible. Assisted with wiping, perineal care, and hand hygiene as needed. (Wore gloves. Changed gloves as needed. Removed and discarded gloves and practiced hand hygiene.)			
27. Observed enema results for amount, color, consistency, shape, and odor. Called the nurse to observe the results. (Flushed after the nurse observes the results.)			

Postprocedure

28. Provided for comfort.			
29. Ensured that the bed was at a safe and comfortable level. Raised or lowered bed rails. Followed the care plan.			

Procedure—cont'd	S	U	Comments
30. Cleaned up and stored supplies and equipment. Followed center policy for used linens and used supplies.			
31. Placed the call light and other needed items within reach.			
32. Followed the care plan and the person's preferences for privacy measures to maintain. Leaving the privacy curtain, window coverings, and door open or closed were examples.			
33. Completed a safety check of the room.			
34. Practiced hand hygiene.			
35. Reported and recorded your care and observations.			

Assisting the Person to Empty an Ostomy Pouch

Name: ______________________ Date: ____________________________

Quality of Life	S	U	Comments
• Knocked before entering the person's room.			
• Addressed the person by name.			
• Introduced yourself by name and title.			
• Explained the procedure before starting and during the procedure.			
• Protected the person's rights during the procedure.			
• Handled the person gently during the procedure.			

Preprocedure	S	U	Comments
1. *Followed Delegation Guidelines:*			
a. *Bowel Needs*			
b. *Emptying Ostomy Pouches*			
Saw *Promoting Safety and Comfort:*			
a. *Bowel Needs*			
b. *Emptying Ostomy Pouches*			
2. Practiced hand hygiene and got the following supplies:			
• Toilet paper			
• Premoistened wipes			
• Plastic bag (for wipes)			
• Gloves			
3. Arranged the following in the person's bathroom. Made a cuff on the plastic bag (if used). (Folded down the top portion of the bag.) Placed the bag within reach. Placed a few sheets of toilet paper in the toilet bowl. This helped to prevent splashing when the pouch was emptied.			
4. Practiced hand hygiene.			
5. Identified the person. Checked the ID bracelet against the assignment sheet. Used two identifiers. Also called the person by name.			
6. Provided for privacy.			

Procedure	S	U	Comments
7. Put on gloves.			
8. Assisted the person to the bathroom. Closed the bathroom door for privacy.			
9. Helped the person sit on the toilet and moved garments out of the way. Made sure the person was comfortable.			
10. Had the person spread legs.			
11. Positioned the pouch between the legs and over the toilet.			
12. Held the pouch outlet over the toilet. Opened the clip or clamp and gently pinched the sides to open the outlet.			
13. Allowed the pouch to empty. If necessary, slid your thumb and index finger down the outside of the pouch to push out stools.			
14. Observed the color, amount, consistency, and odor of stools. Flushed the toilet.			

Procedure—cont'd	S	U	Comments
15. Cleaned the inside of the pouch outlet with toilet paper or a premoistened wipe. Made sure the inside was thoroughly clean. Discarded toilet paper into the toilet. Discarded the wipe into the plastic bag.			
16. Cleaned the outside of the pouch outlet. Cleaned the clip (clamp) if soiled. Made sure the outside and the clip (clamp) were thoroughly clean. Used toilet paper or a premoistened wipe. Discarded toilet paper into the toilet. Discarded the wipe into the plastic bag.			
17. Closed the pouch outlet with the clip (clamp). Followed the manufacturer's instructions.			
18. Removed and discarded the gloves. Practiced hand hygiene. Applied clean gloves.			
19. Assisted the person with hand hygiene.			
20. Tied or sealed the plastic bag (if used). Followed agency policy for disposal.			
21. Removed and discarded gloves. Practiced hand hygiene.			
22. Helped the person back to bed.			

Postprocedure			
23. Provided for comfort.			
24. Made sure the bed was at a safe and comfortable level. Raised or lowered the bed rails. Followed the care plan.			
25. Placed the call light and other needed items within reach.			
26. Followed the care plan and the person's preferences for privacy measures to maintain. Leaving the privacy curtain, window coverings, and door open or closed were examples.			
27. Completed a safety check of the room.			
28. Practice hand hygiene.			
29. Reported and recorded your care and observations.			

Preparing the Person for a Meal

Name: ______________________ Date: ______________________

Quality of Life	S	U	Comments
• Knocked before entering the person's room.			
• Addressed the person by name.			
• Introduced yourself by name and title.			
• Explained the procedure before starting and during the procedure.			
• Protected the person's rights during the procedure.			
• Handled the person gently during the procedure.			

Preprocedure

	S	U	Comments
1. Followed *Delegation Guidelines: Preparing for Meals*. Saw *Promoting Safety and Comfort: Preparing for Meals*.			
2. Practiced hand hygiene and got the following supplies:			
• Supplies for oral hygiene			
• Supplies for elimination			
• Supplies for hand hygiene—hand-wipes or soap, water, washcloth, and towel			
• Supplies for transfer if needed			
• Gloves			
3. Arranged items in the person's room.			
4. Practiced hand hygiene.			
5. Identify the person. Check the identification (ID) bracelet against the assignment sheet. Use two identifiers. Also call the person by name.			
6. Provided for privacy.			

Procedure

	S	U	Comments
7. Made sure eyeglasses and hearing aids were in place.			
8. Assisted with oral hygiene. Made sure dentures were in place. Wore gloves and practiced hand hygiene after removing and discarding gloves.			
9. Assisted with elimination as needed. Made sure the person was clean and dry if incontinent. Wore gloves and practiced hand hygiene after removing and discarding the gloves.			
10. Assisted with hand hygiene. Wore gloves and practiced hand hygiene after removing and discarding them.			
11. Cleaned up and stored supplies and equipment (Wore gloves. Changed gloves as needed.)			
a. Discarded disposable items.			
b. Followed agency procedures to clean and disinfect reusable equipment. Returned supplies and equipment to their proper place.			
c. Followed agency policy for used linens.			
d. Cleaned and dried the over-bed table. Dried with paper towels. Discarded paper towels. Left items off of the over-bed table if it will be used for the meal. Or positioned the over-bed table with needed items if the person preferred a meal in the dining room.			
e. Removed and discarded gloves. Practiced hand hygiene.			

Procedure—cont'd	S	U	Comments
12. *For the person who ate in bed.*			
a. Raised the head of the bed to a comfortable position—Fowler's (45–60 degrees) or high-Fowler's (60–90 degrees). (Note: Some state competency tests require that the person sit upright at least 45 degrees to eat, others require 75 to 90 degrees.)	_____	_____	_____
b. Adjusted the over-bed table in front of the person.	_____	_____	_____
13. *For the person who sat in a chair.*			
a. Positioned the person in a chair or wheelchair.	_____	_____	_____
b. Adjusted the over-bed table in front of the person.	_____	_____	_____
14. For the person who ate in dining area, assisted the person to the dining area.	_____	_____	_____
Postprocedure			
15. *For the person who ate in the room:*			
a. Provided for comfort.	_____	_____	_____
b. Straightened the room. Eliminated unpleasant noise, odors, or equipment.	_____	_____	_____
c. Placed the call light and other needed items within reach.	_____	_____	_____
d. Followed the care plan and the person's preferences for privacy measures to maintain. Leaving the privacy curtain, window coverings, and door open or closed were examples.	_____	_____	_____
e. Completed a safety check of the room.	_____	_____	_____
16. Practiced hand hygiene.	_____	_____	_____
17. Reported and recorded your care and observations.	_____	_____	_____

Serving Meal Trays

Name: ______________________ Date: ______________________

Quality of Life	S	U	Comments
• Knocked before entering the person's room.			
• Addressed the person by name.			
• Introduced yourself by name and title.			
• Explained the procedure before starting and during the procedure.			
• Protected the person's rights during the procedure.			
• Handled the person gently during the procedure.			

Preprocedure

	S	U	Comments
1. Followed *Delegation Guidelines: Serving Meal Trays.* Saw *Promoting Safety and Comfort: Serving Meal Trays.*			
2. Practiced hand hygiene.			
3. Prepared the person for a meal if not already done.			

Procedure

	S	U	Comments
4. Checked items on the tray with the dietary card. Made sure the tray was complete and had necessary adaptive equipment (assistive devices).			
5. Identified the person. Checked the ID (identification) bracelet against the dietary card. Used two identifiers. Also called the person by name.			
6. Placed the tray within the person's reach. Adjusted the over-bed table as needed (if used).			
7. Removed food covers. Opened cartons, cut food into bite-sized pieces, buttered bread, and so on as needed. Seasoned food as the person preferred and the care plan allowed.			
8. Placed the napkin, adaptive equipment (assistive devices), and eating utensils within reach. Helped the person apply a clothes protector (towel or napkin) if needed.			
9. Placed the call light within reach if the person was eating in their room.			
10. Did the following when the person was done eating.			
a. Measured and recorded fluid intake if ordered.			
b. Noted the amount and type of foods eaten.			
c. Checked for and removed any food in the mouth (pocketing). Wore gloves. Practiced hand hygiene after removing and discarding them.			
d. Removed the item used to protect clothing if worn. Followed agency policy for used linens. Discarded a disposable napkin.			
e. Removed the tray.			
f. Cleaned spills. Cleaned and dried the over-bed table if used. Dried with paper towels. Discarded the paper towels.			
g. Changed soiled clothing. Followed agency policy for removed clothing.			
h. Assisted with oral hygiene and hand hygiene. Provided for privacy. Wore gloves. Practiced hand hygiene after removing and discarding the gloves.			
i. Helped the person return to bed if needed.			

Postprocedure

11. Provided for comfort. ______ ______ ______________________
12. Placed the call light and other needed items within reach. ______ ______ ______________________
13. Raised or lowered bed rails. Followed the care plan. ______ ______ ______________________
14. Completed a safety check of the room. ______ ______ ______________________
15. Followed center policy for used linens. ______ ______ ______________________
16. Practiced hand hygiene. ______ ______ ______________________
17. Reported and recorded your observations. ______ ______ ______________________

NATCEP™ VIDEO VIDEO CLIP

Feeding the Person

Name: ______________________ Date: ______________________

Quality of Life	S	U	Comments
• Knocked before entering the person's room.			
• Addressed the person by name.			
• Introduced yourself by name and title.			
• Explained the procedure before starting and during the procedure.			
• Protected the person's rights during the procedure.			
• Handled the person gently during the procedure.			

Preprocedure

	S	U	Comments
1. Followed *Delegation Guidelines: Feeding the Person.* Saw *Promoting Safety and Comfort:*			
• *Serving Meals*			
• *Feeding the person*			
2. Practiced hand hygiene.			
3. Positioned the person in a comfortable position for eating—seated in a chair or in Fowler's (45–60 degrees) or high-Fowler's (60–90 degrees). (Note: Some state competency tests require at least 45 degrees, others require 75–90 degrees.)			
4. Got the tray. Placed the tray on the over-bed table or dining table where the person could reach it.			

Procedure

	S	U	Comments
5. Checked items on the tray with the dietary card. Made sure the tray was complete.			
6. Identified the person. Checked the ID (identification) bracelet with the dietary card. Used two identifiers. Also called the person by name.			
7. Draped a napkin across the person's chest and underneath the chin or applied a clothes protector or towel.			
8. Cleaned the person's hands. (NOTE: Some state competency tests require soap and water, others allow hand sanitizer or a hand wipe.)			
9. Placed the chair where you could sit comfortably. Sat facing the person at eye level.			
10. Told the person what foods and fluids were on the tray.			
11. Prepared food for eating. Cut food into bite-sized pieces. Seasoned foods as the person preferred and as the care plan allowed.			
12. Served foods in the order the person preferred. Identified foods as you served them. Alternated between solid and liquid foods. Used a spoon for safety. Allowed enough time to chew and swallow. Did not rush the person.			

Procedure—cont'd	S	U	Comments
13. Offered fluids (water, coffee, tea, or other fluid). (Note: Some state competency tests require that a drink is offered for at least every two to threee bites of food.) Used straws (if allowed) for liquids if the person could not drink out of a glass or cup. Had one straw for each liquid. Provided short straws if the person was weak. Followed the care plan for using straws.			
14. Followed the care plan if the person had dysphagia. Gave thickened liquids with a spoon if needed.	______	______	______
15. Checked the person's mouth before offering more food or fluids. Made sure the mouth was empty between bites and swallows. Asked if the person was ready for the next bite or drink.	______	______	
16. Wiped the person's hands, face, and mouth as needed during the meal. Used a napkin or hand wipe.	______	______	______
17. Talked with the person in a pleasant manner.	______	______	______
18. Encouraged the person to eat as much as possible.	______	______	______
19. Wiped the person's mouth with a napkin or a hand wipe. Discarded the napkin or hand wipe.	______	______	______
20. Noted how much and which foods were eaten.	______	______	______
21. Measured and recorded fluid intake if ordered.	______	______	______
22. Removed the item used to protect clothing if worn. Followed agency policy for used linens. Discarded a disposable napkin.	______	______	
23. Removed the tray.	______	______	______
24. Took the person to their room (if in a dining area). Cleaned and dried the over-bed table (if used in the person's room). Dried with paper towels. Discarded the paper towels.	______	______	______
25. Assisted with oral hygiene and hand hygiene. Provided for privacy. Wore gloves. Practiced hand hygiene after removing and discarding the gloves.	______	______	______
Postprocedure			
26. Provided for comfort.	______	______	______
27. Raised or lowered bed rails. Followed the care plan.	______	______	______
28. Placed the call light and other needed items within reach.	______	______	______
29. Followed the care plan and the person's preferences for privacy measures to maintain. Leaving the privacy curtain, window coverings, and door open or closed were examples.	______	______	______
30. Completed a safety check of the room.	______	______	______
31. Returned the food tray to the food cart.	______	______	______
32. Practiced hand hygiene.	______	______	______
33. Reported and recorded your observations.	______	______	______

NATCEP™ VIDEO

Measuring Intake and Output

Name: ______________________ Date: ______________________

Quality of Life

S U Comments

- Knocked before entering the person's room.
- Addressed the person by name.
- Introduced yourself by name and title.
- Explained the procedure before starting and during the procedure.
- Protected the person's rights during the procedure.
- Handled the person gently during the procedure.

Preprocedure

1. Followed *Delegation Guidelines: Intake and Output*. Saw *Promoting Safety and Comfort: Intake and Output*.
2. Practiced hand hygiene and got the following supplies:
   - Intake and output (I&O) record
   - Two graduates:
   - A graduate for intake
   - A graduate for output
   - Needed supplies for urinary or bowel elimination
   - Gloves
   - Paper towels or disposable waterproof pad
3. Arranged items in the person's room.
4. Practiced hand hygiene.
5. Identified the person. Checked the identification (ID) bracelet against the I&O record. Used two identifiers. Also called the person by name.
6. Provided for privacy.

Procedure

7. Put on gloves.
8. Measured intake.
   a. Poured liquid remaining in the container into the graduate used to measure intake. Avoided spills and splashes on the outside of the graduate.
   b. Placed the graduate on a flat surface. Measured the amount at eye level.
   c. Checked the serving amount on the I&O record. Or checked the serving size of each container.
   d. Subtracted the remaining amount from the full serving amount. Noted the amount.
   e. Poured fluid in the graduate back into the container.
   f. Repeated steps for each liquid.
      1) Poured liquid remaining in the container into the graduate used to measure intake. Avoided spills and splashes on the outside of the graduate.
      2) Placed the graduate on a flat surface. Measured the amount at eye level on a flat surface.
      3) Checked the serving amount on the I&O record. Or checked the serving size of each container.
      4) Subtracted the remaining amount from the full serving amount. Noted the amount.

Procedure—cont'd	S	U	Comments
5) Poured fluid in the graduate back into the container.			
g. Added the amounts from each liquid together.			
h. Recorded the time and amount on the I&O record.			
i. Discarded the excess liquids. Followed agency procedures to clean the graduate. Returned the graduate to its proper place.			
9. Assisted with elimination if needed. Measured output.			
a. Poured fluid into the graduate used to measure output. Avoided spills and splashes on the outside of the graduate.			
b. Placed the device on a paper towel (or disposable waterproof pad) on a flat surface. Measured the amount at eye level.			
c. Disposed of fluid in the toilet. Avoided splashes.			
d. Rinsed the graduate. Poured the rinse into the toilet and flush. Followed agency procedures for cleaning and disinfection. Returned the graduate to its proper place.			
e. Rinsed the voiding receptacle or other container. Poured the rinse into the toilet and flush. Followed agency procedures for cleaning and disinfection. Returned the item to its proper place.			
f. Removed and discarded the gloves. Practiced hand hygiene.			
g. Recorded the output amount on the person's I&O record.			

Postprocedure

10. Provided for comfort.			
11. Placed the call light and other items within reach.			
12. Followed the care plan and the person's preferences for privacy measures to maintain. Leaving the privacy curtain, window coverings, and door open or closed were examples.			
13. Completed a safety check of the room.			
14. Practiced hand hygiene.			
15. Reported and recorded your care and observations.			

NATCEP™

Providing Drinking Water

Name: ______________________ Date: ______________________

Quality of Life	S	U	Comments
• Knocked before entering the person's room.			
• Addressed the person by name.			
• Introduced yourself by name and title.			
• Explained the procedure before starting and during the procedure.			
• Protected the person's rights during the procedure.			
• Handled the person gently during the procedure.			
Preprocedure			
1. Followed *Delegation Guidelines: Providing Drinking Water*. Saw *Promoting Safety and Comfort: Providing Drinking Water*.			
2. Obtained a list of persons who have special fluid orders from the nurse. Or used your assignment sheet.			
3. Practiced hand hygiene and got the following supplies:			
• Cart			
• Ice chest filled with ice			
• Cover for ice chest			
• Scoop			
• Paper towels			
• Water mugs			
• Water pitcher filled with cold water (optional depending on agency procedure)			
• Towel for the scoop (if there is no scoop holder)			
4. Covered the cart with paper towels. Arranged equipment on top of the paper towels.			
Procedure			
5. Took the cart to the person's room door. Did not take the cart into the room.			
6. Checked the person's fluid orders. Used the list from the nurse.			
7. Practiced hand hygiene.			
8. Identified the person. Checked the ID (identification) bracelet against the fluid order sheet or your assignment sheet. Used two identifiers. Also called the person by name.			
9. Took the mug from the person's over-bed table. Emptied it into the bathroom sink.			
10. Determined if a new mug was needed.			
11. Used the scoop to fill the mug with ice. Did not let the scoop touch the mug, lid, or straw.			
12. Placed the ice scoop holder or on a clean towel.			
13. Filled the mug with water. Got water from the room sink, or bathroom sink or used the water pitcher on the cart.			
14. Placed the mug on the over-bed table. Made sure the mug was within the person's reach.			

Postprocedure

15. Provided for comfort. ______ ______ ______
16. Placed the call light and other needed items within reach. ______ ______ ______
17. Completed a safety check of the room. ______ ______ ______
18. Practiced hand hygiene. ______ ______ ______
19. Repeated for each resident.
    a. Took the cart to the person's room door. Did not take the cart into the room. ______ ______ ______
    b. Checked the person's fluid orders. Used the list from the nurse. ______ ______ ______
    c. Practiced hand hygiene. ______ ______ ______
    d. Identified the person. Checked the ID bracelet against the fluid order sheet or your assignment sheet. Used two identifiers. Also called the person by name. ______ ______ ______
    e. Took the mug from the person's over-bed table. Emptied it into the bathroom sink. ______ ______ ______
    f. Determined if a new mug was needed. ______ ______ ______
    g. Used the scoop to fill the mug with ice. Did not let the scoop touch the mug, lid, or straw. ______ ______ ______
    h. Placed the ice scoop in the scoop holder or on a clean towel. ______ ______ ______
    i. Filled the mug with water. Got water from the room sink, or the bathroom sink or the water pitcher on the cart. ______ ______ ______
    j. Placed the mug on the over-bed table. Made sure the mug was within the person's reach. ______ ______ ______

Postprocedure

20. Provided for comfort. ______ ______ ______
21. Placed the call light and other needed items within reach. ______ ______ ______
22. Completed a safety check of the room. ______ ______ ______
23. Practiced hand hygiene. ______ ______ ______

NATCEP™ VIDEO VIDEO CLIP

Taking a Temperature With an Electronic Thermometer

Name: ______________________ Date: ______________________

Quality of Life	S	U	Comments
• Knocked before entering the person's room.			
• Addressed the person by name.			
• Introduced yourself by name and title.			
• Explained the procedure before starting and during the procedure.			
• Protected the person's rights during the procedure.			
• Handled the person gently during the procedure.			

Preprocedure

	S	U	Comments
1. Followed *Delegation Guidelines: Taking Temperatures*. Saw *Promoting Safety and Comfort: Taking Temperatures*.			
2. For an oral temperature, asked the person not to eat, drink, smoke, or chew gum for at least 15 to 20 minutes before the measurement or as required by agency policy.			
3. Practiced hand hygiene and got the following supplies:			
• Thermometer—standard electronic or tympanic membrane, or temporal artery			
• Probe for a standard electronic thermometer (blue–oral or axillary; red– rectal)			
• Probe covers			
• Toilet paper and lubricant as directed by the nurse (rectal temperature)			
• Towel and laundry bag (axillary temperature)			
• Gloves as needed			
4. Plugged the probe into the thermometer if using a standard electronic thermometer.			
5. Arranged items in the person's room if needed.			
6. Practiced hand hygiene.			
7. Identified the person. Checked the ID (identification) bracelet against the assignment sheet. Used two identifiers. Also called the person by name.			
8. Provided for privacy.			

Procedure

	S	U	Comments
9. Positioned the person.			
a. For an oral, rectal, axillary, or tympanic membrane temperature—Had the person sit or lie down.			
b. For a rectal temperature—Assisted the person into a semi-prone or side-lying position.			
10. Put on the gloves if contact with blood, body fluids, secretions, or excretions was likely.			
11. Inserted the probe into the probe cover.			
12. *For an oral temperature:*			
a. Had the person open the mouth and raise the tongue.			
b. Placed the covered probe at the base of the tongue and to one side.			
c. Had the person lower the tongue and close the mouth.			

Procedure—cont'd	S	U	Comments
d. Started the thermometer. Held the probe in place until the thermometer indicated that the temperature was measured. A tone or a flashing or steady light was common.	______	______	______
13. *For a rectal temperature:*			
a. Lubricated the end of the covered probe.	______	______	______
b. Exposed the anal area.	______	______	______
c. Raised the upper buttock.	______	______	______
d. Inserted the probe ½ inch into the rectum.	______	______	______
e. Started the thermometer if needed. Held the probe in place until thermometer indicated the temperature was measured. A tone or a flashing or steady light was common.	______	______	______
14. *For an axillary temperature:*			
a. Helped the person remove an arm from the gown. Did not expose the person.	______	______	______
b. Dried the axilla with a towel. Followed agency policy for used linens.	______	______	______
c. Placed the covered probe in the center of the axilla.	______	______	______
d. Placed the person's arm over the chest.	______	______	______
e. Started the thermometer if needed. Held the probe in place until thermometer indicated that the temperature was measured. A tone or a flashing or steady light was common.	______	______	______
15. *For a tympanic membrane temperature:*			
a. Asked the person to turn the head so the ear was in front of you.	______	______	______
b. Pulled up and back on the adult's ear to straighten the ear canal. If child was aged 4 years, or less, the nurse may have had you pull the ear down and back.	______	______	______
c. Inserted the covered probe gently.			
d. Started the thermometer if needed. Held the probe in place until thermometer indicated that the temperature was measured. A tone or a flashing or steady light was common. ______	______	______	______
16. *For a temporal artery temperature:*			
a. Placed the device in the center of the forehead.	______	______	______
b. Pressed the scan button.	______	______	______
c. Slid the device right or left across the temporal artery. Used the side of the head that was exposed. Kept the thermometer flat on the forehead and in contact with the skin.	______	______	______
d. Released the scan button when the thermometer reached the hairline.	______	______	______
17. Removed the probe from the site. Read the temperature on the display.	______	______	______
18. Pressed the eject button to discard the cover.	______	______	______
19. Noted the person's name, temperature, and temperature site on your notepad or assignment sheet.	______	______	______
20. Returned the probe to the holder.	______	______	______
21. Helped the person put the gown back on (axillary temperature). For a rectal temperature:			
a. Wiped the anal area with toilet paper to remove lubricant.	______	______	______
b. Covered the person.	______	______	______
c. Disposed of used toilet paper.	______	______	______
d. Removed and discarded the gloves. Practiced hand hygiene.	______	______	______

Postprocedure

22. Provided for comfort. _______ _______ _______
23. Followed the care plan and the person's preferences for privacy measures to maintain. Leaving the privacy curtain, window coverings, and door open or closed were examples. _______ _______ _______
24. Placed the call light and other needed items within reach. _______ _______ _______
25. Completed a safety check of the room. _______ _______ _______
26. Practiced hand hygiene. _______ _______ _______
27. Returned the thermometer to the charging unit. Follow agency policy for disinfection. _______ _______ _______
28. Reported and recorded the temperature. Noted the temperature site when reporting and recording. Reported an abnormal temperature at once. _______ _______ _______

NATCEP™ VIDEO VIDEO CLIP

Taking a Radial Pulse

Name: ______________________ Date: ______________________

Quality of Life	S	U	Comments
• Knocked before entering the person's room.			
• Addressed the person by name.			
• Introduced yourself by name and title.			
• Explained the procedure before starting and during the procedure.			
• Protected the person's rights during the procedure.			
• Handled the person gently during the procedure.			

Preprocedure	S	U	Comments
1. Followed *Delegation Guidelines: Taking Pulses.* Saw *Promoting Safety and Comfort: Taking Pulses.*			
2. Practiced hand hygiene.			
3. Identified the person. Checked the ID (identification) bracelet against the assignment sheet. Used two identifiers. Also called the person by name.			
4. Provided for privacy.			

Procedure	S	U	Comments
5. Had the person sit or lie down.			
6. Located the radial pulse on the thumb side of the person's wrist. Used your first two or three middle fingertips.			
7. Noted if the pulse was strong or weak, regular or irregular.			
8. Counted the pulse for 30 seconds. Multiplied the number of beats by 2 for the number of pulses in 60 seconds (1 minute).			
9. Counted the pulse for 1 minute if:			
a. Directed by the nurse and care plan.			
b. Required by agency policy.			
c. The pulse was irregular.			
d. Required for your state competency test.			
10. Noted the following on your notepad or assignment sheet.			
a. The person's name			
b. Pulse site			
c. Pulse rate			
d. Pulse strength			
e. If the pulse was regular or irregular			

Postprocedure	S	U	Comments
11. Provided for comfort.			
12. Placed the call light and other needed items within reach.			
13. Followed the care plan and the person's preferences for privacy measures to maintain. Leaving the privacy curtain, window coverings, and door open or closed were examples.			
14. Completed a safety check of the room.			
15. Practiced hand hygiene.			
16. Reported and recorded the pulse rate and your observations. Reported an abnormal pulse at once.			

Taking an Apical Pulse and an Apical-Radial Pulse

Name: ____________________ Date: ____________________

Quality of Life	S	U	Comments
• Knocked before entering the person's room.			
• Addressed the person by name.			
• Introduced yourself by name and title.			
• Explained the procedure before starting and during the procedure.			
• Protected the person's rights during the procedure.			
• Handled the person gently during the procedure.			
Preprocedure			
1. Followed *Delegation Guidelines: Taking Pulses*. Saw *Promoting Safety and Comfort:*			
a. *Using a Stethoscope.*			
b. *Taking Pulses.*			
2. Asked a coworker to help you (for an apical-radial pulse).			
3. Practiced hand hygiene and got the following supplies:			
• Stethoscope			
• Antiseptic wipes			
4. Practiced hand hygiene.			
5. Identified the person. Checked the ID (identification) bracelet against the assignment sheet. Used two identifiers. Also called the person by name.			
6. Provided for privacy.			
Procedure			
7. Cleaned the stethoscope earpieces and chest-piece with an antiseptic wipe. Discarded the wipe.			
8. Had the person sit or lie down.			
9. For an apical pulse			
a. Exposed the upper part of the left chest. Exposed a female's breasts only to the extent necessary.			
b. Warmed the diaphragm in your palm.			
c. Placed the stethoscope earpieces in your ears. The bends of the tips pointed forward.			
d. Found the apical pulse. Placed the diaphragm 2 to 3 inches to the left of the breastbone.			
e. Counted the pulse for 1 minute. (Counted each lub-dub as 1 beat). Noted if it was regular or irregular.			
10. For an apical-radial pulse:			
a. Exposed the upper part of the left chest. Exposed a female's breasts only to the extent necessary.			
b. Warmed the diaphragm in your palm.			
c. Placed the stethoscope earpieces in your ears. The bends of the tips pointed forward.			

Procedure—cont'd	S	U	Comments
d. Found the apical pulse. Placed the diaphragm 2 to 3 inches to the left of the breastbone. Your coworker found the radial pulse.			
e. Gave the signal to begin counting.			
f. Counted the apical pulse for 1 minute. Your coworker counted the radial pulse for 1 minute.			
g. Gave the signal to stop counting. Asked your coworker for the radial pulse rate.			
11. Covered the person. Removed the stethoscope earpieces from your ears.			
12. For an apical-radial pulse, subtracted the radial pulse from the apical pulse for the pulse deficit.			
13. Noted the person's name and pulse site(s), pulse rate(s), and pulse deficit on your notepad or assignment sheet. Noted if the pulse was regular or irregular.			

Postprocedure

	S	U	Comments
14. Provided for comfort.			
15. Placed the call light and other needed items within reach.			
16. Followed the care plan and the person's preferences for privacy measures to maintain. Leaving the privacy curtain, window coverings, and door open or closed were examples.			
17. Completed a safety check of the room.			
18. Cleaned the stethoscope earpieces and chest-piece with an antiseptic wipe. Discarded the wipe.			
19. Practiced hand hygiene.			
20. Returned the stethoscope to its proper place. Follow agency policy for disinfection.			
21. Reported and recorded your care and observations. Noted if the pulse was regular or irregular. Recorded the pulse rate with *Ap* for apical. For an apical-radial pulse, recorded the apical and radial pulse rates and the pulse deficit. Reported an abnormal pulse rate at once.			

NATCEP™ VIDEO VIDEO CLIP

Counting Respirations

Name: ____________________ Date: ____________________

Procedure	S	U	Comments
1. Followed *Delegation Guidelines: Counting Respirations.*	______	______	____________
2. Counted respirations after taking the pulse. (Did this if the person tended to change the breathing pattern when being watched.) Kept your fingers or stethoscope over the pulse site.	______	______	____________
3. Did not tell the person you were counting respirations.	______	______	____________
4. Counted chest rises. Each rise and fall of the chest was one respiration.	______	______	____________
5. Noted the following:			
a. If respirations were regular	______	______	____________
b. If both sides of the chest rose equally	______	______	____________
c. The depth of the respirations	______	______	____________
d. If the person had any pain or difficulty breathing	______	______	____________
e. An abnormal respiratory pattern	______	______	____________
6. Counted respirations for 30 seconds. Multiplied the number by 2 for the number of respirations in 60 seconds (1 minute).	______	______	____________
7. Counted respirations for 1 minute if:			
a. Directed by the nurse and care plan.	______	______	____________
b. Required by agency policy.	______	______	____________
c. They were abnormal or irregular.	______	______	____________
d. Required for your state competency test.	______	______	____________
8. Noted the person's name, respiratory rate, and other observations on your notepad or assignment sheet.	______	______	____________

Postprocedure

Postprocedure	S	U	Comments
9. Provided for comfort.	______	______	____________
10. Placed the call light and other needed items within reach.	______	______	____________
11. Followed the care plan and the person's preferences for privacy measures to maintain. Leaving the privacy curtain, window coverings, and door open or closed were examples.	______	______	____________
12. Completed a safety check of the room.	______	______	____________
13. Practiced hand hygiene.	______	______	____________
14. Reported and recorded the respiratory rate and your observations. Reported abnormal respirations at once.	______	______	____________

NATCEP™ VIDEO VIDEO CLIP

Measuring Blood Pressure With an Aneroid Manometer

Name: ____________________ Date: ____________________

Quality of Life	S	U	Comments
• Knocked before entering the person's room.			
• Addressed the person by name.			
• Introduced yourself by name and title.			
• Explained the procedure before starting and during the procedure.			
• Protected the person's rights during the procedure.			
• Handled the person gently during the procedure.			

Preprocedure

	S	U	Comments
1. Followed *Delegation Guidelines: Measuring Blood Pressure*. Saw *Promoting Safety and Comfort:*			
a. *Using a Stethoscope*			
b. *Blood Pressure Equipment*			
2. Practiced hand hygiene and got the following supplies:			
• Aneroid sphygmomanometer			
• Stethoscope			
• Antiseptic wipes			
3. Practiced hand hygiene.			
4. Identified the person. Checked the ID (identification) bracelet against the assignment sheet. Used two identifiers. Also called the person by name.			
5. Provided for privacy.			

Procedure

	S	U	Comments
6. Had the person sit or lie down.			
7. Positioned the person's arm level with the heart. The palm was up.			
8. Cleaned the stethoscope earpieces and chest-piece with an antiseptic wipe. Warmed the diaphragm in your palm. Discarded the wipe.			
9. Stood no more than 3 feet away from the manometer.			
10. Exposed the upper arm.			
11. Squeezed the cuff to expel any air. Closed the valve on the bulb.			
12. Found the brachial artery at the inner aspect of the elbow. (The brachial artery is on the little finger side of the arm.) Used your fingertips.			
13. Located the arrow on the cuff. Aligned the arrow on the cuff over the brachial artery. Wrapped the cuff around the upper arm at least 1 inch above the elbow. It was even and snug.			
14. Placed the stethoscope earpieces in your ears. Placed the stethoscope's diaphragm over the brachial artery. Did not place it under the cuff.			
15. Use Method 1, 2, or 3 as directed by your instructor or the nurse. These methods guided how much to inflate the cuff and at what point to listen for the systolic pressure.			
16. Found the radial pulse for Methods 1 and 2.			

Procedure—cont'd	S	U	Comments
17. *Method 1:*			
a. Inflated the cuff until you could no longer feel the pulse. Noted this point.	______	______	______
b. Inflated the cuff 30 mm Hg beyond the point where you last felt the pulse.	______	______	______
18. *Method 2:*			
a. Inflated the cuff until you no longer felt the pulse. Noted this point.	______	______	______
b. Inflated the cuff 30 mm Hg beyond the point where you last felt the pulse.	______	______	______
c. Deflated the cuff slowly. Noted the point where you felt the pulse.	______	______	______
d. Waited 30 seconds.	______	______	______
e. Inflated the cuff 30 mm Hg beyond the point where you felt the pulse return.	______	______	______
19. *Method 3:*			
a. Inflated the cuff 160 to 180 mm Hg.	______	______	______
b. Deflated the cuff if you heard a blood pressure (BP) sound. Reinflated the cuff to 200 mm Hg if needed.	______	______	______
20. Deflated the cuff at an even rate of 2 to 4 mL/s. Slowly turned the valve counterclockwise to deflate the cuff. If the manometer needle stopped dropping and the cuff was not deflating, you needed to turn the valve more.	______	______	______
21. Noted the point where you heard the first sound. This was the systolic reading.	______	______	______
22. Continued to deflate the cuff. Noted the point where the sound disappeared (the last sound heard). This was the diastolic reading.	______	______	______
23. Deflated the cuff completely. Removed it from the person's arm. Removed the stethoscope earpieces from your ears.	______	______	______
24. Noted the person's name and BP on your notepad or assignment sheet.	______	______	______
25. Returned the cuff to the case or the wall holder.	______	______	______

Postprocedure

26. Provided for comfort.	______	______	______
27. Placed the call light and other needed items within reach.	______	______	______
28. Followed the care plan and the person's preferences for privacy measures to maintain. Leaving the privacy curtain, window coverings, and door open or closed were examples.	______	______	______
29. Completed a safety check of the room.	______	______	______
30. Cleaned the earpieces and chest-piece with an antiseptic wipe. Discarded the wipe.	______	______	______
31. Practiced hand hygiene.	______	______	______
32. Returned the equipment to its proper place. Follow agency policy for disinfection.	______	______	______
33. Reported and recorded the BP. Noted which arm was used. Reported an abnormal BP at once.	______	______	______

Measuring Blood Pressure With an Electronic Manometer

Name: ____________________ Date: ____________________

Quality of Life	S	U	Comments
• Knocked before entering the person's room.			
• Addressed the person by name.			
• Introduced yourself by name and title.			
• Explained the procedure before starting and during the procedure.			
• Protected the person's rights during the procedure.			
• Handled the person gently during the procedure.			

Preprocedure	S	U	Comments
1. Followed *Delegation Guidelines: Measuring Blood Pressure.*			
2. Practiced hand hygiene and got the following supplies:			
• Electronic BP monitor			
• BP cuff for use with the device (in the correct size for the person)			
3. Practiced hand hygiene.			
4. Identified the person. Checked the ID (identification) bracelet against the assignment sheet. Used two identifiers. Also called the person by name.			
5. Provided for privacy.			

Procedure	S	U	Comments
6. Had the person sit or lie down.			
7. Positioned the person's arm level with the heart.			
8. Exposed the upper arm. The palm was up.			
9. Squeezed the cuff to expel any air.			
10. Turned on the electronic BP manometer.			
11. Connected the cuff to the manometer's connection tubing.			
12. Found the brachial artery at the inner aspect of the elbow. (The brachial artery is on the little finger side of the arm.) Used your fingertips.			
13. Located the arrow on the cuff. Aligned the arrow on the cuff over the brachial artery. Wrapped the cuff around the upper arm at least 1 inch above the elbow. It was even and snug.			
14. Pressed the start button on the device. Left the cuff in place while the device measured the BP. Asked the person to be still.			
15. Removed the cuff after the BP was measured. The BP was displayed on the device.			
16. Noted the person's name and BP on your notepad or assignment sheet.			
17. Followed the agency policy for where to store the cuff (in the person's room or with the BP manometer).			

Postprocedure

18. Provided for comfort. ______ ______ ____________
19. Placed the call light and other needed items within reach. ______ ______ ____________
20. Followed the care plan and the person's preferences for privacy measures to maintain. Leaving the privacy curtain, window coverings, and door open or closed were examples. ______ ______ ____________
21. Completed a safety check of the room. ______ ______ ____________
22. Practiced hand hygiene. ______ ______ ____________
23. Returned the equipment to its proper place. ______ ______ ____________
24. Reported and recorded the BP. Noted which arm was used. Reported an abnormal BP at once. ______ ______ ____________

NATCEP™ VIDEO VIDEO CLIP

Performing Range-of-Motion Exercises

Name: ______________________ Date: ______________________

Quality of Life	S	U	Comments
• Knocked before entering the person's room.	____	____	____
• Addressed the person by name.	____	____	____
• Introduced yourself by name and title.	____	____	____
• Explained the procedure before starting and during the procedure.	____	____	____
• Protected the person's rights during the procedure.	____	____	____
• Handled the person gently during the procedure.	____	____	____
Preprocedure			
1. Followed *Delegation Guidelines: Range-of-Motion Exercises*. Saw *Promoting Safety and Comfort: Range-of-Motion Exercises*.	____	____	____
2. Practiced hand hygiene.	____	____	____
3. Identified the person. Checked the ID (identification) bracelet against the assignment sheet. Used two identifiers. Also called the person by name.	____	____	____
4. Obtained a bath blanket.	____	____	____
5. Provided for privacy.	____	____	____
6. Raised the bed for body mechanics. Bed rails were up if used. Lowered the bed rail near you if up.	____	____	____
Procedure			
7. Positioned the person supine or in a position of comfort that allows for joint movement.	____	____	____
8. Covered the person with a bath blanket. Fanfolded top linens to the foot of the bed.	____	____	____
9. Exercised the neck *if allowed by your agency and if the nurse instructed you to do so.*	____	____	____
a. Placed your hands over the person's ears to support the head. Supported the jaw with your fingers.	____	____	____
b. Flexion—brought the head forward. The chin touched the chest.	____	____	____
c. Extension—straightened the head.	____	____	____
d. Hyperextension—brought the head backward until the chin pointed up. (Straightened the head to continue other exercises.)	____	____	____
e. Rotation—turned the head from side to side.	____	____	____
f. Lateral flexion—moved the head to the right and to the left.	____	____	____
g. Repeated flexion, extension, hyperextension, rotation, and lateral flexion 5 times—or the number of times stated on the care plan.	____	____	____
10. Exercised the shoulder.			
a. Supported the wrist with one hand. Supported the elbow with the other hand.	____	____	____
b. Flexion—raised the arm straight in front and over the head.	____	____	____
c. Extension—brought the arm down to the side.	____	____	____
d. Hyperextension—moved the arm behind the body. (Did this if the person was in a straight-backed chair or was standing. Brought the arm back to the side of the body to continue other exercises.)	____	____	____

e. Abduction—moved the straight arm away from the side of the body. ______ ______ ______

f. Adduction—moved the straight arm to the side of the body. ______ ______ ______

g. Internal rotation—bent the elbow. Placed it at the same level as the shoulder. Moved the forearm and hand so the fingers pointed down. ______ ______ ______

h. External rotation—moved the forearm and hand so the fingers pointed up. ______ ______ ______

i. Repeated flexion, extension, hyperextension, abduction, adduction, and internal and external rotation five times—or the number of times stated on the care plan. ______ ______ ______

11. Exercised the elbow.

a. Supported the person's wrist with one hand. Supported the elbow with your other hand. ______ ______ ______

b. Flexion—bent the arm so the same-side shoulder was touched. ______ ______ ______

c. Extension—straightened the arm. ______ ______ ______

d. Repeated flexion and extension five times—or the number of times stated on the care plan. ______ ______ ______

12. Exercised the forearm.

a. Continued to support the wrist and elbow. ______ ______ ______

b. Pronation—turned the hand so the palm was down. ______ ______ ______

c. Supination—turned the hand so the palm was up. ______ ______ ______

d. Repeated pronation and supination five times—or the number of times stated on the care plan. ______ ______ ______

13. Exercised the wrist.

a. Supported the wrist with both of your hands. ______ ______ ______

b. Flexion—bent the hand down. ______ ______ ______

c. Extension—straightened the hand. ______ ______ ______

d. Hyperextension—bent the hand back. (Straightened the hand to continue other exercises.) ______ ______ ______

e. Radial flexion—turned the hand toward the thumb. ______ ______ ______

f. Ulnar flexion—turned the hand toward the little finger. ______ ______ ______

g. Repeated flexion, extension, hyperextension, and radial and ulnar flexion five times—or the number of times stated on the care plan. ______ ______ ______

14. Exercised the thumb.

a. Supported the person's hand with one hand. Supported the thumb with your other hand. ______ ______ ______

b. Abduction—moved the thumb out from the inner part of the index finger. ______ ______ ______

c. Adduction—moved the thumb back next to the index finger. ______ ______ ______

d. Opposition—touched each fingertip with the thumb. ______ ______ ______

e. Flexion—bent the thumb into the hand. ______ ______ ______

f. Extension—moved the thumb out to the side of the fingers. ______ ______ ______

g. Repeated abduction, adduction, opposition, flexion, and extension five times—or the number of times stated on the care plan. ______ ______ ______

15. Exercised the fingers.

a. Abduction—spread the fingers and the thumb apart. ______ ______ ______

Procedure—cont'd	S	U	Comments
b. Adduction—brought the fingers and thumb together.	______	______	____________
c. Flexion—made a fist.	______	______	____________
d. Extension—straightened the fingers so the fingers, hand, and arm were straight.	______	______	____________
e. Repeated abduction, adduction, flexion, and extension five times—or the number of times stated on the care plan.	______	______	____________
16. Exercised the hip.			
a. Supported the leg. Placed one hand under the knee. Placed your other hand under the ankle.	______	______	____________
b. Flexion—raised the leg.	______	______	____________
c. Extension—straightened the leg.	______	______	____________
d. Hyperextension—moved the leg behind the body. (Did this if the person was standing. Brought the leg back to the side of the body to continue other exercises.)	______	______	____________
e. Abduction—moved the leg away from the body.	______	______	____________
f. Adduction—moved the leg toward the other leg.	______	______	____________
g. Internal rotation—turned the leg inward.	______	______	____________
h. External rotation—turned the leg outward.	______	______	____________
i. Repeated flexion, extension, hyperextension, abduction, adduction, and internal and external rotation five times—or the number of times stated on the care plan.	______	______	____________
17. Exercised the knee.			
a. Supported the knee. Placed one hand under the knee. Placed your other hand under the ankle.	______	______	____________
b. Flexion—bent the knee.	______	______	____________
c. Extension—straightened the knee.	______	______	____________
d. Repeated flexion and extension of the knee five times—or the number of times stated on the care plan.	______	______	____________
18. Exercised the ankle.			
a. Supported the foot and ankle. Placed one hand under the foot. Placed your other hand under the ankle.	______	______	____________
b. Dorsiflexion—pulled the foot upward. Pushed down on the heel at the same time.	______	______	____________
c. Plantar flexion—turned the foot down. Or pointed the toes.	______	______	____________
d. Repeated dorsiflexion and plantar flexion five times—or the number of times stated on the care plan.	______	______	____________
19. Exercised the foot.			
a. Continued to support the foot and ankle.	______	______	____________
b. Pronation—turned the outside of the foot up and the inside down.	______	______	____________
c. Supination—turned the inside of the foot up and the outside down.	______	______	____________
d. Repeated pronation and supination five times—or the number of times stated on the care plan.	______	______	____________
20. Exercised the toes.			
a. Flexion—curled the toes.	______	______	____________
b. Extension—straightened the toes.	______	______	____________
c. Abduction—spread the toes apart.	______	______	____________
d. Adduction—pulled the toes together.	______	______	____________
e. Repeated flexion, extension, abduction, and adduction five times—or the number of times stated on the care plan.	______	______	____________

Procedure—cont'd	S	U	Comments
21. Covered the leg. Raised the bed rail if used.			
22. Went to the other side. Lowered the bed rail near you if up.			
23. Repeated exercises.			
a. Exercised the shoulder.			
1) Supported the wrist with one hand. Supported the elbow with the other hand.			
2) Flexion—raised the arm straight in front and over the head.			
3) Extension—brought the arm down to the side.			
4) Hyperextension—moved the arm behind the body. (Did this if the person was in a straight-backed chair or was standing. Brought the arm back to the side of the body to continue other exercises.)			
5) Abduction—moved the straight arm away from the side of the body.			
6) Adduction—Moved the straight arm to the side of the body.			
7) Internal rotation—bent the elbow. Placed it at the same level as the shoulder. Moved the forearm and hand so the fingers pointed down.			
8) External rotation—moved the forearm and hand so the fingers pointed up.			
9) Repeated flexion, extension, hyperextension, abduction, adduction, and internal and external rotation five times—or the number of times stated on the care plan.			
b. Exercised the elbow.			
1) Supported the person's wrist with one hand. Supported the elbow with your other hand.			
2) Flexion—bent the arm so the same-side shoulder was touched.			
3) Extension—straightened the arm.			
4) Repeated flexion and extension five times—or the number of times stated on the care plan.			
c. Exercised the forearm.			
1) Continued to support the wrist and elbow.			
2) Pronation—turned the hand so the palm was down.			
3) Supination—turned the hand so the palm was up.			
4) Repeated pronation and supination five times—or the number of times stated on the care plan.			
d. Exercised the wrist.			
1) Supported the wrist with both of your hands.			
2) Flexion—bent the hand down.			
3) Extension—straightened the hand.			
4) Hyperextension—bent the hand back.			
5) Radial flexion—turned the hand toward the thumb.			
6) Ulnar flexion—turned the hand toward the little finger.			
7) Repeated flexion, extension, hyperextension, and radial and ulnar flexion five times—or the number of times stated on the care plan.			
e. Exercised the thumb.			

Procedure—cont'd	S	U	Comments
1) Supported the person's hand with one hand. Supported the thumb with your other hand.	______	______	______
2) Abduction—moved the thumb out from the inner part of the index finger.	______	______	______
3) Adduction—moved the thumb back next to the index finger.	______	______	______
4) Opposition—touched each fingertip with the thumb.	______	______	______
5) Flexion—bent the thumb into the hand.	______	______	______
6) Extension—moved the thumb out to the side of the fingers.	______	______	______
7) Repeated abduction, adduction, opposition, flexion, and extension five times—or the number of times stated on the care plan.	______	______	______
f. Exercised the fingers.			
1) Abduction—spread the fingers and the thumb apart.	______	______	______
2) Adduction—brought the fingers and the thumb together.	______	______	______
3) Flexion—made a fist.	______	______	______
4) Extension—straightened the fingers so the fingers, hand, and arm were straight.	______	______	______
5) Repeated abduction, adduction, flexion, and extension five times—or the number of times stated on the care plan.	______	______	______
g. Exercised the hip.			
1) Supported the leg. Placed one hand under the knee. Placed your other hand under the ankle.	______	______	______
2) Flexion—raised the leg.	______	______	______
3) Extension—straightened the leg.	______	______	______
4) Hyperextension—moved the leg behind the body. (Did this if the person was standing. Brought the leg back to the side of the body to continue other exercises.)	______	______	______
5) Abduction—moved the leg away from the body.	______	______	______
6) Adduction—moved the leg toward the other leg.	______	______	______
7) Internal rotation—turned the leg inward.	______	______	______
8) External rotation—turned the leg outward.	______	______	______
9) Repeated flexion, extension, hyperextension, abduction, adduction, and internal and external rotation five times—or the number of times stated on the care plan.	______	______	______
h. Exercised the knee.			
1) Supported the knee. Placed one hand under the knee. Placed your other hand under the ankle.	______	______	______
2) Flexion—bent the knee.	______	______	______
3) Extension—straightened the knee.	______	______	______
4) Repeated flexion and extension of the knee five times—or the number of times stated on the care plan.	______	______	______
i. Exercised the ankle.			
1) Supported the foot and ankle. Placed one hand under the foot. Placed your other hand under the ankle.	______	______	______
2) Dorsiflexion—pulled the foot upward. Pushed down on the heel at the same time.	______	______	______

Procedure—cont'd	S	U	Comments
3) Plantar flexion—turned the foot down. Or pointed the toes.	______	______	______
4) Repeated dorsiflexion and plantar flexion five times—or the number of times stated on the care plan.	______	______	______
j. Exercised the foot.			
1) Continued to support the foot and ankle.	______	______	______
2) Pronation—turned the outside of the foot up and the inside down.	______	______	______
3) Supination—turned the inside of the foot up and the outside down.	______	______	______
4) Repeated pronation and supination five times—or the number of times stated on the care plan.	______	______	______
k. Exercised the toes.			
1) Flexion—curled the toes.	______	______	______
2) Extension—straightened the toes.	______	______	______
3) Abduction—spread the toes apart.	______	______	______
4) Adduction—put the toes together.	______	______	______
5) Repeated flexion, extension, abduction, and adduction five times—or the number of times stated on the care plan.	______	______	______
24. Covered the person with the top linens. Removed the bath blanket. Folded and returned the bath blanket to its proper place. Or followed agency policy for used linens.	______	______	______
Postprocedure			
25. Provided for comfort.	______	______	______
26. Lowered the bed to a safe and comfortable level. Followed the care plan.	______	______	______
27. Placed the call light and other needed items within reach.	______	______	______
28. Followed the care plan and the person's preferences for privacy measures to maintain. Leaving the privacy curtain, window coverings, and door open or closed were examples.	______	______	______
29. Completed a safety check of the room	______	______	______
30. Practiced hand hygiene.	______	______	______
31. Reported and recorded your care and observations.	______	______	______

Assisting With Ambulation

Name: ______________________ Date: ______________________

Quality of Life	S	U	Comments
• Knocked before entering the person's room.	____	____	____
• Addressed the person by name.	____	____	____
• Introduced yourself by name and title.	____	____	____
• Explained the procedure before starting and during the procedure.	____	____	____
• Protected the person's rights during the procedure.	____	____	____
• Handled the person gently during the procedure.	____	____	____

Preprocedure

	S	U	Comments
1. Followed *Delegation Guidelines: Assisting with Ambulation*. Saw *Promoting Safety and Comfort: Assisting with Ambulation*.	____	____	____
2. Practiced hand hygiene.	____	____	____
3. Identified the person. Checked the ID (identification) bracelet against the assignment sheet. Used two identifiers. Also called the person by name.	____	____	____
4. Got the following supplies:			
• Slip-resistant shoes or footwear	____	____	____
• Paper or towel to protect bottom linens	____	____	____
• Gait (transfer) belt			
• Walker or cane (if needed)	____	____	____
5. Provided for privacy.	____	____	____

Procedure

	S	U	Comments
6. Adjusted the bed to a safe and comfortable level for the person. Followed the care plan. Locked (braked) the bed wheels.	____	____	____
7. Fanfolded top linens to the foot of the bed.	____	____	____
8. Placed the paper or towel under the person's feet to protect bottom linens. Put the footwear on the person. Or applied footwear when the person was seated on the side of the bed.	____	____	____
9. Helped the person sit on the side of the bed.	____	____	____
10. Ensured that the person's feet were flat on the floor.	____	____	____
11. Ensured that the person was properly dressed.	____	____	____
12. Applied the gait belt at the waist over the clothing.	____	____	____
13. Positioned the walker (if used) in front of the person. Or had the person hold the cane (if used) on the strong side.	____	____	____
14. Helped the person stand. Grasped the gait belt at each side.	____	____	____
15. Stood at the weak side while the person gained balance. Held the belt at the side and back. Grasped the handles or grasped the belt from underneath. Hands were in an upward position (upward grasp).	____	____	____
16. Encouraged the person to stand erect with the head up and back straight.	____	____	____
17. *If using a walker or cane:*			
a. Walker—the walker was 6 to 8 inches in front of the person.	____	____	____
b. Cane—the cane was held on the strong side.			
1) The cane tip was 6 to 10 inches to the side of the strong foot.	____	____	____

Procedure—cont'd	S	U	Comments
18. Helped the person walk. Walked to the side and slightly behind the person on the person's weak side. Provided support with the gait belt. Had the person use the hand rail on their strong side (unless using a walker or cane).	______	______	______
19. *If using a walker or cane:*			
a. Walker—with both hands, the person pushed the walker 6 to 8 inches in front of the feet.	______	______	______
b. Cane:			
1) The cane (on the strong side) was moved forward long with the weak leg. It was even with the weak leg.	______	______	______
2) The strong leg was moved forward past the cane and the weak leg.	______	______	______
20. Encouraged the person to walk normally. The heel struck the floor first. Discouraged shuffling, sliding, or walking on tiptoes.	______	______	______
21. Walked the ordered distance if the person tolerated the activity. Did not rush the person.	______	______	______
22. Helped the person return to bed. Removed the gait belt.	______	______	______
23. Removed the shoes. Removed the paper or towel over the bottom sheet. Discarded the paper or followed agency policy for used linens.	______	______	______
24. Lowered the head of the bed. Helped the person to the center of the bed. Covered the person with the top linens.	______	______	______

Postprocedure

25. Provided for comfort.	______	______	______
26. Lowered the bed to a safe and comfortable level. Raised or lowered bed rails. Followed the care plan.	______	______	______
27. Placed the call light and other needed items within reach.	______	______	______
28. Returned the shoes, gait belt, and walker or cane to their proper place.	______	______	______
29. Followed the care plan and the person's preferences for privacy measures to maintain. Leaving the privacy curtain, window coverings, and door open or closed were examples.	______	______	______
30. Completed a safety check of the room.	______	______	______
31. Practiced hand hygiene.	______	______	______
32. Reported and recorded your care and observations.	______	______	______

Giving a Back Massage

Name: ______________________ Date: ______________________

Quality of Life	S	U	Comments
• Knocked before entering the person's room.			
• Addressed the person by name.			
• Introduced yourself by name and title.			
• Explained the procedure before starting and during the procedure.			
• Protected the person's rights during the procedure.			
• Handled the person gently during the procedure.			

Preprocedure	S	U	Comments
1. Followed *Delegation Guidelines: The Back Massage.* Saw *Promoting Safety and Comfort: The Back Massage.*			
2. Practiced hand hygiene.			
3. Identified the person. Checked the ID (identification) bracelet against the assignment sheet. Used two identifiers. Also called the person by name.			
4. Got the following supplies:			
• Bath blanket			
• Bath towel			
• Lotion			
• Laundry bag			
5. Provided for privacy.			
6. Raised the bed for body mechanics. Bed rails were up if used. Lowered the bed rail near you if up.			

Procedure	S	U	Comments
7. Positioned the person in the prone or side-lying position. The back was toward you.			
8. Covered the person with a bath blanket. Exposed the back, shoulders, and upper arms.			
9. Laid the towel on the bed along the back. Did this if the person was in a side-lying position.			
10. Warmed the lotion.			
11. Explained that the lotion may feel cool and wet.			
12. Applied lotion to the lower back area.			
13. Stroked up from the lower back to the shoulders. Then stroked down over the upper arms. Stroked up the upper arms, across the shoulders, and down the back. Used firm strokes. Kept your hands in contact with the person's skin.			
14. Repeated stroking up from the lower back to the shoulders. Then stroked down over the upper arms. Stroked up the upper arms, across the shoulders, and down the back. Used firm strokes. Kept your hands in contact with the person's skin. Continued this for at least 3 minutes.			
15. Kneaded the back.			
a. Grasped the skin between your thumb and fingers.			
b. Kneaded half of the back. Started at the lower back and moved up to the shoulder. Then kneaded down from the shoulder to the lower back.			
c. Repeated on the other half of the back.			
16. Applied lotion to bony areas. Used circular motions with the tips of your index and middle fingers. *(Did not massage reddened bony areas.)*			

Procedure—cont'd	S	U	Comments
17. Used fast movements to stimulate. Used slow movements to relax the person.	______	______	______
18. Stroked with long, firm movements to end the massage. Told the person you were finishing.	______	______	______
19. Straightened and secured clothing or sleepwear.	______	______	______
20. Covered the person. Removed the towel and bath blanket. Placed them in the laundry bag.	______	______	______

Postprocedure

21. Provided for comfort.	______	______	______
22. Lowered the bed to a safe and comfortable level. Raised or lowered bed rails. Followed the care plan	______	______	______
23. Placed the call light and other needed items within reach.	______	______	______
24. Returned lotion to its proper place. Followed agency policy for used linens.	______	______	______
25. Followed the care plan and the person's preferences for privacy measures to maintain. Leaving the privacy curtain, window coverings, and door open or closed were examples.	______	______	______
26. Completed a safety check of the room.	______	______	______
27. Practiced hand hygiene.	______	______	______
28. Reported and recorded your care and observations.	______	______	______

Preparing the Person's Room

Name: ______________________ Date: ______________________

Procedure	S	U	Comments
1. Followed *Delegation Guidelines: Admissions, Transfers, and Discharges*.			
2. Practiced hand hygiene.			
3. Got the following supplies:			
• Admission kit—wash basin, soap, toothpaste, toothbrush, water mug, and so on.			
• Bedpan and urinal (for a man)			
• Nursing assistant admission checklist			
• Thermometer			
• Stethoscope and blood pressure equipment			
• Pulse oximeter			
• Patient gown or sleepwear (if needed)			
• Towels and washcloth			
• IV (intravenous) pole (if needed)			
• Other items requested by the nurse			
4. Placed the following on the over-bed table.			
• Thermometer			
• Stethoscope and blood pressure equipment			
• Pulse oximeter			
• Nursing assistant admission checklist			
5. Placed the water mug on the bedside stand or over-bed table.			
6. Placed the following in the bedside stand.			
• Admission kit			
• Bedpan and urinal			
• Patient gown or sleepwear			
• Towels and washcloth			
7. *If the person arrived by stretcher:*			
a. Made a surgical bed.			
b. Raised the bed for a transfer from a stretcher.			
8. *If the person was ambulatory or arrived by wheelchair:*			
a. Left the bed closed.			
b. Lowered the bed to a safe and comfortable level as directed by the nurse.			
c. Kept the call light off of the bed.			
9. Attached the call light to the bed linens.			
10. Place an IV pole (if needed) next to the head of the bed.			
11. Practiced hand hygiene.			

Admitting the Person

Name: ______________________ Date: ______________________

Quality of Life	S	U	Comments
• Knocked before entering the person's room.	____	____	____
• Addressed the person by name.	____	____	____
• Introduced yourself by name and title.	____	____	____
• Explained the procedure before starting and during the procedure.	____	____	____
• Protected the person's rights during the procedure.	____	____	____
• Handled the person gently during the procedure.	____	____	____
Preprocedure			
1. Followed *Delegation Guidelines: Admissions, Transfers, and Discharges*. Saw *Promoting Safety and Comfort: Admissions, Transfers, and Discharges*.	____	____	____
2. Practiced hand hygiene.	____	____	____
3. Prepared the room.	____	____	____
Procedure			
4. Practiced hand hygiene.	____	____	____
5. Identified the person. Used two identifiers. Checked the information on the admission form and ID (identification) bracelet.	____	____	____
6. Greeted the person by name. Asked what name the person preferred.	____	____	____
7. Introduced yourself to the person and others present. Gave your name and title. Explained that you assist the nurses in giving care.	____	____	____
8. Introduced the roommate.	____	____	____
9. Provided for privacy. Asked family or friends to leave the room unless the person preferred that someone stay. Told them how much time you needed and directed them to the waiting area.	____	____	____
10. Allowed the person to stay dressed if the condition permitted. Or helped with changing into a patient gown or sleepwear.	____	____	____
11. Provided for comfort. The person was in bed or in a chair as directed by the nurse.	____	____	____
12. Assisted the nurse with assessment.			
a. Measured vital signs and pulse oximetry.	____	____	____
b. Measured weight and height.	____	____	____
c. Collected information for the nursing assistant admission checklist.	____	____	____
13. Oriented the person and family to the area.			
a. Gave names of the nurses and nursing assistants.	____	____	____
b. Explained the purpose of items in the bedside stand.	____	____	____
c. Explained how to use the over-bed table.	____	____	____
d. Showed how to use the call light.	____	____	____
e. Showed the person the bathroom. Explained how to use the call light in the bathroom.	____	____	____
f. Showed how to use the bed, TV, and light controls.	____	____	____
g. Explained how to use the agency's phone. Placed the phone within reach.	____	____	____
h. Explained how to connect to the Internet.	____	____	____
i. Showed the electrical outlets for charging electronic devices.	____	____	____
j. Explained where to find the nurses' station, lounge, chapel, dining room, and other areas.	____	____	____

Procedure—cont'd	S	U	Comments
k. Identified staff—housekeeping, dietary, physical therapy, and others. Also identified students who were in the agency.			
l. Explained when meals and snacks are served.			
m. Explained visiting hours and policies.			
14. Filled the water mug if oral fluids were allowed.			
15. Placed the call light within reach.			
16. Placed other controls and needed items within reach.			
17. Provided a denture container if needed. Labeled it with the person's name, room, and bed number.			
18. Labeled the person's property and personal care items with the person's name (if not completed by the family). Followed agency policy for labeling items.			
19. Completed a clothing and personal belongings list. Followed agency policy for labeling clothing.			
20. Helped the person put away clothes and personal items. Used the closet, drawers, and bedside stand. (The family may have helped with this step.)			

Postprocedure

	S	U	Comments
21. Provided for comfort.			
22. Ensured that the bed was at a safe and comfortable level. Checked that bed rails are raised or lowered as needed. Followed the nurse's direction.			
23. Reminded the person that the call light was nearby to call for staff. Asked if the person had any other needs right away.			
24. Followed the person's preferences for privacy measures to maintain.			
25. Completed a safety check of the room.			
26. Practiced hand hygiene.			
27. Reported and recorded your care and observations.			

NATCEP™ VIDEO VIDEO CLIP

Measuring Weight and Height With a Standing Scale

Name: ______________________ Date: ______________________

Quality of Life	S	U	Comments
• Knocked before entering the person's room.			
• Addressed the person by name.			
• Introduced yourself by name and title.			
• Explained the procedure before starting and during the procedure.			
• Protected the person's rights during the procedure.			
• Handled the person gently during the procedure.			

Preprocedure

	S	U	Comments
1. Followed *Delegation Guidelines: Weight and Height*.			
2. Practiced hand hygiene and got the following supplies:			
• Standing scale			
• Paper towels			
3. Practiced hand hygiene.			
4. Identified the person. Checked the ID (identification) bracelet against the assignment sheet. Used two identifiers. Also called the person by name.			
5. Provided for privacy.			

Procedure

	S	U	Comments
6. Asked the person to void. Assisted as needed.			
7. Placed the paper towels on the scale platform.			
8. Raised the height rod.			
9. Moved the weights to zero (0). The pointer was in the middle.			
10. Had the person remove heavy clothing and footwear. Wearing a gown or sleepwear was best. Assisted as needed. (Note: For some state competency tests, shoes were worn.)			
11. Helped the person stand in the center of the scale. Arms were at the sides. The person did not hold on to anyone or anything.			
12. Moved the lower and upper weights until the balance pointer was in the middle.			
13. Noted the weight on your notepad or assignment sheet.			
14. Asked the person to stand very straight.			
15. Lowered the height rod until it rested on the person's head.			
16. Read the height at the movable part of the height rod. Recorded the height in inches (or in feet and inches) to the nearest ¼ inch.			
17. Noted the height on your notepad or assignment sheet.			
18. Raised the height rod. Helped the person step off of the scale.			
19. Helped the person put on a robe and slip-resistant footwear if the person would be up. Or helped the person back to bed.			
20. Lowered the height rod. Adjusted the weights to zero (0) if this was your agency policy.			

Postprocedure

21. Provided for comfort. ______ ______ ______
22. Ensured that the bed was at a safe and comfortable level. Raised or lowered bed rails. Followed the care plan. ______ ______ ______
23. Placed the call light and other needed items within reach. ______ ______ ______
24. Followed the care plan and the person's preferences for privacy measures to maintain. Leaving the privacy curtain, window coverings, and door open or closed were examples. ______ ______ ______
25. Completed a safety check of the room. ______ ______ ______
26. Discarded the paper towels. ______ ______ ______
27. Practiced hand hygiene. ______ ______ ______
28. Returned the scale to its proper place. ______ ______ ______
29. Reported and recorded the measurements. ______ ______ ______

Measuring Height—The Person Is in Bed

Name: ______________________ Date: ______________________

Quality of Life	S	U	Comments
• Knocked before entering the person's room.			
• Addressed the person by name.			
• Introduced yourself by name and title.			
• Explained the procedure before starting and during the procedure.			
• Protected the person's rights during the procedure.			
• Handled the person gently during the procedure.			
Preprocedure			
1. Followed *Delegation Guidelines: Weight and Height*.			
2. Practiced hand hygiene and got a measuring tape and ruler.			
3. Asked a coworker to help you.			
4. Practiced hand hygiene.			
5. Identified the person. Checked the ID (identification) bracelet against the assignment sheet. Used two identifiers. Also called the person by name.			
6. Provided for privacy.			
7. Raised the bed for body mechanics. Bed rails were up if used. Lowered the bed rails (if up).			
Procedure			
8. Positioned the person supine if the position was allowed. (Some people cannot straighten due to contractures or abnormal curvature of the spine. Followed the nurse's directions for positioning and measurement.)			
9. Positioned the tape measure and ruler.			
a. Had your coworker place and hold the beginning of the tape measure at the person's heel.			
b. Pulled the other end of the tape measure along the person's body. Pulled it until it extended past the head.			
c. Placed the ruler flat across the top of the person's head and across the tape measure. Made sure the ruler was level.			
10. Read the height measurement. This was the point where the lower edge of the ruler touched the tape measure.			
11. Noted the height on your notepad or assignment sheet.			
Postprocedure			
12. Provided for comfort.			
13. Lowered the bed to a safe and comfortable level. Raised or lowered bed rails. Followed the care plan.			
14. Placed the call light and other needed items within reach.			
15. Completed a safety check of the room.			
16. Followed the care plan and the person's preferences for privacy measures to maintain. Leaving the privacy curtain, window coverings, and door open or closed were examples.			
17. Practiced hand hygiene.			
18. Returned equipment to its proper place.			
19. Reported and recorded the height.			

Moving the Person to a New Room

Name: ______________________ Date: ______________________

Quality of Life	S	U	Comments
• Knocked before entering the person's room.			
• Addressed the person by name.			
• Introduced yourself by name and title.			
• Explained the procedure before starting and during the procedure.			
• Protected the person's rights during the procedure.			
• Handled the person gently during the procedure.			
Preprocedure			
1. Followed *Delegation Guidelines: Admissions, Transfers, and Discharges*. Saw *Promoting Safety and Comfort: Admissions, Transfers, and Discharges*.			
2. Practiced hand hygiene and got the following supplies:			
• Wheelchair or stretcher			
• Utility cart			
• Bags for belongings			
• Bath blanket			
3. Asked a coworker to help you.			
4. Practiced hand hygiene.			
5. Identified the person. Checked the ID (identification) bracelet against the assignment sheet. Used two identifiers. Also called the person by name.			
6. Provided for privacy.			
Procedure			
7. Placed the person's belongings in bags if needed. Place belongings and care equipment to be transferred on the cart.			
8. Transferred the person to a wheelchair or a stretcher. Covered the person with the bath blanket.			
9. Transported the person to the new room. Your coworker brought the cart.			
10. Helped transfer the person to the bed or chair. Helped position the person.			
11. Helped arrange the person's belongings and equipment.			
12. Introduced yourself to the receiving nurse by name and title. Reported the following:			
a. How the person tolerated the transfer.			
b. Any observations made during the transfer.			
c. That the nurse from the previous unit would communicate and answer questions about the care.			
13. Practiced hand hygiene.			
Postprocedure			
14. Returned the wheelchair or stretcher and the cart to the storage area.			
15. Reported and recorded the following:			
• The time of the transfer			
• Who helped you with the transfer			
• Where the person was taken			
• How the person was transferred (bed, wheelchair, or stretcher)			

Postprocedure—cont'd	S	U	Comments
• How the person tolerated the transfer	______	______	______
• Who received the person	______	______	______
• Any other observations	______	______	______
16. Removed the bed linens and cleaned the unit if it was your job. Practiced hand hygiene and put on gloves for this step. (The housekeeping staff may have done this step.)	______	______	______
17. Removed and discarded the gloves. Practiced hand hygiene.	______	______	______
18. Made a closed bed.	______	______	______
19. Followed agency policy for used linens.	______	______	______
20. Practiced hand hygiene.	______	______	______

Transferring or Discharging the Person

Name: ______________________ Date: ______________________

Quality of Life	S	U	Comments
• Knocked before entering the person's room.			
• Addressed the person by name.			
• Introduced yourself by name and title.			
• Explained the procedure before starting and during the procedure.			
• Protected the person's rights during the procedure.			
• Handled the person gently during the procedure.			
Preprocedure			
1. Followed *Delegation Guidelines: Admissions, Transfers, and Discharges*. Saw *Promoting Safety and Comfort: Admissions, Transfers, and Discharges*.			
2. Practiced hand hygiene and got the following supplies as needed.			
• Wheelchair			
• Utility cart			
• Bags for belongings			
3. Asked a coworker to help you.			
4. Practiced hand hygiene			
5. Identified the person. Checked the ID (identification) bracelet against the assignment sheet. Used two identifiers. Also called the person by name.			
6. Provided for privacy.			
Procedure			
7. Helped the person dress as needed.			
8. Helped the person pack. Placed belongings in bags if needed. Checked the bathroom and all drawers and closets. Made sure all items were collected.			
9. Checked off the clothing list and personal belongings. Gave the lists to the nurse.			
10. Told the nurse that the person was ready for the final visit. The nurse:			
a. Gave needed prescriptions.			
b. Provided discharge instructions.			
c. Returned valuables from the safe.			
d. Had the person sign the clothing and personal belongings lists.			
11. *If the person left by wheelchair:*			
a. Got a wheelchair and a utility cart for the person's items. Asked a coworker to help you.			
b. Helped the person into the wheelchair.			
c. Took the person to the exit area.			
d. Locked (braked) the wheelchair wheels.			
e. Helped the person into the vehicle.			
f. Helped put the person's items into the vehicle.			
12. *If the person left by ambulance:*			
a. If you left the room, performed the usual postprocedure comfort and safety steps. Returned to assist when the ambulance attendants arrive.			
b. Raised the bed for a transfer to the stretcher. Assist with the transfer as directed.			
13. Practiced hand hygiene.			
14. Returned the wheelchair and cart to the storage area.			
15. Reported and recorded the following:			
• The time of the discharge			

Postprocedure—cont'd	S	U	Comments
• Who helped you with the procedure			
• How the person was transported			
• Who was with the person			
• The person's destination			
• Any other observations			
16. Removed the bed linens and cleaned the unit if it was your job. Practiced hand hygiene and put on gloves for this step. (The housekeeping staff may have done this step.)			
17. Removed and discarded the gloves. Practiced hand hygiene.			
18. Made a closed bed.			
19. Followed agency policy for used linens.			
20. Practiced hand hygiene.			

Preparing the Person for an Examination

Name: ______________________ Date: ______________________

Quality of Life	S	U	Comments
• Knocked before entering the person's room.			
• Addressed the person by name.			
• Introduced yourself by name and title.			
• Explained the procedure before starting and during the procedure.			
• Protected the person's rights during the procedure.			
• Handled the person gently during the procedure.			

Preprocedure	S	U	Comments
1. Followed *Delegation Guidelines: Preparing the Person.* Saw *Promoting Safety and Comfort: Preparing the Person.*			
2. Practiced hand hygiene and got the following supplies:			
• Exam form			
• Flashlight			
• Blood pressure equipment			
• Stethoscope			
• Thermometer			
• Pulse oximeter			
• Scale			
• Tongue depressors (blades)			
• Laryngeal mirror			
• Ophthalmoscope			
• Otoscope			
• Nasal speculum			
• Percussion (reflex) hammer			
• Tuning fork			
• Vaginal speculum (for a female)			
• Tape measure			
• Gloves			
• Water-soluble lubricant			
• Cotton-tipped applicators			
• Specimen containers and labels			
• Disposable bag			
• Kidney basin			
• Towel			
• Bath blanket			
• Tissues			
• Drape (sheet, bath blanket, drawsheet, or paper drape)			
• Paper towels			
• Cotton balls			
• Waterproof underpad			
• Eye chart (Snellen chart)			
• Slides			
• Patient gown			
• Alcohol wipes			
• Wastebasket			
• Container for soiled instruments			
• Marking pencils or pens			
• Laundry bag			
3. Practiced hand hygiene.			
4. Identified the person. Checked the ID (identification) bracelet against the assignment sheet. Used two identifiers. Also called the person by name.			
5. Provided for privacy.			

Procedure

6. Had the person put on the gown. Told the person what clothes to remove and where to put them. Assisted as needed. ______ ______ ______
7. Asked the person to void. Collected a urine specimen, if needed. Provided for privacy. ______ ______ ______
8. Transported the person to the exam room. (Omitted this step when exam was in the person's room.) ______ ______ ______
9. Measured weight and height. Recorded the measurements on the exam form. ______ ______ ______
10. Helped the person onto the exam table. Provided a step stool if necessary. (Omitted this step for an exam in the person's room.) ______ ______ ______
11. Raised the far bed rail (if used). Raised the bed to a safe and comfortable working height. (Omitted this step if an exam table was used.) ______ ______ ______
12. Measured vital signs and pulse oximetry. Recorded them on the exam form. ______ ______ ______
13. Placed a waterproof underpad under the buttocks if not already present. ______ ______ ______
14. Positioned the person as directed. ______ ______ ______
15. Draped the person. ______ ______ ______
16. Raised the bed rail near you (if used). ______ ______ ______
17. Provided adequate lighting. ______ ______ ______
18. Notified the examiner that the person was ready. ______ ______ ______
    a. *If you stayed in the room*—Used the call light and stayed with the person. ______ ______ ______
    b. *If you left the room*—Lowered the bed (if used) to a safe and comfortable level. Provided for comfort and safety. Maintained privacy measures. Practiced hand hygiene. Left the room to notify the examiner. ______ ______

Collecting a Random Urine Specimen

Name: ______________________ Date: ______________________

Quality of Life	S	U	Comments
• Knocked before entering the person's room.			
• Addressed the person by name.			
• Introduced yourself by name and title.			
• Explained the procedure before starting and during the procedure.			
• Protected the person's rights during the procedure.			
• Handled the person gently during the procedure.			

Preprocedure

	S	U	Comments
1. Followed *Delegation Guidelines: Urine Specimens*. Saw *Promoting Safety and Comfort:*			
a. *Collecting and Testing Specimens*			
b. *Urine Specimens*			
2. Practiced hand hygiene and got the following supplies:			
• Laboratory requisition slip			
• Specimen container and lid			
• Voiding device (clean, unused)—bedpan and cover (if used), urinal, commode, or specimen pan			
• Graduate to measure output (if needed)			
• Specimen label			
• Disposable bag (if needed)			
• Plastic bag with a *biohazard* label			
• Gloves			
3. Arranged items in the person's room (bathroom). Opened the plastic bag.			
4. Practiced hand hygiene.			
5. Identified the person. Checked the ID (identification) bracelet against the requisition slip. Compared all information. Also called the person by name. Asked the person to state first and last name and birth date.			
6. Labeled the specimen container in the person's presence.			
7. Provided for privacy.			

Procedure

	S	U	Comments
8. Put on gloves.			
9. Placed the specimen pan on the toilet or commode container if used.			
10. Asked the person to urinate into the voiding device. Had the person put toilet paper in the toilet. Or provided a disposable plastic bag and followed agency policy for disposal. Toilet paper was not put in the bedpan or specimen pan.			
11. Took the voiding device to the bathroom if a bedpan, urinal, or commode was used.			
12. Poured about 120 mL (milliliters) [4 oz (ounces)] into the specimen container.			
13. Secured the lid on the specimen container tightly. Put the container in the plastic bag. Did not let the container touch the outside of the bag.			
14. Measured urine if I&O was ordered. Included the specimen amount.			

Procedure—cont'd	S	U	Comments
15. Disposed the excess urine in the toilet. Avoided splashes. Rinsed equipment. Poured the rinse into the toilet and flushed. Followed agency procedures for cleaning and disinfection. Returned equipment to its proper place.	_____	_____	_____
16. Removed and discarded the gloves. Practiced hand hygiene. Put on clean gloves.	_____	_____	_____
17. Sealed the bag containing the specimen container.	_____	_____	_____
18. Assisted with hand hygiene. Removed and discarded the gloves. Practiced hand hygiene.	_____	_____	_____

Postprocedure			
19. Provided for comfort.	_____	_____	_____
20. Ensured that the bed was at a safe and comfortable level. Raised or lowered bed rails. Followed the care plan.	_____	_____	
21. Placed the call light and other needed items within reach.	_____	_____	_____
22. Followed the care plan and the person's preferences for privacy measures to maintain. Leaving the privacy curtain, window coverings, and door open or closed were examples.	_____	_____	_____
23. Completed a safety check of the room.	_____	_____	_____
24. Practiced hand hygiene.	_____	_____	_____
25. Took the specimen and the requisition slip to the laboratory or storage area. Followed agency policies and procedures for labeling, containment, and transport.	_____	_____	_____
26. Practiced hand hygiene.	_____	_____	_____
27. Reported and recorded your care and observations.	_____	_____	_____

Collecting a Midstream Specimen

Name: ______________________ Date: ______________________

Quality of Life	S	U	Comments
• Knocked before entering the person's room.			
• Addressed the person by name.			
• Introduced yourself by name and title.			
• Explained the procedure before starting and during the procedure.			
• Protected the person's rights during the procedure.			
• Handled the person gently during the procedure.			

Preprocedure

	S	U	Comments
1. Followed *Delegation Guidelines: Urine Specimens*. Saw *Promoting Safety and Comfort:*			
a. *Collecting and Testing Specimens*			
b. *Urine Specimens*			
c. *The Midstream Specimen*			
2. Practiced hand hygiene and got the following supplies:			
• Laboratory requisition slip			
• Midstream specimen kit—specimen container, label, towelettes, sterile gloves			
• Voiding device—bedpan and cover (if used), urinal, commode, or specimen pan if needed			
• Graduate to measure output (if needed)			
• Supplies for perineal care			
• Plastic bag with a *biohazard* label			
• Sterile gloves (if not part of kit and required by agency policy)			
• Disposable gloves			
• Paper towels			
3. Arranged items in the person's room (bathroom). Opened the plastic bag.			
4. Practiced hand hygiene.			
5. Identified the person. Checked the ID (identification) bracelet against the requisition slip. Compared all information. Also called the person by name. Asked the person to state first and last name and birth date.			
6. Provided for privacy.			

Procedure

	S	U	Comments
7. Practiced hand hygiene. Put on gloves.			
8. Provided perineal care. Follow agency policy for used linens. Removed and discarded the gloves. Practiced hand hygiene.			
9. Opened the specimen kit.			
10. Put on the gloves. Applied sterile gloves if required by agency policy.			
11. Opened the packet of towelettes.			
12. Opened the specimen container. Did not touch the inside of the container or the lid. The inside was sterile. Sat the lid down with the inside up.			
13. *For a female*—cleaned the perineal area with the towelettes.			
a. Spread the labia with your thumb and index finger. Used your nondominant hand. (This hand was contaminated and did not touch anything sterile.)			

Procedure—cont'd	S	U	Comments
b. Cleaned down the urethral area from front to back (top to bottom). Used a clean towelette for each stroke. Discarded towelettes after use.			
c. Kept the labia separated to collect the urine specimen.			
d. Asked the person to void into the device.			
e. Passed the specimen container into the urine stream. (Kept labia separated.)			
f. Collected about 30 to 60 mL (1–2 ounces) of urine. [Some agencies required 90 to 120 mL (3–4 oz). Followed agency procedures for the amount to collect.]			
g. Removed the specimen container before the person stopped voiding. Set it on a paper towel. h. Released the labia and allowed the person to finish voiding into the device.			
14. *For a male*—cleaned the penis with towelettes.			
a. Held the penis with your nondominant hand. (This hand was contaminated and did not touch anything sterile.)			
b. Cleaned the penis starting at the meatus. (Retracted the foreskin of the uncircumcised male.) Cleaned in a circular motion. Started at the center and worked outward.			
c. Held the penis (kept the foreskin retracted in the uncircumcised male) until the specimen was collected.			
d. Asked the person to void into the device.			
e. Passed the specimen container into the urine stream. (Kept the foreskin retracted in the uncircumcised male.)			
f. Collected about 30 to 60 mL (1–2 ounces) of urine. [Some agencies required 90 to 120 mL (3–4 oz). Followed agency procedures for the amount to collect.]			
g. Removed the specimen container before the person stopped voiding. Set it on a paper towel.			
h. Released the foreskin and allowed the person to finish voiding into the device.			
15. Removed and discarded soiled gloves. Practiced hand hygiene. Put on clean gloves.			
16. Secured the lid on the specimen container. Touched only the outside of the container and lid. Wiped the outside of the container. Discarded used paper towels.			
17. Labeled the specimen container in the person's presence. Placed the container in the plastic bag. The container did not touch the outside of the bag.			
18. Provided toilet paper after the person was done voiding.			
19. Took the voiding device to the bathroom if a bedpan, urinal, or commode was used.			
20. Measured urine if I&O was ordered. Included the specimen amount.			
21. Disposed the excess urine in the toilet. Avoided splashes. Rinsed equipment. Poured the rinse into the toilet and flushed. Followed agency procedures for cleaning and disinfection. Returned equipment to its proper place.			

Procedure—cont'd	S	U	Comments
22. Removed and discarded the gloves. Practiced hand hygiene. Put on clean disposable gloves.	_____	_____	_____
23. Sealed the bag containing the specimen container.	_____	_____	_____
24. Assisted with hand hygiene. Removed and discarded the gloves. Practiced hand hygiene	_____	_____	_____

Postprocedure

25. Provided for comfort.	_____	_____	_____
26. Made sure that the bed was at a safe and comfortable level. Raised or lowered bed rails. Followed the care plan.	_____	_____	_____
27. Placed the call light and other needed items within reach.	_____	_____	_____
28. Followed the care plan and the person's preferences for privacy measures to maintain. Leaving the privacy curtain, window coverings, and door open or closed were examples.	_____	_____	_____
29. Completed a safety check of the room.	_____	_____	_____
30. Practiced hand hygiene.	_____	_____	_____
31. Took the specimen and the requisition slip to the laboratory or storage area. Followed agency policies and procedures for labeling, containment, and transport.	_____	_____	_____
32. Practiced hand hygiene.	_____	_____	_____
33. Reported and recorded your care and observations.	_____	_____	_____

Collecting a 24-Hour Urine Specimen

Name: ______________________ Date: ______________________

Quality of Life	S	U	Comments
• Knocked before entering the person's room.			
• Addressed the person by name.			
• Introduced yourself by name and title.			
• Explained the procedure before starting and during the procedure.			
• Protected the person's rights during the procedure.			
• Handled the person gently during the procedure.			

Preprocedure

	S	U	Comments
1. Followed *Delegation Guidelines: Urine Specimens*. Saw *Promoting Safety and Comfort:*			
a. *Collecting and Testing Specimens*			
b. *Urine Specimens*			
c. *The 24-Hour Urine Specimen*			
2. Practiced hand hygiene and got the following supplies:			
• Laboratory requisition slip			
• Urine container for a 24-hour collection			
• Voiding device (clean, unused)—bedpan and cover (if used), urinal, commode, or specimen pan			
• Graduate to measure output (if needed)			
• Specimen label			
• Preservative (if needed)			
• Two 24-HOUR URINE labels			
• Funnel (if needed)			
• Basin with ice or an area for refrigeration as directed			
• Disposable bag as needed			
• *Biohazard* label as required by agency policy			
• Gloves			
3. Arranged items in the person's room (bathroom).			
4. Practiced hand hygiene.			
5. Identified the person. Checked the ID (identification) bracelet against the requisition slip. Compared all information. Also called the person by name. Asked the person to state first and last name and birth date.			
6. Labeled the urine container in the person's presence. Placed the labeled container in the bathroom.			
7. Placed one 24-hour urine label in the bathroom. Placed the other near the bed.			
8. Provided for privacy.			

Procedure

	S	U	Comments
9. Put on gloves.			
10. Asked the person to void. A toilet could be used for first void (before the test begins). The person needed a voiding device for urine voided over the next 24 hours. Provided a device. Explained how to use it if needed. A specimen pan was on the front of the toilet or commode container (if used).			
11. Measured urine if I&O were ordered. Discarded (flushed) the urine. Noted the time. This started the 24-hour period.			

Procedure—cont'd	S	U	Comments
12. Followed agency procedures to clean and disinfect equipment. Returned equipment to its proper place.			
13. Removed and discarded the gloves. Practiced hand hygiene. Put on clean gloves.			
14. Assisted with hand hygiene.			
15. Removed and discarded the gloves. Practiced hand hygiene.			
16. Marked the start time on the urine container's label. Marked the time THE test began and the time it was to end (24 hours later) on the room and bathroom labels.			
17. Reminded the person to:			
a. Use the voiding device during the next 24 hours.			
b. Not have a BM when voiding.			
c. Put toilet paper in the toilet. Or provided a disposable bag. Followed the agency policy for disposal.			
d. Put on the call light after voiding.			
18. Practiced hand hygiene before leaving the room. Returned to the room when the person signaled for you. Knocked before entering the room.			
19. Did the following after every voiding.			
a. Practiced hand hygiene. Put on gloves.			
b. Measured urine if I&O was ordered.			
c. Opened the specimen container. Used the funnel or spout on the voiding device to pour urine into the container. Did not spill any urine. Told the nurse if you spilled or discarded the urine because the test would have to be restarted. Secured the lid on the specimen container.			
d. Followed agency procedures to clean and disinfect equipment. Returned equipment to its proper place.			
e. Removed and discarded the gloves. Practiced hand hygiene. Put on clean gloves.			
f. Assisted with hand hygiene.			
g. Removed and discarded the gloves. Practiced hand hygiene.			
h. Followed the nurse's directions for storage of the container for the duration of the test (room temperature, on ice, or refrigerated).			
i. Followed "Postprocedure" steps.			
1) Provided for comfort.			
2) Ensured that the bed was at a safe and comfortable level. Raised or lowered bed rails. Followed the care plan.			
3) Placed the call light and other needed items within reach.			
4) Followed the care plan and the person's preferences for privacy measures to maintain. Leaving the privacy curtain, window coverings, and door open or closed were examples.			
5) Completed a safety check of the room.			
6) Practiced hand hygiene.			
7) Reported and recorded your care and observations.			
20. Did the following at the end of the test.			
a. Asked the person to void at the end of the 24-hour period.			
b. Practiced hand hygiene. Put on gloves.			
c. Measured urine if I&O was ordered.			

Procedure—cont'd	S	U	Comments
d. Opened the specimen container. Used the funnel or spout on the voiding device to pour urine into the container. Did not spill any urine. Told the nurse if you spilled or discarded the urine because the test would have to be restarted. Secured the lid on the specimen container.			
e. Followed agency procedures to clean and disinfect equipment. Returned equipment to its proper place			
f. Removed and discarded the gloves. Practiced hand hygiene. Put on clean gloves.			
g. Assisted with hand hygiene.			
h. Remove and discard the gloves. Practice hand hygiene.			
i. Removed the labels from the room and bathroom.			
j. Noted the end time on the urine container's label.			

Postprocedure

21. Provided for comfort.			
22. Made sure that the bed was at a safe and comfortable level. Raised or lowered bed rails. Followed the care plan.			
23. Placed the call light and other needed items within reach.			
24. Followed the care plan and the person's preferences for privacy measures to maintain. Leaving the privacy curtain, window coverings, and door open or closed were examples.			
25. Completed a safety check of the room.			
26. Practiced hand hygiene.			
27. Took the specimen (labeled urine container) and the requisition slip to the laboratory or storage area. Followed agency policies and procedures for labeling, containment, and transport.			
28. Practiced hand hygiene.			
29. Reported and recorded your care and observations.			

Collecting a Urine Specimen From an Infant or Child

Name: ______________________ Date: ______________________

Quality of Life	S	U	Comments
• Knocked before entering the child's room.			
• Addressed the child by name.			
• Introduced yourself by name and title.			
• Explained the procedure to the child and parents before starting and during the procedure.			
• Protected the child's rights during the procedure.			
• Handled the child gently during the procedure.			

Preprocedure	S	U	Comments
1. Followed *Delegation Guidelines: Urine Specimens*. Saw *Promoting Safety and Comfort:*			
a. *Collecting and Testing Specimens*			
b. *Urine Specimens*			
2. Practiced hand hygiene and got the following supplies:			
• Laboratory requisition slip			
• Collection bag ("wee bag")			
• Plastic bag with a *biohazard* label			
• Specimen container			
• Scissors (if needed)			
• Items for perineal care as directed			
• Diapers			
• Gloves			
3. Arranged items in the child's room.			
4. Practiced hand hygiene.			
5. Identified the child. Checked the ID (identification) bracelet against the requisition slip. Compared all information. Also called the child by name. Asked the parent to state the child's first and last name and birth date.			
6. Provided for privacy.			

Procedure	S	U	Comments
7. Practiced hand hygiene. Put on gloves.			
8. Positioned the child on back. Placed a waterproof underpad below the child if not already present.			
9. Removed and discarded the diaper.			
10. Cleaned and dried the perineal and groin areas. Used towelettes, disposable wipes, or a wash basin, water, soap, washcloths, and towels as directed. The skin was dried well for the adhesive on the bag to stick to the skin.			
11. Removed and discarded the gloves if soiled. (Practiced hand hygiene. Put on clean gloves.)			
12. Flexed the child's knees. Spread the legs.			
13. Removed the adhesive backing from the collection bag. Applied the bag to the perineum.			
14. Diapered the child. As directed, cut a slit in the bottom of a new diaper. Pulled the collection bag through the slit in the diaper. Or positioned the bag to the side out one leg opening.			
15. Removed and discarded the gloves. Practiced hand hygiene.			
16. Raised the head of the crib if allowed. This helped urine collect in the bottom of the bag.			

Procedure—cont'd	S	U	Comments
17. Checked for crib safety. Medical crib rails were raised and locked before leaving the bedside.			
18. Maintained privacy measures as preferred by the child and parents.			
19. Practiced hand hygiene.			
20. Returned to check the child often. Checked the bag for urine. Did the following if the child voided.			
a. Provided for privacy.			
b. Practiced hand hygiene. Put on gloves.			
c. Removed the diaper.			
d. Removed the collection bag gently.			
e. Followed agency procedures to contain the specimen.			
i. Method 1—Transferred the urine to the specimen container. Followed the manufacturer's instructions. Used the drainage tab if one is present.			
ii. Method 2—Pressed the adhesive surfaces of the bag together. Made sure the seal was tight and there were no leaks. Placed the sealed bag in the specimen container.			
iii. Secured the cap on the specimen container tightly.			
f. Cleaned the perineal area. Rinsed and dried well.			
g. Diapered the child.			
h. Removed and discarded the gloves. Practiced hand hygiene.			
21. Labeled the specimen container in the child's presence. Placed it in the plastic bag. Sealed the bag.			

Postprocedure

	S	U	Comments
22. Provided for comfort.			
23. Checked for crib safety. Medical crib rails were raised and locked before leaving the bedside.			
24. Made sure the call light and other needed items were within reach for the parent.			
25. Maintained privacy measures as preferred by the child and parents.			
26. Completed a safety check of the room.			
27. Practiced hand hygiene.			
28. Took the specimen and requisition slip to the laboratory or storage area. Followed agency policies and procedures for labeling, containment, and transport.			
29. Practiced hand hygiene.			
30. Reported and recorded your care and observations.			

Testing Urine With Reagent Strips

Name: ______________________ Date: ______________________

Quality of Life	S	U	Comments
• Knocked before entering the person's room.			
• Addressed the person by name.			
• Introduced yourself by name and title.			
• Explained the procedure before starting and during the procedure.			
• Protected the person's rights during the procedure.			
• Handled the person gently during the procedure.			

Preprocedure

	S	U	Comments
1. Followed *Delegation Guidelines:*. Testing Urine Saw *Promoting Safety and Comfort:*			
a. *Collecting and Testing Specimens*			
b. *Testing Urine*			
2. Practiced hand hygiene and got the following supplies:			
• Reagent (test) strips for the ordered test			
• Equipment for the urine specimen			
• Gloves			
3. Arranged items in the person's room (bathroom).			
4. Practiced hand hygiene.			
5. Identified the person. Checked the ID (identification) bracelet against the assignment sheet. Used two identifiers. Also called the person by name. Asked the person to state first and last name and birth date.			
6. Provided for privacy.			

Procedure

	S	U	Comments
7. Put on gloves.			
8. Collected the urine specimen.			
9. Removed the strip from the bottle. Put the cap tightly on the bottle at once.			
10. Dipped the test strip areas into the urine.			
11. Removed the strip after the correct amount of time. Saw the manufacturer's instructions.			
12. Tapped the strip gently against the container. This removed excess urine.			
13. Waited the required amount of time. Saw the manufacturer's instructions.			
14. Compared the strip with the color chart on the bottle. Read the results.			
15. Discarded disposable items.			
16. Disposed of urine in the toilet. Avoided splashes. Rinsed equipment. Poured the rinse into the toilet and flush. Followed agency procedures for cleaning and disinfection. Returned equipment to its proper place.			
17. Removed and discarded the gloves. Practiced hand hygiene.			

Postprocedure

18. Provided for comfort. _____ _____ __________
19. Ensured that the bed was at a safe and comfortable level. Raised or lowered bed rails. Followed the care plan. _____ _____ __________
20. Placed the call light and other needed items within reach. _____ _____ __________
21. Followed the care plan and the person's preferences for privacy measures to maintain. Leaving the privacy curtain, window coverings, and door open or closed were examples. _____ _____ __________
22. Completed a safety check of the room. _____ _____ __________
23. Practiced hand hygiene. _____ _____ __________
24. Reported and recorded the results and any other observations. _____ _____ __________

Straining Urine

Name: ______________________ Date: ______________________

Quality of Life	S	U	Comments
• Knocked before entering the person's room.			
• Addressed the person by name.			
• Introduced yourself by name and title.			
• Explained the procedure before starting and during the procedure.			
• Protected the person's rights during the procedure.			
• Handled the person gently during the procedure.			

Preprocedure

	S	U	Comments
1. Followed *Delegation Guidelines: Urine Specimens*. Saw *Promoting Safety and Comfort:*			
a. *Collecting and Testing Specimens*			
b. *Urine Specimens*			
2. Practiced hand hygiene.			
3. Got the following supplies before going to the person's room:			
• Laboratory requisition slip			
• Urine strainer			
• Specimen container			
• Specimen label			
• Voiding device (clean, unused)—bedpan and cover (if used), urinal, commode or specimen pan			
• Graduate to measure output (if needed)			
• Two STRAIN ALL URINE labels			
• Plastic bag *biohazard* label			
• Gloves			
4. Arranged items in the person's room (bathroom).			
5. Practiced hand hygiene.			
6. Identified the person. Checked the ID (identification) bracelet against the requisition slip. Compared all information. Also called the person by name. Asked the person to state first and last name and birth date.			
7. Labeled the specimen container in the person's presence.			
8. Provided for privacy.			

Procedure

	S	U	Comments
9. Placed one STRAIN ALL URINE label in the bathroom. Placed the other near the bed.			
10. Provided a voiding device and explained the procedure.			
a. Showed the person the voiding device. Explained its use if needed. Placed the device in the room (bathroom) for use. A specimen pan was on the front of the toilet or commode container (if used). Reminded the person to use the device for urinating.			
b. Explained that all urine would be strained. Asked the person to put on the call light after each voiding.			
11. Allowed the person to void or returned when the person had voided.			
a. *If the person needed to void*—Continued to step 11 to strain the urine after voiding.			

Procedure—cont'd	S	U	Comments
b. *If the person did not need to void*—Practiced hand hygiene before leaving the room. Returned to the room when the person signaled. Knocked before entering. Practiced hand hygiene.			
12. Put on gloves.			
13. Placed the strainer in the graduate.			
14. Poured urine into the graduate. Urine passed through the strainer.			
15. Transferred any crystals, stones, or particles appeared in the strainer into the specimen container.			
16. Secured the lid on the specimen container tightly. Placed the container in the plastic bag. Did not let the container touch the outside of the bag.			
17. Measured urine if I&O was ordered.			
18. Disposed of urine in the toilet. Avoided splashes. Rinsed equipment. Poured the rinse into the toilet and flushed. Followed agency procedures for cleaning and disinfection. Returned equipment to its proper place.			
19. Removed and discarded the gloves. Practiced hand hygiene. Put on clean gloves.			
20. Sealed the bag containing the specimen container.			
21. Assisted with hand hygiene. Removed and discarded the gloves. Practiced hand hygiene.			
Postprocedure			
22. Provided for comfort.			
23. Made sure that the bed was at a safe and comfortable level. Raised or lowered bed rails. Followed the care plan.			
24. Placed the call light and other needed items within reach.			
25. Followed the care plan and the person's preferences for privacy measures to maintain. Leaving the privacy curtain, window coverings, and door open or closed were examples.			
26. Completed a safety check of the room.			
27. Practiced hand hygiene.			
28. Took the specimen container and requisition slip to the laboratory or storage area. Followed agency policies and procedures for labeling, containment, and transport.			
29. Practiced hand hygiene.			
30. Reported and recorded your care and observations.			

Collecting and Testing a Stool Specimen

Name: ____________________ Date: ____________________

Quality of Life

S | U | Comments

- Knocked before entering the person's room.
- Addressed the person by name.
- Introduced yourself by name and title.
- Explained the procedure before starting and during the procedure.
- Protected the person's rights during the procedure.
- Handled the person gently during the procedure.

Preprocedure

1. Followed *Delegation Guidelines: Stool Specimens*. Saw *Promoting Safety and Comfort:*
   a. *Collecting and Testing Specimens*
   b. *Stool Specimens*
2. Practiced hand hygiene and got the following supplies:
   - Laboratory requisition slip
   - Occult blood test kit (if needed)
   - Device to collect the BM (clean, unused)—bedpan and cover (if used), or specimen pan
   - Device for voiding if the person would void—bedpan and cover (if used), commode, urinal, or specimen pan
   - Stool specimen container
   - Specimen label
   - Tongue blade (if needed)
   - Disposable bag
   - Plastic bag with a *biohazard* label
   - Toilet paper
   - Gloves
3. Arranged items in the person's room (bathroom). Opened the plastic bag.
4. Practiced hand hygiene.
5. Identified the person. Checked the ID bracelet against the requisition slip. Compared all information. Also called the person by name. Asked the person to state first and last name and birth date.
6. Labeled the specimen container in the person's presence.
7. Provided for privacy.

Procedure

8. Put on gloves.
9. Had the person void. Provided the voiding device if not using the bathroom. Emptied the device into the toilet. Avoided splashes. Rinsed the device. Poured the rinse into the toilet and flushed. Followed agency procedures for cleaning and disinfection. Returned the device to its proper place. (Changed gloves and practiced hand hygiene as needed.)
10. Put the specimen pan on the back of the toilet or commode if used. Or provided the bedpan.
11. Asked the person to avoid putting toilet paper into the bedpan, commode, or specimen pan. Had the person put toilet paper in the toilet. Or provided a disposable bag and followed agency policy for disposal.

Procedure—cont'd	S	U	Comments
12. Remove and discard the gloves. Practice hand hygiene.			
13. *If the person could be left alone*:			
a. Placed the call light and toilet paper within reach. Asked the person to signal when done.			
b. Maintained privacy measures.			
c. Stayed in the room or left the room and closed the door. Followed the care plan. Was respectful. Provided as much privacy as possible. (Practiced hand hygiene before leaving the room.)			
d. Returned when the person signals. Or checked on the person every 5 minutes. Knocked before entering. Practiced hand hygiene.			
14. Put on clean gloves.			
15. Assisted the person off the toilet or commode (if used). Or removed the bedpan if used. Assisted with wiping and perineal care as needed.			
16. Removed and discarded soiled gloves. Practiced hand hygiene. Put on clean gloves.			
17. Noted the color, amount, consistency, and odor of stools.			
18. Collected the specimen.			
a. Used the spoon attached to the lid to pick up several spoonfuls of stool. Or used a tongue blade to take about two tablespoons of stool to the specimen container. Took the sample from:			
1) The middle of a formed stool			
2) Areas of pus, mucus, or blood and watery areas			
3) The middle and both ends of a hard stool			
b. Secured the lid on the specimen container tightly.			
c. Placed the container in the plastic bag. Did not let the container touch the outside of the bag.			
d. Wrapped the tongue blade in toilet paper. Discarded it into the disposable bag.			
19. Tested the specimen (if needed).			
a. Opened the test kit.			
b. Used a tongue blade to obtain a small amount of stool.			
c. Applied a thin smear of stool on box A on the test paper.			
d. Used another tongue blade to obtain stool from another part of the specimen.			
e. Applied a thin smear of stool on box B on the test paper.			
f. Closed the packet.			
g. Waited 3 to 5 minutes or as required by the manufacturer.			
h. Turned the test packet to the other side. Opened the flap. Applied two drops of developer (from the kit) to boxes A and B. (Also applied one drop of developer to the card's quality control area. This checked that the card was functioning properly.) Followed the manufacturer's instructions.			
i. Read the results within 60 seconds or as required by the manufacturer.			
j. Noted the color changes on your assignment sheet.			
k. Disposed of the test packet.			
l. Wrapped the tongue blades with toilet paper. Then discarded them in the disposable bag.			

Procedure—cont'd	S	U	Comments
20. Disposed excess stool in the toilet. Avoided splashes. Rinsed equipment. Poured the rinse into the toilet and flushed. Followed agency procedures for cleaning and disinfection. Returned equipment to its proper place.			
21. Removed and discarded the gloves. Practiced hand hygiene. Put on clean gloves.			
22. Sealed the bag containing the specimen container.			
23. Assisted with hand hygiene. Removed and discarded the gloves. Practiced hand hygiene.			

Postprocedure

24. Provided for comfort.			
25. Ensured that the bed was at a safe and comfortable level. Raised or lowered bed rails. Followed the care plan.			
26. Placed the call light and other needed items within reach.			
27. Followed the care plan and the person's preferences for privacy measures to maintain. Leaving the privacy curtain, window coverings, and door open or closed were examples.			
28. Completed a safety check of the room.			
29. Practiced hand hygiene.			
30. Delivered the specimen and requisition slip to the laboratory or storage area. Followed agency policies and procedures for labeling, containment, and transport.			
31. Practiced hand hygiene.			
32. Reported and recorded your observations and the test results.			

Collecting a Sputum Specimen

Name: ____________________ Date: ____________________

Quality of Life	S	U	Comments
• Knocked before entering the person's room.			
• Addressed the person by name.			
• Introduced yourself by name and title.			
• Explained the procedure before starting and during the procedure.			
• Protected the person's rights during the procedure.			
• Handled the person gently during the procedure.			

Preprocedure

	S	U	Comments
1. Followed *Delegation Guidelines: Sputum Specimens*. Saw *Promoting Safety and Comfort:*			
a. *Collecting and Testing Specimens*			
b. *Sputum Specimens*			
2. Practiced hand hygiene and got the following supplies:			
• Laboratory requisition slip			
• Sputum specimen container			
• Specimen label			
• Plastic bag with a *biohazard* label			
• Tissues			
• Gloves			
3. Arranged items in the person's room (bathroom). Opened the plastic bag.			
4. Practiced hand hygiene.			
5. Identified the person. Checked the ID (identification) bracelet against the assignment sheet. Compared all information. Also called the person by name. Asked the person to state first and last name and birth date.			
6. Labeled the specimen container in the person's presence.			
7. Provided for privacy. If able, the person used the bathroom for the procedure.			

Procedure

	S	U	Comments
8. Put on gloves.			
9. Asked the person to rinse the mouth out with clear water.			
10. Had the person hold the container. Only the outside was touched.			
11. Asked the person to cover the mouth and nose with tissues when coughing. Followed center policy for used tissues.			
12. Asked the person to take two or three deep breaths and cough up sputum.			
13. Had the person expectorate directly into the container. Sputum did not touch the outside of the container.			
14. Collected one to two tablespoons of sputum.			
15. Secured the lid on the container tightly.			
16. Placed the container in the plastic bag. Did not let the container touch the outside of the bag.			
17. Removed and discarded the gloves. Practiced hand hygiene. Put on clean gloves.			
18. Sealed the bag containing the specimen container.			
19. Assisted with hand hygiene. Removed and discarded the gloves. Practiced hand hygiene.			

Postprocedure

20. Provided for comfort. ______ ______ ____________
21. Ensured that the bed was at a safe and comfortable level. Raised or lowered bed rails. Followed the care plan. ______ ______ ____________
22. Placed the call light and other needed items within reach. ______ ______ ____________
23. Followed the care plan and the person's preferences for privacy measures to maintain. Leaving the privacy curtain, window coverings, and door open or closed were examples. ______ ______ ____________
24. Completed a safety check of the room. ______ ______ ____________
25. Practiced hand hygiene. ______ ______ ____________
26. Delivered the specimen and requisition slip to the laboratory or storage area. Followed agency policies and procedures for labeling, containment, and transport. ______ ______ ____________
27. Practiced hand hygiene. ______ ______ ____________
28. Reported and recorded your care and observations. ______ ______ ____________

VIDEO VIDEO CLIP

Measuring Blood Glucose

Name: ______________________ Date: ______________________

Quality of Life	S	U	Comments
• Knocked before entering the person's room.			
• Addressed the person by name.			
• Introduced yourself by name and title.			
• Explained the procedure before starting and during the procedure.			
• Protected the person's rights during the procedure.			
• Handled the person gently during the procedure.			

Preprocedure

1. Followed *Delegation Guidelines: Measuring Blood Glucose*. Saw *Promoting Safety and Comfort:*
   a. *Collecting and Testing Specimens*
   b. Measuring *Blood Glucose*
2. Practiced hand hygiene and got the following supplies:
   - Sterile lancet in a lancing device
   - Antiseptic wipes
   - Gloves
   - 2 × 2 gauze squares
   - Glucometer
   - Reagent (test) strips. (Used correct ones for the glucometer. Checked expiration date.)
   - Disinfectant
   - Paper towels
   - Warm washcloth (if needed)
3. Followed agency procedures to disinfect the glucometer before use. Followed the manufacturer's instructions for the for the disinfectant. (Wore gloves. Removed gloves and practiced hand hygiene.)
4. Arranged items in the person's room. Place a barrier (paper towel) on the over-bed table if needed
5. Practiced hand hygiene.
6. Identified the person. Checked the ID (identification) bracelet against the assignment sheet. Used two identifiers. Also called the person by name. Asked the person to state first and last name and birth date.
7. Provided for privacy.
8. Raised the bed for body mechanics if needed. Lowered the bed rail near you if needed.

Procedure

9. Practiced hand hygiene. Put on gloves.
10. Prepared the supplies.
    a. Opened the antiseptic wipes.
    b. Prepared the glucometer. Followed the manufacturer's instructions and the prompts on the device.
       i. You entered a user-ID and entered or scanned the person's ID number (ID bracelet).
       ii. Removed a test strip from the bottle. Closed the cap tightly. Inserted a test strip into the glucometer. You may have scanned the bar code on the bottle of test strips. Or compared the code on the bottle of test strips to the code on the glucometer.

Procedure—cont'd	S	U	Comments
c. Prepared the lancet. Followed the manufacturer's instructions for the lancing device.	_____	_____	_____
11. Performed a skin puncture to obtain a drop of blood.	_____	_____	_____
a. Inspected the person's finger. Selected a puncture site.	_____	_____	_____
b. Did the following to increase blood flow to the puncture side.			
1) Warmed the finger. Rubbed it gently or applied a warm washcloth.	_____	_____	_____
2) Massaged the hand and finger toward the puncture site.	_____	_____	_____
3) Lowered the finger below the person's waist.	_____	_____	_____
c. Held the finger with thumb and index finger. Used your nondominant hand. Held the finger.	_____	_____	_____
d. Cleaned the site with antiseptic wipe. *Did not touch the site after cleaning.*	_____	_____	_____
e. Allowed the site to dry.	_____	_____	_____
f. Placed the lancing device against the puncture site.	_____	_____	_____
g. Pushed the button on the lancet to puncture the skin. (Followed the manufacturer's instructions.)	_____	_____	_____
h. Applied gentle pressure below the puncture site.	_____	_____	_____
i. Allowed a large drop of blood to form.	_____	_____	_____
12. Collected and tested the specimen. Followed the manufacturer's instructions and agency policy for the glucometer used.	_____	_____	_____
a. Touched the test strip to the drop of blood. The glucometer tested the sample when enough blood was applied.	_____	_____	_____
b. Applied pressure to the puncture site until the bleeding stopped. Used a gauze square. If able, allowed the person to apply pressure to the site.	_____	_____	_____
c. Read the results on the display. Noted the results on your notepad or assignment sheet. Told the person the results.	_____	_____	_____
d. Turned off the glucometer.	_____	_____	_____
13. Discarded the lancet into the sharps container.	_____	_____	_____
14. Discarded the gauze square and test strip. Followed agency policy.	_____	_____	_____
15. Removed and discarded gloves. Practiced hand hygiene.	_____	_____	_____

Postprocedure

16. Provided for comfort.	_____	_____	_____
17. Lowered the bed to a safe and comfortable level. Raised or lowered bed rails. Followed the care plan.	_____	_____	_____
18. Cleaned up and stored supplies and equipment. (Wore gloves. Changed gloves as needed.)	_____	_____	_____
a. Discarded disposable items.	_____	_____	_____
b. Disinfected the glucometer. Followed agency procedures and the manufacturer's instructions.	_____	_____	_____
c. Followed agency policy for any used linens.	_____	_____	_____
d. Cleaned and dried the over-bed table as needed. Dried with paper towels. Discarded paper towels. Positioned the over-bed table as the person prefers.	_____	_____	_____
e. Removed and discarded gloves. Practiced hand hygiene.	_____	_____	_____

Postprocedure—cont'd	S	U	Comments
19. Placed the call light and other needed items within reach.	______	______	______
20. Followed the care plan and the person's preferences for privacy measures to maintain. Leaving the privacy curtain, window coverings, and door open or closed were examples.	______	______	______
21. Completed a safety check of the room.	______	______	______
22. Practiced hand hygiene.	______	______	______
23. Returned the glucometer to its proper place.	______	______	______
24. Reported and recorded the test results and your observations.	______	______	______

NATCEP™ VIDEO VIDEO CLIP

Applying Elastic Stocking

Name: ______________________ Date: ______________________

Quality of Life	S	U	Comments
• Knocked before entering the person's room.			
• Addressed the person by name.			
• Introduced yourself by name and title.			
• Explained the procedure before starting and during the procedure.			
• Protected the person's rights during the procedure.			
• Handled the person gently during the procedure.			

Preprocedure	S	U	Comments
1. Followed *Delegation Guidelines: Elastic Stockings*. Saw *Promoting Safety and Comfort: Elastic Stockings*.			
2. Practiced hand hygiene and got the following supplies:			
• Elastic stockings in the correct size and length.			
• Bath blanket (if needed)			
3. Identified the person. Checked the ID (identification) bracelet against the assignment sheet. Used two identifiers. Also called the person by name.			
4. Provided for privacy.			
5. Raised the bed for body mechanics. Bed rails were up if used. Lowered the bed rail near you.			

Procedure	S	U	Comments
6. Positioned the person supine.			
7. Fanfolded top linens to the foot of the bed. Or fanfolded linens to the side, toward the other leg. If needed, used a bath blanket to cover the person.			
8. Turned the stocking inside out down to the heel.			
9. Slipped the foot of the stocking over the toes, foot, and heel. Properly positioned the heel pocket on the heel. The toe opening was over or under the toes. Followed the manufacturer's instructions.			
10. Grasped the stocking top. Rolled or pulled the stocking up the leg. It turned right side out as it was rolled or pulled up.			
11. Adjusted the stocking as needed. Made sure the stocking did not cause pressure on the toes.			
12. Removed twists, creases, or wrinkles. Made sure the stocking was even, snug, smooth, and wrinkle free.			
13. Covered the leg. Repeated for the other leg			
a. Turned the stocking inside out down to the heel.			
b. Slipped the foot of the stocking over the toes, foot, and heel. Properly positioned the heel pocket on the heel. The toe opening was over or under the toes. Followed the manufacturer's instructions.			
c. Grasped the stocking top. Rolled or pulled the stocking up the leg. It turned right side out as it was rolled or pulled up.			
d. Adjusted the stocking as needed. Made sure the stocking did not cause pressure on the toes.			
e. Removed twists, creases, or wrinkles. Made sure the stocking was even, snug, smooth, and wrinkle free.			
14. Covered the person. Removed the bath blanket (if used). Folded and returned the bath blanket to its proper place. Or followed agency policy for used linens.			

Postprocedure

15. Provided for comfort.
16. Lowered the bed to a safe and comfortable level. Raised or lowered bed rails. Followed the care plan.
17. Placed the call light and other needed items within reach.
18. Followed the care plan and the person's preferences for privacy measures to maintain. Leaving the privacy curtain, window coverings, and door open or closed were examples.
19. Completed a safety check of the room.
20. Practiced hand hygiene.
21. Reported and recorded your care and observations.

Applying an Elastic Bandage

Name: ______________________ Date: ______________________

Quality of Life	S	U	Comments
• Knocked before entering the person's room.			
• Addressed the person by name.			
• Introduced yourself by name and title.			
• Explained the procedure before starting and during the procedure.			
• Protected the person's rights during the procedure.			
• Handled the person gently during the procedure.			
Preprocedure			
1. Followed *Delegation Guidelines: Elastic Bandages*. Saw *Promoting Safety and Comfort: Elastic Bandages*.			
2. Practiced hand hygiene and got an elastic bandage with closures as directed by the nurse.			
3. Identified the person. Checked the ID bracelet against the assignment sheet. Used two identifiers. Also called the person by name.			
4. Provided for privacy.			
5. Raised the bed for body mechanics. Bed rails were up if used. Lowered the bed rail near you if up.			
Procedure			
6. Helped the person to a comfortable position in good alignment. Exposed the part to bandage.			
7. Made sure the area was clean and dry.			
8. Held the bandage with the roll up. The loose end was on the bottom.			
9. Applied the bandage to the lower (distal) and smallest part of the wrist, foot, ankle, or knee.			
10. Made two circular turns around the part.			
11. Made overlapping spiral turns in an upward (proximal) direction. Each turn overlapped ½ to ¾ of the previous turn. Each overlap was equal.			
12. Applied the bandage smoothly with firm, even pressure. It was not tight.			
13. Ended the bandage with two circular turns.			
14. Secured the bandage in place with the manufacturer's closure. Clips were not under any body part.			
15. Checked the fingers or toes for coldness or cyanosis (bluish color). Asked about pain, itching, numbness, or tingling. Removed the bandage if any were noted. Reported your observations.			
Postprocedure			
16. Provided for comfort.			
17. Lowered the bed to a safe and comfortable level. Raised or lowered bed rails. Followed the care plan.			
18. Placed the call light and other needed items within reach.			
19. Followed the care plan and the person's preferences for privacy measures to maintain. Leaving the privacy curtain, window coverings, and door open or closed were examples.			
20. Completed a safety check of the room.			
21. Practiced hand hygiene.			
22. Reported and recorded your care and observations.			

VIDEO

Applying a Dry, Nonsterile Dressing

Name: ______________________ Date: ______________________

Quality of Life

S U Comments

- Knocked before entering the person's room.
- Addressed the person by name.
- Introduced yourself by name and title.
- Explained the procedure before starting and during the procedure.
- Protected the person's rights during the procedure.
- Handled the person gently during the procedure.

Preprocedure

1. Followed *Delegation Guidelines: Applying Dressings*. Saw *Promoting Safety and Comfort:*
   a. *Wound Care*
   b. *Applying Dressings*
2. Practiced hand hygiene and got the following supplies:
   - Gloves
   - PPE (personal protective equipment) as needed
   - Tape or Montgomery ties
   - Dressings as directed by the nurse
   - 4 × 4 gauze
   - Saline solution as directed by the nurse
   - Cleansing solution as directed by the nurse
   - Adhesive remover (if needed)
   - Dressing set with scissors and forceps
   - Plastic bag with a Biohazard label
   - Bath blanket
3. Arranged your work area. You did not have to reach over or turn your back on your work area.
4. Practiced hand hygiene.
5. Identified the person. Checked the identification (ID) bracelet against the assignment sheet. Used two identifiers. Also called the person by name.
6. Provided for privacy.
7. Raised the bed for body mechanics. Bed rails were up if used. Lowered the bed rail near you if up.

Procedure

8. Helped the person to a comfortable position.
9. Covered the person with a bath blanket. Fanfolded top linens to the foot of the bed.
10. Exposed the affected body part.
11. Made a cuff on the plastic bag. Placed the bag within reach.
12. Practiced hand hygiene.
13. Put on needed PPE. Put on gloves.
14. Removed tape or undid Montgomery ties.
    a. *Tape:* held the skin down. Gently pulled the tape toward the wound. Applied adhesive remover during removal if needed. Followed the manufacturer's instructions.
    b. *Montgomery straps:* undid the straps. Folded the straps away from the wound.
15. Removed any adhesive from the skin. Followed the manufacturer's instructions for adhesive remover use. Cleaned away from the wound.

Procedure—cont'd	S	U	Comments
16. Removed dressings with a gloved hand or forceps. Started with the top dressing and removed each layer. Kept the soiled side from the person's sight. Put dressings in the plastic bag. They did not touch the outside of the bag.			
17. Removed the dressing over the wound very gently. It may have stuck to the wound or drain site. If directed by the nurse, moistened the dressing with saline if it stuck to the wound. Put dressings in the plastic bag. They did not touch the outside of the bag.			
18. Observed the wound, drain site, and wound drainage.			
19. Removed the gloves and put them in a plastic bag. Practiced hand hygiene.			
20. Opened the new dressings.			
21. Put on clean gloves.			
22. Cleaned the wound with saline or other solution as directed by the nurse.			
23. Applied dressings as directed by the nurse. Touched only the outer edges of the dressing. Did not touch the part that had contact with the wound.			
24. Secured the dressings. Used tape or Montgomery straps.			
25. Removed the gloves. Put them in the bag.			
26. Removed and discarded PPE.			
27. Practiced hand hygiene.			
28. Covered the person. Removed the bath blanket. Folded and returned the bath blanket to its proper place. Or followed agency policy for used linens.			

Postprocedure

29. Provided for comfort.			
30. Lowered the bed to a safe and comfortable level. Raised or lowered bed rails. Followed the care plan.			
31. Cleaned up and stored supplies and equipment. (Wore gloves. Changed gloves as needed.)			
a. Discarded used supplies in the bag. Tied the bag closed. Discarded the bag following agency policy. Followed the Blood-borne Pathogen Standard.			
b. Returned equipment and supplies to their proper place. Left extra dressings and tape in the room.			
c. Cleaned and dried your work area. Dried with paper towels. Discarded the paper towels.			
d. Removed and discarded gloves. Practiced hand hygiene.			
32. Placed the call light and other needed items within reach.			
33. Followed the care plan and the person's preferences for privacy measures to maintain. Leaving the privacy curtain, window coverings, and door open or closed were examples.			
34. Completed a safety check of the room.			
35. Practiced hand hygiene.			
36. Reported and recorded your care and observations.			

Applying Heat and Cold Applications

Name: ____________________ Date: ____________________

Quality of Life	S	U	Comments
• Knocked before entering the person's room.			
• Addressed the person by name.			
• Introduced yourself by name and title.			
• Explained the procedure before starting and during the procedure.			
• Protected the person's rights during the procedure.			
• Handled the person gently during the procedure.			

Preprocedure	S	U	Comments
1. Followed *Delegation Guidelines: Hot and Cold Applications; Applying Heat and Cold.* Saw *Promoting Safety and Comfort: Applying Heat and Cold.*			
2. Practiced hand hygiene and got the following supplies:			
a. *For a hot compress:*			
• Basin			
• Water thermometer			
• Small towel, washcloth, or gauze squares			
• Plastic wrap or aquathermia pad			
• Ties, tape, or rolled gauze			
• Bath towel			
• Waterproof underpad			
b. *For a hot soak:*			
• Water basin or arm or foot bath			
• Water thermometer			
• Waterproof underpad			
• Bath blanket			
• Towel			
c. *For a sitz bath:*			
• Disposable sitz bath			
• Water thermometer			
• Two bath blankets, bath towels, and a clean gown			
d. *For an aquathermia pad:*			
• Aquathermia pad and heating unit			
• Distilled water			
• Flannel cover or other cover as directed			
• Ties, tape, or rolled gauze (if needed)			
e. *For a hot or cold pack:*			
• Commercial pack			
• Pack cover			
• Ties, tape, or rolled gauze (if needed)			
f. *For an ice bag, ice collar, ice glove, or ice mask:*			
• Ice bag, collar, glove, or mask			
• Crushed ice			
• Flannel cover or other cover as directed (if needed)			
• Ties, tape, or rolled gauze(if needed)			
• Paper towels			
• Waterproof underpad (if needed)			
g. *For a cold compress:*			
• Large basin with ice			
• Small basin with cold water			
• Gauze squares, washcloths, or small towels			
• Waterproof underpad			

Preprocedure—cont'd	S	U	Comments
3. Arranged items in the person's room.			
4. Practiced hand hygiene.			
5. Identified the person. Checked the ID (identification) bracelet against the assignment sheet. Used two identifiers. Also called the person by name.			
6. Provided for privacy.			

Procedure	S	U	Comments
7. Positioned the person for the procedure.			
8. Placed the waterproof underpad under the body part.			
9. *For a hot compress:*			
a. Filled the basin ½ to 2⁄3 (one-half to two-thirds) full with hot water as directed. Measured water temperature.			
b. Placed the compress in the water and wrung it out.			
c. Applied the compress over the area. Noted the time.			
d. Covered the compress as directed. Did one of the following:			
1) Applied plastic wrap and then a bath towel. Secured the towel in place with ties, tape, or rolled gauze.			
2) Applied an aquathermia pad.			
10. *For a hot soak:*			
a. Filled a container ½ (one-half) full with hot water. Measured water temperature.			
b. Placed the part into the water. Padded the edge of the container with a towel. Noted the time.			
c. Covered the person with a bath blanket for warmth.			
11. *For a sitz bath:*			
a. Placed the sitz bath on the toilet seat.			
b. Filled the sitz bath 2⁄3 (two-thirds) full with water. Measured water temperature.			
c. Secured the gown above the waist.			
d. Helped the person sit on the sitz bath. Noted the time.			
e. Provided for warmth. Placed a bath blanket around the shoulders. Placed another over the legs.			
f. Stayed with the person if they were weak or unsteady.			
12. *For an aquathermia pad:*			
a. Filled the heating unit to the fill line with distilled water.			
b. Opened any hose clamps. Followed the manufacturer's instructions to fill the connecting hoses and pad with water and remove air. Ensured that there were no kinks in the hoses or the pad.			
c. Set the temperature as the nurse directed [usually 105°F (40.5°C)]. Removed the key.			
d. Placed the pad in the cover.			
e. Set the heating unit on the bedside stand. Kept the pad and connecting hoses level with the unit.			
f. Plugged in the unit. Allowed water to warm to the desired temperature.			
g. Applied the pad to the part. Noted the time.			
h. Secured the pad in place with ties, tape, or rolled gauze as needed.			

Procedure—cont'd	S	U	Comments
13. *For a hot or cold pack:*			
a. Squeezed, kneaded, or struck the pack as directed by the manufacturer.			
b. Placed the pack in the cover.			
c. Applied the pack. Noted the time.			
d. Secured the pack in place with ties, tape, or rolled gauze as needed. Some packs were secured with Velcro straps.			
14. *For an ice bag, collar, glove or mask:*			
a. Filled the device with water. Put in the stopper. Turned the device upside down to check for leaks.			
b. Emptied the device.			
c. Filled the device ½ to 2⁄3 (one-half to two-thirds) full with crushed ice or ice chips.			
d. Removed excess air. Bent, twisted, or squeezed the device. Or pressed it against a firm surface.			
e. Placed the cap or stopper on securely.			
f. Dried the device with paper towels.			
g. Placed the device in the cover if needed. Some were designed with a covering and could be applied directly to the skin.			
h. Applied the device. Noted the time.			
i. Secured the device in place with ties, tape, or rolled gauze as needed.			
15. *For a cold compress:*			
a. Placed the small basin with cold water into the large basin with ice.			
b. Placed the compress into the cold water.			
c. Wrung out the compress.			
d. Applied the compress to the part. Noted the time.			
16. Placed the call light and other needed items within reach. Maintained privacy measures as needed and as the person preferred.			
17. Made sure the bed was at a safe and comfortable level. Raised or lowered bed rails. Followed the care plan.			
18. Did the following every 5 minutes:			
a. Checked the person for signs and symptoms of complications. Removed the application if complications occurred. Told the nurse at once.			
b. Checked the application for cooling (hot application) or warming (cold application).			
19. Removed the application at the specified time after 15 to 20 minutes.			

Postprocedure

20. Provided for comfort.			
21. Ensured that the bed was at a safe and comfortable level. Raised or lowered bed rails. Followed the care plan.			
22. Cleaned up and store supplies and equipment. (Wore gloves as needed.)			
a. Discarded disposable items.			
b. Followed agency procedures to clean and disinfect reusable equipment. Returned supplies and equipment to their proper place.			
c. Followed agency policy for used linens.			

Postprocedure—cont'd	S	U	Comments
d. Cleaned and dried the over-bed table if used. Dried with paper towels. Discarded paper towels. Positioned the over-bed table as the person prefers.	______	______	______
e. Removed and discarded gloves. Practiced hand hygiene.	______	______	______
23. Placed the call light and other needed items within reach.	______	______	______
24. Followed the care plan and the person's preferences for privacy measures to maintain. Leaving the privacy curtain, window coverings, and door open or closed were examples.	______	______	______
25. Completed a safety check of the room.	______	______	______
26. Practiced hand hygiene.	______	______	______
27. Reported and recorded your care and observations.	______	______	______

Using a Pulse Oximeter

Name: ______________________ Date: ______________________

Quality of Life	S	U	Comments
• Knocked before entering the person's room.			
• Addressed the person by name.			
• Introduced yourself by name and title.			
• Explained the procedure before starting and during the procedure.			
• Protected the person's rights during the procedure.			
• Handled the person gently during the procedure.			

Preprocedure

	S	U	Comments
1. Followed *Delegation Guidelines: Oxygen Needs, Pulse Oximetry*. Saw *Promoting Safety and Comfort: Pulse Oximetry*.			
2. Practiced hand hygiene and got the following supplies:			
• Oximeter			
• Sensor (if not part of the device)			
• Tape (if needed)			
• Alcohol wipe			
3. Arranged your work area.			
4. Practiced hand hygiene.			
5. Identified the person. Checked the ID (identification) bracelet against the assignment sheet. Used two identifiers. Also called the person by name.			
6. Provided for privacy.			

Procedure

	S	U	Comments
7. Provided for comfort.			
8. If needed disinfected the sensor; followed the manufacturer's instructions. Selected and cleaned the site with an alcohol wipe. Discarded the wipe. If measuring blood pressure, used one arm for blood pressure and a site on the other arm for pulse oximetry.			
9. Clipped or taped the sensor to the site. If necessary, connected the sensor to the oximeter.			
10. Turned on the oximeter.			
11. *For continuous monitoring:*			
a. Set the high and low alarm limits for SpO_2 and pulse rate as directed by the nurse.			
b. Turned on audio and visual alarms.			
12. Checked the apical or radial pulse with the pulse on the display. The pulses should have been about the same. Noted both pulses on your assignment sheet.			
13. Read the SpO_2 on the display. Noted the value on the flow sheet and your assignment sheet.			
14. Left the sensor in place for continuous monitoring. Otherwise, turned off the device and removed the sensor.			

Postprocedure

	S	U	Comments
15. Provided for comfort.			
16. Placed the call light and other needed items within reach.			
17. Followed the care plan and the person's preferences for privacy measures to maintain.			
18. Completed a safety check of the room.			

Postprocedure—cont'd	S	U	Comments
19. Practiced hand hygiene.			
20. Returned the device to its proper place (unless monitoring was continuous). Followed agency policy for disinfection.			
21. Reported and recorded the SpO_2, the pulse rate, and your other observations.			

Assisting With Deep Breathing and Coughing Exercises

VIDEO

Name: ______________________ Date: ______________________

Quality of Life	S	U	Comments
• Knocked before entering the person's room.			
• Addressed the person by name.			
• Introduced yourself by name and title.			
• Explained the procedure before starting and during the procedure.			
• Protected the person's rights during the procedure.			
• Handled the person gently during the procedure.			

Preprocedure

	S	U	Comments
1. Followed *Delegation Guidelines: Deep Breathing and Coughing*. Saw *Promoting Safety and Comfort: Deep Breathing and Coughing*.			
2. Practiced hand hygiene and got gloves if needed.			
3. Identified the person. Checked the ID (identification) bracelet against the assignment sheet. Used two identifiers. Also called the person by name.			
4. Provided for privacy.			
5. Raised the bed for body mechanics. Bed rails were up if used. Lowered the bed rail if up.			

Procedure

	S	U	Comments
6. Helped the person to a comfortable sitting position.			
• Sitting on the side of the bed			
• Semi-Fowler's			
• Fowler's			
7. For deep breathing:			
a. Had the person place the hands over the rib cage.			
b. Had the person inhale through the nose and breathe as deeply as possible.			
c. Asked the person to hold the breath for 2 to 3 seconds.			
d. Asked the person to exhale slowly through pursed lips. Asked the person to exhale until the ribs moved as far down as possible.			
e. Repeated four more times. Had the person take normal breaths as needed before each deep breath. Had the person:			
1) Deep breathe in through the nose.			
2) Hold the breath for 2 to 3 seconds.			
3) Exhale slowly with pursed lips until the ribs moved as far down as possible.			
8. For coughing:			
a. *If the person did not have a productive cough:* Had the person place both hands over the chest or abdominal incision. One hand was on top of the other. Or the person held a pillow or folded towel over the chest or abdominal incision.			
b. *If the person had a productive cough:*			
1) Had the person practice cough etiquette.			
2) Splinted the chest or abdominal incision with your hands or a pillow. Wore gloves.			
c. Had the person take in a deep breath.			
i. Deep breathe in through the nose.			
ii. Hold the breath for 2 to 3 seconds.			

Procedure—cont'd	S	U	Comments
iii. Exhale slowly with pursed lips until the ribs moved as far down as possible.	______	______	______
d. Had the person cough strongly two times with the mouth open.	______	______	______
9. Assisted with hand hygiene. Wore gloves. Removed and discarded gloves. Practiced hand hygiene.	______	______	______
Postprocedure			
10. Provided for comfort.	______	______	______
11. Lowered the bed to a safe and comfortable level. Raised or lowered bed rails. Followed the care plan.	______	______	______
12. Placed the call light and other needed items within reach.	______	______	______
13. Followed the care plan and the person's preferences for privacy measures to maintain. Leaving the privacy curtain, window coverings, and door open or closed were examples.	______	______	______
14. Completed a safety check of the room.	______	______	______
15. Practiced hand hygiene.	______	______	______
16. Reported and recorded your care and observations.	______	______	______

Setting Up Oxygen

Name: ______________________ Date: ______________________

Quality of Life	S	U	Comments
• Knocked before entering the person's room.			
• Addressed the person by name.			
• Introduced yourself by name and title.			
• Explained the procedure before starting and during the procedure.			
• Protected the person's rights during the procedure.			
• Handled the person gently during the procedure.			
Preprocedure			
1. Followed *Delegation Guidelines: Oxygen Needs, Oxygen Set-Up*. Saw *Promoting Safety and Comfort: Oxygen Set-Up*.			
2. Practiced hand hygiene and got the following supplies:			
• Oxygen (O_2) device with connecting tubing			
• Flowmeter			
• Humidifier (if ordered)			
• Distilled water (if using humidifier)			
3. Arranged your work area.			
4. Practiced hand hygiene.			
5. Identified the person. Checked the ID (identification) bracelet against the assignment sheet. Used two identifiers. Also called the person by name.			
Procedure			
6. Made sure the flowmeter was in the OFF position.			
7. Attached the flowmeter to the wall outlet for oxygen.			
8. Filled the humidifier with distilled water.			
9. Attached the humidifier to the bottom of the flowmeter.			
10. Attached the O_2 device and connecting tubing to the humidifier. *Did not set the flowmeter. Did not apply the O_2 device on the person.* Placed the device and tubing in a clean place where the device would not fall to the floor.			
11. Placed the cap securely on the distilled water. Stored the water according to agency policy.			
12. Discarded the packaging from the O_2 device and connecting tubing.			
Post procedure			
13. Provided for comfort.			
14. Placed the call light and other needed items within reach.			
15. Completed a safety check of the room.			
16. Practiced hand hygiene.			
17. Told the nurse when you were done.			
The nurse would then:			
• Turn on the O_2 and set the flow rate.			
• Apply the O_2 device on the person.			

Caring for Eyeglasses

Name: ______________________ Date: ______________________

Quality of Life	S	U	Comments
• Knocked before entering the person's room.	___	___	___
• Addressed the person by name.	___	___	___
• Introduced yourself by name and title.	___	___	___
• Explained the procedure before starting and during the procedure.	___	___	___
• Protected the person's rights during the procedure.	___	___	___
• Handled the person gently during the procedure.	___	___	___
Preprocedure			
1. Followed *Delegation Guidelines: Eyeglasses.* Saw *Promoting Safety and Comfort: Corrective Lenses.*	___	___	___
2. Practiced hand hygiene and got the following supplies:	___	___	
• Eyeglass case	___	___	___
• Cleaning solution or warm water	___	___	___
• Lens cloth or cotton cloth	___	___	___
Procedure			
3. Removed the eyeglasses.			
a. Held the frames in front of the ears.	___	___	___
b. Lifted the frames from the ears. Brought the eyeglasses down away from the face.	___	___	___
4. Cleaned the lenses with cleaning solution or warm water. Cleaned in a circular motion. Dried the lenses with the cloth.	___	___	___
5. *If the person did not wear the glasses:*			
a. Opened the eyeglass case.	___	___	___
b. Folded the glasses. Put them in the case. Did not touch the clean lenses.	___	___	___
c. Placed the eyeglass case in the top drawer of the bedside stand.	___	___	___
6. *If the person wore the eyeglasses:*			
a. Held the frames at each side. Placed them over the ears.	___	___	___
b. Adjusted the eyeglasses so the nosepiece rested on the nose.	___	___	___
c. Returned the eyeglass case to the top drawer in the bedside stand.	___	___	___
Postprocedure			
7. Provided for comfort.	___	___	___
8. Returned the cleaning solution and cloth to their proper place. Discarded a disposable cloth. Or followed agency policy for used linens.	___	___	___
9. Placed the call light and other needed items within reach.	___	___	___
10. Completed a safety check of the room.	___	___	___
11. Practiced hand hygiene.	___	___	___
12. Reported and recorded your care and observations.	___	___	___

Cleaning Baby Bottles

Name: ______________________ Date: ______________________

Preprocedure	S	U	Comments
1. Followed *Delegation Guidelines: Cleaning Baby Bottles*, Saw *Promoting Safety and Comfort: Cleaning Baby Bottles*.	____	____	____
2. Practiced hand hygiene and got the following supplies:	____	____	____
• Bottles, nipples, and caps and any other bottle parts (rings, valves, and so on)	____	____	____
• Wash basin—clean, used only for washing baby-feeding items	____	____	____
• Bottle brush—clean, used only for washing baby-feeding items (used a brush that will not scratch or damage items)	____	____	____
• Dishwashing soap	____	____	____
• Other items used to prepare formula	____	____	____
• Towel	____	____	____
• Gloves (if needed)	____	____	____

Procedure	S	U	Comments
3. Follow agency policy for glove use. Apply gloves if needed.	____	____	____
4. Took apart the bottles. Separated all of the parts—bottles, nipples, caps, and any other parts.	____	____	____
5. Rinsed the bottles, nipples, caps, and other bottle parts in warm or cold running water.	____	____	____
6. Placed the items in the basin.	____	____	____
7. Filled the basin with hot water. Added dishwashing soap.	____	____	____
8. Washed the bottles, nipples, caps, and other bottle parts. Washed any other items used to prepare formula.	____	____	____
9. Cleaned inside baby bottles with the bottle brush.	____	____	____
10. Squeezed hot, soapy water through the nipples.	____	____	____
11. Rinsed all items thoroughly in hot water. Squeezed hot water through the nipples to remove soap.	____	____	____
12. Laid a clean towel on the counter. Or used a drying rack as directed.	____	____	____
13. Stood bottles upside down to drain. Placed nipples, caps, and other items on the towel or the drying rack. Let the items dry.	____	____	____
14. Rinsed the basin and bottle brush well. Let them air-dry after use.	____	____	____
15. Remove and discard gloves if worn. Practiced hand hygiene.	____	____	____
16. Follow agency policies and procedures to sanitize or sterilize items.	____	____	____

Diapering a Baby

Name: ______________________ Date: ______________________

Quality of Life	S	U	Comments
• Knocked before entering the baby's room.			
• Addressed the baby and parents by name.			
• Introduced yourself by name and title.			
• Explained the procedure to the parents before starting and during the procedure.			
• Protected the baby's rights during the procedure.			
• Handled the baby gently during the procedure.			

Preprocedure

	S	U	Comments
1. Followed *Delegation Guidelines: Diapering a Baby*. Saw *Promoting Safety and Comfort: Diapering a Baby*.			
2. Practiced hand hygiene and got the following supplies:			
• Gloves			
• Clean diaper			
• Waterproof changing pad			
• Washcloth and towels or disposable wipes			
• Basin of warm water (if needed)			
• Baby soap (if needed)			
• Laundry bag (if needed)			
• Cream or ointment as directed by the nurse			
3. Arranged items in your work area.			
4. Provide for privacy.			

Procedure

	S	U	Comments
5. Practiced had hygiene. Put on gloves.			
6. Placed the changing pad under the baby.			
7. Unfastened the dirty diaper. Placed diaper pins out of the baby's reach if used.			
8. Wiped the genital area with the front of the diaper. Wiped from the front to the back (top to bottom).			
9. Noted the color and amount of urine and feces. Folded the diaper so urine and feces were inside. Set the diaper aside.			
10. Cleaned the genital area from front to back (top to bottom). Used a wet washcloth, disposable wipes. Washed with mild soap and water for a large amount of feces or if the baby had a rash. Rinsed thoroughly and patted the area dry. Place a used washcloth and towel in the laundry bag. Discarded used wipes.			
11. Remove and discard the gloves. Practice hand hygiene. Put on clean gloves.			
12. Cleaned the circumcision. Follow the nurse's instructions for cord care.			
13. Applied cream or lotion to the genital area and buttocks. Did not use too much. Avoided caking lotion.			
14. Raised the baby's legs. Slid a clean diaper under the buttocks.			
15. Folded a cloth diaper as follows:			
a. *For a boy:* the extra thickness was in the front.			
b. *For a girl:* the extra thickness was in the back.			
c. Brought the diaper between the baby's legs.			
16. Made sure the diaper was snug around the hips and abdomen.			

Procedure—cont'd	S	U	Comments
a. It was loose near the penis if the circumcision had not healed.			
b. It was below the umbilicus if the cord stump had not healed.			
17. Secured the diaper in place. Used the tape strips or Velcro on the disposable diapers. Made sure the tabs stuck in place. Used baby pins or Velcro for cloth diapers. Pins pointed away from the abdomen.			
18. Applied a diaper cover or waterproof pants if cloth diapers were worn.			
19. Placed the baby in the crib, infant seat, or other safe place.			

Postprocedure

	S	U	Comments
20. Cleaned up and stored supplies and equipment. (Wore gloves. Changed gloves as needed.)			
a. Disposed of stools from the cloth diaper into the toilet and flushed. Stored used cloth diapers in a designated covered pail.			
b. Discarded disposable items. Placed a disposable diaper in the trash.			
c. Followed agency procedures to clean and disinfect reusable equipment. Returned supplies and equipment to their proper place.			
d. Followed agency policy for used linens.			
e. Removed and discarded the gloves. Practiced hand hygiene.			
21. Asked the parent what privacy measures to maintain. Followed the parent's preferences.			
22. Completed a safety check of the room.			
23. Practiced hand hygiene.			
24. Reported and recorded your care and observations.			

Giving a Baby a Sponge Bath

Name: ______________________ Date: ______________________

Quality of Life	S	U	Comments
• Knocked before entering the baby's room.			
• Addressed the baby and parents by name.			
• Introduced yourself by name and title.			
• Explained the procedure to the parents before starting and during the procedure.			
• Protected the baby's rights during the procedure.			
• Handled the baby gently during the procedure.			

Preprocedure	S	U	Comments
1. Followed *Delegation Guidelines: Bathing an Infant*. Saw *Promoting Safety and Comfort: Bathing an Infant*.			
2. Practiced hand hygiene and got the following supplies:			
• Baby bathtub			
• Water thermometer			
• Bath towel			
• Two hand towels			
• Receiving blanket			
• Washcloth			
• Items for diaper changing			
• Clean clothing for the baby			
• Cotton balls			
• Baby soap (if needed)			
• Baby shampoo			
• Baby lotion			
• Petrolatum gauze or petrolatum jelly (if needed)			
• Laundry bag			
• Gloves			
3. Arranged items in your work area.			
4. Practiced hand hygiene.			
5. Identified the baby. Checked the ID (identification) bracelet against the assignment sheet. Used two identifiers. Followed agency policy.			
6. Provided for privacy.			

Procedure	S	U	Comments
7. Filled the baby bathtub with 2 to 3 inches of warm water. Water temperature was around 100°F (37.7°C). Measured water temperature with the water thermometer or used the inside of your wrist. The water felt warm and comfortable.			
8. Put on gloves.			
9. Undressed the baby. Left the diaper on.			
10. Washed the baby's eyelids.			
a. Dipped a cotton ball into the water.			
b. Squeezed out excess water.			
c. Washed one eyelid from the inner part to the outer part.			
d. Repeated for the other eye with a new cotton ball.			
11. Moistened the washcloth and made a mitt. Cleaned the outside of the ear and then behind the ear. Repeated for the other ear. Was gentle. Did not use cotton swabs to clean inside of the ears.			
12. Rinsed and squeezed out the washcloth. Made a mitt with the washcloth.			

Procedure—cont'd	S	U	Comments
13. Washed the baby's face. Cleaned inside the nostrils with the washcloth. *Did not use cotton swabs to clean inside the nose.* Patted the face dry.			
14. Picked up the baby. Held the baby over the baby bathtub basin using the football hold. Supported the baby's head and neck with your wrist and hand.			
15. Washed the baby's head.			
a. Squeezed a small amount of water from the washcloth onto the baby's head. Or brought water to the baby's head using a cupped hand.			
b. Applied a small amount of baby shampoo to the head.			
c. Washed the head with circular motions.			
d. Rinsed the head by squeezing water from a washcloth over the baby's head. Or brought water to the baby's head using a cupped hand. Rinsed thoroughly. Did not get soap in the baby's eyes.			
e. Used a small hand towel to dry the head.			
16. Laid the baby on the table.			
17. Removed the diaper.			
18. Washed the front of the body with a washcloth or your hands. Did not get the cord wet. Also washed the arms, hands, fingers, legs, feet, and toes. Washed the genital area and all creases and folds. Rinsed thoroughly. Patted dry.			
19. Followed the nurse's instructions for cord care. Cleaned the circumcision.			
20. Turned the baby to the prone position. Washed the back and buttocks. Used a washcloth or your hands. Rinsed thoroughly. Patted dry.			
21. Applied baby lotion as directed by the nurse.			
22. Applied petrolatum gauze or petrolatum jelly to the penis as the nurse directed.			
23. Applied cream (ointment) to the genital area and buttocks as directed.			
24. Put a clean diaper and clean clothes on the baby.			
25. Wrapped the baby in the receiving blanket. Put the baby in the crib or other safe area.			
Postprocedure			
26. Cleaned up and store supplies and equipment. (Wore gloves. Changed gloves as needed.)			
a. Discarded disposable items			
b. Followed agency procedures to clean and disinfect reusable equipment. Returned supplies and equipment to their proper place.			
c. Followed agency policy for used linens.			
d. Removed and discarded gloves. Practiced hand hygiene.			
27. Asked the parent what privacy measures to maintain. Followed the parent's preferences.			
28. Completed a safety check of the room.			
29. Practiced hand hygiene.			
30. Reported and recorded your care and observations.			

Giving a Baby a Bath in a Baby Bathtub

Name: ______________________ Date: ______________________

Quality of Life	S	U	Comments
• Knocked before entering the baby's room.			
• Addressed the baby and parents by name.			
• Introduced yourself by name and title.			
• Explained the procedure to the parents before starting and during the procedure.			
• Protected the baby's rights during the procedure.			
• Handled the baby gently during the procedure.			

Procedure

	S	U	Comments
1. Did the following:			
a. Followed *Delegation Guidelines: Bathing an Infant.* Saw *Promoting Safety and Comfort: Bathing an Infant.*			
b. Practiced hand hygiene and got the following supplies:			
• Baby bathtub			
• Water thermometer			
• Bath towel			
• Two hand towels			
• Receiving blanket			
• Washcloth			
• Items for diaper changing			
• Clean clothing for the baby			
• Cotton balls			
• Baby soap (if needed)			
• Baby shampoo			
• Baby lotion			
• Petrolatum gauze or petrolatum jelly (if needed)			
• Laundry bag			
• Gloves			
c. Arranged items in your work area.			
d. Practiced hand hygiene.			
e. Identified the baby. Checked the ID (identification) bracelet against the assignment sheet. Used two identifiers. Followed agency policy.			
f. Provided for privacy.			
g. Filled the baby bathtub with 2 to 3 inches of warm water. Water temperature was 100°F to 103°F (37.7°C–40.5°C). Measured water temperature with the water thermometer or used the inside of your wrist. The water felt warm and comfortable.			
h. Put on gloves.			
i. Undressed the baby. Left the diaper on.			
j. Washed the baby's eyelids.			
1) Dipped a cotton ball into the water.			
2) Squeezed out excess water.			
3) Washed one eyelid from the inner part to the outer part.			
4) Repeated for the other eye with a new cotton ball.			
k. Moistened the washcloth and made a mitt. Cleaned the outside of the ear and then behind the ear. Repeated for the other ear. Was gentle. Did not use cotton swabs to clean inside the ears.			
l. Rinsed and squeezed out the washcloth. Made a mitt with the washcloth.			

Procedure—cont'd	S	U	Comments
m. Washed the baby's face. Cleaned inside the nostrils with the washcloth. *Did not use cotton swabs to clean inside the nose.* Patted the face dry.			
n. Picked up the baby. Held the baby over the baby bathtub basin using the football hold. Supported the baby's head and neck with your wrist and hand.			
o. Washed the baby's head.			
1) Squeezed a small amount of water from the washcloth onto the baby's head. Or brought water to the baby's head using a cupped hand.			
2) Applied a small amount of baby shampoo to the head.			
3) Washed the head with circular motions.			
4) Rinsed the head by squeezing water from a washcloth over the baby's head. Or brought water to the baby's head using a cupped hand. Rinsed thoroughly. Did not get soap in the baby's eyes.			
5) Used a small hand towel to dry the head.			
p. Laid the baby on the table.			
q. Removed the diaper.			
2. Held the baby.			
a. Placed one hand under the baby's shoulders. Your thumb was over the baby's shoulder. Your fingers were under the arm.			
b. Supported the buttocks with your other hand. Slid your hand under the thighs. Held the far thigh with your other hand.			
3. Lowered the baby into the water feet first.			
4. Washed the front of the baby's body. Also washed the arms, hands, fingers, legs, feet, and toes. Washed the genital area and all creases and folds.			
5. Washed the baby's back and buttocks. (Hold the baby securely. Keep the baby's face out of the water.)			
6. Rinsed thoroughly.			
7. Lifted the baby out of the water and onto a towel.			
8. Wrapped the baby in the towel. Also covered the baby's head.			
9. Patted the baby dry. Dried all folds and creases.			
10. Applied baby lotion as directed by the nurse.			
11. Applied cream (ointment) to the genital area and buttocks as directed.			
12. Put a clean diaper and clean clothes on the baby.			
13. Wrap the baby in the receiving blanket. Put the baby in the crib or other safe area.			

Postprocedure

14. Cleaned up and stored supplies and equipment. (Wore gloves. Changed gloves as needed.)			
a. Discarded disposable items.			
b. Followed agency procedures to clean and disinfect reusable equipment. Returned supplies and equipment to their proper place.			
c. Followed agency policy for used linens.			
d. Removed and discarded gloves. Practiced hand hygiene.			

Postprocedure—cont'd	S	U	Comments
15. Asked the parent what privacy measures to maintain. Followed the parent's preferences.			
16. Completed a safety check of the room.			
17. Practiced hand hygiene.			
18. Reported and recorded your care and observations.			

Weighing an Infant

Name: ______________________ Date: ______________________

Quality of Life	S	U	Comments
• Knocked before entering the baby's room.	____	____	____
• Addressed the baby and parents by name.	____	____	____
• Introduced yourself by name and title.	____	____	____
• Explained the procedure to the parents before starting and during the procedure.	____	____	____
• Protected the baby's rights during the procedure.	____	____	____
• Handled the baby gently during the procedure.	____	____	____
Preprocedure			
1. Followed *Delegation Guidelines: Weighing Infants.* Saw *Promoting Safety and Comfort: Weighing Infants.*	____	____	____
2. Practiced hand hygiene and got the following supplies:	____	____	____
• Baby scale	____	____	____
• Paper for the scale	____	____	____
• Items for diaper changing	____	____	____
• Gloves	____	____	____
3. Arranged items in your work area.	____	____	____
4. Practiced hand hygiene.	____	____	____
5. Identified the baby. Checked the ID (identification) bracelet against the assignment sheet. Used two identifiers. Followed agency policy.	____	____	____
6. Provided for privacy.	____	____	____
Procedure			
7. Placed the paper on the scale. Adjusted the scale to zero (0).	____	____	____
8. Put on gloves.	____	____	____
9. Undressed the baby and removed the diaper. Cleaned the genital area. Removed and discarded the gloves and practiced hand hygiene. Put on clean gloves.	____	____	____
10. Laid the baby on the scale. Kept one hand over the baby to prevent falling.	____	____	____
11. Read the digital display or moved the weights until the scale was balanced.	____	____	____
12. Noted the measurement.	____	____	____
13. Took the baby off of the scale.	____	____	____
14. Diapered and dressed the baby. Laid the baby in the crib.	____	____	____
Postprocedure			
15. Cleaned up and stored supplies and equipment.	____	____	____
a. Discarded the paper and soiled diaper.	____	____	____
b. Disinfected the scale; followed agency policy.	____	____	____
c. Removed and discarded the gloves. Practiced hand hygiene.	____	____	____
16. Asked the parent what privacy measures to maintain. Followed the parent's preferences.	____	____	____
17. Complete a safety check of the room.	____	____	____
18. Practiced hand hygiene.	____	____	____
19. Returned the scale to its proper place.	____	____	____
20. Reported and recorded your care and observations.	____	____	____

Assisting With Postmortem Care

Name: ______________________ Date: ______________________

Preprocedure	S	U	Comments
1. Followed *Delegation Guidelines: Care of the Body After Death*. Saw *Promoting Safety and Comfort: Care of the Body After Death*.			
2. Practiced hand hygiene and got the following supplies:			
• Postmortem kit [shroud or body bag, gown, ID (identification) tags, gauze squares, safety pins]			
• Disposable bed protectors			
• Wash basin			
• Bath towel and washcloths			
• Denture cup			
• Items for shaving facial hair, as needed			
• Tape			
• Dressings			
• Cotton balls			
• Valuables envelope			
• Gloves			
• Laundry bag			
3. Arranged items in the room.			
4. Provided for privacy.			
5. Raised the bed for body mechanics.			
6. Made sure the bed was flat.			

Procedure	S	U	Comments
7. Put on gloves.			
8. Positioned the body supine. Arms and legs were straight. A pillow was under the head and shoulders. Or raised the head of the bed 15 to 20 degrees, according to agency policy.			
9. Closed the eyes. Gently pulled the eyelids over the eyes. Followed the nurse's directions if the eyes did not stay closed. Moist cotton balls were gently applied over the eyelids.			
10. Inserted dentures or put them in a labeled denture cup. Followed agency policy.			
11. Closed the mouth. If necessary, placed a rolled towel under the chin to keep the mouth closed.			
12. Follow agency policy for rings and jewelry. In some agencies, jewelry is removed except for a wedding ring. Listed any jewelry that was removed. Placed the jewelry and the list in a valuables envelope. Rings that remain in place were secured with a cotton ball and tape after the family viewed the body.			
13. Removed drainage containers.			
14. Removed tubes and catheters with the gauze squares as the nurse directed.			
15. Removed soiled dressings. Replaced them with clean ones.			
16. Shaved facial hair if this was agency policy or desired by the family. Some males normally grow facial hair (beard, mustache). If so, did not shave facial hair.			
17. Bathed soiled areas with plain water. Dried thoroughly.			
18. Placed a bed protector under the buttocks.			
19. Removed and discarded the gloves. Practiced hand hygiene. Put on clean gloves.			

Postprocedure—cont'd	S	U	Comments
20. Put a clean gown on the body. Positioned the body supine. Arms and legs were straight. A pillow was under the head and shoulders. Or the head of the bed was raised 15 to 20 degrees according to agency policy.			
21. Brushed and combed the hair if necessary.			
22. Covered the body to the shoulders with a sheet if the family viewed the body.			
23. Gathered the person's belongings. Put them in a bag labeled with the person's name. Included eyeglasses, hearing aids, and other valuables.			
24. Removed supplies, equipment, and linens. Straightened the room. Provided soft lighting.			
25. Removed and discarded the gloves. Practiced hand hygiene.			
26. Let the family view the body. Provided for privacy. Returned to the room after they left.			
27. Practiced hand hygiene. Put on gloves.			
28. Filled out the ID tags. Tied one to the ankle or to the right big toe.			
29. Placed the body in the body bag or covered it with a sheet. Raised the bed; asked coworkers to help with turning and positioning. Or applied the shroud.			
a. Positioned the shroud under the body.			
b. Brought the top down over the head.			
c. Folded the bottom up over the feet.			
d. Folded the sides over the body.			
e. Pinned or taped the shroud in place.			
30. Attached the second ID tag to the shroud, sheet, or body bag.			
31. Left the denture cup with the body.			
32. Removed and discarded the gloves. Practiced hand hygiene.			

Postprocedure

	S	U	Comments
33. Maintained privacy measures. Leaving the privacy curtain, window coverings, and door closed were examples. Followed the nurse's instructions.			
34. Cleaned the unit after the body was removed if this was your job. Wore gloves for this step.			
35. Removed and discarded the gloves. Practiced hand hygiene.			
36. Reported the following:			
• The time the body was taken by the funeral director			
• What was done with jewelry, other valuables, and personal items			
• What was done with dentures			

Competency Evaluation Review

Preparing for the Competency Evaluation

After completing your state's training program, you need to pass the competency evaluation. The purpose of the competency evaluation is to make sure you can do your job safely. This section will help you prepare for the test.

Competency Evaluation

The competency evaluation has a written test and a skills test. The number (70+) of questions varies with each state. Each question has four answer choices. Although some questions may appear to have more than one possible answer, there is only one best answer. You will have about 1 minute to read and answer each question. Some questions take less time to read and answer. Other questions take longer. You should have enough time to take the test without feeling rushed.

The content of the written test varies depending on your state. Content may include:

- Activities of Daily Living—hygiene, dressing and grooming, nutrition and hydration, elimination, rest/sleep/comfort
- Basic Nursing Skills—infection control, safety/emergency, prevention, technical procedures (e.g., vital signs, bedmaking), data collection and reporting
- Self-care/Independence
- Emotional and Mental Health Needs
- Spiritual and Cultural Needs
- Client's Rights
- Legal and Ethical Behavior
- Being a Member of the Health-Care Team
- Communication

The written test is given as a paper and pencil test. Some test sites may use computers. If you have difficulty reading English, you may request to take an oral test. Some states offer Spanish as an option. Talk with your instructor or employer about details for computer testing or oral testing.

The skills test involves performing five nursing skills that you learned in your training program. These skills are chosen randomly. You do not select the skills. You are allowed about 30 minutes to do the skills.

Taking the Competency Evaluation

To register for the test, you need to complete an application. Your instructor or employer tells you when and where the tests are given. There is a fee for the evaluation. If you work in a nursing center, the employer may pay this fee. If you pay the fee, you may need to purchase a money order or certified check. Make sure your name is on the money order or certified check. Cash and personal checks may not be accepted.

Plan to arrive at the test site about 15 to 30 minutes before the evaluation begins. You will not be admitted if you are late. Know the exact location of the test site and room. Drive or take transportation to the test site a few days or a week before the test. Making a "dry run" lets you know how much time you need to travel, park, and get to the test site. It will also help decrease your anxiety level on the test day.

To be admitted to the test, you need two pieces of identification (ID). The first form of ID is a government-issued document, such as a driver's license or passport. It must have a current photo and your signature. The name on the ID must be the same as the name on your application form. If your name has changed and you have not been able to have the name changed on your identification documents, ask your instructor or employer what to do. The second form of ID must include your name and signature. Examples include a US state- or federal-issued ID, student or work ID, or a US financial institution–issued ID.

Take several sharpened Number 2 pencils to the test. For the skills test you will need a watch with a second hand.

Taking the written test and skills test may take several hours. You may want to bring snacks or lunch and a beverage to the testing site. Eating and drinking are not allowed during the test. However, you may be told where you can eat while waiting for the test.

You cannot bring textbooks, study notes, or other materials into the testing room. The only exception may be a language translation dictionary that you show to the proctor (a person who monitors the test) before the test begins. Cell phones, laptops, calculators, or other electronic devices are not permitted during testing. Children and pets are not allowed in the testing areas.

Studying for the Competency Evaluation

You began to prepare for the written test and skills test during your training program. You learned the basic nursing content and skills needed to provide safe, quality care. The following suggestions can help you study for the competency evaluation.

- Begin to study at least 2 to 3 weeks before the test. Plan to study for 1 to 2 hours each day.
- Decide on a specific time to study. Choose a study time that is best for you. This may be early in the morning before others are awake. It may be in the evening after others go to sleep. Try to choose a time when you are mentally alert.
- Choose a specific area to study in. This area should be quiet, well lit, and comfortable. You should have enough room to write and to spread out your books, notes, and other study aids. The area does not need to be noise free. The testing site is not absolutely quiet. You want to concentrate and not be distracted by the noise around you.
- Collect everything you need before settling down to study. This includes your textbook, notes, paper, highlighters, and pens or pencils.

- Take short breaks when you need them. Take a break when your mind begins to wander or if you feel sleepy.
- Develop a study plan. Write your plan down so you can refer to it. Study one content area before going on to the next. For example, study personal hygiene before going on to vital signs. Do not jump from subject to subject.
- Use a variety of ways to study.
  - Use index cards to help you review abbreviations and terminology. Put the abbreviation or term on the front of the card and place the meaning on the back. Take the cards with you and review them whenever you have a break or are waiting.
  - Record key points. You can listen to the recording while cooking or while riding in the car.
  - Study groups are another way to prepare for a test. Group members can quiz each other.
- To remember what you are learning, try these ideas.
  - Relax when you study. When relaxed, you learn information quickly and recall it with greater ease.
  - Repeat what you are learning. Say it out loud. This helps you remember the idea.
  - Make the information you are learning meaningful. Think about how the information will help you be a good nursing assistant.
  - Write down what you are learning. Writing helps you remember information. Prepare study sheets.
  - Be positive about what you are learning. You remember what you find interesting.
- Suggestions for studying if you have children:
  - When you first come home from work or school, spend time with your children. Then plan study time.
  - Select educational programs on TV that your children can watch as you study.
  - When you take your study breaks, spend time with your children.
  - Ask other adults to take care of the children while you study.
- Take the two practice tests in this section. Each question has the correct answer and the reason why an answer is correct or incorrect. If you practice taking tests, you are more likely to pass them. Take the practice tests under conditions similar to the real test. Work within time limits.
- If your state has a practice test and a candidate handbook, study the content. Some states have practice tests online. Information can be obtained at the NCSBN website: https://www.ncsbn.org/exams/nnaap-and-mace/nnaap-exam.page

Managing Anxiety

Almost everyone dreads taking tests. It is common and normal to experience anxiety before taking a test. If used wisely, anxiety can help you do well. When you are anxious, that means you are concerned. You may be concerned about how prepared you are to take the test. Or you may be concerned about how you will feel about yourself if you do not pass the test. Being concerned usually results in some action. To overcome anxiety before the test:

- Study and prepare for the test. That helps increase your confidence as you recall or clarify what you have learned. Anxiety decreases as confidence increases. When you think you know the information, keep studying. This reinforces your learning.
- Develop a positive mental attitude. You can pass this test. You took tests in your training program and passed them. Praise yourself. Talk to yourself in a positive way. If a negative thought enters your mind, stop it at once. Challenge the mental thought and tell yourself you will pass the test.
- Visualize success. Think about how wonderful you will feel when you are notified that you have passed the test.
- Perform breathing exercises. Breathe slowly and deeply.
- Perform regular exercise. Exercise helps you stay physically fit. It also helps keep you calm.
- Good nourishment helps you think clearly. Eat a nourishing meal before the test. Do not skip breakfast. Vitamin C helps fight short-term stress. Protein and calcium help overcome the effects of long-term stress. Complex carbohydrates (e.g., pasta, nuts, yogurt) can help settle your nerves. Eat familiar foods the day before and the day of the test. Do not eat foods that could cause stomach or intestinal upset.
- Maintain a normal routine the day before the test.
- Get a good night's sleep before the test. Go to bed early enough so you do not oversleep or are too tired to get up. Set your alarm clock properly. You may want to set two alarm clocks.
- Do not "cram" the evening before or the day of the test. Last-minute cramming increases your anxiety. Do something relaxing with family and friends.
- Avoid drinking large amounts of coffee, colas, water, or other beverages. You do not want to be uncomfortable with a full bladder when you take the test.
- Wear comfortable clothes. Dress in layers so that you are prepared for a cold or warm room.
- If you are a female, remember that worry and anxiety can affect your menstrual cycle. Wear a panty liner, sanitary napkin, or tampon if you think your period may start. This eliminates worry about soiling your clothing during the test.
- Allow plenty of time for travel, traffic, and parking.
- Arrive early enough to use the restroom before the test begins.
- Do not talk about the test with others. Their panic or anxiety may affect your self-confidence.
- In the unlikely event that you fail the test, do not panic. There are opportunities for you to take it again.

Taking the Test

Follow these guidelines for taking the test.

- Listen carefully and follow the instructions given by the proctor (a person administering the test).
- When you receive the test, make certain you have all the test pages.

- Read and follow all directions carefully.
- You are not allowed to ask questions about the content of the test questions.
- Do deep breathing and muscle relaxation exercises as needed.
- Cheating of any kind is not allowed. If the proctor sees you giving or receiving any type of assistance, your test booklet is taken and you must leave the testing site.
- If using a computer answer sheet, completely fill in the bubble.
- If you make a mistake, erase the wrong answer completely. Do not make any stray marks on the paper. Not erasing completely or leaving stray marks could cause the computer to misread your answer.
- Do not worry or get anxious if people finish the test before you do. Persons who finish a test early do not necessarily have a better score than those who finish later.
- You cannot take any evaluation materials or notes out of the testing room.

Answering Multiple-Choice Questions

Pace yourself during the test. If you are taking a paper and pencil test, first, answer all the questions that you know. Then go back and answer skipped questions. Sometimes you will remember the answer later. Or another test question may give you a clue to the one you skipped. Spending too much time on a question can cost you valuable time later. To help you answer the questions or statements:

- Always read the questions or statements carefully. Do not scan or glance at questions. Scanning or glancing can cause you to miss important key words. Read each word of the question.
- Before reading the options, decide what the answer is in your own words. Then read all the four options to the question. Select the one best answer.
- Do not read into a question. Take the question as it is asked. Do not add your own thoughts and ideas to the question. Do not assume or suppose "what if." Just respond to the information provided.
- Trust your common sense. If unsure of an answer, select your first choice. Do not change your answer unless you are absolutely sure of the correct answer. Your first reaction is usually correct.
- Look for key words in every question. Sometimes key words are in italics, highlighted, or underlined. Common key words are *always, never, first, except, best, not, correct, incorrect, true, and false.*
- Know which words can make a statement correct (e.g., *may, can, usually, most, at least, sometimes*). The word "except" can make a question a false statement.
- Be careful of answers with these key words or phrases: *always, never, every, only, all, none, at all times, or at no time.* These words and phrases do not allow for exceptions. In nursing, exceptions are generally present. However, sometimes answers containing these words are correct. For example, which of the following is correct and which are incorrect?
    a. Always use a turning sheet.
    b. Never shake linens.
    c. Soap is used for all baths.
    d. The call light must always be attached to the bed.

  The correct answer is b. Incorrect answers are a, c, and d.
- Omit answers that are obviously wrong. Then choose the best of the remaining answers.
- Go back to the questions you skipped. Answer all questions by eliminating or narrowing your choices. Always mark an answer even if you are not sure.
- Review the test a second time for completeness and accuracy before turning it in.
- Make sure you have answered each question. Also check that you have given only one answer for each question.
- Remember, the test is not designed to trick or confuse you. The written competency evaluation tests what you know, not what you do not know. You know more than you are asked.

Computer Testing

The test may be given by computer at the test site. Ask your instructor what computer skills you will need. You usually do not need keyboard or typing skills. You will use a computer mouse to select answers. Also, you will usually receive instruction before the test begins. If you do not have computer experience, practicing on the computer will help to decrease your anxiety.

Computer testing may or may not allow you to return to previous questions. If you plan to take the test by computer, ask your instructor for alternative test-taking strategies.

Textbook Chapters Review

Note: This review covers selected chapters only based on Competency Evaluation requirements.

CHAPTER 1 HEALTH CARE AGENCIES

Health-Care Agency Purposes

- Health promotion
- Disease prevention
- Detection and treatment of disease
- Rehabilitation and restorative care

Hospitals

- Hospitals provide emergency care, surgery, nursing care, x-ray procedures and treatments, and laboratory testing.
- Hospitals also provide respiratory, physical, occupational, speech, and other therapies.
- Persons cared for in hospitals are called *patients*. Hospital patients have acute, chronic, or terminal illnesses.

Rehabilitation and Subacute Care Agencies

- Medical and nursing care is provided for people who do not need hospital care but are too sick to go home.

Long-Term Care Centers

- Persons who live in long-term care centers are called residents.
- Long-term care is for residents who do not need hospital care but cannot care for themselves at home.
- Centers provide medical and nursing, dietary, recreational, rehabilitative, and social services. Housekeeping and laundry services are also provided.
- Residents are older or disabled.
- Skilled nursing facilities provide more complex care.
- Some residents are recovering from illness, injury, or surgery.
- Some residents return home when well enough. Some residents need nursing care until death.
- Memory care units provide care for residents with Alzheimer disease or other dementias.

Assisted Living Facilities

- Housing, personal care, support services, health care, and social activities are provided in a homelike setting for persons needing help with daily activities.

Other Health Agencies

- Other health agencies include mental health centers, home care, hospice, and health-care systems.

The Health Team

- Many health-care workers with skills and knowledge contribute to total care.
- The team works together to provide coordinated care to meet each person's needs.
- The team is usually lead by a registered nurse (RN).

The Nursing Team

- The nursing team provides quality care to people.
- Care is coordinated by an RN.

Nursing Assistants

- Nursing assistants report to the licensed nurse supervising their work.
- Delegated tasks are performed under the supervision of a licensed nurse.
- Nursing assistant training and competency evaluation must be successfully completed.

Meeting Standards

Survey Process

- Surveys are done to see if agencies meet standards for licensure, certification, and accreditation.
- A license is issued by the state. A center must have a license to operate and provide care.
- Certification is required to receive Medicare and Medicaid funds.
- Accreditation is voluntary. It signals quality and excellence.

Your Role

- Provide quality care
- Protect the person's rights
- Provide for the person's and your own safety
- Help keep the center clean and safe
- Conduct yourself in a professional manner
- Have good work ethics
- Follow agency policies and procedures
- Answer questions honestly and completely

CHAPTER 1 REVIEW QUESTIONS

Circle the BEST answer

1. Which educational requirement applies to nursing assistants?
   a. Must pass a nursing assistant training program and a competency evaluation
   b. Needs to complete a 2-, 3-, or 4-year program and pass a licensure examination
   c. Should have advanced skills and certification to assist in the care of hospice patients
   d. Must learn how to teach people how to make and maintain healthy lifestyle changes

2. Who would the nursing assistant contact if a patient has a question about the medical diagnosis?
   a. Nurse practitioner
   b. RN
   c. Physician's assistant
   d. Physician
3. What is the most important goal of the health team?
   a. Support and respect each other
   b. Treat and cure disease
   c. Provide quality care
   d. Follow the instructions of the RN

Answers to these questions are on p. 577.

CHAPTER 2 THE PERSON'S RIGHTS

- Centers must protect and promote residents' rights. Residents must be free to exercise their rights without interference. If residents are not able to exercise their rights, legal representatives do so for them.

The Omnibus Budget Reconciliation Act of 1987 (OBRA)

- OBRA is a federal law.
- OBRA requires that nursing centers provide care in a manner and in a setting that maintains or improves each person's quality of life, health, and safety.
- OBRA requires nursing assistant training and competency evaluation.
- Resident rights are a major part of OBRA.

Information

- The right to information includes:
  - o Access to all records about the person, including medical records, incident reports, contracts, and financial records
  - o Information about the person's health condition
  - o Information about the person's doctor, including name, specialty, and contact information
- Report any request for information to the nurse

Refusing Treatment

- The person has the right to refuse treatment.
- A person who does not give consent or refuses treatment cannot be treated against their wishes.
- The center must find out what the person is refusing and why.
- Advance directives are part of the right to refuse treatment.
- Report any treatment refusal to the nurse.

Privacy and Confidentiality

- Residents have the right to:
  - o Personal privacy. The person's body is not exposed unnecessarily. Only staff directly involved in care and treatments are present. The person must give consent for others to be present. A person has the right to use the bathroom in private. Privacy is maintained for all personal care measures.
  - o Visit with others in private—in areas where others cannot see or hear them. This includes phone calls.
  - o Send and receive mail without others interfering. No one can open mail the person sends or receives without their consent. Unopened mail is given to the person within 24 hours of delivery to the center.
- Information about the person's care, treatment, and condition is kept confidential. So are medical and financial records. Consent is needed to release information to other agencies or persons.

Personal Choice

- Residents have the right to make their own choices. They can:
  - o Choose their own doctors.
  - o Take part in planning and deciding their care and treatment.
  - o Choose activities, schedules, and care based on their preferences.
  - o Choose when to get up and go to bed, what to wear, how to spend their time, and what to eat.
  - o Choose friends and visitors inside and outside the center.

Grievances

- Residents have the right to voice concerns, questions, and concerns about treatment or care.
- The center must try to correct the matter promptly.
- No one can punish the person in any way for voicing the grievance.

Work

- The person is not required to work or perform services for the center.
- The person has the right to work or perform services if he or she wants to.
- Residents volunteer or are paid for their services.

Taking Part in Resident Groups

- The person has the right to:
  - o Form and take part in resident and family groups.
  - o Take part in social, cultural, religious, and community events. The resident has the right to help in getting to and from events of their choice.

Personal Items

- The resident has the right to:
  - o Keep and use personal items, such as clothing and some furnishings.
  - o Have their property treated with care and respect. Items are labeled with the person's name.
- Protect yourself and the center from being accused of stealing a person's property. Do not go through a person's closet, drawers, purse, or other space without

the person's knowledge and consent. If you have to inspect closets and drawers, follow center policy for reporting and recording the inspection.

Freedom From Abuse, Mistreatment, and Neglect

- Residents have the right to be free from:
  - Verbal, sexual, physical, or mental abuse.
  - Involuntary seclusion—separating a person from others against their will, confining a person to a certain area, or keeping the person away from their room without consent.
- No one can abuse, neglect, or mistreat a resident. This includes center staff, volunteers, staff from other agencies or groups, other residents, family members, friends, visitors, and legal representatives.
- Nursing centers must investigate suspected or reported cases of abuse.

Freedom From Restraint

- Residents have the right to not have body movements restricted by restraints or drugs.
- Restraints are used only if required to treat the person's medical symptoms or if necessary to protect the person or others from harm. If a restraint is required, a doctor's order is needed.

Quality of Life

- Residents must be cared for in a manner that promotes dignity and self-esteem. Physical, psychological, and mental well-being must be promoted. Review Box 2.3 (p. 17), Promoting Dignity and Privacy-OBRA Required Actions, in the Textbook.
- Centers must provide activity programs that promote physical, intellectual, social, spiritual, and emotional well-being.
- Residents have the right to a safe, clean, comfortable, and homelike setting. The center must provide a setting and services that meet the person's needs and preferences. The setting and staff must promote the person's independence, dignity, and well-being.

Ombudsman Program

- The Older Americans Act requires a long-term care ombudsman program in every state.
- Ombudsmen are employed by a state agency. They are not nursing center employees. Some are volunteers.
- Ombudsmen protect the health, safety, welfare, and rights of residents. They also may investigate and resolve concerns, provide support to resident and family groups, and help the center manage difficult problems.
- OBRA requires that nursing centers post the names, addresses, and phone numbers of local and state ombudsmen where the residents can easily see it.
- Because a family member or resident may share a concern with you, you must know the state and center policies and procedures for contacting an ombudsman.

CHAPTER 2 REVIEW QUESTIONS

Circle the BEST answer

1. Which circumstance is a violation of a resident's rights?
   a. Resident refuses a treatment.
   b. Resident makes a private telephone call.
   c. Resident chooses an activity to attend.
   d. Resident is shunned after voicing a grievance.
2. What is the primary purpose for the OBRA requirements for nursing assistant training and competency evaluation?
   a. Nursing assistants are trained to provide care that improves or maintains quality of life, health, and safety.
   b. Nursing assistants have an easier time getting a job after undergoing the training and competency evaluation.
   c. Nursing care facilities can receive insurance, Medicare and Medicaid funding if nursing assistants are trained.
   d. Nursing care facilities can contain costs by hiring nursing assistants who have completed OBRA-approved programs.
3. Which situation best demonstrates that the person is exercising his rights to take part in planning and deciding their care?
   a. Family is told about the benefits and risks of the treatments.
   b. Person asks about the expected outcome of the treatment.
   c. Doctor advises the patient that there is no cure for his condition.
   d. Nurse gives the patient and family written information about treatments.
4. Which action should be taken if a person volunteers to do some chores around the center?
   a. Tell the person that he can get extra medical supplies in exchange for this work
   b. Ask the family if the person is qualified and able to do the assigned chores
   c. Tell the person that he does not need to do any chores because he is paying for services
   d. Include the volunteer work in the care plan as it fulfills a desire or need to work

Answers to these questions are on p. 577.

CHAPTER 3 THE NURSING ASSISTANT

Federal and State Laws

Nurse Practice Acts

- Each state has a nurse practice act. It regulates nursing practice in that state.

Nursing Assistants

- A state's nurse practice act is used to decide what nursing assistants can do. Some nurse practice acts also regulate nursing assistant roles, functions, education, and certification requirements. Some states have separate laws for nursing assistants.
- Nursing assistants must be able to function with skill and safety. They can have their certification, license, or registration denied, revoked, or suspended.

The Omnibus Budget Reconciliation Act of 1987 (OBRA)

- The purpose of OBRA, a federal law, is to improve the quality of life of nursing center residents.
- OBRA sets minimum training and competency evaluation requirements for nursing assistants. Each state must have a nursing assistant training and competency evaluation program (NATCEP). A nursing assistant must successfully complete the NATCEP to work in a nursing center, hospital, long-term care unit, or home care agency receiving Medicare funds.
- OBRA requires at least 75 hours of instruction. Some states have more hours. At least 16 hours of supervised training in a laboratory or clinical setting are required.
  - The competency evaluation has a written test and a skills test.
  - The written test has multiple-choice questions.
  - The number of questions varies from state to state.
  - The skills test involves performing certain skills learned in the training program.
- OBRA requires a nursing assistant registry in each state. It is an official record that lists persons who have successfully completed the NATCEP.
- Retraining and a new competency evaluation program are required for nursing assistants who have not worked for 24 months. To work in another state, nursing assistants must meet that state's NATCEP.
- Each state's NATCEP must meet OBRA requirements.

Roles and Responsibilities

- Nurse practice acts, OBRA, state laws, and legal and advisory opinions direct what nursing assistants can do.
- The range of functions for nursing assistants varies among states and agencies. Before performing a nursing task make sure that:
  - The state allows nursing assistants to do that task.
  - It is in the job description.
  - You have the necessary education and training.
  - A nurse is available to answer questions and to supervise the task.
- Rules for nursing assistants to follow are given in Box 3.1 (p. 26), Rules for Nursing Assistants, in the Textbook.
  - You are an assistant to the nurse.
  - A nurse assigns and supervises your work.
  - You report observations about the person's physical and mental status to the nurse. Report changes in the person's condition or behavior at once.
  - The nurse decides what should be done for a person. You do not make these decisions.
  - Review directions and the care plan with the nurse before going to the person.
  - Perform only those nursing tasks that you are trained to do.
  - Ask a nurse to supervise you if you are not comfortable performing a nursing task.
  - Perform only the nursing tasks that your state and job description allow.
- State laws and rules limit nursing assistant functions. State laws differ. Know what you can do in the state in which you are working.
- Role limits for nursing assistants are given in Box 3.2 (p. 26), Role Limits, in the Textbook.
  - Never give drugs.
  - Never insert tubes or objects into body openings. Do not remove tubes from the body.
  - Never take oral or telephone orders from doctors.
  - Never tell the person or family the person's diagnosis or treatment plans.
  - Never diagnose or prescribe treatments or drugs for anyone.
  - Never supervise others, including other nursing assistants.
  - Never ignore an order or request to do something. This includes nursing tasks that you can do, those you cannot do, and those that are beyond your legal limits.

Nursing Assistant Standards

- OBRA defines the basic range of functions for nursing assistants.
- All NATCEPs include those functions. Some states allow other functions.
- Review Box 3.3 (p. 27), Nursing Assistant Standards, in the Textbook.

Job Description and Job Titles

- Always obtain a written job description when you apply for a job. Do not take a job that requires you to:
  - Act beyond the legal limits of your role.
  - Function beyond your training limits.
  - Perform acts that are against your morals or religion.
- For job purposes, agencies often use other titles for nursing assistants who have completed the NATCEP and are on a state registry. Your job title depends on the setting and your roles and functions in the agency.

CHAPTER 3 REVIEW QUESTIONS

Circle the BEST answer

1. Which question is a surveyor most likely to ask you about maintaining your clinical competency?
   a. Have you submitted your information to the nursing assistant registry?
   b. Have you ever allowed anyone to use your nursing assistant certificate?
   c. What kind of work did you do before you became a nursing assistant?
   d. How long have you been working for this agency?
2. Which action would the nursing assistant take when a resident asks about the medical condition?
   a. Tell the nurse about the resident's request
   b. Give the resident a copy of the medical record
   c. Ignore the question and quickly change the subject
   d. Explain that nursing assistants cannot give information
3. Which action would the nursing assistant take when a family phones in a resident's medical information?
   a. Write down the information and promptly give it to the doctor
   b. Politely give name and title, ask the person to wait, and promptly find the nurse
   c. Politely ask the family member to call back later or to call the doctor
   d. Politely give the nurse's name and tell the family to call later and ask for that nurse

4. When would a nursing assistant refuse to do a task?
   a. The task is not in the job description.
   b. The task is within the legal limits of the role.
   c. The directions for the task are clear.
   d. A nurse is available for questions and supervision.

Answers to these questions are on p. 577.

CHAPTER 4 DELEGATION

Who Can Delegate

- Registered nurses (RNs) can delegate tasks to nursing assistants. In some states, licensed practical nurses/licensed vocational nurses (LPNs/LVNs) can delegate tasks to nursing assistants.
- An Advanced Practice Registered Nurse (APRN) can delegate to RNs, LPNs/LVNs, and nursing assistants.
- A nurse's delegation decisions must protect the person's health and safety. The delegating nurse is legally accountable to the person; accountable for delegation decisions; and accountable for safe and correct task completion.
- Nursing assistants cannot delegate. You cannot delegate any task to other nursing assistants or to any other worker.

The Delegation Process

- Delegation decisions must protect the person's health and safety.
- If you perform a task that places the person at risk, you may face serious legal problems.
- Step 1—Assessment and Planning. The nurse assesses the person's needs and then decides if it is safe to delegate the task.
- Step 2—Communication. The nurse must give clear and complete directions about the task and you must understand the directions to give safe care. After the task, you report and record the care that was given.
- Step 3—Surveillance and Supervision. The nurse observes the care you give and makes sure you complete the task correctly. The nurse must follow up on problems or concerns; for example, you did not correctly perform the task or the person's condition has changed.
- Step 4—Evaluation and Feedback. The nurse decides if the delegation was successful by observing if the task was done correctly and the outcome and the person's response were as expected. The nurse should provide feedback to the nursing assistant about what was done correctly and what errors should be corrected.

The Five Rights of Delegation

- *The right task.* Is the task in your job description? Does your state allow you to do the task? Were you trained to do the task?
- *The right circumstances.* Do you have experience with the task given the person's condition and needs? Do you understand the purpose of the task? Can you safely perform the task? Do you have the equipment and supplies? Do you know how to use the equipment and supplies?
- *The right person.* Do you have the training and experience to perform the task safely? Do you have concerns about performing the task?
- *The right directions and communication.* Did the nurse give clear directions and instructions. Did the nurse allow questions and help you set priorities? Do you understand what the nurse expects?
- *The right supervision.* Is the nurse available to answer questions. Is the nurse available if the person's condition changes or if problems occur? Did the nurse evaluate the results?

Your Role in Delegation

- When you agree to perform a delegated task on a person, you must protect the person from harm. You are responsible for your own actions. You must complete the task safely. You must ask for help if you have questions or are unsure. Report to the nurse what you did and the observations you made.
- You should refuse to perform a task when:
  - The task is beyond the legal limits of your role.
  - The task is not in your job description.
  - You were not trained to do the task.
  - The task could harm the person.
  - The person's condition has changed.
  - You do not know how to use the supplies or equipment.
  - Directions are not ethical or legal.
  - Directions are against agency policies.
  - Directions are unclear or incomplete.
  - A nurse is not available for supervision.
- Never ignore an order or refuse a task because you do not like it or do not want to do it. Tell the nurse about your concerns.

CHAPTER 4 REVIEW QUESTIONS

Circle the BEST answer

1. A nurse delegates a task that you did not learn in your training; however, the task is in your job description. Which response is best?
   a. "I must refuse, because I don't know how to do that task."
   b. "I did not learn that task in my training. Can you show me how to do it?"
   c. "I will ask the other nursing assistant to watch me do the task."
   d. "I will ask the other nursing assistant to do the task for me."
2. The nursing assistant is busy with a new resident. It is time for another resident's bath. What would the nursing assistant do first?
   a. Tell the nurse about the delay in the resident's bath
   b. Tell the resident that he will be helped to bathe later
   c. Delegate the bath to another nursing assistant
   d. Ask another assistant to help with the new resident

3. Which task would the nursing assistant refuse to do?
   a. Help another nursing assistant transfer a person
   b. Encourage residents to wake up and eat breakfast
   c. Take vitals signs for another nursing assistant
   d. Bathe a resident who appears to be very ill

Answers to these questions are on p. 577.

CHAPTER 5 ETHICS AND LAWS

Ethical Aspects

- Ethics is the knowledge of what is right conduct and wrong conduct. It also deals with choices or judgments about what should or should not be done. An ethical person does not cause a person harm.
- Ethical behavior involves not being prejudiced or biased. To be prejudiced or biased means to make judgments and have views before knowing the facts. You should not judge a person by your values and standards. Also, do not avoid persons whose standards and values differ from your own.
- Ethical problems involve making choices. You must decide what is the right thing to do.

Codes of Ethics

- Professional groups have codes of ethics. A **code of ethics** has rules, or standards of conduct, for group members to follow.
- Rules of conduct for nursing assistants can be found in Box 5.1 (p. 41), Code of Conduct for Nursing Assistants, in the Textbook.

Boundaries

- **Professional boundaries** separate helpful actions and behaviors from those that are not helpful.
- A **boundary crossing** is a brief act of overinvolvement with the person to meet the person's needs, such as giving a crying patient a hug.
- A **boundary violation** is an act or behavior that meets your needs, not the person's. The act or behavior is unethical. Boundary violations include abuse, keeping secrets with a person, or giving a lot of personal information about yourself to another.
- **Professional sexual misconduct** is an act, behavior, or comment that is sexual in nature. It is sexual misconduct even if the person consents or makes the first move.
- To maintain professional boundaries, review Box 5.2 (p. 42), Professional Boundaries. Be alert to **boundary signs** (acts, behaviors, or thoughts that warn of a boundary crossing or violation).

Legal Aspects

- Ethics is about what you *should or should not do*. Laws tell you what you *can and cannot do*.
- **Negligence** is an unintentional wrong. The negligent person did not act in a reasonable and careful manner, and the person or person's property was harmed. The person causing harm did not mean to cause harm.
- **Malpractice** is negligence by a professional person.
- You are legally responsible (liable) for your own actions. The nurse is liable as your supervisor.
- **Defamation** is injuring a person's name and reputation by making false statements to a third person. **Libel** is making false statements in print, writing (including e-mails and texts), or through pictures or drawings. **Slander** is making false statements orally. Never make false statements about a patient, resident, family member, coworker, or any other person.
- **False imprisonment** is the unlawful restraint or restriction of a person's freedom of movement. It involves threatening to restrain a person, restraining a person, and preventing a person from leaving the agency.
- **Invasion of privacy** is violating a person's right not to have their name, photo, or private affairs exposed or made public without giving consent. Review Box 5.3 (p. 44), Protecting the Right to Privacy, in the Textbook.
- The Health Insurance Portability and Accountability Act (HIPAA) of 1996 protects the privacy and security of a person's health information. **Protected health information** refers to identifying information and information about the person's health care that is maintained or sent in any form (paper, electronic, oral). Direct any questions about the person or the person's care to the nurse.
- **Fraud** is saying or doing something to trick, fool, or deceive a person. The act is fraud if it does or could cause harm to a person or the person's property.
- **Assault** is intentionally attempting or threatening to touch a person's body without the person's consent. The person fears bodily harm.
- **Battery** is touching a person's body without their consent. Protect yourself from being accused of assault and battery. Explain to the person what you are going to do and get the person's consent.

Wrongful Use of Electronic Communication

- Electronic communications include e-mail, text messages, faxes, websites, video sites, and social media sites. Video and social media sites include Facebook, LinkedIn, YouTube, Instagram, Pinterest, blogs and comments to blog postings, chat rooms, bulletin boards, and so on.
- Wrongful use of electronic communications can result in job loss and loss of your certification (license, registration) for:
  - Defamation
  - Invasion of privacy
  - HIPAA violations
  - Violating the right to confidentiality
  - Patient or resident abuse
  - Unprofessional or unethical conduct

Informed Consent

- A person has the right to decide what will be done to their body and who can touch their body. Consent is informed when the person clearly understands all aspects of treatment.
- Persons who cannot give consent are persons who are under the legal age or are mentally incompetent.

Unconscious, sedated, or confused persons cannot give consent. Informed consent is given by a responsible party—wife, husband, daughter, son, or legal representative.
- You are never responsible for obtaining written consent.

Reporting Abuse

- **Abuse** is
  - The willful infliction of injury, unreasonable confinement, intimidation, or punishment that results in physical harm, pain, or mental anguish. Intimidation means to make afraid with threats of force or violence.
  - Depriving the person (or the person's caregiver) of the goods or services needed to attain or maintain well-being.
- Abuse also includes involuntary seclusion.
- **Vulnerable adults** are persons aged 18 years or older who have disabilities or conditions that make them at risk to be wounded, attacked, or damaged. They have problems caring for or protecting themselves due to:
  - A mental, emotional, physical, or developmental disability
  - Brain damage
  - Changes from aging
- All residents are vulnerable. Older persons and children are at risk for abuse.
- **Elder abuse** is any knowing, intentional, or negligent act by a caregiver or another person to an older adult. It may include physical abuse, neglect, verbal abuse, involuntary seclusion, financial exploitation or misappropriation, emotional or mental abuse, sexual abuse, or abandonment. Review Box 5.6 (p. 49), Signs of Elder Abuse, in the Textbook.
- Federal and state laws require the reporting of elder abuse.
- If you suspect a person is being abused, report your observations to the nurse.
- **Child abuse or neglect** is the intentional harm or mistreatment of a child younger than 18 years. It includes the failure of the parent or caregiver to act which creates immediate risk or results in death, serious physical or emotional harm, sexual abuse, or exploitation. Review Table 5.2 (p. 51), Signs of Child Abuse and Neglect, in the Textbook.
- **Intimate partner violence is** physical violence, sexual violence, stalking, or psychological aggression by a current or former partner. Review Box 5.7 (p. 53), Warning Signs of Intimate Partner Violence, in the Textbook.

CHAPTER 5 REVIEW QUESTIONS

Circle the BEST answer

1. What would the nursing assistant do when a resident offers a gift certificate for being kind and giving good care?
   a. Say "thank you for thinking of me" and accept the gift
   b. Ask the nurse what to do about the gift
   c. Thank the resident and explain that a gift is not necessary
   d. Accept the gift and ask the resident not to mention it to anyone
2. Which action violates the person's privacy?
   a. Texting about the person's condition to his family member
   b. Discussing the person's treatment with the supervising nurse
   c. Reading the content of the person's mail aloud at his request
   d. Allowing the person to visit with others with the door closed
3. What should the nursing assistant do for a suspicion that an older person is being abused?
   a. Report the situation to the health department.
   b. Notify the nurse and discuss the observations.
   c. Notify the doctor about the suspected abuse.
   d. Ask the family why they are abusing the person.
4. A resident needs help going to the bathroom, but the nursing assistant does not answer the call light promptly. The resident gets up without help, falls, and breaks a leg. This is an example of
   a. Negligence
   b. Defamation
   c. False imprisonment
   d. Slander
5. Which member of the health-care team has committed defamation?
   a. Nurse implies that a physical therapist uses drugs.
   b. Doctor tells the nurse that the patient has a mental illness.
   c. Nursing assistant reports seeing a person steal money from a patient.
   d. Dietician tells the patient that she needs to lose some weight.
6. Which advice would the nursing assistant give to another nursing assistant who says that she is a victim of intimate partner violence?
   a. Report the circumstances and violent events to the supervising nurse
   b. Get to a safe place and never speak or interact with the violent partner
   c. Go to a doctor and have injuries checked and documented
   d. Call the police and report everything that happened including injuries
7. Which circumstance is a threat of false imprisonment?
   a. You gently tell a resident that you will restrain him if he continues to take his roommate's belongings.
   b. You restrain a resident according to the doctor's order and follow the RN's instructions for giving care.
   c. You tell the resident that the bathroom door must be slightly open, so that you can maintain his safety.
   d. You prevent a resident who has dementia and wandering behaviors from going outside by himself.
8. To prevent being accused of assault and battery, which action should the nursing assistant take before touching the person?
   a. Always be polite and consider the other person's needs
   b. Explain to the resident what plan is and get consent
   c. Ask the nurse to verify the goals of care and the tasks to be done
   d. Review the steps of the procedure and then follow through

Answers to these questions are on p. 577.

CHAPTER 6 STUDENT AND WORK ETHICS

- **Professionalism** involves following laws, being ethical, having good work ethics, and having the skills to do your work.
- **Work ethics** deals with behavior in the workplace. Work ethics also applies to students in nursing assistant training and competency evaluation programs (NATCEPs).
- To be a successful student, practice good work ethics in the classroom and clinical setting and in your relationships with instructors and fellow students.

Health, Hygiene, and Appearance

- To give safe and effective care, you must be physically and mentally healthy. You need a balanced diet, sleep and rest, good body mechanics, and exercise on a regular basis. Smoking, drugs, and alcohol can affect performance and safety.
- Personal hygiene needs careful attention. Bathe daily, use deodorant or antiperspirant, and brush your teeth often. Shampoo often. Keep fingernails clean, short, and neatly shaped.
- Review Box 6.1 (p. 58), Professional Appearance, in the Textbook.

Teamwork

- Practice good work ethics—work when scheduled, be cheerful and friendly, perform delegated tasks, be kind to others, and be available to help others.
- Be ready to work when your shift starts. Arrive on your nursing unit a few minutes early. Stay the entire shift. When it is time to leave, report off duty to the nurse.
- Gossiping is unprofessional and hurtful. To avoid being a part of gossip:
  - Remove yourself from where people are gossiping.
  - Do not make or repeat any comment that can hurt another person or the agency.
  - Do not make or write false statements about another person.
  - Do not talk about residents, family members, patients, visitors, coworkers, or the agency at home or in social settings.
- **Confidentiality** means trusting others with personal and private information. The person's information is shared only among staff involved in their care. Agency, family, and coworker and student information is also confidential.
- Your speech and language must be professional.
  - Do not swear or use foul, vulgar, or abusive language.
  - Do not use slang.
  - Speak softly, gently, and clearly.
  - Do not shout or yell.
  - Do not fight or argue with a person, family member, visitor, or coworker.
- A courtesy is a polite, considerate, or helpful comment or act.
  - Address others by Miss, Mrs., Ms., Mr., or Doctor. Use the name that the person prefers.
  - Say "please" and "thank you." Say "I'm sorry" when you make a mistake or hurt someone.
  - Let residents, families, and visitors enter elevators first.
  - Be thoughtful—compliment others, give praise.
  - Wish the person and family well when they leave the center.
  - Hold doors open for others.
  - Help others willingly when asked.
  - Do not take credit for another person's deeds. Give the person credit for the action.
- Keep personal matters out of the workplace.
  - Make personal phone calls during meals and breaks.
  - Do not let family and friends visit you on the unit.
  - Do not use the agency's computers and other equipment for personal use.
  - Do not take agency supplies for personal use.
  - Do not discuss personal problems at work.
  - Control your emotions.
  - Do not borrow money from or lend money to coworkers.
  - Do not sell things or engage in fundraising at work.
  - Do not have wireless phones or personal pagers on while at work.
  - Do not text message.
- Leave for and return from breaks and meals on time. Tell the nurse when you leave and return to the unit.
- Protect yourself and others from harm.
  - Understand the roles, functions, and responsibilities in your job description.
  - Follow agency rules, policies, and procedures in the employee handbook or policy and procedure manual.
  - Know what is right and wrong conduct and what you can and cannot do.
  - Follow the nurse's directions and instructions and question unclear directions and things you do not understand. Ask for any training you might need.
  - Help others willingly when asked.
  - Report accurately. This includes measurements, observations, the care given, the person's concerns, and any errors.
  - Accept responsibility for your actions. Admit when you are wrong or make mistakes. Do not blame others. Do not make excuses for your actions. Learn what you did wrong and why. Always try to learn from your mistakes.
  - Handle the person's property carefully and prevent damage.
  - Always follow safety measures.
- Planning your work involves setting priorities. Decide:
  - Which person has the greatest or most life-threatening needs.
  - What task the nurse or person needs done first.
  - What tasks need to be done at a certain time.

- What tasks need to be done when your shift starts.
  - What tasks need to be done at the end of your shift.
  - How much time it takes to complete a task.
  - How much help you need to complete a task.
  - Who can help you and when.
- Priorities change as the person's needs change.

Managing Stress

- These guidelines can help you reduce or cope with stress.
  - Exercise regularly
  - Get enough sleep or rest
  - Eat healthy
  - Plan personal and quiet time for yourself
  - Use common sense about what you can do
  - Do one thing at a time
  - Do not judge yourself harshly
  - Give yourself praise
  - Have a sense of humor
  - Talk to the nurse if your work or a person is causing too much stress
- Conflict in the workplace can cause stress and care can be compromised. Resolving conflict involves six steps: (1) define the problem, (2) collect information about the problem, (3) identify possible solutions, (4) carry out the best solution, and (6) evaluate the results.
- Communication and good work ethics help prevent and resolve conflicts.
- **Burnout** is a job stress resulting in physical or mental exhaustion and doubts about your abilities or the value of your work. Managing stress can prevent burnout.

Harassment

- **Harassment** means to trouble, torment, offend, or worry a person by one's behavior or comments.
- Harassment is illegal: it can be sexual or it can involve age, race, ethnic background, religion, or disability.
- You must respect others. Do not offend others by your gestures, remarks, or use of touch. Do not offend others with jokes, photos, or other pictures.

CHAPTER 6 REVIEW QUESTIONS

Circle the BEST answer

1. Which member of the health-care team is demonstrating good work ethics?
   a. Nurse works when scheduled, but never works extra shifts.
   b. Nursing assistant is consistently cheerful and friendly.
   c. Nurse declines to assist others to complete their tasks.
   d. Nursing assistant refuses to do tasks that are not assigned.
2. A nursing assistant is gossiping about a coworker. You should
   a. Listen but do not contribute or comment
   b. Discuss the gossipers with a trusted coworker
   c. Remove yourself from where gossip is occurring
   d. Repeat the comment to trusted coworkers
3. Which health-care team member has failed to maintain confidentiality about others?
   a. Nurse talks about a patient's diagnosis with a friend of the patient's family.
   b. Nursing assistant never talks about patients in the elevator, hallway, or dining area.
   c. Physician discusses the diagnosis and treatment with the patient and his wife.
   d. Nursing assistant walks away when encountering people in a private conversation.
4. Which nursing assistant is using professional speech and language?
   a. Nursing assistant A swears when she accidentally drops a patient's food tray on the floor, "Darn it!"
   b. Nursing assistant B shouts, "I know you can't hear me, but I am here to help you get out of bed!"
   c. Nursing assistant C loudly says, "You can't see your mother right now, she didn't sleep well last night."
   d. Nursing assistant D clearly and softly says, "Mr. Smith, I am going to help you with your bath."
5. Which behavior contributes to the nursing assistant's personal health?
   a. Eating a balanced meal before going to the clinical setting
   b. Sleeping and napping whenever there is extra time
   c. Exercising to build strength to independently lift patients
   d. Drinking alcohol and socializing to relax and unwind
6. Which student is correctly using the phone to attend to personal matters?
   a. Tells instructor that cell phone is on for family emergencies
   b. Makes personal cell phone calls during meal or break time
   c. Turns cell phone on to silent and discretely carries it in a pocket
   d. Uses cell phone only to text and connect to the Internet

Answers to these questions are on p. 577.

CHAPTER 7 THE PERSON AND FAMILY

Caring for the Person

- The whole person needs to be considered when you provide care—physical, social, psychological, and spiritual parts. These parts are woven together and cannot be separated.
- Follow these rules to address persons with dignity and respect.
  - Call persons by their titles—Mrs. Dennison, Mr. Smith, Miss Turner, or Dr. Gonzalez.
  - Do not call persons by their first names unless they ask you to.
  - Do not call persons by any other name unless they ask you to.
  - Do not call persons Grandma, Papa, Sweetheart, Honey, or other names.
  - Persons' gender identity may differ from the biological sex. Use persons preferred name and pronouns.

Basic Needs

- A **need** is something necessary or desired for maintaining life and mental well-being.
- According to Maslow, basic needs must be met for a person to survive and function. Needs are arranged in order of importance, lower level to higher level.
  - *Physiological or physical needs*—are required for life. They are oxygen, food, water, elimination, rest, and shelter.
  - *Safety and security needs*—relate to feeling safe from harm, danger, and fear.
  - *Love and belonging needs*—relate to love, closeness, affection, and meaningful relationships with others. Family, friends, and the health team can meet love and belonging needs.
  - *Self-esteem needs*—relate to thinking well of oneself and to seeing oneself as useful and having value. People often lack self-esteem when ill, injured, older, or disabled.
  - *The need for self-actualization*—involves learning, understanding, and creating to the limit of a person's capacity. Rarely, if ever, is it totally met.

Culture and Religion

- **Culture** is the characteristics of a group of people. People come from many cultures, races, and nationalities. Family practices, food choices, hygiene habits, clothing styles, and language are part of their culture. The person's culture also influences health beliefs and practices.
- **Religion** relates to spiritual beliefs, needs, and practices. A person's religion influences health and illness practices. Many may want to pray and observe religious practices. Assist residents to attend religious services as needed. If a person wants to see a spiritual leader or adviser, tell the nurse. Provide privacy during the visit.
- A person may not follow all the beliefs and practices of their culture or religion. Some people do not practice a religion.
- Respect and accept the person's culture and religion. Learn about practices and beliefs different from your own. Do not judge a person by your own standards.

Communicating With the Person

- For effective communication between you and the person, you must:
  - Understand and respect the patient or resident as a person.
  - View the person as a physical, psychological, social, and spiritual human being.
  - Appreciate the person's problems and frustrations.
  - Respect the person's rights.
  - Respect the person's religion and culture.
  - Give the person time to understand the information that you give.
  - Repeat information as often as needed.
  - Ask questions to see if the person understood you.
  - Be patient. People with memory problems may ask the same question many times.
  - Include the person in conversations when others are present.

Verbal Communication

- When talking with a person, follow these rules:
  - Face the person. Look directly at the person.
  - Position yourself at the person's eye level.
  - Control the loudness and tone of your voice.
  - Speak clearly, slowly, and distinctly.
  - Do not use slang or vulgar words.
  - Repeat information as needed.
  - Ask one question at a time and wait for an answer.
  - Do not shout, whisper, or mumble.
  - Be kind, courteous, and friendly.
- Use written words if the person cannot speak or hear but can read. Keep written messages brief and concise. Use a black felt pen on white paper and print in large letters.
- Some persons cannot speak or read. Ask questions that have "yes" or "no" answers. A picture board may be helpful.

Nonverbal Communication

- Gestures, facial expressions, posture, body movements, touch, and smell are used to convey messages. Nonverbal messages more accurately reflect a person's feelings than words do. A person may say one thing but act another way. Watch the person's eyes, hand movements, gestures, posture, and other actions.
- Touch conveys comfort, caring, love, affection, interest, trust, concern, and reassurance. Touch should be gentle. Touch means different things to different people. Some people do not like to be touched. To use touch, follow the care plan. Maintain professional boundaries.
- People send messages through their **body language**—facial expressions, gestures, posture, hand and body movements, gait, eye contact, and appearance. Your body language should show interest, enthusiasm, caring, and respect for the person. Often you need to control your body language. Control reactions to odors from body fluids, secretions, or excretions.

Communication Methods

- *Listening* means to focus on verbal and nonverbal communication. You use sight, hearing, touch, and smell. To be a good listener:
  - Face the person.
  - Have good eye contact with the person.
  - Lean toward the person. Do not sit back with your arms crossed.
  - Respond to the person. Nod your head and ask questions.
  - Avoid communication barriers.
- *Paraphrasing* is restating the person's message in your own words.
- *Direct questions* focus on certain information. You ask the person something you need to know.
- *Open-ended questions* lead or invite the person to share thoughts, feelings, or ideas. The person chooses what to talk about.
- *Clarifying* lets you make sure that you understand the message. You can ask the person to repeat the message, say you do not understand, or restate the message.

- *Focusing* deals with a certain topic. It is useful when a person wanders in thought.
- *Silence* is a very powerful way to communicate. Silence gives time to think, organize thoughts, choose words, and gain control. Silence on your part shows caring and respect for the person's situation and feelings.

Communication Barriers

- *Language*. You and the person must use and understand the same language.
- *Cultural differences*. A person from another country may attach different meanings to verbal and nonverbal communication than what you intended.
- *Changing the subject*. Someone changes the subject when the topic is uncomfortable.
- *Giving your opinions*. Opinions involve judging values, behaviors, or feelings. Let others express feelings and concerns without adding your opinion. Do not make judgments or jump to conclusions.
- *Talking a lot when others are silent*. Talking too much is usually because of nervousness and discomfort with silence.
- *Failure to listen*. Do not pretend to listen. It shows lack of caring and interest. You may miss reports of pain, discomfort, or other symptoms that you must report to the nurse.
- *Pat answers*. "Don't worry." "Everything will be okay." These make the person feel that you do not care about their concerns, feelings, and fears.
- *Illness and disability*. Speech, hearing, vision, cognitive function, and body movements may be affected. Verbal and nonverbal communication is affected.
- *Age*. Values and communication styles vary among age groups.

Persons With Special Needs

- Common courtesies and manners apply to any person with a disability. Review Box 7.2 (p. 74), Disability Etiquette, in the Textbook.
- The person who is comatose is unconscious and cannot respond to others. Often the person can hear and feel touch and pain. Assume that the person hears and understands you. Use touch and give care gently. Practice these measures.
  - o Knock before entering the person's room.
  - o Tell the person your name, the time, and the place every time you enter the room.
  - o Give care on the same schedule every day.
  - o Explain what you are going to do.
  - o Tell the person when you are finishing care.
  - o Use touch to communicate care, concern, and comfort.
  - o Tell the person what time you will be back to check on him or her.
  - o Tell the person when you are leaving the room.

Family and Friends

- If you need to give care when visitors are there, protect the person's right to privacy. Politely ask the visitors to leave the room when you give care. A partner or family member may help you if the patient or resident consents.
- Treat family and visitors with courtesy and respect.
- Do not discuss the person's condition with family and friends. Refer questions to the nurse. A visitor may upset or tire a person. Report your observations to the nurse.

Behavior Issues

- Many people do not adjust well to illness, injury, and disability. They have some of the following behaviors.
  - o *Anger*. Verbal outbursts, shouting, and rapid speech are common. Some people are silent. Others are uncooperative. Nonverbal signs include rapid movements, pacing, clenched fists, and a red face. Glaring and getting close to you when speaking are other signs. Violent behaviors can occur.
  - o *Demanding behavior*. Nothing seems to please the person. The person is critical of others.
  - o *Self-centered behavior*. The person cares only about their own needs. The needs of others are ignored. The person becomes impatient if needs are not met.
  - o *Aggressive behavior*. The person may swear, bite, hit, pinch, scratch, or kick. Protect the person, others, and yourself from harm.
  - o *Withdrawal*. The person has little or no contact with family, friends, and staff. Some people are generally not social and prefer to be alone.
  - o *Inappropriate sexual behavior*. Some people make inappropriate sexual remarks or touch others in the wrong way. These behaviors may be on purpose. Or they are caused by disease, confusion, dementia, or drug side effects.
- You cannot avoid persons with unpleasant behaviors, but you can learn ways to respond. Review Box 7.4 (p. 80), Managing Difficult Behavior, in the Textbook.

CHAPTER 7 REVIEW QUESTIONS

Circle the BEST answer

1. Which circumstance is the best example of providing holistic care?
   a. Nursing assistant cheerfully talks to the resident while helping with morning hygiene and eating breakfast.
   b. Nursing assistant reminds the resident to wear the hearing aid and join others in the singing at church service.
   c. Nursing assistant respectfully listens to the resident explain how to prepare for the morning bath.
   d. Nursing assistant assists the resident to go to the chapel and quietly waits while morning prays are recited.
2. Which method would the nursing assistant use to address the residents in a long-term care center?
   a. Be friendly, cheerful and polite and use gender neutral pronouns: they, them
   b. Use terms of endearment (Honey, Dear) to show affection
   c. Call everyone by their first name to create a casual atmosphere
   d. Use title and surname, unless the resident prefers something else

3. Based on Maslow's theory of basic needs, which person's needs must be met first?
   a. Person desires to talk about her grandson.
   b. Person requests to leave the dining room.
   c. Person wants mail sorted and opened.
   d. Person needs assistance to drink more water.
4. What is the best strategy when caring for people who have a variety of different cultural backgrounds?
   a. Expect that people from different cultures will follow the doctor's advice.
   b. Give excellent care because people from all cultures expect good service.
   c. Disregard the person's culture because other care issues are more important.
   d. Learn about other cultures because culture affects health beliefs and practices.
5. What is the nursing assistant's responsibility in relation to a person's religion and spiritual beliefs?
   a. Ask the person how religion influences his health practices.
   b. Assist a person to attend religious services in the nursing center.
   c. Advise the person to find comfort from religion during illness.
   d. Follow and agree with all the beliefs of the person's religion.
6. What should the nursing assistant do first when a person is angry and shouting?
   a. Stay calm and professional
   b. Raise voice so the person can hear
   c. Instruct the person to stop yelling
   d. Ask the nurse to deal with the person
7. Which action would the nursing assistant take when a person tries to scratch and kick?
   a. Protect self from harm
   b. Firmly, but gently hold the person
   c. Leave until the person calms down
   d. Refuse to care for the person
8. Which nursing assistant is using poor communication skills?
   a. Nursing assistant A positions self at the person's eye level.
   b. Nursing assistant B speaks slowly, clearly, and distinctly.
   c. Nursing assistant C speaks while walking away from person.
   d. Nursing assistant D asks one question at a time.
9. Which nursing assistant is using good listening behavior?
   a. Nursing assistant A starts talking before the person is finished.
   b. Nursing assistant B is texting while the person is talking.
   c. Nursing assistant C leans slightly toward the person who is talking.
   d. Nursing assistant D slouches and crosses arms as the person talks.
10. In which circumstance would the nursing assistant use silence?
   a. Nursing assistant is irritated because the resident is rude.
   b. The resident wants to share happy news with everyone.
   c. Nursing assistance does not know the answer to the resident's question.
   d. The resident is upset and needs to gain control.
11. Which nursing assistant needs additional reminders to properly communicate with a person who speaks a foreign language?
   a. Nursing assistant A gestures and says, "Sir, please sit down."
   b. Nursing assistant B points to a picture of a comb.
   c. Nursing assistant C shouts, "I am here to help you."
   d. Nursing assistant D repeats the message in a different way.
12. When caring for a person who is comatose, which action would the nursing assistant perform?
   a. Talk about normal events that are happening around the unit
   b. Do not say anything because the person cannot understand
   c. Use touch to communicate care, comfort, and concern
   d. Work quickly and quietly to avoid extra stimulation
13. When a person is in a wheelchair, which action would the nursing assistant perform?
   a. Lean on armrests of the wheelchair while talking to the person
   b. Sit or squat to talk to a person in a wheelchair or chair
   c. Announce obstacles while pushing the person in a wheelchair
   d. Encourages a person in a wheelchair with a friendly pat on the head
14. Which action would the nursing assistant take when family is visiting and hygienic care needs to be completed?
   a. Do any care that does not expose the body
   b. Politely ask the family to leave the room
   c. Defer the care until the next day
   d. Invite the family to help with the care

Answers to these questions are on p. 577.

CHAPTER 8 HEALTH TEAM COMMUNICATIONS

Communication

- For good communication:
  - Use words that mean the same thing to you and the receiver of the message.
  - If you do not know a term, ask what it means.
  - Be brief and concise.
  - Give information in a logical and orderly manner.
  - Give facts and be specific.

The Medical Record

- The **medical record, or chart, is** the permanent, legal account of the person's condition and response to treatment and care. Medical records can be written or stored electronically. The electronic health record or electronic medical record is the electronic version of the person's medical record. It is a permanent legal document.
- The medical record is a way for the health team to share information about the person. Agencies have policies about medical records and who can see them.

Some agencies allow nursing assistants to read and/or record observations in medical records. Follow your agency's policies.
- Medical records can include the person's admission record, advanced directives, health history, graphic and flow sheets for recording measurements and observations, diagnostic reports, and progress reports. See Table 8.1 (p. 86), Parts of the Medical Record, in the Textbook for additional information.
- The Kardex or care summary is a summary of the person's medical record. The summary can be electronic or on paper as a card file.
- The **nursing process** is the method nurses use to plan and deliver nursing care. It has five steps: assessment, analysis, planning, implementation, and evaluation.
- **Assessment** involves collecting information about the person. A health history is taken. A registered nurse (RN) assesses the person's body systems and mental systems. Although the nursing assistant does not assess, you play a key role in assessment. You make many observations as you give care and talk to the person.
- **Observation** is using the senses of sight, hearing, touch, and smell to collect information.
- Basic observations are outlined in Box 8.3 (p. 90), Basic Observations, in the Textbook. See Box 8.2 (p. 89), Observations to Report at Once, in the Textbook:
  - A change in the person's ability to respond
  - A change in the person's mobility
  - Reports of sudden, severe pain
  - A sore or reddened area on the person's skin
  - Reports of a sudden change in vision
  - Reports of pain or difficulty breathing
  - Abnormal respirations
  - Reports of or signs of difficulty swallowing
  - Vomiting
  - Bleeding
  - Dizziness
  - Vital signs outside the normal ranges
- **Objective data (signs)** are seen, heard, felt, or smelled by an observer. For example, you can feel a pulse.
- **Subjective data (symptoms)** are things a person tells you about that you cannot observe through your senses. For example, you cannot see the person's nausea.
- The nurse uses assessment data to **analyze** and identify health problem that can be treated by nursing measures.
- The nurse will then conduct **planning** to set priorities and goals for the person's care.
- **Nursing interventions** or **implementations** are the actions taken by the nursing team to help the person reach a goal.
- The nursing diagnoses, goals, and actions for each goal are recorded in the **nursing care plan**. The care plan is a communication tool. Each agency has a care plan tool.
- The RN may conduct a care conference with the health-care team to share information and ideas about the person's care.
- The nurse will **evaluate** the planning and implementation based on the person's progress toward the stated goal.
- The nurse may delegate tasks to the nursing assistant via the assignment sheet during any step of the nursing process.

Reporting and Recording

- The health team communicates by reporting and recording.

Reporting

- You report care and observations to the nurse. Report to the nurse:
  - Whenever there is a change from normal or a change in the person's condition. Report these changes at once.
  - When the nurse asks you to do so.
  - When you leave the unit for meals, breaks, or other reasons.
  - Before the end-of-shift report.
- Follow the rules of reporting.
  - Be prompt, thorough, and accurate.
  - Give the person's name and room and bed numbers.
  - Give the time your observations were made or the care was given.
  - Report only what you observed or did yourself.
  - Report care measures that you expect the person to need.
  - Report expected changes in the person's condition.
  - Give reports as often as the person's condition requires or when the nurse asks you to.
  - Report any changes from normal or changes in the person's condition at once.
  - Use your written notes to give a specific, concise, and clear report.

Recording

- When recording or documenting, communicate clearly and thoroughly what you observed, what you did, and the person's response.
- The general rules for recording on paper are:
  - Always use ink. Use the color required by the center.
  - Include the date and time for every recording.
  - Make sure writing is readable and neat.
  - Use only agency-approved abbreviations.
  - Use correct spelling, grammar, and punctuation.
  - Do not use ditto marks.
  - Never erase or use correction fluid. Follow agency procedure for correcting errors.
  - Sign all entries with your name and title as required by agency policy.
  - Do not skip lines.
  - Make sure each form has the person's name and other identifying information.
  - Record only what you observed and did yourself.
  - Never chart a procedure, treatment, or care measure until after it is completed.
  - Be accurate, concise, and factual. Do not record judgments or interpretations.
  - Record in a logical and sequential manner.
  - Be descriptive. Avoid terms with more than one meaning.
  - Use the person's exact words whenever possible. Use quotation marks to show that the statement is a direct quote.
  - Chart any changes from normal or changes in the person's condition. Also chart that you informed the

nurse (include the nurse's name), what you told the nurse, and the time you made the report.
  - Do not omit information.
  - Record safety measures. For example, reminding a person not to get out of bed.
- Review the 24-hour clock, Fig. 8.7 (p. 94), and Box 8.4 (p. 94), 24-Hour Clock.
- Review Box 8.5 (p. 95), Rules for Reporting, and Box 8.6 (p. 97), Rules for Recording.

Computers and Other Electronic Devices

- Computers contain vast amounts of information about a person. Therefore the right to privacy must be protected. If allowed access, you must follow the agency's policies.
- Review Box 8.7 (p. 98), Electronic Devices, in the Textbook.

Phone Communications

- Guidelines for answering phones:
  - Answer the call after the first ring if possible.
  - Do not answer the phone in a rushed or hasty manner.
  - Give a courteous greeting. Identify the nursing unit and your name and title.
  - When taking a message, write down the caller's name, phone number (with area code and extension), date and time, and who the message is for.
  - Repeat the message and phone number back to the caller.
  - Ask the caller to "Please hold" if necessary.
  - Do not lay the phone down or cover the receiver with your hand when not speaking to the caller. The caller may hear confidential information.
  - Return to a caller on hold within 30 seconds.
  - Do not give confidential information to any caller.
  - Transfer a call if appropriate. Tell the caller you are going to transfer the call. Give the name and phone number in case the call gets disconnected or the line is busy.
  - End the conversation politely.
  - Give the message to the appropriate person.

CHAPTER 8 REVIEW QUESTIONS

Circle the BEST answer

1. Which nursing assistant needs a reminder about the rules of good communication?
   a. Nursing assistant A uses words with more than one meaning.
   b. Nursing assistant B use words that are familiar to the person.
   c. Nursing assistant C gives facts in a brief and concise manner.
   d. Nursing assistant D gives information in a logical and orderly manner.
2. Which recording reflects application of the rules of recording?
   a. Morning care was provided by another nursing assistant.
   b. Resident felt sad and depressed after the visitor left.
   c. Resident had abdominal pane; nurse A was advised.
   d. 1200: Resident ate 75% of meal and drank 300 mL of milk.
3. Which report to the nurse correctly incorporates the rules for reporting?
   a. Room 102 is asking for pain medication and a sedative.
   b. Mr. Smith was having problems breathing about an hour ago.
   c. Mrs. Jones refused to shower, but she washed her face and hands.
   d. Sorry, I forgot to tell you I was going on break; my son called me.
4. Which observation needs to be reported at once?
   a. Person has a bad taste in his mouth.
   b. Person passed a large amount of brown stool.
   c. Person has a reddened area on lower back.
   d. Person independently accomplished his hygiene.
5. Which data are subjective?
   a. The person has pain in his abdomen.
   b. The person's pulse is 76.
   c. The person's urine is dark amber.
   d. The person's breath has an odor.

Answers to these questions are on p. 577.

CHAPTER 9 MEDICAL TERMINOLOGY

Medical Terminology and Abbreviations

- Medical terminology and abbreviations are used in health care. Someone may use a word or phrase that you do not understand. If so, ask the nurse to explain its meaning.
- Review Table 9.1 (p. 103), Table 9.2 (p. 105), Table 9.3 (p. 106) Word Elements, and Table 9.6 (p. 110), Common Health-Care Terms and Phrases, in the Textbook.
- Use only the abbreviations accepted by the center. If you are not sure that an abbreviation is acceptable, write the term out in full. See the inside back cover of the Textbook for common abbreviations.

CHAPTER 9 REVIEW QUESTIONS

Circle the BEST answer

1. In which area would the nursing assistant be extra gentle when washing a child who has a severe sunburn on the posterior surface of the body?
   a. Face and neck
   b. Back and buttocks
   c. Hands and feet
   d. Top of the head
2. Which term best describes the location of the xiphoid process?
   a. Lateral chest
   b. Proximal to neck
   c. Medial chest
   d. Distal to abdomen
3. Which of these four patients is going to require the most time to complete the care?
   a. Patient A needs to be nil per os (NPO) after midnight.
   b. Patient B requires total assistance with activities of daily living (ADLs).
   c. Patient C requires vital signs q4 hours.
   d. Patient D has a urinary tract infection and needs intake and output measurements.

CHAPTER 11 GROWTH AND DEVELOPMENT

- **Growth** is the physical changes that are measured and occur in a steady and orderly manner.
- **Development** relates to changes in mental, emotional, and social function.
- Growth and development occur in a sequence, order, and pattern. Review the stages of growth and development detailed in the Textbook.
- Middle adulthood (aged 40–65 years). At this stage, developmental tasks are adjusting to physical changes, having grown children, developing leisure-time activities, and adjusting to aging parents.
- Late adulthood (aged 65 years and older). At this stage, developmental tasks are adjusting to decreased strength and loss of health, adjusting to retirement and reduced income, coping with a partner's death, developing new friends and relationships, and preparing for one's own death.

CHAPTER 11 REVIEW QUESTIONS

Circle the BEST answer

1. Based on the principle of growth and development "simple to complex," which activity would the nursing assistant expect a baby to display first?
   a. Running
   b. Walking
   c. Standing
   d. Sitting
2. During weekly home visits to an elderly person, the nursing assistant notices that a 3-month-old grandchild is alert, but not cooing, smiling, or interacting with others. Which action would the nursing assistant take?
   a. Ask the primary caregiver if the baby is ill or tired
   b. Report the observation to the supervising nurse
   c. Do nothing, the baby is not the assistant's responsibility
   d. Try smiling, playing, and stimulating the baby
3. What is a developmental task of late adulthood?
   a. Accepting changes in appearance
   b. Adjusting to decreased strength
   c. Developing a satisfactory sex life
   d. Performing self-care

Answers to these questions are on p. 577.

CHAPTER 12 THE OLDER PERSON

- Aging is normal. Normal changes occur in body structure and function. Psychological and social changes also occur. The risk for illness or injury increases with aging.

Psychological and Social Changes

- Physical reminders of growing old affect self-esteem and may threaten self-image, self-worth, and independence.
- People adjust to aging in their own way. How they cope depends on their health status, life experiences, finances, education, and social support systems.
- *Retirement*. Many people enjoy retirement. Others are in poor health and have medical bills that can make retirement difficult.
- *Reduced income*. Retirement usually means reduced income. Reduced income may force lifestyle changes. One example is the person avoids health care or needed drugs.
- *Social relationships*. Social relationships change throughout life. Companionship with people of the same age is important. Hobbies, religious and community events, and new friends provide enjoyment.
- *Children as caregivers*. Some older persons feel more secure when children care for them. Others feel unwanted and useless. Some lose dignity and self-respect. Tensions may occur among the child, parent, and other household members.
- *Death and grieving*. Death of an adult child or a partner can cause immense grief. Emotional needs will be great. The person may be left with few family and friends to provide support.

Physical Changes

- Body processes slow down. Energy level and body efficiency decline.
- *The integumentary system*. The skin loses its elasticity, strength, and fatty tissue layer. Wrinkles appear. Dry skin occurs and may cause itching. The skin is fragile and easily injured. The person is more sensitive to cold. Nails become thick and tough. White or gray hair is common. Hair thins. Facial hair may occur in women. Hair is drier.
- *The musculoskeletal system*. Muscle and bone strength are lost. Bones become brittle and break easily. Vertebrae shorten. Joints become stiff and painful. Mobility decreases. There is a gradual loss of height.
- *The nervous system*. Confusion and dizziness may occur. Responses are slower. The risk for falls increases. Forgetfulness increases. Memory is shorter. Events from long ago are remembered better than recent ones. Older persons have a harder time falling asleep. Sleep periods are shorter. Older persons wake often during the night and have less deep sleep. Less sleep is needed. They may rest or nap during the day. They may go to bed early and get up early.
- *The senses*. Hearing and vision losses occur. Taste and smell dull. Touch and sensitivity to pain, and pressure are reduced.
- *The circulatory system*. The heart muscle weakens. Arteries narrow and are less elastic.
- Fatigue occurs. Poor circulation occurs in many body parts.
- *The respiratory system*. Respiratory muscles weaken. Lung tissue becomes less elastic. Difficult or labored breathing may occur with activity. The person may lack strength to cough and clear the airway of secretions.
- *The digestive system*. Less saliva is produced. The person may have difficulty swallowing (dysphagia). Appetite decreases. Indigestion may occur. Loss of teeth and ill-

fitting dentures cause chewing problems and digestion problems. Flatulence and constipation can occur.
- *The urinary system*. Bladder muscles weaken. Urinary frequency or urgency may occur. Urinary tract infections are risks. Many older persons have to urinate at night. Urinary incontinence may occur. In men, the prostate gland enlarges. This may cause difficulty urinating or frequent urination.
- *The reproductive system*. In men, testosterone decreases. An erection takes longer. Orgasm is less forceful. Women experience menopause. Female hormones of estrogen and progesterone decrease. The uterus, vagina, and genitalia shrink (atrophy). Vaginal walls thin. There is vaginal dryness. Arousal takes longer. Orgasm is less intense.

Housing Options
- A person's home holds memories, and it is a link to neighbors and communities and brings pride and self-esteem.
- Most older people live in their own homes. Others need help from family or community agencies. Review Box 12.3 (p. 153), In-Home and Community-Based Services, in the Textbook.

Nursing Centers
- The person needing nursing center care may suffer some or all these losses.
  - Loss of identity as a productive member of a family and community
  - Loss of possessions—home, household items, car, and so on
  - Loss of independence
  - Loss of real-world experiences—shopping, traveling, cooking, driving, hobbies
  - Loss of health and mobility
- The person may feel useless, powerless, and hopeless. The health team helps the person cope with loss and improve the quality of life. Treat the person with dignity and respect. Also practice good communication skills. Follow the care plan.

CHAPTER 12 REVIEW QUESTIONS
Circle the BEST answer

1. Which nursing assistant is verbalizing a myth about aging and older people?
   a. Nursing assistant A says, "Older people are always so lonely; nobody cares it's sad."
   b. Nursing assistant B says, "Everybody occasionally forgets something; not just the elderly."
   c. Nursing assistant C says, "My Grandma is crabby, but she was always unhappy."
   d. Nursing assistant D says, "A small percentage of the elderly live in nursing centers."
2. Which care measure would the nursing assistant use when caring for an older person with changes in the integumentary system?
   a. Assist the person to shower daily and use soap to remove body odor
   b. Keep the feet warm by using a heating pad on the lowest setting.
   c. Set the thermostat on a low setting and provide sweaters and socks
   d. Apply lotion and creams to prevent dryness of the skin and itching
3. Which care measure would the nursing assistant perform to assist an older person who has changes of the musculoskeletal system related to aging?
   a. Assist with range-of-motion (ROM) exercises as ordered
   b. Encourage person to use stairs and jog to build muscles
   c. Tell the person to perform own care to maintain mobility
   d. Feed a diet that is high in calories for energy
4. Which behavior would the nursing assistant expect to observe for a person who has age-related changes of the nervous system?
   a. Person's speech is slurred.
   b. Person may refuse to eat.
   c. Person may be forgetful.
   d. Person has trouble breathing.
5. Which older person needs to have thickened liquids as a care measure for a change in the digestive system?
   a. Person has a decreased appetite.
   b. Person has lost several teeth.
   c. Person is having flatulence.
   d. Person is having trouble swallowing.
6. How will age-related changes of the urinary system impact the amount of time that the nursing assistant will spend caring for and assisting the person?
   a. Person will have pain, and this will frequently need to be reported to the nurse.
   b. Person will need frequent vital signs that need to be recorded and reported.
   c. Person will frequently use the call bell for assistance to go to the bathroom.
   d. Person will desire and need extra amounts of fluid especially in the evening.

Answers to these questions are on p. 577.

CHAPTER 13 THE PERSON'S UNIT
- A person's unit is the space, furniture, and equipment used by the person in the agency. Centers for Medicare & Medicaid Services (CMS) requires that resident units be as personal and homelike as possible.
- Keep the person's room clean, neat, safe, and comfortable. Follow the rules in Box 13.1 (p. 160), Maintaining the Person's Unit, and Long-Term Care and Home Care: The Person's Unit, (p. 161) in the Textbook.

Comfort
- Age, illness, and activity affect comfort.
- Temperature, ventilation, noise, odors, and lighting are factors that are controlled to meet the person's needs.

Temperature and Ventilation

- Older persons and those who are ill may need higher temperatures for comfort. Ventilation systems provide fresh air and move air within the room.
- To protect older and ill persons from drafts, make sure the person wears enough clothing, offer a lap cover when sitting in a chair and cover the legs, use a bath blanket when providing care, and move the person from drafty areas.

Odors

- To reduce odors in nursing centers:
  - Empty, clean, and disinfect bedpans, urinals, commodes, and kidney basins promptly.
  - Check to make sure toilets are flushed.
  - Check incontinent people often.
  - Clean persons who are wet or soiled from urine, feces, vomitus, or wound drainage.
  - Change wet or soiled linens and clothing promptly.
  - Keep laundry containers closed.
  - Follow agency policy for wet or soiled linens and clothing.
  - Dispose of incontinence and ostomy products promptly.
  - Provide good hygiene to prevent body and breath odors.
  - Use room deodorizers as needed and as allowed by agency policy.
- If you smoke, practice handwashing after handling smoking materials and before giving care. Pay attention to your uniforms, hair, and breath because of smoke odors.

Noise

- To decrease noise:
  - Control your voice.
  - Handle equipment carefully.
  - Keep equipment in good working order.
  - Answer phones, call lights, and intercoms promptly.

Lighting

- Adjust lighting to meet the person's needs. Glares, shadows, and dull lighting can cause falls, headaches, and eyestrain. A bright room is cheerful. Dim light is better for relaxing and rest. Persons with poor vision need bright light. Always keep light controls within the person's reach.

Room Furniture and Equipment

- Rooms are furnished and equipped for safety and to meet basic needs.

The Bed

- Beds are raised to give care. This reduces bending and reaching.
- Bed wheels are locked at all times except when moving the bed.
- Use bed rails as the nurse and care plan direct.
- Basic bed positions:
  - *Flat*—the usual sleeping position.
  - *Fowler's position*—a semi-sitting position. The head of the bed is raised between 45 and 60 degrees.
  - *High Fowler's position*—a semi-sitting position. The head of the bed is raised 60 to 90 degrees.
  - *Semi-Fowler's position*—the head of the bed is raised 30 degrees. Some agencies define semi-Fowler's position as when the head of the bed is raised 30 degrees and the knee portion is raised 15 degrees. Know the definition used by your agency.
  - *Trendelenburg's position*—the head of the bed is lowered and the foot of the bed is raised. A doctor orders the position.
  - *Reverse Trendelenburg's position*—the head of the bed is raised and the foot of the bed is lowered. A doctor orders the position.

Bed Safety

- *Entrapment* means getting caught, trapped, or entangled in spaces created by bed rails, the mattress, the bed frame, or the headboard and footboard. Head, neck, or chest entrapment can cause serious injuries and deaths. Always check for entrapment. If a person is caught, trapped, or entangled, try to release the person. Call for the nurse at once.

The Over-Bed Table

- Only clean and sterile items are placed on the table. Never place bedpans, urinals, or soiled linens on the over-bed table or on top of the bedside stand.
- Clean the table and bedside stand after using them for a work surface and before serving meal trays.

Privacy Curtains

- Always pull the curtain completely around the bed before giving care. Privacy curtains do not block sound or conversations.

The Call System

- Always keep the call light within the person's reach—in the room, bathroom, and shower or tub room. You must:
  - Place the call light on the person's strong side.
  - Remind the person to signal when help is needed.
  - Answer call lights promptly.
  - Answer bathroom and shower or tub room call lights at once.
- Persons with limited hand mobility may need special communication measures.
- Be careful when using the intercom. Remember confidentiality. Persons nearby can hear what you and the person say.

The Bathroom

- Grab bars are by the toilet so persons can use them to get on and off the toilet.
- Some toilet seats are raised to make transfers easier and for persons with joint problems.
- A call light or button is within reach of the toilet if the person needs assistance.
- Towel racks, toilet paper, soap, paper towels, and a wastebasket should be within reach.

Closet and Drawer Space

- The person must have free access to the closet and its contents. You must have the person's permission to open or search closets or drawers.
- Agency staff can inspect a person's closet or drawers if hoarding is suspected. The person is informed of the inspection and is present when it takes place. Have a coworker present when you inspect a person's closet.

CHAPTER 13 REVIEW QUESTIONS

Circle the BEST answer

1. Which person and situation create the greatest risk for entrapment?
   a. An older person is sitting in a wheelchair and visiting with family.
   b. An obese person is learning to use the trapeze over the bariatric bed.
   c. A small, frail older person is confused and very restless in bed.
   d. A frail older person is sitting in the dining room and refuses to eat.
2. Which bed position would most people prefer for sleeping?
   a. Semi-Fowler's
   b. Flat
   c. Trendelenburg
   d. High Fowler's
3. Which task is a nursing assistant responsibility?
   a. Clean the bedside stand after using it for a work surface.
   b. Routinely check closets and drawers for unsafe items.
   c. Encourage independent residents not to use call lights.
   d. Clean upholstered furniture and rugs every day.
4. Which person needs additional measures to be protected from drafts?
   a. Person is wearing a sleeveless t-shirt and a short skirt.
   b. Person is sitting in a wheelchair with a lab robe over legs.
   c. Person is covered with a bath blanket during morning hygiene.
   d. Person is provided an extra blanket while taking a nap.
5. Which action would the nursing assistant perform to reduce odors?
   a. Empty and clean commodes at the end of the shift
   b. Keep laundry containers open in well-ventilated areas
   c. Use circulating fans to move air and disperse odors
   d. Clean persons who are wet or soiled from urine or feces
6. Which nursing assistant needs to be counseled about the call lights?
   a. Nursing assistant A ensures that the call light is within the person's reach.
   b. Nursing assistant B places the call light on the person's strong side.
   c. Nursing assistant C only answers the call lights of assigned residents.
   d. Nursing assistant D promptly answers a bathroom call light.
7. Which action would the nursing assistant take before inspecting a resident's closet for suspected hoarding food?
   a. Tell the resident that hoarding violates agency policy.
   b. Inspect the closet when the resident is not in the room.
   c. Tell the family to check the closet for unwanted items.
   d. Ask the resident for permission to inspect the closet.

Answers to these questions are on p. 577.

CHAPTER 14 SAFETY

Accident Risk Factors

- *Age.* Older persons and children are at risk for injuries.
- *Awareness of surroundings.* Confused or disoriented persons may not understand what is happening to them or around them.
- *Agitated and aggressive behaviors.* Pain, confusion, fear, and decreased awareness of surroundings can cause these behaviors.
- *Vision loss.* Persons can fall or trip over items. Some have problems reading labels on containers.
- *Hearing loss.* Persons may not hear warning signals or fire alarms and will not move to safety.
- *Impaired smell and touch.* Illness and aging affect smell and touch. The person may not detect smoke or gas or may be unaware of injury. Burns are a risk.
- *Impaired mobility.* Some diseases and injuries affect mobility. A person may recognize danger but be unable to move to safety. Some persons are paralyzed. Some persons cannot walk or propel wheelchairs.
- *Drugs.* Drugs have side effects. Reduced awareness, confusion, and disorientation can occur. Report behavior changes and the person's concerns.

Identifying the Person

- You must give the right care to the right person. To identify the person:
  - Compare identifying information on the assignment sheet or treatment card with that on the identification (ID) bracelet.
  - Call the person by name when checking the ID bracelet. Just calling the person by name is not enough to identify him or her. Confused, disoriented, drowsy, hard-of-hearing, or distracted persons may answer to any name.
- Use at least two identifiers. Agencies have different requirements. Some may require the person to state and spell their name and give a birth date. Others require using the person's ID number. Always follow agency policy.

Preventing Burns

- Smoking, spilled hot liquids, very hot water, and electrical devices are common causes of burns. See Box 14.1 (p. 180), Preventing Burns, in the Textbook for safety measures to prevent burns.

Preventing Poisoning

- Drugs and household products are common poisons. Poisoning in adults may be from carelessness, confusion, or poor vision when reading labels. To prevent poisoning:
  - Make sure patients and residents cannot reach hazardous materials.
  - Follow agency policy for storing personal care items.
- See Box 14.2 (p. 181), Preventing Poisoning, in the Textbook for safety measures to prevent poisoning.

Preventing Suffocation

- **Suffocation** is when breathing stops from the lack of oxygen. Death occurs if the person does not start breathing.
- To prevent suffocation, review Box 14.5 (p. 187), Preventing Suffocation, in the Textbook.

Choking

- Choking or foreign-body airway obstruction occurs when a foreign body (e.g., food or toy) obstructs the airway. Air cannot pass through the air passages into the lungs. The body does not get enough oxygen. This can lead to death.
- Choking often occurs during eating. A large, poorly chewed piece of meat is a common cause. Other common causes include laughing and talking while eating.
- With *mild airway obstruction*, some air moves in and out of the lungs. The person is conscious. Usually the person can speak. Often, forceful coughing can remove the object.
- With *severe airway obstruction*, the conscious person clutches at the throat—the "universal sign of choking." The person has difficulty breathing. Some persons cannot breathe, speak, or cough. The person appears pale and cyanotic (bluish color). Air does not move in and out of the lungs. If the obstruction is not removed, the person will die. Severe airway obstruction is an emergency.
- Use abdominal thrusts to relieve severe choking. Chest thrusts are used for very obese persons and pregnant women.
- Call for help when a person has an obstructed airway. Report and record what happened, what you did, and the person's response.

Preventing Equipment Accidents

- All equipment is unsafe if broken, not used correctly, or not working properly. Inspect all equipment before use. Review Box 14.7 (p. 192), Preventing Equipment Accidents, in the Textbook.

Hazardous Chemicals

- A hazardous chemical is any chemical in the workplace that can cause harm. Hazardous substances include latex, mercury, disinfectants, and cleaning agents.
- Hazardous substance containers must have a warning label. If a label is removed or damaged, do not use the substance. Take the container to the nurse. Do not leave the container unattended.
- Check the material safety data sheet (MSDS) before using a hazardous substance, cleaning up a leak or spill, or disposing of the substance. Tell the nurse about a leak or spill right away. Do not leave a leak or spill unattended. Review Box 14.8 (p. 194), Hazardous Chemical Safety Measures, in the Textbook.

Disasters

- A **disaster** is a sudden catastrophic event. The agency has procedures for disasters that could occur in your area. Follow them to keep patients, residents, visitors, staff, and yourself safe.
- Natural disasters include tornadoes, hurricanes, blizzards, earthquakes, volcanic eruptions, floods, and some fires.
- Man-made disasters include auto, bus, train, and airplane accidents. They also include fires, bombings, nuclear power plant accidents, gas or chemical leaks, explosions, and wars.
- Follow agency protocol for a bomb threat or if you find an item that looks or sounds strange.

Fire Safety

- Faulty electrical equipment and wiring, overloaded electrical circuits, and smoking are major causes of fires.
- Safety measures are needed where oxygen is used and stored.
- Review Box 14.9 (p. 195), Fire Prevention Measures, in the Textbook.
- Know your center's policies and procedures for fire emergencies. Know where to find fire alarms, fire extinguishers, and emergency exits. Remember the word *RACE*.
  - **R—*rescue*.** Rescue persons in immediate danger. Move them to a safe place.
  - **A—*alarm*.** Sound the nearest fire alarm.
  - **C—*confine*.** Close doors and windows. Turn off oxygen or electrical items.
  - **E—*extinguish*.** Use a fire extinguisher on a small fire.
- Remember the word *PASS* for using a fire extinguisher.
  - **P—*pull*** the safety pin.
  - **A—*aim*** low. Aim at the base of the fire.
  - **S—*squeeze*** the lever. This starts the stream of water.
  - **S—*sweep*** back and forth. Sweep side to side at the base of the fire.
- Do not use elevators during a fire.

Elopement

- Elopement is when a resident leaves the agency without staff knowledge. The Centers for Medicare and Medicaid Services (CMS) requires that an agency's emergency preparedness plan address elopement.

- The agency must:
  - Identify persons at risk for elopement.
  - Monitor and supervise persons at risk.
  - Address elopement in the person's care plan.
  - Have a plan to find a missing patient or resident.

Workplace Violence

- **Workplace violence** is violent acts (including assault or threat of assault) directed toward persons at work or while on duty. Review Box 14.10 (p. 201), Workplace Violence—Risk Factors and Safety Measures, in the Textbook.

CHAPTER 14 REVIEW QUESTIONS

Circle the BEST answer

1. Which action would the nursing assistant take on seeing a water spill in the hallway?
   a. Notify housekeeping to wipe up the spill.
   b. Wipe up the spill right away.
   c. Report the spill to the nurse.
   d. Ask all residents to walk around the spill.
2. Which action would the nursing assistant take when an electrical outlet in a person's room does not work?
   a. Tell the administrator about the problem.
   b. Tell the resident to avoid using the outlet.
   c. Put a "do not use" sign over the outlet.
   d. Follow the policy for reporting the problem.
3. Which resident has the greatest risk for accidents?
   a. Resident A walks with a cane.
   b. Resident B uses a hearing aid.
   c. Resident C is confused and agitated.
   d. Resident D uses eyeglasses for reading.
4. Which action would the nursing assistant use for the prevention of burns?
   a. For children, serve hot liquids in sippy cups.
   b. Turn cold water on first; turn hot water off first.
   c. Turn the heating pad to lowest setting during sleep.
   d. Tell older people to stay indoors on sunny days.
5. Which nursing assistant has performed an action that puts the person at risk for suffocation?
   a. Nursing assistant A makes sure the person's dentures fit properly.
   b. Nursing assistant B checks the care plan before giving liquids.
   c. Nursing assistant C leaves the child alone in the bathtub.
   d. Nursing assistant D puts the person in Fowler's position.
6. Which person is showing signs of a severe airway obstruction?
   a. Person A says something is in his throat.
   b. Person B has wheezing and coughing.
   c. Person C is cyanotic and cannot speak.
   d. Person D is forcefully coughing.
7. What is the "universal sign of choking"?
   a. Clutching at the chest
   b. Clutching at the throat
   c. Not being able to talk
   d. Not being able to breathe
8. Which environment has been safely prepared for a resident who must use supplemental oxygen?
   a. NO SMOKING signs are placed on the resident's door and near the bed.
   b. Candles are arranged in a distant corner of the room.
   c. Wool blankets are used for warmth instead of heaters.
   d. Smoking materials are stored with other personal property.
9. Which action would the nursing assistant take first on discovering a fire in the nursing center?
   a. Rescue persons in immediate danger
   b. Sound the nearest fire alarm
   c. Close doors and turn off oxygen
   d. Use a fire extinguisher on a small fire
10. Which action is incorrect when using a fire extinguisher to extinguish a small fire?
    a. Pull the safety pin on the fire extinguisher
    b. Aim at the top of the flames
    c. Squeeze the lever to start the stream
    d. Sweep the stream back and forth

Answers to these questions are on p. 577.

CHAPTER 15 PREVENTING FALLS

- Falls are a leading cause of injuries and deaths among older persons. A history of falls increases the risk of falling again.
- Causes for falls are weakness and walking problems, poor lighting, cluttered floors, throw rugs, needing to use the bathroom, out-of-place furniture, wet and slippery floors, bathtubs, and showers. Review Box 15.1 (p. 208), Fall Risk Factors, in the Textbook.
- Agencies have fall prevention programs. Review Box 15.2 (p. 210), Measures to Prevent Falls and Injuries in the Textbook. The person's care plan also lists measures specific for the person.
- Position change alarms alert staff when the person is moving from the bed or chair.

Bed Rails

- A **bed rail** *(siderail)* is a device that serves as a guard or barrier along the side of the bed.
- The nurse and care plan tell you when to raise bed rails. They are needed by persons who are unconscious or sedated with drugs. Some confused and disoriented people need them. When bed rails are needed, always keep them up except when giving bedside nursing care.
- Bed rails present hazards. When bed rails are raised, the person cannot get out of bed. They can fall when trying to climb over the rails. Or the person can get caught, trapped, entangled, or strangled.
- Bed rails are considered restraints if the person cannot get out of bed or lower them without help.
- Bed rails are only used for the treatment of medical symptoms. The need for bed rails is carefully noted in the person's medical record and the care plan. If a

person uses bed rails, check the person often. Record when you checked the person and your observations.

- To prevent falls:
  - Never leave the person alone when the bed is raised.
  - Lower the bed to its lowest position after giving care.
  - If a person does not use bed rails and you need to raise the bed, ask a coworker to stand on the far side of the bed to protect the person from falling.
  - If you raise the bed to give care, always raise the far bed rail if you are working alone.
  - Be sure the person who uses raised bed rails has access to items on the bedside stand and over-bed table. The call light and personal items should be within the person's reach.

Handrails and Grab Bars

- Handrails give support to persons who are weak or unsteady when walking.
- Grab bars (safety bars) provide support for sitting down or getting up from a toilet. They also are used when standing in the shower and for getting in and out of the shower or tub.

Wheel Locks

- Bed wheels are locked at all times except when moving the bed.
- Wheelchair and stretcher wheels are locked when transferring a person.

Transfer/Gait Belts

- Use a **transfer belt (gait belt)** to support a person who is unsteady or disabled. Always follow the manufacturer's instructions. Apply the belt over clothing and under the breasts. The belt buckle is never positioned over the person's spine. Tighten the belt so it is snug. You should be able to slide your open, flat hand under the belt. Tuck the excess strap under the belt. Remove the belt after the procedure.
- Check with the nurse and care plan before using a transfer/gait belt if the person has:
  - A colostomy, ileostomy, gastrostomy, or urostomy
  - Chronic obstructive pulmonary disease
  - An abdominal wound, incision, or drainage tube
  - A chest wound, incision, or drainage tube
  - Monitoring equipment
  - A hernia
  - Other conditions or care equipment involving the chest or abdomen

The Falling Person

- If a person starts to fall, do not try to prevent the fall. You could injure yourself and the person. Ease the person to the floor and protect the person's head.
- Do not let the person get up before the nurse checks for injuries. An incident report is completed after all falls.

CHAPTER 15 REVIEW QUESTIONS

Circle the BEST answer

1. Which observation should the nursing assistant report to the nurse as a risk for falls for an older home health patient?
   a. Rooms are simply furnished.
   b. Kitchen items are hard to reach.
   c. There is a shower with safety bars.
   d. There is a narrow staircase with handrails.
2. What does the nursing assistant need to clarify with the nurse for a person who needs to be observed as a fall prevention measure?
   a. When and where should the person receive meals.
   b. How frequently does the person need to be checked.
   c. How long are visitors allowed to stay with person.
   d. Is the color-code risk for fall band on the person.
3. A person selects clothes and dresses self. Which selection is unsafe?
   a. Slip-resistant footwear is worn.
   b. Long sleeve shirt is buttoned.
   c. Pants are too long.
   d. Belt is fastened.
4. In which circumstance would it be correct to raise the bed rails?
   a. The nurse says that medical symptoms warrant the use of bed rails.
   b. Change of shift report indicates that the person should be restrained as needed for safety.
   c. The person tries to strike out at staff during morning hygiene.
   d. The family asks that the bed rails be raised because the person might fall out of bed.
5. Which nursing assistant is promoting safety and comfort during the use of a transfer/gait belt?
   a. Nursing assistant A positions the quick release buckle at the person's back.
   b. Nursing assistant B asks the person to stand up to apply the belt around the waist.
   c. Nursing assistant C applies the belt so that it hangs loosely outside the clothing.
   d. Nursing assistant D lets the excess strap dangle so that the grandchild can hold it.
6. What would the nursing assistant do when a person becomes faint in the hallway and begins to fall?
   a. Stand back so that the person will not grab as he falls
   b. Catch the person before he falls and call for assistance
   c. Take the person back to the room so the nurse can check him
   d. Ease the person to the floor and protect the person's head

Answers to these questions are on p. 577.

CHAPTER 16 RESTRAINT ALTERNATIVES AND RESTRAINTS

- The Centers for Medicare & Medicaid Services (CMS) has rules for using restraints. These rules protect the person's right to be free from restraints.

- Restraints may be used for a brief time to treat a medical symptom that would require restraint use or for the immediate physical safety of the person or others. Restraints may be used only when less restrictive measures fail to protect the person or others. They must be discontinued as soon as possible.
- The Centers for Medicare & Medicaid Services (CMS) uses these terms.
  - A **physical restraint** is any manual method or physical or mechanical device, material, or equipment attached to or near the person's body that they cannot remove easily and that restricts freedom of movement or normal access to one's body.
  - A **chemical restraint** is a drug that is used for discipline or convenience and not required to treat medical symptoms. The drug or dosage is not a standard treatment for the person's condition.
  - A **restraint** is the restriction of voluntary movement or the control of behavior.
  - A **restraint alternative** is measures used instead of restraint to manage a potentially harmful situation.
  - **Seclusion** is confining a person to a room or area and preventing the person from leaving.
- Federal, state, and accrediting agencies have guidelines about restraint use. They do not forbid restraint use. All other appropriate alternatives must be considered or tried first.
- Every agency has policies and procedures about restraints. They include identifying persons at risk for harm, harmful behaviors, restraint alternatives, and proper restraint use. Staff training is required.

Restraint Alternatives

- Knowing and treating the cause for harmful behaviors can prevent restraint use. There are many alternatives to restraints. See Box 16.2 (p. 223), Restraint Alternatives.

Safe Restraint Use

- Restraints are used only when necessary to treat a person's medical symptoms—physical, emotional, or behavioral problems. Sometimes restraints are needed to protect the person or others.

Physical and Chemical Restraints

- *Physical restraints* are applied to the chest, waist, elbows, wrists, hands, or ankles. They confine the person to a bed or chair. Or they prevent movement of a body part. Some furniture or barriers prevent free movement.
- Drugs or drug dosages are *chemical restraints* if they:
  - Control behavior or restrict movement.
  - Are not standard treatment for the person's condition.

Risks From Restraints

- Restraints can cause many complications. Injuries occur as the person tries to get free of the restraint. Injuries also occur from using the wrong restraint, applying it wrong, or keeping it on too long. Cuts, bruises, and fractures are common. The most serious risk is death from strangulation. Review Box 16.3 (p. 223), Risks From Restraint Use, in the Textbook.

Legal Aspects

- *Restraints must protect the person.* A restraint is used only when it is the best safety measure for the person.
- *A doctor's order is required.* The doctor gives the reason for the restraint, what body part to restrain, what to use, and how long to use it.
- *The least restrictive method is used.* It allows the greatest amount of movement or body access possible.
- *Restraints are used only after other measures fail to protect the person.* Box 16.2 (p. 223), Restraint Alternatives, in the Textbook lists alternatives to restraint use.
- *Unnecessary restraint is false imprisonment.* An unneeded restraint may lead to false imprisonment charges.
- *Informed consent is required.* The person must understand the reason for the restraint. If the person cannot give consent, their legal representative is given the information. The doctor or nurse provides the necessary information and obtains consent.

Safety Guidelines

- Review Box 16.4 (p. 225), Safety Measures for Using Restraints, in the Textbook.
- *Observe for increased confusion and agitation.* Provide repeated explanations and reassurance. Spending time with the person has a calming effect.
- *Protect the person's quality of life.* Restraints are used only for a brief time. You must meet the person's physical, emotional, and social needs.
- *Follow the manufacturer's instructions to safely apply and secure the restraints.* The person must be comfortable and able to move the restrained part to a limited and safe extent.
- *Apply restraints with enough help to protect the person and staff from injury.*
- *Observe the person at least every 15 minutes or as often as directed by the nurse and the care plan.* Injuries and deaths can result from improper restraint use and poor observation.
- *Remove or release the restraint, reposition the person, and meet basic needs at least every 2 hours or as often as noted in the care plan.* The restraint is removed for at least 10 minutes. Provide for food, fluid, comfort, safety, hygiene, and elimination needs and give skin care. Perform range of motion (ROM) exercises or help the person walk.

Reporting and Recording

- Report and record the following:
  - Type of restraint applied
  - Body part or parts restrained
  - Safety measures taken
  - Time you applied the restraint
  - Time you removed or released the restraint

- o Care given when restraint was removed
- o Person's vital signs
- o Skin color and condition
- o Condition of the extremities
- o Pulse felt in the restrained part
- o Changes in the person's behavior
- Report these concerns to the nurse at once: Reports of discomfort; a tight restraint; difficulty breathing; or pain, numbness, or tingling in the restrained part.

CHAPTER 16 REVIEW QUESTIONS

Circle the BEST answer

1. Which care measure would be considered an alternative to restraints?
   a. Tucking the sheets tightly, so that the person does not fall out of bed
   b. Raising the bed rails to prevent getting up without calling for assistance
   c. Putting the bed close to the wall so that the person will not fall out
   d. Having a companion or family member sit at the person's bedside
2. Which nursing assistant has used a restraint as a convenience?
   a. Nursing assistant A puts the person in a chair with a laptop tray for meals.
   b. Nursing assistant B raises a bed rail so that the person can use it to move in bed.
   c. Nursing assistant C puts the person in a belt restraint during shift change.
   d. Nursing assistant D places a mitt restraint according to the care plan.
3. What is the first thing the nursing assistant should do on seeing that a person is being strangled by the restraint?
   a. Run to the nurses' station to get the nurse
   b. Release the restraint or cut it with scissors
   c. Call the Rapid Response Team or the doctor
   d. Start cardiopulmonary resuscitation and rescue breathing
4. How often should the person with a restraint be observed?
   a. At least every 15 minutes
   b. At least every 30 minutes
   c. Once every hour
   d. Once every 2 hours
5. How often do restraints need to be removed?
   a. At least every hour
   b. At least every 2 hours
   c. Once every 3 hours
   d. Once every 4 hours
6. Which documentation related to restraints is correct?
   a. Person was restrained for bad behavior until he calmed down.
   b. Restraints were in place for the entire shift, with no problems.
   c. Restraints removed for 10 minutes and fluids offered at 1400.
   d. Vital signs were deferred because both arms were restrained.

Answers to these questions are on p. 577.

CHAPTER 17 PREVENTING INFECTION

- An **infection** is a disease state resulting from the invasion and growth of microbes in the body. Infection is a major safety hazard.
- Following certain practices and procedures prevents the spread of infection **(infection control)**.

Microorganisms

- A **microorganism (microbe)** is a small *(micro)* living plant or animal *(organism)*.
- Some microbes are harmful and can cause infections **(pathogens)**. Others do not usually cause infection **(nonpathogens)**.

Multidrug-Resistant Organisms

- *Multidrug-resistant organisms (MDROs)* can resist the effects of antibiotics. Such organisms are able to change their structures to survive in the presence of antibiotics. The infections they cause are harder to treat.
- MDROs are caused by prescribing antibiotics when they are not needed (overprescribing). Not taking antibiotics for the prescribed days is also a cause.
- Two common types of MDROs are resistant to many antibiotics.
  - o *Methicillin-resistant Staphylococcus aureus (MRSA)*
  - o *Vancomycin-resistant Enterococcus (VRE)*

Infection

- **A local infection** is in a body part.
- **A systemic infection** involves the whole body.
- Older persons may not show the normal signs and symptoms of infection. The person may have only a slight fever or no fever at all. Redness and swelling may be very slight. The person may not complain of pain. Confusion and delirium may occur.
- Infections can become life threatening before the older person has obvious signs and symptoms. Be alert to minor changes in the person's behavior or condition.
- Report any concerns to the nurse at once. Review Box 17.1 (p. 238), Infection—Signs and Symptoms, in the Textbook.

Health Care–Associated Infection

- A **health care–associated infection (HAI)** is an infection that develops in a person who has received health care in any setting where health care is given. Hospitals, nursing centers, clinics, and home care settings are examples. Review Box 17.2 (p. 248), Health Care–Associated Infections—Examples, in the Textbook.
- The health team must prevent the spread of HAIs by:
  - o Medical asepsis. This includes hand hygiene.
  - o Surgical asepsis.
  - o Standard Precautions.
  - o Transmission-Based Precautions.
  - o Bloodborne Pathogen Standard.

Medical Asepsis

- **Asepsis** is the absence of disease-producing microbes.

- **Medical asepsis (clean technique)** refers to the practices used to:
  - o Reduce the number of microbes
  - o Prevent microbes from spreading from 1 person or place to another person or place.

Common Aseptic Practices

- To prevent the spread of microbes, wash your hands:
  - o After elimination.
  - o After changing tampons or sanitary pads.
  - o After contact with your own or another person's blood, body fluids, secretions, or excretions. This includes saliva, vomitus, urine, feces, vaginal discharge, mucus, semen, wound drainage, pus, and respiratory secretions.
  - o After coughing, sneezing, or blowing your nose.
  - o Before and after handling, preparing, or eating food.
  - o After smoking.
- Also do the following:
  - o Provide all persons with their own linens and personal care items.
  - o Cover your nose and mouth when coughing, sneezing, or blowing your nose.
  - o If without tissues, cough or sneeze into your upper arm. Do not cough or sneeze into your hands.
  - o Bathe, wash hair, and brush your teeth regularly.
  - o Wash fruits and raw vegetables before eating or serving them.
  - o Wash cooking and eating utensils with soap and water after use.

Hand Hygiene

- *Hand hygiene is the easiest and most important way to prevent the spread of infection.* Practice hand hygiene before and after giving care. Review Box 17.3 (p. 243), Rules of Hand Hygiene in Health Care Settings, in the Textbook.

Supplies and Equipment

- Most health-care equipment is disposable. Bedpans, urinals, wash basins, water pitchers, and drinking cups are multiuse items and should be labeled with the person's name, room number and bed number. Do not "borrow" these items for another person.
- Nondisposable items are cleaned and then disinfected. Then they are sterilized.

Other Aseptic Measures

- Review Box 17.5 (p. 249), Aseptic Measures, in the Textbook.

Bloodborne Pathogen Standard

- The health team is at risk for exposure to human immunodeficiency virus (HIV) and the hepatitis B virus (HBV). HIV and HBV are blood-borne pathogens found in the blood.
- The Bloodborne Pathogen Standard is intended to protect you from exposure.
- Staff at risk for exposure to HIV and HBV receive free training.
- *Hepatitis B vaccination.* You can receive the hepatitis B vaccination within 10 working days of being hired. The agency pays for it. If you refuse the vaccination, you must sign a statement. You can have the vaccination at a later date.

Laundry

- OSHA requires these measures for contaminated laundry.
  - o Handle it as little as possible.
  - o Wear gloves or other needed PPE.
  - o Bag contaminated laundry where it is used.
  - o Mark laundry bags or containers with the *biohazard* symbol for laundry sent off-site.
  - o Place wet, contaminated laundry in leakproof containers before transport. The containers are color coded in red or have the *biohazard* symbol.

Equipment

- Contaminated equipment and work surfaces are cleaned and decontaminated with a proper disinfectant:
  - o On completing tasks
  - o At once when there is obvious contamination
  - o At the end of the work shift if the surfaces have been contaminated since the last cleaning

Exposure Incidents

- An **exposure incident** is any eye, mouth, other mucous membrane, nonintact skin, or parenteral contact with blood or OPIM (other potentially infectious materials).
- Report exposure incidents at once. Medical evaluation, follow-up, and required tests are free. Your blood is tested for HIV and HBV. Confidentiality is important.

Personal Protective Equipment (PPE)

- OSHA requires these measures for PPE: gloves, goggles, face shields, masks, laboratory coats, gowns, shoe covers, and surgical caps.
  - o Remove PPE before leaving the work area.
  - o Remove PPE when a garment becomes contaminated.
  - o Place used PPE in marked areas or containers when being stored, washed, decontaminated, or discarded.
  - o Wear gloves when you expect contact with blood or OPIM.
  - o Wear gloves when handling or touching contaminated items or surfaces.
  - o Replace worn, punctured, or contaminated gloves.
  - o Do not wash or decontaminate disposable gloves for reuse.
  - o Discard utility gloves that show signs of cracking, peeling, tearing, or puncturing. Utility gloves are decontaminated for reuse if the process will not ruin them.

Work Practice Controls

- *Work practice controls* reduce employee exposure in the workplace. All tasks involving blood or OPIM are done in ways to limit splatters, splashes, and sprays.
  - o Do not eat, drink, smoke, apply cosmetics or lip balm, or handle contact lenses in areas of occupational exposure.
  - o Do not store food or drinks where blood or OPIM are kept.

- o Practice hand hygiene after removing gloves.
- o Wash hands as soon as possible after skin contact with blood or OPIM.
- o Do not recap, bend, or remove needles by hand.
- o Do not shear or break needles.
- o Discard needles and sharp instruments (razors) in containers that are closable, puncture resistant, and leakproof. Containers are color coded in red and have the *biohazard* symbol.

Surgical asepsis

- **Surgical asepsis (sterile technique)** are the practices used to remove all microbes.
- Surgical asepsis is required any time the skin or sterile tissues are entered. Review Box 17.6 (p. 253), Surgical Asepsis—Principles and Practices.

CHAPTER 17 REVIEW QUESTIONS

Circle the BEST answer

1. Which action would the nursing assistant take to prevent HAIs?
   a. Wear sterile gloves when caring for people with infections
   b. Perform hand hygiene before and after giving care
   c. Get the hepatitis B vaccination series
   d. Immediately report an exposure incident
2. In which circumstance would the use of an alcohol-based hand sanitizer be acceptable?
   a. After assisting with wound care
   b. After taking a person's vital signs
   c. After cleaning up diarrheal feces
   d. After known exposure to *Clostridium difficile*
3. Which nursing assistant is correctly following the procedure for handwashing?
   a. Nursing assistant A stands away from the sink and clothes do not touch the sink.
   b. Nursing assistant B raises hands above elbows toward the faucet.
   c. Nursing assistant C quickly washes hands by rubbing palms several times.
   d. Nursing assistant D dries hands with a paper towel; then uses towel to turn off faucet.
4. Which person has a HAI?
   a. Nursing assistant develops a cold after her son gets a cold at school.
   b. Person develops a urinary infection because catheter care was not performed.
   c. Nursing assistant gets hepatitis after getting stuck with a dirty needle.
   d. Person becomes HIV positive after unprotected sex with several partners.
5. Which member of the health-care team is following work practice controls to prevent blood-borne pathogen exposure?
   a. Nurse recaps needle before putting it in the sharps box.
   b. Nursing assistant throws a disposable razor in the trash can.
   c. Doctor performs hand hygiene after removing gloves.
   d. Nursing assistant applies lip balm in a procedure area.

Answers to these questions are on p. 577.

CHAPTER 18 ISOLATION PRECAUTIONS

- Infection control is the practices and procedures that prevent the spread of infection. A goal is to isolate (contain) and prevent the spread of pathogens.
- The Centers for Disease and Control and Prevention's (CDC's) isolation precautions guideline has two tiers of precautions.
  - o Standard Precautions
  - o Transmission-Based Precautions

Standard Precautions

- Standard Precautions reduce the risk of spreading pathogens and known and unknown infections. Standard Precautions are used for all persons whenever care is given. They prevent the spread of infection from:
  - o Blood.
  - o All body fluids, secretions, and excretions even if blood is not visible. Sweat is not known to spread infections.
  - o Nonintact skin (skin with open breaks).
  - o Mucous membranes.
- Review Box 18.1 (p. 259), Standard Precautions, in the Textbook.

Transmission-Based Precautions

- Some infections require Transmission-Based Precautions. Review Box 18.3 (p. 262), Transmission-Based Precautions, in the Textbook.
- Agency policies may differ from those in the Textbook. The rules in Box 18.2 (p. 261), Rules for Transmission-Based Precautions, in the Textbook are a guide for giving safe care.

Gloves

- Wear gloves whenever contact with blood, body fluids, secretions, excretions, mucous membranes, and nonintact skin is likely. Wearing gloves is the most common protective measure used with Standard Precautions and Transmission-Based Precautions. Remember the following when using gloves:
  - o Outer surface of gloves is considered contaminated.
  - o Gloves are easier to put on when your hands are dry.
  - o Do not tear gloves when putting them on.
  - o Remove and discard torn, cut, or punctured gloves at once. Practice hand hygiene. Then put on a new pair.
  - o Apply a new pair for every person.
  - o Wear gloves once. Discard them after use.
  - o Put on clean gloves just before touching mucous membranes or nonintact skin.

- Put on new gloves whenever gloves become contaminated with blood, body fluids, secretions, or excretions. A task may require more than one pair of gloves.
- Change gloves whenever moving from a contaminated body site to a clean body site.
- Change gloves if interacting with the person involves touching portable computer keyboards or other mobile equipment that is transported from room to room.
- Put on gloves last when worn with other PPE.
- Make sure gloves cover your wrists. If you wear a gown, gloves cover the cuffs.
- Remove gloves so the inside part is on the outside. The inside is clean.
- Practice hand hygiene after removing gloves.

- Latex allergies are common and can cause skin rashes. Difficulty breathing and shock are more serious problems. Report skin rashes and breathing problems at once. If you or a resident has a latex allergy, wear latex-free gloves.

Personal Protective Equipment (PPE)

- The PPE needed—gloves, a gown, a mask, and goggles or a face shield—depends on the task, the procedures, care measures, and the type of Transmission-Based Precautions used. The nurse will tell you what equipment is needed.
- Gowns must completely cover you from your neck to mid-thigh or below. The gown front and sleeves are considered contaminated. A wet gown is contaminated. Gowns are used once. When removing a gown, roll it inside out into a bundle.
- Masks are disposable. A wet or moist mask is contaminated. When removing a mask, touch only the ties or elastic bands. The front of the mask is contaminated.
- The front of goggles or a face shield is contaminated. Use the device's ties, headband, or earpieces to remove the device.

Donning and Removing PPE

- According to the CDC, PPE is donned in the following order.
  - Gown
  - Mask or respirator
  - Eyewear (goggles or face shield)
  - Gloves
- Removing PPE (removed at the doorway before leaving the person's room):
  - *Method 1*
    1. Gloves
    2. Eyewear (goggles or face shield)
    3. Gown
    4. Mask or respirator (respirator is removed after leaving the person's room and closing the door)
    5. Wash hands or use an alcohol-based hand sanitizer immediately after removing all PPE
  - *Method 2*
    1. Gown and gloves
    2. Eyewear (goggles or face shield)
    3. Mask or respirator (respirator is removed after leaving the person's room and closing the door)
    4. Wash hands or use an alcohol-based hand sanitizer immediately after removing all PPE
- Review Figs. 18.6, 18.7, 18.8, and 18.9 (pp. 266, 267, 269–270, 271), Donning and Removing PPE, in the Textbook.
- Practice hand hygiene after removing PPE. Practice hand hygiene between steps if your hands become contaminated. Then practice hand hygiene again after removing all PPE.
- NOTE: Some state competency tests require hand hygiene after removing each PPE item. And some states use a different order for donning and removing PPE. Follow the procedures used in your state and agency.
- Some very severe and deadly infections require additional PPE and special training.

Bagging Items

- Contaminated items, linens, and trash are bagged to remove them from the person's room. Leakproof plastic bags are used. They have the *biohazard* symbol. Double-bagging is not needed unless the outside of the bag is wet, soiled, or may be contaminated.

Collecting Specimens

- Follow agency procedures to collect, store, and transport specimens (e.g., blood, body fluids, secretions, and excretions) when a person is on Transmission-Based Precautions. Specimens are transported to the laboratory in biohazard specimen bags.

CHAPTER 18 REVIEW QUESTIONS

Circle the BEST answer

1. What is the most common measure that would be used in caring for any person who needs Standard or Transmission-Based Precautions?
   a. Respiratory hygiene
   b. Using shoe covers
   c. Donning gloves
   d. Wearing a mask
2. When would the nursing assistant perform hand hygiene?
   a. After donning a gown.
   b. When the mask is contaminated.
   c. When the gown is contaminated.
   d. After removing PPE.
3. Which nursing assistant is using PPE correctly?
   a. Nursing assistant A removes PPE when it becomes contaminated.
   b. Nursing assistant B wears gloves during all encounters with patients.
   c. Nursing assistant C removes contaminated gloves in the nurses' station.
   d. Nursing assistant D wears PPE because her uniform has a stain.
4. When does the nursing assistant need to change gloves?
   a. When taking the dirty linen off the bed and then putting it in the laundry hamper.
   b. When emptying the bedpan and then flushing and cleaning the toilet.
   c. When giving perineal care and then the person asks to have feet cleaned.
   d. When helping a person brush the teeth and then she needs to rinse and spit.

5. In which circumstance would the nursing assistant anticipate the need to don a mask?
   a. Transporting a person on droplet precautions to the x-ray department
   b. Entering the room of a person on droplet precautions to assist with hygiene
   c. Entering the room of a person on contact precautions to deliver a meal tray
   d. Taking vital signs on a person who needs standard precautions

Answers to these questions are on p. 577.

CHAPTER 19 SAFE HANDLING AND POSITIONING

Principles of Body Mechanics

- The strongest and largest muscles are in the shoulders, upper arms, hips, and thighs. Use these muscles to lift and move persons and heavy objects.
- For good body mechanics:
  - Bend your knees and squat to lift a heavy object. Do not bend from your waist.
  - Hold items close to your body and base of support.
- Review Box 19.2 (p. 277), Rules for Body Mechanics, in the Textbook.

Work-Related Injuries

- **Musculoskeletal disorders (MSDs)** are injuries and disorders of the muscles, tendons, ligaments, joints, and cartilage.
- The Occupational Safety and Health Administration (OSHA) identifies MSD risk factors as:
  - Force: the amount of physical effort needed to perform a task.
  - Repeating action: doing the same motions or series of motions continually or frequently.
  - Awkward postures: assuming positions that place stress on the body.
  - Heavy lifting: manually lifting people who cannot lift themselves.
- According to the US Department of Labor, nursing assistants have high risk for MSDs.
- Always report a work-related injury as soon as possible. Early attention can help prevent the problem from becoming worse. Review Box 19.3 (p. 277), Guidelines for Safe Handling, in the Textbook.

Positioning the Person

- The person must be positioned correctly at all times. Regular position changes and good alignment promote comfort and well-being. Breathing is easier. Circulation is promoted. Pressure injuries and contractures are prevented.
- Whether in bed or in a chair, the person is repositioned at least every 2 hours. To safely position a person:
  - Use good body mechanics.
  - Ask a coworker to help you if needed.
  - Explain the procedure to the person.
  - Be gentle when moving the person.
  - Provide for privacy.
  - Use pillows as directed by the nurse for support and alignment.
  - Provide for comfort after positioning.
  - Place the call light within reach after positioning.
  - Complete a safety check before leaving the room.
- **Fowler's position** is a semi-sitting position. In **semi-Fowler's** position, the head of the bed is raised 30 degrees, but some agencies define semi-Fowler's position as raising the head of the bed 30 degrees and the knee portion 15 degrees. In **high Fowler's** position, the head of the bed is raised between 60 and 90 degrees.
- The **supine position (dorsal recumbent position)** is the back-lying position.
- In the **prone position**, the person lies on the abdomen with the head turned to one side.
- A person in the **lateral position (side-lying position)** lies on one side or the other.
- The **semi-prone side position** is a left side-lying position. The upper (right) leg is sharply flexed so it is not on the lower (left) leg. The lower (left) arm is behind the person.
- Persons who sit in chairs must hold their upper bodies and heads erect. For good alignment:
  - The person's back and buttocks are against the back of the chair.
  - Feet are flat on the floor or wheelchair footplates. Never leave feet unsupported.
  - Backs of the knees and calves are slightly away from the edge of the seat.

CHAPTER 19 REVIEW QUESTIONS

Circle the BEST answer

1. Which muscles would the nursing assistant use to lift and move residents and heavy objects?
   a. Muscles in the lower arms, hands, and fingers offer dexterity.
   b. Muscles in the lower legs and upper back are the most efficient.
   c. Muscles in the shoulders, upper arms, hips, and thighs are the strongest.
   d. Muscles in the chest, abdomen, and lower back are the largest.
2. Which nursing assistant is not using good body mechanics?
   a. Nursing assistant A bends knees and squats to lift a heavy object.
   b. Nursing assistant B bends over at waist to lift a heavy object.
   c. Nursing assistant C holds heavy items close to body and base of support.
   d. Nursing assistant D bends at hips and knees but does not bend back.
3. Which person is most likely to benefit from being placed in the Fowler's position?
   a. A person with a respiratory disorder who has difficulty breathing.
   b. A person who is comatose and has a contracture of the right forearm.
   c. A person who has fragile skin and is at risk for a pressure injury.
   d. A person who has a work-related musculoskeletal back injury.

4. How does the nursing assistant adjust the head of the bed to achieve a high Fowler's position?
   a. Raises to 30 degrees
   b. Raises between 30 and 45 degrees
   c. Raises between 45 and 60 degrees
   d. Raises between 60 and 90 degrees

Answers to these questions are on p. 577.

CHAPTER 20 MOVING THE PERSON

Preventing Work-Related Injuries

- Good body mechanics alone will not prevent injury. The Occupational Safety and Health Administration (OSHA) recommends
  - o Minimizing manual lifting in all cases.
  - o Eliminating manual lifting whenever possible.
- Careful planning is needed to move the person safely. You must know the person's physical abilities, the number of staff needed, what procedure to use, and the equipment needed.

Protecting the Skin

- Protect the person's skin from friction and shearing. Both cause infection and pressure injuries. To reduce friction and shearing:
  - o Use friction-reducing devices such as a turning sheet, turning pads, large, reusable waterproof underpads, and slide sheets.

Moving Persons in Bed

- Know how much help and what equipment or friction-reducing devices are needed.
- Review Box 20.1 (p. 288), Guidelines for Moving Persons in Bed, in the Textbook.

Raising the Person's Head and Shoulders

- You can raise the person's head and shoulders easily and safely by locking arms with the person (do not pull on the person's arm or shoulder).
- Have help with older persons and with those who are heavy or hard to move.

Moving the Person Up in Bed

- Two or more staff members are needed to move heavy, weak, and very old persons up in bed. Always protect the person and yourself from injury.

Moving the Person Up in Bed With an Assist Device

- Assist devices are used to reduce shearing and friction. Such assist devices include a drawsheet (flat sheet folded in half), turning pad, slide sheet, and large, reusable waterproof underpads.
- Assist devices are used to move most patients and residents, and at least two staff members are needed to position and use the assist device.
- Moving the person to the side of the bed. You (assistance from coworkers, as needed) move the person in segments by placing your hands and arms underneath the person. Move the upper body first (while supporting the person's neck), then the lower body, and finally the legs and feet.

Turning Persons

- Turning persons onto their sides helps prevent complications from bed rest. Procedures and care measures often require the side-lying position. After the person is turned, position them in good alignment. Use pillows as directed to support the person in the side-lying position.
- **Logrolling** is turning the person as a unit, in alignment, with one motion. The spine is kept straight.

Sitting on the Side of the Bed (Dangling)

- Many persons become dizzy or faint when getting out of bed too fast. They may need to sit on the side of the bed for 1 to 5 minutes before walking or transferring. Some persons increase activity in stages—bed rest, to dangling, to sitting in a chair, to walking.
- While dangling, the person coughs and deep breathes. Encourage the person to move the legs in circles to stimulate circulation.
- If dizziness or faintness occurs, lay the person down. Report this to the nurse.

Repositioning in a Chair or Wheelchair

- The person can slide down into the chair. For good alignment and safety, the person's back and buttocks must be against the back of the chair.
- Follow the nurse's directions and the care plan for the best way to reposition a person in a chair or wheelchair. Do not pull the person from behind the chair or wheelchair.
- If the chair reclines, have a coworker assist, recline the chair, put an assist device under the person, and use the assist device to move the person up.
- If the person is in a wheelchair and has strength to assist, lock the wheels of the wheelchair and move the footrests to the sides. Position a transfer belt around the person, stand in front of the person, block the person's knees with your knees, and grasp the transfer belt with both hands. Ask the person to push with their feet and arms on the count of 3 and move the person back into the wheelchair while the person pushes with their feet and arms.

CHAPTER 20 REVIEW QUESTIONS

Circle the BEST answer

1. Which care measure is the best to reduce friction and shearing while moving the person in bed?
   a. Use the bed controls to move the bed
   b. Ask the person to slide himself
   c. Link arms with person and pull him across
   d. Use a slide board or slide sheet

2. Which factors are used to determine the number of staff required to safely move a person?
   a. Person's height, weight, cognitive function, and physical abilities
   b. Person's age, health status, and desire for independence
   c. Person's strength in the extremities and ability to balance
   d. Person's medical diagnosis and willingness to cooperate
3. In which circumstance would the nursing assistant decide to logroll the person?
   a. Person gets dizzy when he first sits up to dangle.
   b. Person is recovering from spinal injury.
   c. Person can reach across grasp the siderail with coaching.
   d. Person needs limited assistance according to the care plan.

Answers to these questions are on p. 577.

CHAPTER 21 TRANSFERRING THE PERSON

- A transfer is how a person safely moves to and from a surface.
- The amount of help needed and the method used vary with the person's ability.

Wheelchair and Stretcher Safety

- Wheelchairs are used for persons who cannot walk or who have severe problems walking. Stretchers are used to transfer persons who are seriously ill, cannot sit up, or must stay in a lying position.
- Review Box 21.1 (p. 305), Wheelchair and Stretcher Safety, in the Textbook.

Stand and Pivot Transfers

- Some persons can stand and pivot (to turn one's body from a set standing position). Use this transfer if the person's legs are strong enough to bear weight and the person is cooperative and can follow directions and assist in the transfer.
- Transfer belts (gait belts) are used to support persons during transfers and to reposition persons in chairs and wheelchairs.

Chair or Wheelchair Transfers

- Arrange the room so there is enough space for a safe transfer. Correct placement of the chair, wheelchair, or other device also is needed for a safe transfer.
- Have the person wear slip-resistant footwear for transfers.
- Lock the wheels of the bed, wheelchair, stretcher, or other assist device.
- The person must not put their arms around your neck when assisting the person to stand.
- After the transfer, position the person in good alignment.
- For bed to chair or wheelchair transfers, the strong side moves first. Help the person out of bed on their strong side. When transferring the person from the chair or wheelchair back to bed, the same rules apply. Help the person from the wheelchair to the bed on their strong side. If the person is weak on one side, position the chair or wheelchair so that the person's strong side is nearest the bed. The strong side moves first.

Transferring To and From the Toilet

- Transferring the person to and from the toilet is often hard because bathrooms are small. If the wheelchair can fit in the bathroom, place it next to the toilet and use the stand and pivot transfer from the wheelchair to the toilet.

Lateral Transfers

- A lateral transfer moves a person between two horizontal surfaces, such as from a bed to a stretcher. The person slides from one surface to the other.
- Use friction-reducing devices to protect the skin from friction and shearing during lateral transfers.
- When moving a person from a bed to a stretcher, use a friction-reducing device and at least two or three staff members to assist. If the person weighs more than 200 lbs. (90.7 kg), a lateral transfer device, or a mechanical ceiling lift is used.
- Persons who cannot help themselves are transferred with mechanical lifts. So are persons who are too heavy for the staff to transfer.
- Before using a mechanical lift, you must be trained in its use. The sling, straps, hooks, and chains must be in good repair. The person's weight must not exceed the lift's capacity. At least two staff members are needed. Always follow the manufacturer's instructions for using the lift.
- Falling from the lift is a common fear. To promote the person's mental comfort, always explain the procedure before you begin. Also show the person how the lift works.

CHAPTER 21 REVIEW QUESTIONS

Circle the BEST answer

1. Which action would the nursing assistant use to transfer a person from the bed to a wheelchair?
   a. Help the person put on slip-resistant footwear after seated in the wheelchair.
   b. Encourage the person to put their arms around the assistant's neck to rise to a standing position.
   c. Apply a vest restraint and check it for a snug fit before helping the person to stand.
   d. Ensure that the wheels are locked on the bed and wheelchair before transferring the person.
2. Which action is correct for transferring from the bed to the wheelchair when the person has a weak left side and a strong right side?
   a. Place the wheelchair on the left side of bed before transfer
   b. Lower the weak side into the wheelchair first
   c. Get the person out of bed on the strong side
   d. Use the weak side for balance and the strong side for strength

3. When using a mechanical lift, what is an important safety feature to remember?
   a. The wheels of the lift should always be unlocked.
   b. Persons who are very thin are at risk to slip through the straps.
   c. In a narrow space, the lift is stable in a narrow position.
   d. Keep the base in the wide (open) position as much as possible.

Answers to these questions are on p. 577.

CHAPTER 22 BEDMAKING

- Clean, dry, and wrinkle-free linens promote comfort and help to prevent skin breakdown and pressure injuries.
- To keep beds neat and clean:
  - Change linens whenever they become wet, soiled, or damp.
  - Straighten linens whenever loose or wrinkled and at bedtime.
  - Check for and remove food and crumbs after meals and snacks.
  - Check linens for dentures, eyeglasses, hearing aids, sharp objects, and other items.
  - Follow Standard Precautions and the Bloodborne Pathogen Standard.

Types of Beds

- Beds are made in these ways.
  - A closed bed is not in use or the bed is ready for a new resident. Top linens are not folded back.
  - An open bed is in use. Top linens are fanfolded back so the person can get into bed. A closed bed becomes an open bed by fanfolding back the top linens.
  - An occupied bed is made with the person in it.
  - A surgical bed is made to transfer a person from a stretcher. This bed is also made for persons who arrive by ambulance.

Linens

- When handling linens and making beds:
  - Practice medical asepsis.
  - Always hold linens away from your body and uniform. Your uniform is considered dirty.
  - Never shake linens.
  - Place clean linens on a clean surface.
  - Never put clean or used linens on the floor.
- Collect enough linens. Do not bring unneeded linens to the person's room. Once in the room, extra linens are considered contaminated. They cannot be used for another person.
- Roll each piece of used linens away from you. The side that touched the person is inside the roll and away from you.

Making Beds

- When making beds, safety and medical asepsis are important. Use good body mechanics. Follow the rules for safe resident handling, moving, and transfers. Practice hand hygiene before handling clean linens and after handling used linens. To save time and energy, make beds with a coworker.
- Review Box 22.2 (p. 329), Bedmaking Guidelines, in the Textbook.
- Closed beds are made for nursing center residents who are up and away from the bed for all or most of the day. Change linens as needed. For beds awaiting new residents or patients, the entire bed requires clean linens after the bed system has been cleaned and disinfected.
- The closed bed becomes an open bed by fanfolding back the top linens so the person can get into bed with ease.
- An occupied bed is made while the person stays in bed. Keep the person in good alignment. Follow restrictions or limits in the person's movement or position. Explain each procedure step to the person before it is done. This is important even if the person cannot respond to you.

CHAPTER 22 REVIEW QUESTIONS

Circle the BEST answer

1. Which aspect of bedmaking is most likely to be of interest to a surveyor who is observing at a health-care facility?
   a. How nursing assistants make a mitered corner?
   b. How nursing assistants transport linens?
   c. How nursing assistants position the pillow on the bed?
   d. How nursing assistants center bed linen?
2. Which item would the nursing assistant obtain first when collecting a stack of linen to change a soiled bed?
   a. Bottom sheet
   b. Top sheet
   c. Pillowcase
   d. Mattress pad
3. Which action would the nursing assistant use when changing a soiled bed?
   a. Wear gloves when removing soiled linens from the bed
   b. Reach across bed and roll soiled linens toward body
   c. Gather soiled linens in a tight ball in the middle of the bed
   d. Pull soiled linens from bed directly into a laundry bag
4. Which action would the nursing assistant take to keep beds neat and clean?
   a. Encourage residents to leave their rooms after the beds are made.
   b. Check for and remove food and crumbs after meals.
   c. Ask the nurse if closed or open bed method is preferred.
   d. Change linens whenever the residents want them changed.

5. Which nursing assistant needs to be reminded about the bedmaking guidelines?
   a. Nursing assistant A practices medical asepsis when handling linens.
   b. Nursing assistant B holds linens away from her body and uniform.
   c. Nursing assistant C shakes linens to remove crumbs and food
   d. Nursing assistant D put soiled linens in the used laundry bin.

Answers to these questions are on p. 577.

CHAPTER 23 ORAL HYGIENE

Oral Hygiene

- Oral hygiene keeps the mouth and teeth clean. It prevents mouth odors and infections, increases comfort, and makes food taste better. Mouth care also reduces the risk for cavities and periodontal disease.
- Ask the person about their preferences for when and how often oral hygiene is performed. Follow the care plan.
- Follow Standard Precautions and the Bloodborne Pathogen Standard.

Brushing and Flossing Teeth

- Flossing removes plaque and tartar from the teeth as well as food from between the teeth.
- Flossing is recommended at least once a day and can be done when the person desires.
- You need to floss for persons who cannot do so themselves.
- Some persons need help gathering and setting up equipment for oral hygiene. Perform oral care for persons who are weak, cannot move their arms, or are too confused to brush their teeth.

Mouth Care for the Unconscious Person

- Unconscious persons have dry mouths and crusting on the tongue and mucous membranes. Oral hygiene keeps the mouth clean and moist. It also helps prevent infection.
- Use sponge swabs to apply the cleaning agent. To prevent cracking of the lips, apply a lubricant to the lips. Follow the care plan.
- To prevent aspiration for the unconscious person:
  - Position the person on their side with the head turned well to the side.
  - Use only a small amount of fluid to clean the mouth.
  - Do not insert dentures. Dentures are not worn when the person is unconscious.
- When giving oral hygiene, keep the person's mouth open with a bite block or a plastic tongue depressor.
- Mouth care is given at least every 2 hours. Follow the care plan.

Denture Care

- Mouth care is given and dentures are cleaned as often as natural teeth. Dentures are usually removed at bedtime. Some persons remove dentures at mealtime. Remind people not to wrap dentures in tissues or napkins at mealtime, as they could be discarded accidentally.
- Dentures are slippery when wet. Hold them firmly. During cleaning, hold them over a sink that is half-filled with water and lined with a towel. Use a cleaning agent and follow the manufacturer's instructions.
- Hot water causes dentures to lose their shape. If dentures are not worn after cleaning, store them in a container with cool water or a denture soaking solution.
- Label the denture cup with the person's name, room number, and bed number. Report lost or damaged dentures to the nurse at once. Losing or damaging dentures is negligent conduct.
- Many people do not like being seen without their dentures. Privacy is important. If you clean dentures, return them to the person as quickly as possible.
- Persons with partial dentures have some natural teeth. They need to brush and floss the natural teeth.

Reporting and Recording

- Dry, cracked, swollen, or blistered lips
- Mouth or breath odor
- Redness, swelling, irritation, sores, or white patches in the mouth or on the tongue
- Bleeding, swelling, or redness of the gums
- Loose teeth
- Rough, sharp, or chipped areas on dentures
- Loose-fitting dentures

CHAPTER 23 REVIEW QUESTIONS

Circle the BEST answer

1. When would the nursing assistant offer to help with oral hygiene for a person who lacks appetite and is eating less and less?
   a. At night, just before he goes to bed
   b. Before he goes to the dining room for meals
   c. In the morning as soon as he gets up
   d. After he has finished eating meals or snacks
2. Which information related to oral hygiene, would the nursing assistant report and record?
   a. Lips are dry, cracked, swollen, and blistered.
   b. Position and angle of the toothbrush preferred by patient.
   c. Amount of time spent on assisting the patient with hygiene.
   d. Number and location of fillings that the patient has.
3. Which nursing assistant needs a reminder about how to do mouth care for a person who is unconscious?
   a. Nursing assistant A uses a small amount of fluid to clean the mouth.
   b. Nursing assistant B uses her fingers to keep the person's mouth open.
   c. Nursing assistant C explains each step of care before proceeding.
   d. Nursing assistant D gives mouth care at least every 2 hours.

4. What is the rationale for cleaning dentures over a sink half-filled with water and lined with a towel?
   a. This action prevents breakage if they are accidentally dropped.
   b. Dentures fit more comfortably into the mouth if they are wet.
   c. Food particles, mucous and plaque must be scrubbed and rinsed off.
   d. Dentures will warp or loose shape if they are too dry.

Answers to these questions are on p. 577.

CHAPTER 24 DAILY HYGIENE AND BATHING

- Besides cleansing, good hygiene prevents body and breath odors. It is relaxing and increases circulation.
- Many factors affect daily hygiene needs—perspiration (sweating), elimination, vomiting, drainage from wounds or body openings, bed rest, and activity.

Daily Care

- Most people have hygiene routines and habits. Hygiene measures are often done before and after meals and at bedtime. You assist with hygiene whenever it is needed. Protect the person's right to privacy and to personal choice.

Bathing

- Bathing cleans the skin. The mucous membranes of the genital and anal areas are cleaned as well. A bath is refreshing and relaxing. Circulation is stimulated and body parts exercised. Talk to the person while assisting with hygiene and make observations.
- Review Box 24.2 (p. 359), Rules for Bathing, in the Textbook.
- Review Promoting Safety and Comfort: Bathing (p. 361) in the Textbook
- Soap dries the skin. Therefore older persons usually need a complete bath or shower twice a week. Partial baths are taken the other days. Some bathe daily but not with soap. Thorough rinsing is needed when using soap. Lotions and oils keep the skin soft.
- Water temperature for complete bed baths and partial bed baths is between 110°F and 115°F. Older persons have fragile skin and need lower water temperatures. Measure water temperature according to agency policy.
- Report and record:
  - o The color of the skin, lips, nail beds, and sclera (whites of the eyes)
  - o If the skin appears pale, grayish, yellow (jaundice), or bluish (cyanotic)
  - o The location and description of rashes
  - o Skin texture—smooth, rough, scaly, flaky, dry, moist
  - o Diaphoresis—profuse (excessive) sweating
  - o Bruises or open areas
  - o Pale or reddened areas, particularly over bony parts
  - o Drainage or bleeding from wounds or body openings
  - o Swelling of the feet and legs
  - o Corns or calluses on the feet
  - o Skin temperature
  - o Reports of pain or discomfort

The Complete Bed Bath

- The complete bed bath involves washing the person's entire body in bed. Wash around the person's eyes with water. Do not use soap. Gently wipe from the inner to the outer aspect of the eye. Use a clean part of the washcloth for each stroke. Ask the person if you should use soap to wash the face. Let the person wash the genital area if they is able.
- Give a back massage after the bath. Apply deodorant or antiperspirant, lotion, and powder as requested. Comb and brush the hair. Empty and clean the wash basin.

The Partial Bath

- The partial bath involves bathing the face, hands, axillae (underarms), back, buttocks, and perineal area. You assist the person as needed. Most need help washing the back.

Tub Baths and Showers

- Falls, burns, and chilling from water are risks. Review Box 24.2 (p. 359), Rules for Bathing, and Promoting Safety and Comfort: Tub Baths and Showers (p. 370), in the Textbook.
- A tub bath can cause a person to feel faint, weak, or tired. The person may need a bathing lift, a tub with a side entry door, or a mechanical lift to get in and out of the tub.
- Some people can use a regular shower. Have the person use the grab bars for support during the shower. Use a bath mat if the shower does not have slip-resistant surfaces. Never let weak or unsteady persons stand in the shower. They may need to use shower chairs, shower stalls or cabinets, or shower trolleys. Some shower rooms have two or more stations. Protect the person's privacy. Properly screen and cover the person.
- Water temperature for tub baths and showers is usually 105°F (40.5°C).
- Report and record dizziness and light-headedness.
- Clean and disinfect the tub or shower before and after use.

Perineal Care

- Perineal care involves cleaning the genital and anal areas. It is done daily during the bath and whenever the area is soiled with urine or feces. The person does perineal care if able.
- *Perineal* and *perineum* are not common terms. Most people understand *privates, private parts, crotch, genitals,* or *the area between the legs*. Use terms the person understands.
- Standard Precautions, medical asepsis, and the Bloodborne Pathogen Standard are followed.
- Work from clean to the dirty—commonly called cleaning from "front to back." On a female, clean from the urethra (cleanest) to the anal (dirtiest) area. On a male, start at the meatus of the urethra and work outward.

- Use warm water. Use washcloths, towelettes, cotton balls, or swabs according to agency policy. Rinse thoroughly. Pat dry. Water temperature is usually 105°F to 109°F.
- Report and record:
  - Bleeding, redness, swelling, irritation, discharge
  - Reports of pain, burning, or other discomfort
  - Signs of urinary or fecal incontinence
  - Signs of skin breakdown
  - Odors

CHAPTER 24 REVIEW QUESTIONS

Circle the BEST answer

1. In hospitals, what is the most common time for bathing?
   a. After breakfast
   b. Before going to bed
   c. After procedures
   d. Before being discharged
2. What is the water temperature for a complete bed bath?
   a. 102°F to 108°F (38.9°C–42.2°C)
   b. 110°F to 115°F (43.3°C–46.1°C)
   c. 115°F to 120°F (46.1°C–48.9°C)
   d. 120°F to 125°F (48.9°C–51.6°C)
3. What can happen if the nursing assistant is not careful when applying powder after a bath or shower to a person who has a respiratory disorder?
   a. Powder will worsen the dryness of the skin.
   b. Powder will cake when the person sweats.
   c. Powder could cause a skin rash with severe itching.
   d. Powder, if inhaled, could irritate the lungs and the airways.
4. Which nursing measure would the nursing assistant use when washing a person's eyes?
   a. Have the person rinse the eyes with cool water
   b. Avoid the eye area unless given specific instructions
   c. Gently wipe from the outer to the inner aspect of the eye
   d. Use a clean part of the washcloth for each stroke
5. Which action would the nursing assistant use when giving female perineal care?
   a. Cleanse the anal area first with a paper towel
   b. Cleanse from the urethra to the anal area
   c. Have the person soak in tub of warm water
   d. Coach the person as she performs self-care
6. Which action would the nursing assistant use when giving male perineal care?
   a. Use the bag bath method
   b. Ask the person to retract the foreskin
   c. Start at the meatus and work outward
   d. Clean the scrotum first; it is cleaner than the penis

Answers to these questions are on p. 577.

CHAPTER 25 GROOMING

- Hair care, shaving, and nail and foot care prevent infection and promote comfort.

Hair Care

- You assist patients and residents with brushing and combing hair and with shampooing as needed and according to the care plan.

Brushing and Combing Hair

- Encourage residents to brush and comb their own hair but assist as needed.
- Daily brushing and combing prevent tangled and matted hair.
- When brushing and combing hair, start at the scalp and brush or comb to the hair ends.
- Never cut hair for any reason.
- Special measures are needed for curly, coarse, and dry hair. Check the care plan.
- When giving hair care, place a towel across the person's back and shoulders to protect garments from falling hair. If the person is in bed, give hair care before changing the linens and pillowcase.

Shampooing

- Shampooing frequency depends on the person's needs and preferences.
- Keep shampoo away from and out of eyes. Have the person hold a washcloth over the eyes.
- Wear gloves if the person has scalp sores, nits, lice, or other hair or scalp problems.
- Follow Standard Precautions and the Bloodborne Pathogen Standard.
- Water temperature is usually 105°F.
- Hair is dried and styled as soon as possible after the shampooing.
- During shampooing, report and record:
  - Scalp sores
  - Flaking
  - Itching
  - Presence of nits or lice
  - Hair falling out in patches; patches of hair loss
  - Very dry or very oily hair
  - Matted or tangled hair
  - How the person tolerated the procedure

Shaving

- Shaving is common for facial hair, underarms, and legs.
- Electric shaver or safety razors are used. Some persons have their own shavers. Do not use safety razors on persons with healing problems or persons taking anticoagulant drugs. Older persons with wrinkled skin are at risk for nicks and cuts. Safety razors are not used to shave them or persons with dementia.
- Wash and comb mustaches and beards daily and as needed. Ask the person how to groom his mustache or beard. Never shave or trim a mustache or a beard.
- Many women shave their legs and underarms. This practice varies among cultures. Legs and underarms are shaved after bathing when the skin is soft.
- Review Box 25.1 (p. 388), Rules for Shaving, in the Textbook.

Nail and Foot Care

- Nail and foot care prevent infection, injury, and odors.
- Nails are easier to trim and clean right after soaking or bathing.
- Use nail clippers to cut fingernails. Never use scissors. Use extreme caution to prevent damage to nearby tissues.
- Some agencies do not let nursing assistants cut or trim toenails. Follow agency policy.
- Follow Standard Precautions and the Bloodborne Pathogen Standard.
- Report and record:
  - o Dry, reddened, irritated, or callused areas
  - o Breaks in the skin
  - o Corns on top of and between the toes
  - o Blisters
  - o Very thick nails
  - o Loose nails
- You do not cut or trim toenails if a person has diabetes or poor circulation to the legs and feet or takes drugs that affect blood clotting. Also, do not cut or trim toenails if the person has nail fungus, very thick nails, or ingrown toenails. The nurse or podiatrist cuts toenails and provides foot care for these persons.
- When doing foot care, check between the toes for cracks and sores. If left untreated, a serious infection could occur.
- The feet of persons with decreased sensation or circulatory problems may easily burn because they do not feel hot temperatures.
- After soaking, apply lotion to the feet. Because the lotion can cause slippery feet, help the person put on slip-resistant footwear before you transfer the person or let the person walk.

CHAPTER 25 REVIEW QUESTIONS

Circle the BEST answer

1. Which aspect of grooming is a surveyor most likely to observe for?
   a. Personal grooming supplies are stored in the bathroom.
   b. Female residents are wearing nail polish.
   c. Shared items, such as nail clippers, are stored in the proper place.
   d. Residents have their hair combed and styled.
2. What should the nursing assistant do if a person's hair is matted and tangled?
   a. Shampoo the hair first and then use a wide-tooth comb
   b. Get the nurse's permission to cut the hair at the tangled area
   c. Brush through the matting and tangling from the hair ends to the scalp
   d. Wet the hair, apply conditioner, and wait for the hair shaft to soften
3. Which instruction is the nurse most likely to give when the nursing assistant reports observing small white oval shapes and tan-colored insects that are about the size of a sesame seed in the person's hair?
   a. Wash the person's hair twice and use generous amounts of shampoo
   b. Always wear gloves whenever performing any care for the person
   c. Report to the employee health clinic for exposure to infection
   d. Wash combs, hair brushes, and hairclips in hot water
4. When should the nursing assistant wear gloves for shampooing a person's hair?
   a. The person has oily hair.
   b. The person has sores on the scalp.
   c. The person likes a long scalp massage.
   d. The person has very thin hair.
5. Which adverse outcome could occur, when a new and inexperienced nursing assistant uses a blade razor to shave a person who is taking an anticoagulant medication?
   a. The hair is brittle and breaks under the razor blade.
   b. The skin is fragile and easily torn during shaving.
   c. Shaving will be uncomfortable, because the hair is coarse.
   d. A nick or a cut could cause serious bleeding.
6. Which action would the nursing assistant perform before beginning to shave facial hair with a safety razor?
   a. Brush out the whiskers and hair
   b. Gently rub the face with a towel
   c. Apply lotion or aftershave
   d. Apply a warm moist towel
7. Which nursing assistant needs a reminder about the rules and guidelines for grooming?
   a. Nursing assistant A uses scissors to trim the fingernails and toenails.
   b. Nursing assistant B brushes out tangles before shampooing the hair.
   c. Nursing assistant C stores the person's eyeglasses before combing hair.
   d. Nursing assistant D reports to the nurse that the person has corn on the toe.
8. What is included in the daily care of mustaches and beards?
   a. Clipping
   b. Combing
   c. Trimming
   d. Shaving
9. For a person who has diabetes, which aspect of grooming is not part of a nursing assistant duties?
   a. Trimming the toenails
   b. Shampooing the hair
   c. Assisting with shaving
   d. Styling the hair
10. Which piece of equipment is used to trim a person's fingernails?
    a. Scissors
    b. Nail clippers
    c. An emery board
    d. A nail file

Answers to these questions are on p. 577.

CHAPTER 26 CHANGING GARMENTS

Changing Garments

- Garments are changed after the bath and whenever wet or soiled or on admission or discharge.
- To assist with dressing and undressing, you need this information from the nurse and the care plan.
  - o How much help the person needs
  - o Which side is the person's unaffected side (strong side)
  - o If certain garments are needed
- What observations to report and record:
  - o How much help was given
  - o How the person tolerated the procedure
  - o Comments or concerns by the person
  - o Changes in the person's behavior
  - o When to report observations
  - o What patient or resident concerns to report at once
- When changing clothing:
  - o Provide for privacy. Do not expose the person.
  - o Encourage the person to do as much as possible.
  - o Let the person choose what to wear. Make sure the right undergarments are chosen.
  - o Make sure garments and footwear are the correct size.
  - o Remove clothing from the strong (unaffected) side first.
  - o Put clothing on the weak (affected) side first.
  - o Support the arm or leg when removing or putting on a garment.
  - o Move or handle the body gently. Do not force a joint beyond its range of motion or to the point of pain.
- When changing gowns, remove the gown from the strong arm first while supporting the weak arm. Put a clean gown on the weak arm first and then the strong arm.
- To change the gown of a person with an intravenous (IV) bag, gather the sleeve of the arm with the IV bag and slide it over the IV site and tubing. Remove the IV bag, draw it through the sleeve, and rehang the IV bag. Gather the sleeve of the clean gown, remove the IV bag, slide the sleeve over the IV bag, and then rehang the bag. Slide the sleeve over the tubing, hand, arm, and IV site. Do not pull on the tubing.
- Have the nurse check the flow rate after changing the gown of a person with an IV. If the person is on an IV pump, do not change the gown; ask the nurse for instructions.

CHAPTER 26 REVIEW QUESTIONS

Circle the BEST answer

1. Which nursing assistant needs a reminder about assisting residents to dress and undress?
   a. Nursing assistant A provides privacy when residents are changing clothes.
   b. Nursing assistant B helps residents to don street clothes for the day.
   c. Nursing assistant C encourages the residents to choose what to wear.
   d. Nursing assistant D stretches the residents' clothes so they are easier to put on.
2. Which action would be the best to use in assisting a person with Alzheimer disease to get dressed?
   a. Assist him to dress at the same time every day
   b. Ask him what he would like to wear
   c. Assist him to find his long johns
   d. Give him a button hook dressing aid
3. What is the primary purpose of labeling residents' clothing and shoes on the inside?
   a. To ensure that residents are wearing their own clothes
   b. To help confused residents recognize their items
   c. To respect and preserve dignity of residents
   d. To prevent theft of residents' personal items
4. Which action would you take when assisting a person who is lying in bed to remove his pants but he is unable to lift his hips and buttocks?
   a. Ask a coworker to lift him up
   b. Tug on his pants one side at a time
   c. Assist him to stand up
   d. Turn him toward you
5. Which nursing assistant has performed the correct action while changing the gown of a person who has an IV?
   a. Nursing assistant A turns the IV pump off to thread the tubing through the sleeve.
   b. Nursing assistant B places the IV bag on the bed while assisting the patient with the gown.
   c. Nursing assistant C asks the nurse to check the IV flow rate after the gown is changed.
   d. Nursing assistant D cuts off the standard gown and obtains a clean gown with snap fasteners.

Answers to these questions are on p. 577.

CHAPTER 27 URINARY NEEDS

Normal Urination

- The healthy adult produces about 1500 mL of urine a day.
- The frequency of urination is affected by amount of fluid intake, habits, availability of toilet facilities, activity, work, and illness. People usually void at bedtime, after sleep, and before meals. Some people void every 2 to 3 hours. The need to void at night disturbs sleep. Some persons need help getting to the bathroom and others use bedpans, urinals, or commodes. Review Box 27.1 (p. 411), Rules for Normal Urination, in the Textbook.

Observations

- Observe urine for color, clarity, odor, amount, particles, and blood. Normal urine is pale yellow, straw colored, or amber. It is clear with no particles. A faint odor is normal.
- Some foods and drugs affect urine color. Ask the nurse to observe urine that looks or smells abnormal.
- Report the following urinary problems.
  - o **Dysuria**—painful or difficult urination
  - o **Enuresis**—involuntary loss or leakage of urine during sleep: bedwetting
  - o **Hematuria**—blood in the urine
  - o **Nocturia**—frequent urination at night

- **Oliguria**—scant amount of urine; less than 500 mL in 24 hours
- **Polyuria**—abnormally large amounts of urine
- **Urinary frequency**—voiding at frequent intervals
- **Urinary retention**—not being able to completely empty the bladder
- **Urinary incontinence**—involuntary loss or leakage of urine
- **Urinary urgency**—the need to void at once

Assisting with a Bedpan, Urinal, or Commode

- Follow Standard Precautions and the Bloodborne Pathogen Standard when handling bedpans, urinals, commodes, and their contents.
- Bedpans are used when the person cannot be out of bed.
- Urinals for men or women can be used standing, sitting, or lying down (supine or lateral position). Female urinals are shaped to fit snugly under the urethra. See Delegation Guidelines: Urinals (p. 416) in the Textbook. Remind people not to place urinals on over-bed tables and bedside stands.
- Commodes are chairs or wheelchairs with an opening for a container. Persons unable to walk to the bathroom often use commodes. See Delegation Guidelines: Commodes (p. 418) in the Textbook.
- Thoroughly clean and disinfect bedpans, urinals, and commodes after use.

Urinary Incontinence

- **Urinary incontinence** is the involuntary loss or leakage of urine.
- If urinary incontinence is a new problem, tell the nurse at once.
- Incontinence is embarrassing. Garments are wet and odors develop. Skin irritation, infection, and pressure injuries are risks. The person's pride, dignity, and self-esteem are affected. Social isolation, loss of independence, and depression are common.
- Good skin care and dry garments and clean linens are essential. Promoting normal urinary elimination prevents incontinence in some people. Other people may need bladder training.
- Review Box 27.3 (p. 421), Urinary Incontinence: Nursing Measures, in the Textbook.
- Caring for persons with incontinence is stressful. Remember, the person does not choose to be incontinent. If you find yourself becoming short tempered and impatient, talk to the nurse at once. Kindness, empathy, understanding, and patience are needed.

Applying Incontinence Products

- Incontinence products are used to keep the person dry. Most are disposable and only used once.
- Incontinence products include a complete incontinence brief, a pad and undergarment, pull-on underwear, or a belted undergarment. Follow the manufacturer's instructions for applying incontinence products.
- Observations to report and record:
  - Reports of pain, burning, irritation, or the need to void
  - Signs and symptoms of skin breakdown, including redness, irritation, blisters, and reports of pain, burning, itching, or tingling
  - The amount of urine and urine color
  - Blood in the urine
  - Leakage or a poor product fit
- Review Box 27.4 (p. 424), Applying Incontinence Products, in the Textbook.

Bladder Training

- Bladder training helps some persons with urinary incontinence. Control of urination is the goal. Bladder control promotes comfort and quality of life. It also increases self-esteem.
- You assist with bladder training as directed by the nurse and the care plan. The care plan may include one of the following: bladder rehabilitation, prompted voiding, habit training/scheduled voiding, or catheter clamping.

CHAPTER 27 REVIEW QUESTIONS

Circle the BEST answer

1. Which observation is abnormal and needs to be reported to the nurse?
   a. Urine is straw colored.
   b. Urine is a pale yellow color.
   c. Urine is an amber color.
   d. Urine is a bright red color.
2. Which observation needs to be promptly reported to the nurse?
   a. Person is having new onset of urinary urgency.
   b. Person has been assisted to the commode three times.
   c. Person needs a larger size of incontinence underwear.
   d. Person voided a large amount of yellow urine after lunch.
3. Which liquid may contribute to bladder irritation and temporary incontinence?
   a. Water
   b. Low-fat milk
   c. Coffee
   d. Apple juice
4. Which person is demonstrating functional incontinence?
   a. Confused person cannot find the bathroom.
   b. Older woman passes urine when she sneezes.
   c. Older man has dribbling and a weak stream.
   d. Person is being treated for a urinary tract infection.
5. What is the goal of bladder training?
   a. To allow the person to use the toilet
   b. To improve perineal hygiene
   c. To gain control of urination
   d. To decrease dependence on staff

Answers to these questions are on p. 577.

CHAPTER 28 URINARY CATHETERS

- A catheter is a tube used to drain or inject fluid through a body opening. A urinary catheter is inserted through the urethra into the bladder and is used to drain urine.
- The types of catheters are a **straight catheter**, which is used to drain the urine and then removed, and an **indwelling catheter (retention or Foley catheter)**, which is left in the bladder and drains urine constantly into a drainage bag. A **suprapubic catheter** is surgically inserted into the bladder through an incision above (supra) the pubis bone (pubic).

Catheter Care

- The risk of a urinary tract infection (UTI) is high. Review Box 28.1 (p. 433), Indwelling Catheter Care, in the Textbook.
- The catheter must not pull at the insertion site. Hold the catheter securely during catheter care. Then properly secure the catheter. Also make sure the tubing is not under the person. Besides obstructing urine flow, lying on the tubing is uncomfortable. It can also cause skin breakdown.
- Follow Standard Precautions and the Bloodborne Pathogen Standard.
- Report and record:
  - o Reports of pain, burning, irritation, or the need to void (report at once)
  - o Crusting, abnormal drainage, or secretions
  - o The color, clarity, and odor of urine
  - o Particles in the urine
  - o Blood in the urine
  - o Cloudy urine
  - o Urine leaking at the insertion site
  - o Drainage system leaks

Urine Drainage Systems

- A closed urinary drainage system is used for indwelling catheters. Infections can occur if microbes enter the drainage system. The two types of drainage bags are standard drainage bags and leg bags.
- The standard drainage bag hangs from the bed frame, chair, or wheelchair. It must not touch the floor. The bag is always kept lower than the person's bladder. Do not hang the drainage bag on a bed rail.
- If the drainage system is disconnected accidentally, tell the nurse at once. Do not touch the ends of the catheter or tubing. Do the following:
  - o Practice hand hygiene. Put on gloves.
  - o Wipe the end of the drainage tube with an antiseptic wipe.
  - o Wipe the end of the catheter with another antiseptic wipe.
  - o Do not put the ends down. Do not touch the ends after you clean them.
  - o Connect the drainage tubing to the catheter.
  - o Discard the wipes into a biohazard bag.
  - o Remove the gloves. Practice hand hygiene.
- Check with the nurse and care plan about when to empty and measure the urine in the drainage bag. Follow Standard Precautions and the Bloodborne Pathogen Standard.
- A leg bag is a drainage system that attaches to the thigh or calf. Empty and measure a leg bag when it is half full.
- Report and record:
  - o The amount of urine measured
  - o The color, clarity, and odor of urine
  - o Particles in the urine
  - o Blood in the urine
  - o Cloudy urine
  - o Reports of pain, burning, irritation, or the need to urinate
  - o Drainage system leaks

Removing Indwelling Catheters

- Before removing an indwelling catheter, be sure that your state allows you to perform this procedure, the procedure is in your job description, you know how to use the supplies and equipment, and you review the procedure with the nurse.
- The balloon of an indwelling catheter is inflated with water injected with a syringe. A syringe is also used to remove the water. Before removing the indwelling catheter, learn the size of the balloon before deflating it. If the balloon is 5 mL in size, you must withdraw 5 mL of water with the syringe. Do not remove the catheter if water remains in the balloon. Call the nurse.
- Report and record the following observations:
  - o The amount of urine in the drainage bag
  - o The color, clarity, and odor of urine
  - o Particles in the urine
  - o Blood in the urine
  - o How the person tolerated the procedure
  - o Reports of pain, burning, irritation, or the need to void

Condom Catheters

- Condom catheters are often used for incontinent men. They are also called external catheters, Texas catheters, and urinary sheaths.
- These catheters are changed daily after perineal care.
- To apply a condom catheter, follow the manufacturer's instructions. Thoroughly wash and dry the penis before applying the catheter.
- Some condom catheters are self-adhering. Other catheters are secured in place with elastic tape in a spiral manner. Never use adhesive tape to secure catheters. It does not expand. Blood flow to the penis is cut off, injuring the penis.
- When removing or applying a condom catheter, report and record the following observations:
  - o Reddened or open areas on the penis
  - o Swelling of the penis
  - o Color, clarity, and odor of urine
  - o Particles in the urine
  - o Blood in the urine
  - o Cloudy urine
- Do not apply a condom catheter if the penis is red, is irritated, or shows signs of skin breakdown. Report your observations to the nurse at once.

CHAPTER 28 REVIEW QUESTIONS

Circle the BEST answer

1. Which nursing assistant is correctly managing the urinary drainage system?
   a. Nursing assistant A places the bag on the floor under the person's bed.
   b. Nursing assistant B places the drainage bag on the bed during a stretcher transfer.
   c. Nursing assistant C places the bag on the person's lap while the wheelchair is moving.
   d. Nursing assistant D keeps the drainage bag lower than the person's bladder.
2. Which action would the nursing assistant take if the urinary drainage system accidentally becomes disconnected?
   a. Call the nurse right away
   b. Use antiseptic wipes to clean the ends of the tubing
   c. Put on gloves and clamp the tubing
   d. Put the ends of the tubing on paper towels
3. Which action would the nursing assistant use before removing an indwelling catheter?
   a. Gently tug to see if the catheter will come out
   b. Wipe the meatus and catheter with an antiseptic wipe
   c. Remove the water from balloon with a syringe
   d. Use a syringe and inflate balloon with 10 mL of air
4. How often are condom catheters changed?
   a. Condom catheters are changed daily.
   b. Condom catheters are changed at the end of each shift.
   c. Whenever the tape becomes loose.
   d. When the penis is sore or red.

Answers to these questions are on p. 577.

CHAPTER 29 BOWEL NEEDS

Normal Bowel Elimination

- Bowel movements (BMs) vary from person to person—daily, two to three times a day, every 2 to 3 days. Time of day also varies.
- Carefully observe stools before disposing of them. Observe and report the color, amount, consistency, odor, and shape of stools. Also observe and report the presence of blood or mucus, the time the person had the BM, the frequency of BMs, and any reports of pain or discomfort.

Factors Affecting Bowel Elimination

- *Privacy*. Bowel elimination is a private act.
- *Habits*. Many people have a BM after breakfast. Some read. Defecation is easier when a person is relaxed.
- *Diet—high-fiber foods*. Fiber helps prevent constipation.
- *Diet—other foods*. Some foods cause constipation. Other foods cause frequent stools or diarrhea.
- *Fluids*. Drinking six to eight glasses of water daily promotes normal bowel elimination. Warm fluids—coffee, tea, hot cider, warm water—increase peristalsis.
- *Activity*. Exercise and activity maintain muscle tone and stimulate peristalsis.
- *Drugs*. Drugs can prevent constipation or control diarrhea. Some have diarrhea or constipation as side effects.
- *Disability*. Some people cannot control BMs. A bowel training program is needed.
- *Aging*. Older persons are at risk for constipation. Some older persons lose bowel control and have fecal incontinence.
- To provide comfort and safety during bowel elimination, review Box 29.1 (p. 452), Safety and Comfort—Bowel Needs, in the Textbook. Follow Standard Precautions and the Bloodborne Pathogen Standard.

Common Problems

- Common problems include constipation, fecal impaction, diarrhea, fecal incontinence, and flatulence.
- **Constipation** is the passage of a hard, dry stool.
- Common causes of constipation are a low-fiber diet and ignoring the urge to defecate. Other causes include decreased fluid intake, inactivity, drugs, aging, and certain diseases.
- Dietary changes, fluids, and activity prevent or relieve constipation. So do stool softeners, laxatives, suppositories, and enemas.
- A **fecal impaction** is the prolonged retention and buildup of feces in the rectum.
- Fecal impaction results if constipation is not relieved. The person cannot defecate. Liquid feces pass around the hardened fecal mass in the rectum. The liquid feces seep from the anus.
- Signs and symptoms of fecal impaction include: abdominal discomfort, abdominal distention, nausea, cramping, and rectal pain. Older persons have poor appetite or confusion. Some persons have a fever. Report these signs and symptoms to the nurse.
- Checking for and removing a fecal impaction can be dangerous, because the vagus nerve can be stimulated, resulting in a slowing of the heart rate. Check with your state and agency policies to determine if you may perform this procedure.
- **Diarrhea** is the frequent passage of liquid stools.
- The need to have a BM is urgent. Some people cannot get to a bathroom in time. Abdominal cramping, nausea, and vomiting may occur.
- Assist with elimination needs promptly, dispose of stools promptly, and give good skin care. Liquid stools irritate the skin. So does frequent wiping with toilet paper. Skin breakdown and pressure injuries are risks.
- Follow Standard Precautions and the Bloodborne Pathogen Standard when in contact with stools.
- Report signs of diarrhea at once. Ask the nurse to observe the stool.
- **Fecal incontinence** is the inability to control the passage of feces and gas through the anus.
- Fecal incontinence affects the person emotionally. Frustration, embarrassment, anger, and humiliation are common. The person may need:
  - Bowel training
  - Help with elimination after meals and every 2 to 3 hours
  - Incontinence products to keep garments and linens clean
  - Good skin care

- **Flatulence** is the excessive formation of gas or air in the stomach and intestines.
- Causes include swallowing air while eating and drinking and bacterial action in the intestines. Other causes may be gas-forming foods, constipation, bowel and abdominal surgeries, and drugs that decrease peristalsis.
- If flatus is not expelled, the intestines distend (swell or enlarge from the pressure of gases). Abdominal cramping or pain, shortness of breath, and a swollen abdomen occur. "Bloating" is a common complaint. Exercise, walking, moving in bed, and the left side–lying position often produce flatus. Enemas and drugs may be ordered.

Bowel Training

- Bowel training has two goals.
  - To gain control of BMs.
  - To develop a regular pattern of elimination. Fecal impactions, constipation, and fecal incontinence are prevented.
- Factors that promote elimination are part of the care plan and bowel training program.

Suppositories

- A suppository is a cone-shaped, solid drug that is inserted into a body opening. A rectal suppository is inserted into the rectum. Suppositories melt at body temperature.
- A BM occurs about 30 minutes after inserting a suppository.
- Check with your state and agency policies to determine if you can insert a suppository.

Enemas

- An **enema** is the introduction of fluid into the rectum and lower colon.
- Doctors order enemas to:
  - Remove feces.
  - Relieve constipation, fecal impaction, or flatulence.
  - Clean the bowel of feces before certain surgeries and diagnostic procedures.
- Review Box 29.2 (p. 455), Giving Enemas, in the Textbook.
- The preferred position for an enema is the left side–lying position.
- A cleansing enema is used to clean the bowel of feces and flatus and to relieve constipation and fecal impaction. Cleansing enemas take effect in 10 to 20 minutes.
- A small-volume enema irritates the bowel and distends the rectum, causing a BM. The person should retain the enema solution until they need to have a BM, which usually takes 1 to 5 minutes or as long as 10 minutes.
- An oil-retention enema relieves constipation and fecal impaction by softening the feces and lubricating the rectum so the feces can pass. The oil is retained for 30 minutes to 1 to 3 hours.

The Person With an Ostomy

- Sometimes part of the intestines is removed surgically. An ostomy is sometimes necessary. An **ostomy** is a surgically created opening for the elimination of body wastes. The opening is called a **stoma**. The person wears an ostomy pouch over the stoma to collect stools and flatus.
- Stools irritate the skin. Skin care prevents skin breakdown around the stoma. The skin is washed and dried. Then a skin barrier is applied around the stoma. It prevents stools from having contact with the skin. The skin barrier is part of the ostomy pouch or a separate device.
- The pouch has an adhesive backing that is applied to the skin. Sometimes pouches are secured to ostomy belts.
- The pouch is changed every 3 to 7 days and when it leaks. Frequent pouch changes can damage the skin.
- An ostomy pouch is emptied when it is about one-third (1/3) to one-half (1/2) full with feces or gas. Depending on the person, ostomy type, and ostomy location, pouches are usually emptied two to six times a day. Many pouches have a drain at the bottom that closes with a clip, clamp, or wire closure. The drain is opened to empty the pouch. The drain is wiped with toilet tissue before it is closed.
- Observations to report and record include signs of skin breakdown, color, amount, consistency, and odor of stools, and reports of pain or discomfort.

CHAPTER 29 REVIEW QUESTIONS

Circle the BEST answer

1. Which habit is most likely to contribute to constipation?
   a. Eats whole grain cereal and fruit for breakfast
   b. Spends most of the day sitting in a chair
   c. Drinks six to eight glasses of water daily.
   d. Has two cups of coffee in the morning
2. Which food is gas forming and will therefore stimulate peristalsis?
   a. Biscuit
   b. Cottage cheese
   c. Chocolate
   d. Cabbage
3. How often should the nursing assistant help a person who has fecal incontinence to go to the bathroom?
   a. Whenever you have extra time
   b. After meals and every 2 to 3 hours
   c. In the morning and at bedtime
   d. Every 30 minutes while awake
4. What is the preferred position for an enema?
   a. Left side–lying position
   b. Prone position
   c. Supine position
   d. Trendelenburg's position

Answers to these questions are on p. 577.

CHAPTER 30 NUTRITION

- A poor diet and poor eating habits:
  - Increase the risk for disease and infection.
  - Cause chronic illnesses to become worse.

- o Cause healing problems.
- o Increase the risk of accidents and injuries.

Basic Nutrition

- **Nutrition** is the process involved in the ingestion, digestion, absorption, and use of foods and fluids by the body. Good nutrition is needed for growth, healing, and body functions.
- A *nutrient* is a substance that is ingested, digested, absorbed, and used by the body.
- A *calorie* is the fuel or energy value of food.

Dietary Guidelines for Americans

- The Dietary Guidelines help people attain and maintain a healthy weight, reduce the risk of chronic disease, and promote overall health. The Dietary Guidelines focus on consuming fewer calories, making informed food choices, and being physically active.

MyPlate

- The MyPlate symbol, issued by the US Department of Agriculture, helps you make wise food choices by balancing calories, increasing certain foods such as fruits and vegetables, and reducing certain foods with excess salt and sugar.

Nutrients

- A well-balanced diet ensures an adequate intake of essential nutrients.
- *Protein*—is needed for tissue growth and repair. Sources include meat, fish, poultry, eggs, milk and milk products, cereals, beans, peas, and nuts.
- *Carbohydrates*—provide energy and fiber for bowel elimination. They are found in fruits, vegetables, breads, cereals, and sugar.
- *Fats*—provide energy, add flavor to food, and help the body use certain vitamins. Sources of healthy fats include salmon, avocados, and olive oil. Unhealthy fats usually come from animal sources (meats and dairy foods).
- *Vitamins*—are needed for certain body functions. The body stores vitamins A, D, E, and K. The vitamin C and the B complex vitamins are not stored and must be ingested daily.
- *Minerals*—are needed for bone and tooth formation, nerve and muscle function, fluid balance, and other body processes.
- *Water*—is needed for all body processes.
- Review Tables 30.2 (p. 471), Common Vitamins, and 30.3 (p. 471), Common Minerals, in the Textbook.

Special Diets

The Sodium-Controlled Diet

- A sodium-controlled diet decreases the amount of sodium in the body. The diet involves:
  - o Omitting high-sodium foods. Review Box 30.1 (p. 475), High-Sodium Foods, in the Textbook.
  - o Not adding salt when eating.
  - o Limiting the amount of salt used in cooking.
  - o Diet planning.

Diabetes Meal Planning

- Diabetes meal planning is for people with diabetes. It involves the person's food preferences and calories needed. It also involves eating meals and snacks at regular times.
- Serve the person's meals and snacks on time to maintain a certain blood sugar level.
- Always check the tray to see what was eaten. Tell the nurse what the person did and did not eat. If not all the food was eaten, a between-meal nourishment is needed. The nurse tells you what to give. Tell the nurse about changes in the person's eating habits.

The Dysphagia Diet

- **Dysphagia** means difficulty swallowing. Food thickness is changed to meet the person's needs.

Food Intake

- Food intake is measured in different ways. Follow agency policy for the method use.
- *Percentage of food eaten*. Some agencies measure the percent of the whole meal tray. Other agencies measure the percent of each food item eaten.
- *Calorie counts*. Note what the person ate and how much. A nurse or dietitian converts the portion amounts into calories.

CHAPTER 30 REVIEW QUESTIONS

Circle the BEST answer

1. Which snack would be best for a person who is on a sodium-controlled diet?
   a. Apple slices and plain almonds
   b. Biscuit and peanut butter
   c. Pretzels and tomato juice
   d. Cheese and crackers
2. Which item needs to be taken off the tray when a person is on a clear liquid diet?
   a. Gelatin
   b. Iced-tea
   c. Broth
   d. Milk
3. Which food needs to be removed from the tray if the person is on a bland diet?
   a. Chicken breast
   b. Plain rice
   c. White bread
   d. French fries
4. Which mineral would be important for persons with anemia, those who have sustained a blood loss or women during the reproductive years?
   a. Iron
   b. Calcium
   c. Potassium
   d. Magnesium

Answers to these questions are on p. 577.

CHAPTER 31 MEETING NUTRITION NEEDS

Factors Affecting Eating and Nutrition

- *Culture*. Culture influences dietary practices, food choices, and food preparation.
- *Religion*. Selecting, preparing, and eating food often involves religious practices. A person may follow all, some, or none of the dietary practices of their faith.
- *Finances*. People with limited incomes often buy cheaper carbohydrate foods. Their diets often lack protein and certain vitamins and minerals.
- *Appetite*. Illness, drugs, anxiety, pain, and depression can cause loss of appetite ***(anorexia)***. Unpleasant sights, thoughts, and smells are other causes.
- *Personal choice*. Food likes and dislikes are influenced by foods served in the home. Food preferences tend to expand with age and social experiences.
- *Body reactions*. Foods that cause allergic reactions, such as a rash, swelling, or itching, are usually avoided. Some reactions are life threatening. *Food intolerance (food sensitivity)* occurs when there are problems digesting certain foods. Nausea, vomiting, diarrhea, indigestion, gas, or headaches may occur.
- *Illness*. Appetite usually decreases during illness and recovery from injuries. However, nutritional needs are increased.
- *Drugs*. Drugs can cause loss of appetite, confusion, nausea, constipation, impaired taste, or changes in gastrointestinal (GI) function. They can cause inflammation of the mouth, throat, esophagus, and stomach.
- *Chewing problems*. Mouth, teeth, and gum problems can affect chewing. Examples include oral pain, dry or sore mouth, gum disease, and dentures that fit poorly. Broken, decayed, or missing teeth also affect chewing, especially the meat group.
- *Swallowing problems*. Stroke, pain, confusion, dry mouth, and diseases of the mouth, throat, and esophagus can affect swallowing.
- *Disability*. Disease or injury can affect the hands, wrists, and arms. Adaptive equipment lets the person eat independently.
- *Impaired cognitive function*. Impaired cognitive function may affect the person's ability to use eating utensils. And it may affect eating, chewing, and swallowing.
- *Age*. Many GI changes occur with aging. Taste and smell dull. Appetite decreases. Secretion of digestive juices decreases. Fried and fatty foods may cause indigestion. Foods providing soft bulk are often ordered for chewing problems or constipation. Calorie needs are lower because energy and activity levels are lower.

Centers for Medicare & Medicaid Services (CMS) Dietary Requirements

- CMS has requirements for food served in nursing centers.
  - Each person's nutritional and dietary needs are met.
  - Each person's religious and cultural needs and preferences are met.
  - The person's diet is well balanced. It is nourishing and tastes good. Food is well seasoned.
  - Food is appetizing. It has an appealing aroma and is attractive.
  - Hot food is served hot. Cold food is served cold.
  - Food is served promptly.
  - Food is prepared to meet each person's needs. Some people need food cut, ground, or chopped. Others have special diets.
  - Other foods are offered if the person refused the food served. Substituted food must have a similar nutritional value to the first foods served.
  - Each person receives at least three meals a day. A bedtime snack is offered.
  - The center provides needed adaptive equipment and utensils.

Dysphagia means difficulty *(dys)* swallowing *(phagia)*. A *slow swallow* means that the person has difficulty getting enough food and fluids for good nutrition and fluid balance. An *unsafe swallow* means that food enters the airway (aspiration). ***Aspiration*** is breathing fluid, food, vomitus, or an object into the lungs.

- You may need to feed a person with dysphagia. To promote the person's comfort:
  - Know the signs and symptoms of dysphagia. Review Box 31.1 (p. 481), Dysphagia—Signs and Symptoms, in the Textbook.
  - Feed the person according to the care plan.
  - Follow the ordered diet; fluid thickeners are used to meet the person's needs.
  - Follow aspiration precautions (see Box 31.1, p. 481, Aspiration Precautions, in the Textbook) and the care plan.
  - Report changes in how the person eats.
  - Report choking, coughing, or difficulty breathing during or after meals. Also report abnormal breathing or respiratory sounds. Report these observations at once.

Preparing the Person for Meals

- Preparing residents for meals promotes their comfort.
  - Assist with elimination needs.
  - Provide oral hygiene. Make sure dentures are in place.
  - Make sure eyeglasses and hearing aids are in place.
  - Make sure incontinent persons are clean and dry.
  - Position the person in a comfortable position.
  - Reduce or remove unpleasant odors, sights, and sounds.
  - Follow the care plan for pain-relief measures.
  - Assist the person with hand hygiene.
- Food is served in containers that keep foods at the correct temperature. Hot food is kept hot. Cold food is kept cold.
- Prompt serving keeps food at the correct temperature.

Feeding the Person

- Serve food and fluid in the order the person prefers. Offer fluids during the meal.
- Use teaspoons to feed the person.
- Persons who need to be fed are often angry, humiliated, and embarrassed. Some are depressed or refuse to eat.

Let them do as much as possible. If strong enough, let them hold milk or juice glasses. Never let them hold hot drinks.
- Tell the visually impaired person what is on the tray. Describe what you are offering. For persons who feed themselves, use the numbers on the clock for the location of foods.
- Many people pray before eating. Allow time and privacy for prayer.
- Meals provide social contact with others. Engage the person in pleasant conversations. Sit facing the person. Allow time to chew and swallow. The person will eat better if not rushed. Wipe the person's hands, face, and mouth as needed during the meal.
- Report and record:
  - The amount and kind of food eaten
  - Reports of nausea or dysphagia
  - Signs and symptoms of dysphagia
  - Signs and symptoms of aspiration
- Many special diets involve between-meal snacks. These snacks are served on arrival on the nursing unit. Follow the same considerations and procedures for serving meal trays and feeding persons.

CHAPTER 31 REVIEW QUESTIONS

Circle the BEST answer

1. Which person needs to have thickened liquids?
   a. Person A has dysphagia and frequently chokes and coughs during a meal.
   b. Person B has diabetes and needs consistent calories throughout the day.
   c. Person C has heart problems and blood pressure is higher than normal.
   d. Person D has constipation, is inactive, and prefers low-fiber foods.
2. What would the nursing assistant do when feeding a person?
   a. Feed all of the protein foods first
   b. Offer fluids at the end of the meal
   c. Hand the person a spoon and check on him frequently
   d. Wipe the person's hands, face, and mouth as needed
3. Which action would the nursing assistant use to assist a person who is visually impaired during mealtime?
   a. Draw a map of how the food is arranged on the plate.
   b. Use the numbers on a clock to indicate the location of food.
   c. Talk about your favorite foods and share recipes.
   d. Let the person smell the food as each bite is offered.

Answers to these questions are on p. 577.

CHAPTER 32 FLUID NEEDS

Fluid Balance

- Fluid balance is needed for health. The amount of fluid taken in **(intake)** and the amount of fluid lost **(output)** must be approximately equal. If fluid intake exceeds fluid output, body tissues swell with water **(edema)**.
- **Dehydration** is a decrease in the amount of water in body tissues. Fluid output exceeds intake. Review Table 32.1 (p. 493), Dehydration and Fluid Overload, in the Textbook.

Normal Fluid Requirements

- An adult needs 1500 mL of water daily to survive. About 2000 to 2500 mL of fluid per day is needed for normal fluid balance. Water requirements increase with hot weather, exercise, fever, illness, and excess fluid loss.
- Older persons may have a decreased sense of thirst. Their bodies need water, but they may not feel thirsty. Offer fluids according to the care plan.

Electrolytes

- Sodium, potassium, calcium, and magnesium are some electrolytes. Electrolytes are needed for:
  - Fluid balance
  - Acid-base (pH) balance (see Chapter 10)
  - Movement of nutrients into the cells and wastes out of the cells
  - Nerve, muscle, heart, and brain function

Special Fluid Orders

- The doctor may order the amount of fluid a person can have in 24 hours. Intake and output (I&O) measurements may be ordered by the doctor or nurse.
- *Encourage fluids.* The person drinks an increased amount of fluid.
- *Restrict fluids.* Fluids are limited to a certain amount.
- *Nothing by mouth (NPO).* The person cannot eat or drink.
- *Thickened liquids.* All liquids are thickened, including water.

Intake and Output

- All fluids taken by mouth are measured and recorded—such as water and milk. So are foods that melt at room temperature—ice cream, sherbet, custard, pudding, gelatin, and Popsicles.
- Output includes urine, vomitus, diarrhea, and wound drainage.

Measuring Intake and Output

- To measure I&O, you need to know:
  - 1 cubic centimeter (cc) equals 1 mL.
  - 1 teaspoon equals 5 mL.
  - 1 ounce (oz) equals 30 mL.
  - 1 cup equals 240 mL
  - A pint is about 500 mL.
  - A quart is about 1000 mL.
  - 1 L equals 1000 mL.
  - The serving sizes of bowls, dishes, cups, pitchers, glasses, and other containers.
- An I&O record is kept at the bedside. Record I&O measurements in the correct column. Amounts are

totaled at the end of the shift. The totals are recorded in the person's chart. They are also shared during the end-of-shift report.

- The urinal, commode, bedpan, or specimen pan is used for voiding. Remind the person not to void in the toilet. Also remind the person not to put toilet paper into the receptacle.

Providing Drinking Water

- Patients and residents need fresh drinking water each shift. Follow the agency's procedure for providing fresh water.
- Water mugs and pitchers can spread microbes. To prevent the spread of microbes:
  - o Label the water mug with the person's name and room and bed number.
  - o Do not touch the rim or inside of the mug or lid.
  - o Do not let the ice scoop touch the mug, lid, or straw.
  - o Place the ice scoop in the holder or on a towel, not in the ice container or dispenser.
  - o Keep ice chest closed when not in use.
  - o Make sure the person's water mug is clean and free of cracks and chips. Provide a new mug as needed.

CHAPTER 32 REVIEW QUESTIONS

Circle the BEST answer

1. Which person has a sign or symptom of dehydration?
   a. Person A has a swollen leg.
   b. Person B has dark amber urine.
   c. Person C has trouble swallowing.
   d. Person D has an intake of 2000 mL.
2. Which item is recorded as intake for a person who requires I&O measurements?
   a. Ice cream
   b. Apple slices
   c. Toast
   d. Strawberry jam
3. Which quantity would the nursing assistant record when a person drank a pint of milk at lunch?
   a. 250 mL of milk
   b. 350 mL of milk
   c. 500 mL of milk
   d. 750 mL of milk
4. Which quantity would the nursing assistant for record for intake when person ate all of the soup from a 6 ounces bowl?
   a. 50 mL
   b. 120 mL
   c. 180 mL
   d. 200 mL
5. Which person is most likely to need frequent oral hygiene?
   a. Person A is on "encourage fluids."
   b. Person B needs "restricted fluids."
   c. Person C needs "thickened fluids."
   d. Person D is on "regular fluids."

Answers to these questions are on p. 578.

CHAPTER 34 VITAL SIGNS

Vital Signs

- The vital signs of body function are temperature, pulse, respirations, blood pressure, and, in some agencies, pain or pulse oximetry.
- Accuracy is essential when you measure, record, and report vital signs. If unsure of your measurements, promptly ask the nurse to take them again.
- Report the following at once:
  - o Any vital sign that is changed from a prior measurement
  - o Vital signs above or below the normal range

Body Temperature

- Thermometers are used to measure temperature. It is measured using the Fahrenheit (F) and centigrade or Celsius (°C) scales.
- Temperature sites are the mouth, rectum, axilla (underarm), tympanic membrane (ear), and temporal artery (forehead).
- Review Box 34.2 (p. 519), Temperature Sites, in the Textbook.
- Normal range for body temperatures depends on the site.
  - o Oral: 97.6°F to 99.6°F (36.5°C–37.5°C)
  - o Rectal: 98.6°F to 100.4°F (37.0°C–38.0°C)
  - o Axillary: 96.6°F to 98.6°F (36.0°C–37.0°C)
- Older persons have lower body temperatures than younger persons.

Thermometers

- Electronic thermometers include:
  - o Standard electronic thermometers with a blue probe for oral and axillary temperatures and red probes for rectal temperatures. A disposable cover protects the probe.
  - o Tympanic membrane thermometer, which measures body temperature at the tympanic membrane in the ear.
  - o Temporal artery thermometer, which measures body temperature at the temporal artery in the forehead.
  - o Digital thermometers, which measure body temperature at the oral, axillary, or rectal sites.
- Other thermometers include disposable thermometers which are used for oral temperatures and glass thermometers. Glass thermometers are less common but may be used in home settings. When using glass thermometers, rectal temperatures require 2 minutes, oral requires 2 to 3 minutes, and axillary requires 5 to 10 minutes.

Taking Temperatures

- *The oral site.* Place the thermometer under the person's tongue and to the side.
- *The rectal site.* Lubricate the tip end of the rectal thermometer. Privacy is important.
- *The axillary site.* The axilla must be dry. Place the probe in the center of the axilla and place the person's arm over the chest to hold the probe in place.

- Tympanic membrane thermometers are inserted gently into the ear. Pull the adult ear up and back to straighten the ear canal.
- Temporal thermometers. Use the exposed side of the head. Do not use the side that was on a pillow.

Pulse

- The adult pulse rate is between 60 and 100 beats per minute. Report these abnormal rates to the nurse at once.
  - *Tachycardia*—the heart rate is more than 100 beats per minute.
  - *Bradycardia*—the heart rate is less than 60 beats per minute.
- The rhythm of the pulse should be regular. Report and record an irregular pulse rhythm.
- Report and record if the pulse force is strong, full, bounding, weak, thready, or feeble.

Taking Pulses

- The radial pulse is used for routine vital signs. Place the first two or three fingers against the radial pulse. Do not use your thumb to take a pulse. Count the pulse for 30 seconds and multiply by 2 if the agency policy permits. If the pulse is irregular, count it for 1 minute. Report and record if the pulse is regular or irregular, strong or weak.
- The apical pulse is located 2 to 3 inches to the left of the sternum. A stethoscope is used to measure the apical or the apical-radial pulse. Count the apical pulse for 1 minute.

Respirations

- The healthy adult has 12 to 20 respirations per minute. Respirations are normally quiet, effortless, and regular. Both sides of the chest rise and fall equally.
- Count respirations when the person is at rest. Count respirations right after taking a pulse.
- Count respirations for 30 seconds and multiply the number by 2 if the agency policy permits. If an abnormal pattern is noted, count the respirations for 1 minute.
- Report and record:
  - The respiratory rate
  - Equality and depth of respirations
  - If the respirations were regular or irregular
  - If the person has pain or difficulty breathing
  - Any respiratory noises
  - An abnormal respiratory pattern

Blood Pressure

Normal and Abnormal Blood Pressures

- Blood pressure has normal ranges.
  - *Systolic pressure* (upper number)—90 mm Hg and higher but lower than 120 mm Hg
  - *Diastolic pressure* (lower number)—60 mm Hg and higher but lower than 80 mm Hg
- **Hypertension**—blood pressure measurements that remain above a systolic pressure of 140 mm Hg or a diastolic pressure of 90 mm Hg. Report any systolic measurement above 120 mm Hg. Also report a diastolic pressure above 80 mm Hg.
- **Hypotension**—when the systolic blood pressure is below 90 mm Hg and the diastolic pressure is below 60 mm Hg. Report a systolic pressure below 90 mm Hg. Also report a diastolic pressure below 60 mm Hg.
- Review Box 34.5 (p. 539), Guidelines for Measuring Blood Pressure, in the Textbook.

CHAPTER 34 REVIEW QUESTIONS

Circle the BEST answer

1. Which method would the nursing assistant use when the nurse asks for the temperature of a confused older person?
   a. Oral electronic probe thermometer
   b. Axillary glass thermometer
   c. Temporal artery thermometer
   d. Rectal glass thermometer
2. Which pulse rate should the nursing assistant report at once?
   a. A pulse rate of 52 beats per minute
   b. A pulse rate of 60 beats per minute
   c. A pulse rate of 76 beats per minute
   d. A pulse rate of 100 beats per minute
3. Which nursing assistant needs a reminder about how to take a pulse?
   a. Nursing assistant A counts an irregular pulse for 1 minute.
   b. Nursing assistant B uses the thumb to check the radial pulse rate.
   c. Nursing assistant C locates the radial pulse to count the rate.
   d. Nursing assistant D uses a stethoscope to take an apical pulse.
4. Which blood pressure should the nursing assistant report?
   a. 120/80 mm Hg
   b. 88/62 mm Hg
   c. 110/70 mm Hg
   d. 92/68 mm Hg

Answers to these questions are on p. 578.

CHAPTER 35 EXERCISE AND ACTIVITY

Bed Rest

- Bed rest means restricting the person to bed for health reasons.
- Bed rest is ordered to:
  - Reduce oxygen needs.
  - Reduce pain.
  - Reduce swelling.
  - Promote healing.

Complications From Bed Rest

- Pressure injuries, constipation, and fecal impactions can result. Urinary tract infections and renal calculi (kidney stones) can occur. So can blood clots and pneumonia.
- The musculoskeletal system is affected by lack of exercise and activity. These complications must be prevented to maintain normal movement.

- o A **contracture** is caused by abnormal shortening of a muscle; this results in decreased motion and joint stiffness. Common sites are the fingers, wrists, elbows, toes, ankles, knees, and hips. The site is deformed and disabled.
- o **Atrophy** is the decrease in size or the wasting away of tissue. Tissues shrink in size.
- **Orthostatic hypotension (postural hypotension)** is abnormally low blood pressure when the person stands up suddenly. The person can experience dizziness, weakness, or see spots before the eyes. Fainting can occur. To prevent orthostatic hypotension, have the person change slowly from a lying or sitting position to a standing position.

Positioning

- Supportive devices are often used to support and maintain the person in a certain position.
  - o *Bed boards*—are placed under the mattress to prevent the mattress from sagging.
  - o *Footboards*—are placed at the foot of mattresses to prevent plantar flexion that can lead to footdrop.
  - o *Trochanter rolls*—prevent the hips and legs from turning outward (external rotation).
  - o *Hip abduction wedges*—keep the hips abducted (apart).
  - o *Hand rolls or hand grips*—prevent contractures of the thumb, fingers, and wrist.
  - o *Splints*—keep the elbows, wrists, thumbs, fingers, ankles, and knees in normal position.
  - o *Bed cradles*—keep the weight of top linens off the feet and toes.

Range-of-Motion Exercises

- **Range-of-motion (ROM)** exercises involve moving the joints through their complete range of motion without causing pain. They are usually done at least two times a day.
  - o *Active ROM*—exercises are done by the person.
  - o *Passive ROM*—you move the joints through their range of motion.
  - o *Active-assistive ROM*—the person does the exercises with some help.
- Review Box 35.1 (p. 548), Range-of-Motion Exercises, in the Textbook.
- ROM exercises can cause injury if not done properly. Practice these rules.
  - o Exercise only the joints the nurse tells you to exercise.
  - o Expose only the body part being exercised.
  - o Use good body mechanics.
  - o Support the part being exercised at all times
  - o Move the joint slowly, smoothly, and gently.
  - o Do not force a joint beyond its present range of motion or to the point of pain.
  - o Ask the person if there is pain or discomfort.
  - o Stop if you meet resistance or suspect pain. Tell the nurse.
  - o Perform ROM exercises to the neck only if allowed by your agency and if the nurse instructs you to do so.

Ambulation

- **Ambulation** is the act of walking.
- Follow the care plan when helping a person walk. Use a gait (transfer) belt if the person is weak or unsteady. The person uses handrails along the wall. Always check the person for orthostatic hypotension.
- When you help the person walk, walk to the side and slightly behind the person on the person's weak side. Encourage the person to use the handrail on their strong side.

Walking Aids

- A cane is held on the strong side of the body. The cane tip is about 6 to 10 inches to the side of the foot. It is about 6 to 10 inches in front of the foot on the strong side. The grip is level with the hip. To walk:
  - o Step A: The cane is moved forward 6 to 10 inches.
  - o Step B: The weak leg (opposite the cane) is moved forward even with the cane.
  - o Step C: The strong leg is moved forward and ahead of the cane and the weak leg.
- A walker gives more support than a cane. Wheeled walkers are common. They have wheels on the front legs and rubber tips on the back legs. The person pushes the walker about 6 to 8 inches in front of the feet.
- Crutches are used when the person cannot use one leg or when one or both legs need to gain strength. Tips are checked. Bolts are tightened. Person should wear slip-resistant shoes. Crutches should be placed within the person's reach.
- Braces support weak body parts, prevent or correct deformities, or prevent joint movement. A brace is applied over the ankle, knee, or back. Skin and bony points under braces are kept clean and dry. Report redness or signs of skin breakdown, and pain or discomfort at once. The care plan tells you when to apply and remove a brace.

CHAPTER 35 REVIEW QUESTIONS

Circle the BEST answer

1. Which nursing measure would the nursing assistant use to prevent orthostatic hypotension?
   a. Move the person from the supine position to the standing position
   b. Check the person's vital signs after you help the person to stand up
   c. Move a person slowly from the lying or sitting position to a standing position
   d. Keep the person in bed if they usually feel dizzy when getting up
2. The nursing assistant is reviewing the assignment sheet to plan the work. Which person is likely to need the most help throughout the day?
   a. Person A is on strict bed rest.
   b. Person B is on bed rest.
   c. Person C is on bed rest with commode privileges.
   d. Person D is on bed rest with bathroom privileges.

3. Which piece of equipment would the nursing assistant obtain when the nurse says to use a trochanter roll to help maintain a person's body alignment?
   a. Rubber ball
   b. Splint
   c. Bath blanket
   d. Bed cradle
4. How does a person with a weak left leg hold a cane?
   a. The cane is grasped with the right hand.
   b. The cane is held on the left side.
   c. The cane is with the dominant hand
   d. The cane is held in the nondominant hand

Answers to these questions are on p. 578.

CHAPTER 36 COMFORT, REST, AND SLEEP

- Comfort is a state of well-being. Person has no physical or emotional pain.
- Pain or discomfort means to ache, hurt, or be sore. Pain is subjective. You must rely on what the person says.
- Pain is often considered a vital sign. Report pain and your observations to the nurse.

Factors Affecting Pain

- *Past experience.* The severity of pain, its cause, how long it lasted, and if relief occurred all affect the person's current response to pain.
- *Anxiety.* Pain and anxiety are related. Pain can cause anxiety. Anxiety increases how much pain the person feels. Reducing anxiety helps lessen pain.
- *Rest and sleep.* Pain seems worse when a person is tired or restless. Pain often seems worse at night.
- *Attention.* The more a person thinks about pain, the worse it seems.
- *Personal and family duties.* Often pain is ignored because of responsibilities related to job, school, children, partner, or parents. Some deny pain if a serious illness is feared.
- *The value or meaning of pain.* To some people, pain is a sign of weakness. Or it may signal the need for tests or treatment. For some persons, pain means avoiding work, daily routines, and certain people. Some people like attention and pampering by others.
- *Support from others.* Dealing with pain is often easier when family and friends offer comfort and support. Facing pain alone can be difficult.
- *Culture.* Culture affects pain responses. Non–English-speaking persons may have problems describing pain.
- *Illness.* Some diseases cause decreased pain sensations.
- *Age.* Older persons may have chronic pain that masks new pain. They may deny or ignore new pain, thinking that it is related to a known problem. Or they may deny or ignore pain because they are afraid of what it may mean. For persons who cannot tell you about pain, changes in usual behavior may signal pain. Loss of appetite also signals pain. Report any changes in a person's usual behavior to the nurse.

Signs and Symptoms

- Rely on what the person tells you. Promptly report any information you collect about pain. Use the person's exact words when reporting and recording pain.
- The nurse needs the following information.
  - *Location.* Where is the pain?
  - *Onset and duration.* When did the pain start? How long has it lasted?
  - *Intensity.* Ask the person to rate the pain. Use a pain scale.
  - *Description.* Ask the person to describe the pain.
  - *Factors causing pain.* Ask what the person was doing before the pain started and when it started.
  - *Factors affecting pain.* Ask what makes the pain better and what makes it worse.
  - *Vital signs.* Increases often occur with acute pain. They may be normal with chronic pain.
  - *Other signs and symptoms.* Dizziness, nausea, vomiting, weakness, numbness, and tingling.
- Review Box 36.3 (p. 567), Pain: Signs and Symptoms, and Box 36.4 (p. 569), Comfort and Pain—Relief Measures, in the Textbook.

The Back Massage

- The back massage can promote comfort and relieve pain. It relaxes muscles and stimulates circulation.
- A good time to give a massage is after baths and showers and with evening care. Massages last 3 to 5 minutes.
- Observe the skin for breaks, bruises, reddened areas, and other signs of skin breakdown.
- Lotion reduces friction during the massage. It is warmed before applying.
- Use firm strokes. Keep your hands in contact with the person's skin.
- After the massage, apply some lotion to the elbows, knees, and heels.
- Back massages are dangerous for persons with certain heart diseases, back injuries, back and other surgeries, skin diseases, and some lung disorders. Check with the nurse and the care plan before giving back massages to persons with these conditions.
- Do not massage reddened bony areas. Reddened areas signal skin breakdown and pressure injuries. Massage can lead to more tissue damage.
- Wear gloves if the person's skin is not intact. Always follow Standard Precautions and the Bloodborne Pathogen Standard.
- Report and record skin breakdown, redness, bruising, and breaks in the skin.

Rest

- *Rest* means to be calm, at ease, and relaxed with no anxiety or stress. Rest may involve inactivity. Or the person does things that are calming and relaxing.
- Promote rest by meeting physical, safety, and security needs.
  - Thirst, hunger, pain or discomfort, and elimination needs can affect rest. A comfortable position and

good alignment are important. A quiet setting promotes rest.
    - The person must feel safe from falling or other injuries. The person is secure with the call light within reach. Understanding the reasons for care and knowing how care is given also help the person feel safe.
- Many persons have rituals or routines before resting. Follow them whenever possible.
- Love and belonging are important for rest. Visits or calls from family and friends may relax the person. Reading cards and letters may also help.
- Meet self-esteem needs.
- Some persons are refreshed after a 15- or 20-minute rest. Others need more time.
- Ill or injured persons need to rest more often. Do not push the person beyond their limits.

Sleep

- Sleep is a basic need. Tissue healing and repair occur during sleep. Sleep lowers stress, tension, and anxiety. It refreshes and renews the person. The person regains energy and mental alertness. The person thinks and functions better after sleep.

Factors Affecting Sleep

- *Illness*. Illness increases the need for sleep.
- *Nutrition*. Sleep needs increase with weight gain. Foods with caffeine prevent sleep.
- *Exercise*. Exercise can help people to sleep better.
- *Usual sleep settings*. Changes in usual sleep settings (e.g., bed, pillow, lighting) can interfere with sleep.
- *Drugs and other substances*. Sleeping pills promote sleep. Drugs for anxiety, depression, and pain can induce sleep. Some drugs may cause nightmares or interfere with normal sleep patterns. Caffeine can prevent sleep.
- *Lifestyle changes*. Changes in daily routines may affect sleep.
- *Emotional problems*. Fear, worry, depression, and anxiety affect sleep.
- *Age*. The amount of sleep needed decreases with age.

Sleep Disorders

- **Insomnia** is a chronic condition in which the person cannot sleep or stay asleep all night.
- **Sleep deprivation** means that the amount and quality of sleep are inadequate. Function and alertness are decreased.
- **Sleepwalking** is when the person leaves the bed and walks about. If a person is sleepwalking, protect the person from injury. Guide sleepwalkers back to bed. They startle easily. Awaken them gently.

Promoting Sleep

- To promote sleep, allow a flexible bedtime, provide a comfortable room temperature, and have the person void before going to bed. Review Box 36.7 (p. 574), Promoting Sleep, in the Textbook for other measures.

CHAPTER 36 REVIEW QUESTIONS

Circle the BEST answer

1. Which question would the nursing assistant ask when a person reports pain?
    a. Where is the pain?
    b. Has this pain happened before?
    c. When did you take the last pain pill?
    d. Why does it hurt?
2. Which observation should be investigated as a possible nonverbal signal of pain?
    a. Illness
    b. Mental alertness
    c. Loss of appetite
    d. Hyperactivity
3. Which nursing assistant needs a reminder about the procedure for giving a back massage?
    a. Nursing assistant A uses long firm strokes to stimulate circulation.
    b. Nursing assistant B gives the massage after the bath.
    c. Nursing assistant C observes the skin before beginning the massage.
    d. Nursing assistant D uses cold lotion for the massage.
4. What is the priority concern when caring for a person who occasionally sleepwalks?
    a. Risk for falls
    b. Startles easily
    c. Fatigue
    d. Memory loss
5. Which action would promote sleep for a person?
    a. Offer the person coffee and cookies
    b. Accompany the person on a walk
    c. Encourage usual bedtime rituals
    d. Tell the person to go to bed

Answers to these questions are on p. 578.

CHAPTER 37 ADMISSIONS, TRANSFERS, AND DISCHARGES

- Admission is the official entry of a person into a health-care setting. It can cause anxiety and fear in patients, residents, and families.
- Transfer is moving the person to another health-care setting or moving the person to a new room within the agency.
- Discharge is the official departure of a person from a health-care setting.
- During the admission process:
    - Identifying information is obtained from the person or family.
    - The person is given an identification (ID) number and bracelet.
    - The person signs admitting papers and a general consent form.
- You prepare the person's room before the person arrives.

Admitting the Person

- Admission is your first chance to make a good impression. You must:
    - Greet the person by name and title. Use the admission records to find out the person's name.

  - Introduce yourself by name and title to the person, family, and friends.
  - Make roommate introductions.
  - Act in a professional manner.
  - Treat the person with dignity and respect.
- During the admission procedure the nurse may ask you to:
  - Collect some information for the nursing assistant admission checklist.
  - Measure the person's weight and height.
  - Measure the person's vital signs.
  - Obtain a urine specimen (if needed).
  - Complete a clothing and personal belongings list.
  - Orient the person to the room, nursing unit, and agency.

Weight and Height

- When weighing a person, follow the manufacturer's instructions and center procedures for using the scales. Follow these guidelines when measuring weight and height.
  - The person wears only a gown or sleepwear. No footwear is worn.
  - The person voids before being weighed and a dry incontinence product is worn if needed.
  - Weigh the person at the same time of day. Before breakfast is the best time.
  - Use the same scale for daily, weekly, and monthly weights.
  - Balance the scale at zero before weighing the person.

Moving the Person to a New Room

- Sometimes a person is moved to a new room because of a change in condition or care needs, the person requests a room change, or roommates do not get along. Support and reassure the person moving to a new room.
- The person is transported by wheelchair, stretcher, or the bed.

Transfers and Discharges

- When transferred or discharged, the person leaves the agency. The person goes home or to another health-care setting.
- Transfers and discharges are usually planned in advance by the health team.
- For discharges, the health team teaches the person and family about diet, exercise, and drugs. They also teach them about procedures and treatments and arrange for home care, equipment, and therapies as needed.
- The nurse tells you when to start the transfer or discharge procedure. Usually a wheelchair is used. If leaving by ambulance, a stretcher is used.
- If a person wants to leave the agency without the doctor's permission, tell the nurse at once. The nurse or social worker handles the matter.

CHAPTER 37 REVIEW QUESTIONS

Circle the BEST answer

1. What is the best response when the nursing assistant is preparing a person to transfer to another long-term facility that will be closer to family and the person seems tearful?
   a. "You should be cheerful; you will get to see your family."
   b. "Don't cry; everything is going to be just fine."
   c. "You seem sad; is there anything that I can do for you?"
   d. "I am sure that the new facility will be much nicer than this one."
2. What would the nursing assistant do when a person is admitted?
   a. Greet the person by name and title
   b. Go get a coworker if the person is obese
   c. Ask the family to take responsibility for valuables
   d. Ask the nurse how much time to spend on the admission process
3. Which action is correct when weighing the person?
   a. Have the person void before being weighed
   b. Tell the person not to eat until after being weighed
   c. Balance the scale at zero after weighing every person
   d. Have the person wear shoes when being weighed
4. What would the nursing assistant do when a person wants to leave the hospital without the doctor's permission?
   a. Persuade the person to stay
   b. Tell the nurse at once
   c. Call hospital security
   d. Stay with the person and close the door

Answers to these questions are on p. 578.

CHAPTER 39 COLLECTING AND TESTING SPECIMENS

Collecting Specimens

- When collecting specimens:
  - Follow the rules for medical asepsis.
  - Follow Standard Precautions and the Bloodborne Pathogen Standard.
  - Use a clean container for each specimen.
  - Use the correct container.
  - Do not touch the inside of the container or the inside of the lid.
  - Identify the person.
  - Label the container in the person's presence.
  - Collect the specimen at the correct time.

Urine Specimens

- There are different types of urine specimens: random, midstream, 24-hour, catheter or urine from an infant or child. The purpose of the specimen and the collection process will vary. When you are asked to obtain a urine specimen you need to know:
  - Type of voiding device—bedpan, urinal, commode, or toilet with specimen pan

- The type of specimen needed
- What time to collect the specimen
- What special measures are needed
- If you need to test the specimen
- If measuring I&O is ordered
- Straining urine is done when stones (calculi) are present or suspected.
- Urine can be tested with a reagent strip to detect: urine pH, blood (hematuria), glucose (glucosuria), ketones, infection, and protein.

Stool Specimens

- Stools are studied for fat, microbes, worms, blood, and other abnormal contents.
- Stool specimens should not be contaminated with urine or toilet paper.
  - Take the sample from:
  - The middle of a formed stool.
  - Areas of pus, mucus, or blood and watery areas.
  - The middle and both ends of a hard stool.
  - To detect occult blood, a thin smear of stool is applied to the test kit. Developer is added and color changes are noted.

Sputum Specimens

- Sputum is collected in the morning. Have the person rinse the mouth with water first. If tuberculosis is known or suspected, wear a respirator mask for your protection.

Blood Glucose Testing

- Blood glucose testing is used for persons with diabetes.
- If you are delegated to perform glucose testing, first know if your state and agency allow you to perform the procedure.
- Information that you need from the nurse includes:
  - What sites to avoid for a skin puncture
  - When to collect and test the specimen—usually before meals and at bedtime
  - If the person receives drugs that affect blood clotting

CHAPTER 39 REVIEW QUESTIONS

Circle the BEST answer

1. Which equipment does the nursing assistant need to obtain when the nurse instructs to test the person's urine for glucose and ketones?
   a. Glucometer
   b. Bottle of reagent strips
   c. Occult blood kit
   d. Syringe
2. Which person needs to drink 2000 to 3000 mL of water per day?
   a. Child who is wearing a urine collection bag ("wee bag").
   b. Person who is collecting urine for a 24-hour urine specimen.
   c. Person who is having all urine strained for stones.
   d. Older adult who needs to produce a midstream urine specimen.
3. Which type of specimen may require suctioning?
   a. Urine
   b. Stool
   c. Blood
   d. Sputum
4. What would the nursing assistant do when asked to perform blood glucose testing on a person who takes a medication that affects blood clotting?
   a. Decline to do the procedure
   b. Apply firm pressure until bleeding stops
   c. Puncture the middle fleshy part of the finger
   d. Perform the procedure very quickly

Answers to these questions are on p. 578.

CHAPTER 40 THE PERSON HAVING SURGERY

- Surgery may be inpatient, requiring a hospital stay, or same-day surgery, also called outpatient, 1-day, or ambulatory surgery. The person is prepared for what happens before, during, and after surgery.

Preoperative Care

- The person may have special tests such as chest x-ray or electrocardiogram (ECG). Nutrition and fluids may be restricted 6 to 8 hours before surgery.
- Personal care before surgery includes:
  - A complete bath, shower, or tub bath and shampoo. A special soap or shampoo may be ordered to reduce the number of microbes and the risk of infection.
  - Makeup, nail polish, and fake nails are removed.
  - Hair accessories, wigs, and hairpieces are removed, and a surgical cap keeps the hair out of the face and the operative site.
- Being NPO causes thirst and a dry mouth. The person must not swallow any water during oral hygiene.
- Dentures, eyeglasses, contact lenses, hearing aids, and other prostheses are removed.
- Often elastic stockings and sequential compression devices are put on before transport to the OR.

Postoperative Care

- The person's room must be ready. Make a surgical bed, place supplies in the room, and move furniture out of the way for a stretcher.
- Your role in postoperative care depends on the person's condition. Vital signs, including and pulse oximetry, are taken. The nurse tells you how often to check the person. Review Box 40.2 (p. 627), Postoperative Complications and Observations, in the Textbook.
- The person is repositioned every 1 to 2 hours to prevent respiratory and circulatory complications. Turning may be painful. Provide support and use smooth, gentle motions.

- Coughing and deep breathing exercises help prevent respiratory complications.
- Circulation must be stimulated for blood flow in the legs. If blood flow is sluggish, blood clots may form.
- Report the following at once:
  - Swollen area of a leg.
  - Pain or tenderness in a leg. This may occur only when standing or walking.
  - Warmth in the part of the leg that is swollen or painful.
  - Red or discolored skin.

Leg Exercises

- Leg exercises promote venous blood flow and help prevent thrombi. They are usually done five times, at least every 1 or 2 hours, while the person is awake.
  - Make circles with the toes. This rotates the ankles.
  - Dorsiflex and plantar flex the feet.
  - Flex and extend one knee and then the other.
  - Raise and lower the leg off the bed. Repeat with the other leg.

Elastic Stockings

- Elastic stockings exert pressure on the veins. The pressure promotes venous blood return to the heart. The stockings help prevent blood clots in the leg veins.
- Elastic stockings are also called AE (antiembolism or antiembolic) stockings or TED (thromboembolic disease) hose.
- The nurse measures the person for the correct size of elastic stockings. Most stockings have an opening near the toes that is used to check circulation, skin color, and skin temperature.
- The person usually has two pairs of stockings. One pair is washed; the other pair is worn.
- Stockings should not have twists, creases, or wrinkles after you apply them. Twists can affect circulation. Creases and wrinkles can cause skin breakdown.
- Loose stockings do not promote venous blood return to the heart. Stockings that are too tight can affect circulation. Tell the nurse if the stockings are too loose or too tight.

CHAPTER 40 REVIEW QUESTIONS

Circle the BEST answer

1. Which postoperative complication is associated with the nursing assistant's observation and report of a swollen calf that is red, warm to the touch, and painful?
   a. Hypovolemia
   b. Thrombus
   c. Dehiscence
   d. Pneumonia
2. What is the main purpose of the toe opening on the elastic stockings?
   a. It is used to determine the correct size of the elastic stockings.
   b. Opening allows for movement of toes and gives access for hygiene for feet.
   c. Opening allows access to smooth creases or wrinkles after application.
   d. It is used to check circulation, skin color, and temperature in the toes.
3. Which task will the nurse assign to the nursing assistant before a person is transported from postanesthesia care unit?
   a. Take vital signs with pulse oximeter reading every 5 minutes
   b. Position the person in high Fowler's to improve breathing
   c. Stay with the person because he will not be able to call for help
   d. Make a surgical bed, raise the bed, and lower the side rails

Answers to these questions are on p. 578.

CHAPTER 41 WOUND CARE

- A **wound** is a break in the skin or mucous membrane.
- The wound is a portal of entry for microbes. Infection is a major threat. Wound care involves preventing infection and further injury to the wound and nearby tissues.

Skin Tears

- A **skin tear** is a break or rip in the skin.
- Skin tears are caused by friction, shearing, pulling, or pressure on the skin. Bumping a hand, arm, or leg on any hard surface can cause a skin tear. Beds, bed rails, chairs, wheelchair footplates, and tables are dangers. So is holding the person's arm or leg too tight, removing tape or adhesives, bathing, dressing, and other tasks. Buttons, zippers, jewelry, or long or jagged finger or toenails can also cause skin tears.
- Skin tears are painful. They are portals of entry for microbes. Wound complications can develop. Tell the nurse at once if you cause or find a skin tear.
- Review Box 41.1 (p. 638), Preventing Skin Tears, in the Textbook.

Circulatory Ulcers

- *Circulatory ulcers (vascular ulcers)* are open sores on the lower legs or feet. They are caused by decreased blood flow through the arteries or veins.
- Review Box 41.2 (p. 639), Preventing Circulatory Ulcers, in the Textbook.
- *Venous ulcers (stasis ulcers)* are open sores on the lower legs or feet. They are caused by poor blood flow through the veins. The heels and inner aspect of the ankles are common sites for venous ulcers.
- *Arterial ulcers* are open wounds on the lower legs or feet caused by poor arterial blood flow. They are found between the toes, on top of the toes, and on the outer side of the ankle.
- A *diabetic foot ulcer* is an open wound on the foot caused by complications from diabetes.

- With nerve damage, the person can lose sensation in a foot or leg. The person may not feel pain, heat, or cold. Therefore the person may not feel a cut, blister, burn, or other trauma to the foot. Infection and a large sore can develop. Blood flow to the foot decreases; tissues and cells do not get oxygen and nutrients. A sore does not heal properly. Tissue death (gangrene) can occur. Review Box 41.3 (p. 640), Diabetes Foot Care, in the Textbook.

Prevention and Treatment
- Check the person's feet and legs every day. Report any sign of a problem to the nurse at once. Follow the care plan to prevent and treat circulatory ulcers.
- Complications of wounds include hemorrhage and infection
- Report wound observations. Review Box 41.4 (p. 643), Wound Observations in the Textbook.
- Some agencies let you apply simple, dry, nonsterile dressings to simple wounds. Follow the rules in Box 41.5 (p. 645), Applying Dressings, in the Textbook.

CHAPTER 41 REVIEW QUESTIONS
Circle the BEST answer
1. Which action would the nursing assistant perform to prevent skin tears?
   a. Use an assist device to move and turn the person in bed
   b. Firmly hold a confused person to prevent sudden movements
   c. Refuse to help people who wear rings, watches, bracelets
   d. Tell a confused person to cooperate with care
2. How often would the nursing assistant inspect the feet of a person who is diabetic?
   a. Every 4 hours
   b. Every day
   c. Once a week
   d. Once a month
3. What is the main purpose for using elastic stockings?
   a. To prevent circulatory ulcers
   b. To reduce skin tears
   c. To decrease risk for excoriation
   d. To eliminate wound infection

Answers to these questions are on p. 578.

CHAPTER 42 PRESSURE INJURIES
- A **pressure injury** is defined by the National Pressure Ulcer Advisory Panel as localized damage to the skin and/or underlying soft tissue.
- Pressure injuries usually occur over a bony prominence—for example, shoulder blades, elbows, hips, spine, sacrum, knees, ankles, heels, and toes.
- Pressure, shearing, and friction are common causes of skin breakdown and pressure injuries. Risk factors include breaks in the skin, poor circulation to an area, moisture, dry skin, and irritation by urine and feces. Review Box 42.1 (p. 654), Pressure Injury Risk Factors, in the Textbook.

Persons at Risk
- Persons at risk for pressure injuries are those who:
  - Are confined to a bed or chair.
  - Need some or total help in moving.
  - Are agitated or have involuntary muscle movements.
  - Have loss of bowel or bladder control.
  - Are exposed to moisture.
  - Have poor nutrition or poor fluid balance.
  - Have limited awareness.
  - Have problems sensing pain or pressure.
  - Have circulatory problems.
  - Are obese or very thin.
  - Have a medical device.
  - Have a healed pressure injury.

Pressure Injury Stages
- Pressure injuries range from reddened intact skin to tissue loss with bone exposure.
- Fig. 42.9 (pp. 656-657) in the Textbook shows the stages of pressure injuries.

Prevention and Treatment
- Good nursing care, cleanliness, and skin care are essential. Managing moisture, good nutrition and fluid balance, and relieving pressure also are key measures.
- Preventing pressure injuries is much easier than trying to heal them. Review Box 42.2 (p. 659), Preventing Pressure Injuries, in the Textbook.
- The person at risk for pressure injuries may be placed on a foam, air, alternating air, gel, or water mattress.
- Protective devices are often used to prevent and treat pressure injuries and skin breakdown. Protective devices include:
  - Bed cradle
  - Heel and elbow protectors
  - Heel and foot elevators
  - Gel or fluid-filled pads and cushions
  - Special beds
  - Other equipment—pillows, trochanter rolls, and footboards

CHAPTER 42 REVIEW QUESTIONS
Circle the BEST answer
1. Which medical device could cause a pressure injury?
   a. Trochanter roll
   b. Oxygen tubing
   c. Foot elevator
   d. Fluid-filled pad
2. Which device would be the best to use to prevent shearing?
   a. Alternating air mattress
   b. Bed cradle
   c. Drawsheet
   d. Pillow

3. Which action would help to prevent a mucosal membrane injury?
   a. Frequently checking on a person who is placed on a bedpan
   b. Reporting redness and irritation at the urinary meatus
   c. Reminding person who is sitting to shift position every 15 minutes
   d. Keeping the head of the bed at 30 degrees or less according to care plan
4. A person likes to sit in a wheelchair in the dayroom. Which action will help to prevent shearing?
   a. Encouraging the person to recline back in the chair
   b. Locking the wheels after person is positioned
   c. Positioning the person's feet on the footrests
   d. Making sure that the armrests are well padded

Answers to these questions are on p. 578.

CHAPTER 43 HEAT AND COLD APPLICATIONS

Heat Applications

- Heat relieves pain, relaxes muscles, promotes healing, reduces tissue swelling, and decreases joint stiffness.

Complications

- High temperatures can cause burns. Report pain, excessive redness, and blisters at once. Also observe for pale skin.
- Metal implants pose risks. Pacemakers and joint replacements are made of metal. Do not apply heat to an implant area.
- Heat is not applied to a pregnant woman's abdomen. The heat can affect fetal growth.

Moist and Dry Heat Applications

- In moist heat applications, water is in contact with the skin. Moist heat applications include hot compresses, hot soaks, sitz baths, and hot packs.
- Dry heat applications do not use water, allowing the application to stay at the desired temperature longer. Aquathermia pads, some hot packs, and warming therapy pads are dry heat applications.

Cold Applications

- Cold applications reduce pain, prevent swelling, and decrease circulation and bleeding. Cold is useful right after an injury.
- Complications include pain, burns, blisters, and poor circulation. Burns and blisters occur from intense cold. They also occur when dry cold is in direct contact with the skin.

Applying Heat and Cold

- Protect the person from injury during heat and cold applications. Review Box 43.1 (p. 668), Applying Heat and Cold, in the Textbook.

CHAPTER 43 REVIEW QUESTIONS

Circle the BEST answer

1. What is a common use for heat applications?
   a. Abdominal pain
   b. Wound infections
   c. Musculoskeletal injuries
   d. Postsurgical pain
2. Which response is expected when heat is applied to an area?
   a. Skin becomes red and warm.
   b. Skin is pale, white, or gray.
   c. Person begins to shiver.
   d. Area is excessively red.

Answers to these questions are on p. 578.

CHAPTER 44 OXYGEN NEEDS

Altered Respiratory Function

- Hypoxia means that cells do not have enough oxygen.
- Restlessness, dizziness, and disorientation are early signs of hypoxia.
- Report signs and symptoms of hypoxia to the nurse at once. Hypoxia is life threatening.
- Review Box 44.1 (p. 675), Altered Respiratory Function, in the Textbook.

Abnormal Respirations

- Adults normally have 12 to 20 respirations per minute. They are quiet, effortless, and regular. Both sides of the chest rise and fall equally.
- Abnormal patterns are listed below. Report these observations at once.
  - **Tachypnea**—rapid breathing. Respirations are 20 or more per minute.
  - **Bradypnea**—slow breathing. Respirations are fewer than 12 per minute.
  - **Apnea**—lack or absence of breathing.
  - **Hypoventilation**—respirations are slow, shallow, and sometimes irregular.
  - **Hyperventilation**—respirations are rapid and deeper than normal.
  - **Dyspnea**—difficult, labored, painful breathing.
  - **Cheyne-Stokes respirations**—respirations gradually increase in rate and depth. Then they become shallow and slow. Breathing may stop for 10 to 20 seconds.
  - **Orthopnea**—breathing deeply and comfortably only when sitting.
  - **Biot's respirations**—rapid and deep respirations followed by 10 to 30 seconds of apnea.
  - **Kussmaul respirations**—very deep and rapid respirations.

Pulse Oximetry

- Pulse oximetry measures the oxygen concentration in arterial blood.
- A sensor attaches to a finger, toe, earlobe, nose, or forehead.
- Avoid swollen sites and sites with skin breaks. Bright light, poor blood flow to the fingers, fake nails, nail polish, and movements can affect the measurements.

Promoting Oxygenation

- Breathing is usually easier in semi-Fowler's and Fowler's positions. Persons with difficulty breathing often prefer the **orthopneic position** (sitting up and leaning over a table to breathe).
- Deep breathing moves air into most parts of the lungs. Coughing removes mucus. Deep breathing and coughing are usually done every 1 to 2 hours while the person is awake. They help prevent pneumonia and atelectasis (the collapse of a portion of the lung).
    - The incentive spirometer is a device used to improve lung function and prevent complications. Your role may be to assist or remind the person to use the spirometer. See Delegation Guidelines: Incentive Spirometry (p. 682) in the Textbook.

Oxygen Devices

- A nasal cannula allows eating and drinking. Tight prongs can irritate the nose. Pressure on the ears and cheekbones is possible.
- There are different kinds of face masks that cover the nose and mouth. Talking and eating are hard to do with a mask. Listen carefully. Moisture can build up under the mask. Keep the face clean and dry. Masks are removed for eating. Usually oxygen is given by cannula during meals.

Oxygen Flow Rates

- When giving care and checking the person, always check the flow rate. Tell the nurse at once if it is too high or too low. A nurse or respiratory therapist will adjust the flow rate.

Oxygen Safety

- You do not give oxygen. You assist the nurse in providing safe care.
- Always check the oxygen level when you are with or near persons using oxygen systems that contain a limited amount of oxygen. Oxygen tanks and liquid oxygen systems are examples. Report a low oxygen level to the nurse at once.
- Follow the rules for fire and the use of oxygen in Chapter 14 (p. 197) in the Textbook.
- Never remove the oxygen device. However, turn off the oxygen flow if there is a fire.
- Make sure the oxygen device is secure but not tight.
- Check for signs of irritation from the oxygen device—behind the ears, under the nose, around the face, and on the cheekbones.
- Keep the face clean and dry when a mask is used.
- Never shut off the oxygen flow.
- Do not adjust the flow rate unless allowed by your state and agency.
- Tell the nurse at once if the flow rate is too high or too low.
- Tell the nurse at once if the humidifier is not bubbling.
- Secure tubing to the person's garment. Follow agency policy.
- Make sure there are no kinks in the tubing.
- Make sure the person does not lie on any part of the tubing.
- Report signs of hypoxia, respiratory distress, or abnormal breathing to the nurse at once.
- Give oral hygiene as directed. Follow the care plan.
- Make sure the oxygen device is clean and free of mucus.
- Make sure the oxygen tank is secure in its holder.

CHAPTER 44 REVIEW QUESTIONS

Circle the BEST answer

1. Which piece of equipment will the nurse ask you to obtain for a person who has orthopnea?
    a. Oxygen face mask
    b. Over-the-bed table
    c. Box of tissues
    d. Incentive spirometer
2. What is the normal respiratory rate for adults?
    a. 8 to 10 respirations per minute
    b. 12 to 20 respirations per minute
    c. 10 to 12 respirations per minute
    d. 20 to 24 respirations per minute
3. What is the best description of dyspnea?
    a. Breathing appears difficult, labored, or painful.
    b. Breathing is slow with 12 or fewer respirations per minute.
    c. Breathing is rapid with 24 or more respirations per minute.
    d. Breathing seems absent or barely measurable.
4. For which action would the nursing assistant intervene when helping a new nursing assistant who is performing a pulse oximeter reading on a person?
    a. Tells the person that the sensor clips on snugly, but pain is not expected
    b. Places the blood pressure cuff and the pulse oximeter on the same arm
    c. Checks the fingers and toes for swelling, skin breaks or nail polish
    d. Checks the SpO_2 and pulse rate and records information on the flow sheet
5. What is the purpose of using a pinwheel and helping a child to blow bubbles during play activities?
    a. Encourages and promotes deep breathing
    b. Distracts the child from the oxygen therapy
    c. Prevents hyperventilation
    d. Strengths chest muscles

Answers to these questions are on p. 578.

CHAPTER 46 REHABILITATION NEEDS

- A **disability** is any lost, absent, or impaired physical or mental function.
- **Rehabilitation** is the process of restoring the person to the highest possible level of physical, psychological, social, and economic function. The focus is on improving abilities. This promotes function at the highest level of independence.
- **Restorative nursing care** is care that helps persons regain health and strength for safe and independent

living. Restorative nursing measures promote healing, self-care, elimination, positioning, mobility, communication, and cognitive function.

Rehabilitation and the Whole Person

- Rehabilitation takes longer in older persons. Changes from aging affect healing, mobility, vision, hearing, and other functions. Chronic health problems can slow recovery.

Physical Aspects

- Rehabilitation starts when the person first seeks health care. Complications, such as contractures and pressure injuries, are prevented.
- *Elimination.* Bowel or bladder training may be needed. Fecal impaction, constipation, and fecal incontinence are prevented.
- *Self-care.* Self-care for activities of daily living (ADL) is a major goal. Self-help devices are often needed.
- *Mobility.* The person may need to learn how to move in bed and how to perform transfers. Crutches, a walker, a cane, a brace, or a wheelchair may be needed.
- *Nutrition.* The person may need a dysphagia diet or enteral nutrition.
- *Communication.* Speech therapy and communication devices may be helpful.

Psychological and Social Aspects

- A disability can affect function and appearance. Self-esteem and relationships may suffer. The person may feel less than whole, useless, unattractive, unclean, or undesirable. The person may deny the disability. The person may expect therapy to correct the problem. The person may be depressed, angry, and hostile.
- Successful rehabilitation depends on the person's attitude. The person must accept their limits and be motivated. The focus is on abilities and strengths. Despair and frustration are common. Progress may be slow.
- Remind persons of their progress. They need help accepting disabilities and limits. Give support, reassurance, and encouragement. Spiritual support helps some people. Psychological and social needs are part of the care plan.

The Rehabilitation Team

- Rehabilitation is a team effort. The person is the key member. The health team and family help the person set goals and plan care. The focus is to help the person regain function and independence.

Your Role

- Every part of your job focuses on promoting the person's independence. Preventing decline in function also is a goal. Review Box 46.2 (p. 706), Assisting With Rehabilitation Needs, in the Textbook.

Quality of Life

- To promote quality of life:
  - Protect the right to privacy.
  - Protect the right to be free from abuse and mistreatment.
  - Learn to deal with your anger and frustration.
  - Encourage activities.
  - Provide a safe setting.
  - Show patience, understanding, and sensitivity.

CHAPTER 46 REVIEW QUESTIONS

Circle the BEST answer

1. Which qualifications would signify a promotion from nursing assistant to the position of restorative aide?
   a. Special training in restorative nursing and rehabilitation skills
   b. Experience in caring for people who have rehabilitation needs
   c. Review and study of material on how to perform rehabilitation duties
   d. Establishment of seniority and longevity at a rehabilitation facility
2. What would the nursing assistant do if a person with a disability expressed angry or hostility while being encouraged and directed to wash the face and perform additional self-care?
   a. Take over and perform the hygienic care
   b. Tell the person that care will continue after he has calmed down
   c. Be patient and talk to the nurse if the behavior continues
   d. Firmly inform that a nursing assistant's job is to encourage self-care
3. Which response is best when a person attempts to tie the shoelace, but the knot doesn't hold, and the shoelace comes untied?
   a. "Tying your shoelaces is not that hard; try again."
   b. "Here, let me do it for you. I'm sorry that it's so hard for you."
   c. "You used the wrong kind of knot, try to remember what to do."
   d. "That was a good try and you had a nice hold on the laces."
4. Which action would the home health nursing assistant take on seeing a family member hit and yell at a disabled person?
   a. Check the person to see if there are any serious injuries
   b. Call the police and report the abusive behavior
   c. Talk to the nurse and describe observations and behaviors
   d. Tell the family member to leave at once and do not come back
5. Which nursing measure would the nursing assistant use when a person has a weak left arm?
   a. Place the call light on the left side
   b. Place the call light on the right side
   c. Give sympathy and pity
   d. Instruct to call out loudly for assistance

Answers to these questions are on p. 578.

CHAPTER 47 HEARING, SPEECH, AND VISION PROBLEMS

Hearing Loss

- Hearing loss is not being able to hear the normal range of sounds associated with normal hearing. Deafness is hearing loss in which it is impossible for the person to understand speech through hearing alone.
- Obvious signs and symptoms of hearing loss include:
  - Speaking too loudly
  - Leaning forward to hear
  - Turning and cupping the better ear toward the speaker
  - Straining to understand a conversation
  - Answering questions or responding inappropriately
  - Asking others to repeat themselves, speak louder, or to speak more slowly and clearly
  - Having trouble hearing over the phone
  - Finding it hard to follow conversations when two or more people are talking
  - Turning up the TV, radio, or music volume so loud that others complain
- Persons with hearing loss may wear hearing aids or lip-read (speech-read). They watch facial expressions, gestures, and body language. Some people learn American Sign Language (ASL). Others may have hearing assistance dogs.
- Review Box 47.3 (p. 714), Measures to Promote Hearing, in the Textbook.
- Hearing aids are battery operated. If they do not seem to work properly:
  - Check if the hearing aid is on. It has an on and off switch.
  - Check the battery position.
  - Insert a new battery if needed.
  - Clean the hearing aid. Follow the nurse's direction and the manufacturer's instructions.
- Hearing aids are turned off when not in use. The battery is removed.
- Handle and care for hearing aids properly. If lost or damaged, report it to the nurse at once.
- Review Box 47.4 (p. 714), Hearing Aids—Care Measures, in the Textbook.

Speech Disorders

Aphasia

- **Aphasia** is the total or partial loss of the ability to use or understand language.
- *Expressive aphasia* relates to difficulty expressing or sending out thoughts. Thinking is clear. The person knows what to say but has difficulty or cannot speak the words.
- *Receptive aphasia* relates to difficulty understanding language. The person has trouble understanding what is said or read. People and common objects are not recognized.
- *Global aphasia* is a difficulty in speaking and understanding language.

Eye Disorders

- *Cataract*. Cataract is a clouding of the lens in the eye. Signs and symptoms include cloudy, blurry, or dimmed vision. Persons may also be sensitive to light and glares or see halos around lights. Poor vision at night and double vision in one eye are other symptoms. Surgery is the only treatment.
- *Age-related macular degeneration (AMD)*. AMD blurs central vision needed for reading, sewing, driving, and seeing faces and fine detail. Treatment may stop or slow the disease progress.
- *Diabetic retinopathy*. Diabetic retinopathy causes blood vessels in the retina to become damaged. Usually both eyes are affected. It is a leading cause of blindness. Control of diabetes, blood pressure, and cholesterol can help to decrease risk or worsening of diabetic retinopathy.
- *Glaucoma*. Glaucoma results when fluid builds up in the eye and causes pressure on the optic nerve. The optic nerve is damaged. Vision loss with eventual blindness occurs. Drugs and surgery can control glaucoma and prevent further damage to the optic nerve. Prior damage cannot be reversed.
- See Box 47.6 (p. 716), Vision Problems—Signs and Symptoms, in the Textbook.

Impaired Vision and Blindness

- Blindness is absence of sight. The legally blind person sees at 20 feet what a person with normal vision sees at 200 feet.
- Review Box 47.7 (p. 721), Caring for Persons who are Blind or Visually Impaired Persons, in the Textbook.

Corrective Lenses

- Clean eyeglasses daily and as needed.
- Protect eyeglasses from loss or damage. When not worn, put them in their case.
- Contact lenses are cleaned, removed, and stored according to the manufacturer's instructions.

CHAPTER 47 REVIEW QUESTIONS

Circle the BEST answer

1. Which nursing assistant needs a reminder about measures that promote hearing?
   a. Nursing assistant A pauses slightly between sentences.
   b. Nursing assistant B speaks clearly, distinctly, and slowly.
   c. Nursing assistant C uses facial expressions and gestures to give clues.
   d. Nursing assistant D chats with the person while making the bed.
2. Which action would the nursing assistant perform for a person who uses a hearing aid and is preparing to go to bed?
   a. Turn the hearing aid off, then put it in the ear canal
   b. Discard the battery and store the hearing aid
   c. Place the hearing aid in the storage case
   d. Clean the hearing aid and assist with repositioning

3. Which nursing assistant needs a reminder about caring for a person who is blind?
   a. Nursing assistant A identifies self when entering the room.
   b. Nursing assistant B cleans up and stores personal items in the closet.
   c. Nursing assistant C describes people, places, and things thoroughly.
   d. Nursing assistant D asks how much the person can see.
4. Which condition occurs when fluid buildup in the eye causes pressure on the optic nerve?
   a. Cataract
   b. Cerumen
   c. Glaucoma
   d. Tinnitus

Answers to these questions are on p. 578.

CHAPTER 48 CANCER, IMMUNE SYSTEM, AND SKIN DISORDERS

Cancer

- Cancer is the second leading cause of death in the United States. Risk factors include: age, tobacco, radiation, infections, immunosuppressive drugs, alcohol, hormones, diet and obesity, and environment.
- Review Box 48.1 (p. 728), Cancer—Signs and Symptoms, in the Textbook.
- Treatments include surgery, radiation therapy, chemotherapy, hormone therapy, immune therapy, targeted therapy, stem cell transplants, and complementary and alternative medicine.
- Persons with cancer have many needs. They include:
  - Pain relief or control
  - Rest and exercise
  - Fluids and nutrition
  - Preventing skin breakdown
  - Preventing bowel problems (constipation, diarrhea)
  - Dealing with treatment side effects
  - Psychological and social needs
  - Spiritual needs
  - Sexual needs
- Anger, fear, and depression are common. Some surgeries are disfiguring. The person may feel unwhole, unattractive, or unclean.
- Talk to the person. Do not avoid the person because you are uncomfortable. Use touch and listening to show that you care.

Immune System Disorders

- The immune system protects the body from microbes, cancer cells, and other harmful substances. It defends against threats inside and outside the body.

HIV/AIDS

- Acquired immunodeficiency syndrome (AIDS) is caused by the human immunodeficiency virus (HIV). The virus is spread through body fluids—blood, semen, vaginal secretions, rectal fluids, and breast milk. HIV is not spread by air, saliva, tears, sweat, sneezing, coughing, insects, casual contact, closed mouth or social kissing, or toilet seats.
- Persons with AIDS are at risk for pneumonia, tuberculosis, Kaposi's sarcoma (a cancer), nervous system disorders, mental health disorders, and dementia.
- To protect yourself and others from HIV, follow Standard Precautions and the Bloodborne Pathogen Standard.
- Review Box 48.4 (p. 734), Caring for the Person With AIDS, in the Textbook.
- Older persons also get AIDS. They get and spread HIV through sexual contact and intravenous (IV) drug use. Aging and some diseases can mask the signs and symptoms of AIDS. Older persons are less likely to be tested for HIV/AIDS.

Skin Disorders—Shingles

- Shingles is caused by the same virus that causes chicken pox. A rash or blisters can occur. Pain is mild to intense and itching is a common complaint.
- Shingles is most common in persons older than 50 years. Persons at risk are those who have had chicken pox as children and who have weakened immune systems. Shingles lesions are infectious until they crust over.
- Treatments include antiviral and pain-relief drugs. A vaccine is available to prevent shingles.

CHAPTER 48 REVIEW QUESTIONS

Circle the BEST answer

1. Which personal protective equipment is the most important to maintain safety when caring for a person who is receiving chemotherapy?
   a. Shoe covers
   b. Gown
   c. Mask
   d. Gloves
2. Which observation, noted while assisting the patient with bathing, would the home health nursing assistant report to the nurse as a possible sign of skin cancer?
   a. Sees an irregular shaped mole that is oozing on the back
   b. Applies lotion to lower extremities for dry, flaky skin
   c. Notes that toenails are long, thickened, and dirty
   d. Observes that the skin underneath the breasts is moist
3. Which body fluid is most likely to be a source of HIV?
   a. Breast milk
   b. Tears
   c. Saliva
   d. Sweat
4. Which nursing assistant should inform the nurse about a personal condition that would affect being assigned to care for a person who has shingles in the infectious stage?
   a. Nursing assistant A has a child who had the chicken pox vaccination.
   b. Nursing assistant B is taking antibiotics for a respiratory infection.
   c. Nursing assistant C recently found out that she is pregnant.
   d. Nursing assistant D has an elderly parent who had the shingles vaccination.

Answers to these questions are on p. 578.

CHAPTER 49 NERVOUS SYSTEM AND MUSCULOSKELETAL DISORDERS

Nervous System Disorders

Stroke

- Stroke is also called a brain attack or cerebrovascular accident (CVA). Stroke is caused by bleeding in the brain (cerebral hemorrhage) or by a blood clot in the brain.
- Review Box 49.1 (p. 741), Stroke: Signs and Symptoms, in the Textbook.
- The effects of stroke include:
  - Loss of face, hand, arm, leg, or body control
  - **Hemiplegia**—paralysis on one side of the body
  - Changing emotions (crying easily or mood swings, sometimes for no reason)
  - Difficulty swallowing (dysphagia)
  - Aphasia or slowed or slurred speech
  - Changes in sight, touch, movement, and thought
  - Impaired memory
  - Urinary frequency, urgency, or incontinence
  - Loss of bowel control or constipation
  - Depression and frustration
  - Behavior changes
- The health team helps the person regain the highest possible level of function. Review Box 49.2 (p. 742), Stroke Care Measures, in the Textbook.

Parkinson Disease

- Parkinson disease is a slow, progressive disorder with no cure. Persons older than 60 years are at risk. Signs and symptoms become worse over time. They include:
  - *Tremors*—often start in one finger and spread to the whole arm. Pill-rolling movements—rubbing the thumb and index finger—may occur. The person may have trembling in the hands, arms, legs, jaw, and face.
  - *Rigid, stiff muscles*—in the arms, legs, neck, and trunk.
  - *Slow movements*—the person has a slow, shuffling gait.
  - *Stooped posture and impaired balance*—it is hard to walk. Falls are a risk.
  - *Mask-like expression*—the person cannot blink and smile. A fixed stare is common.
  - *Speech changes*—the person may have slurred, monotone, and soft speech.
- Other signs and symptoms that develop over time include swallowing and chewing problems, constipation, and bladder problems. Sleep problems, depression, emotional changes (fear, insecurity), memory loss and slow thinking can occur.
- Drugs are ordered to treat and control the disease. Exercise and physical therapy improve strength, posture, balance, and mobility. Therapy is needed for speech and swallowing problems. The person may need help with eating and self-care. Safety measures are needed to prevent falls and injury.

Multiple Sclerosis

- Multiple sclerosis (MS) is a chronic disease. The myelin (which covers nerve fibers) in the brain and spinal cord is destroyed. Nerve impulses are not sent to and from the brain in a normal manner. Functions are impaired or lost. There is no cure.
- Symptoms usually start between the ages of 15 and 60 years. Signs and symptoms may include vision problems, muscle weakness that usually starts on one side of the body, and balance and coordination problems. Tingling, prickling, or numb sensations may occur. Partial or complete paralysis and pain may occur. Other problems include fatigue; hearing loss; tremors; dizziness; depression; bladder function; sexual function; and changes in speech, concentration, attention, memory, and judgment.
- Persons with MS are kept active and independent as long as possible. Skin care, hygiene, and ROM exercises are important. So are turning, positioning, and deep breathing and coughing. Bowel and bladder elimination are promoted. Injuries and complications from bed rest are prevented.

Amyotrophic Lateral Sclerosis

- Memory and intellect are usually unaffected; but affected nerve cells in the brain and spinal cord stop sending messages to the voluntary muscles. The muscles weaken, waste away (atrophy), and twitch. The person cannot move the arms, legs, and body. Muscles for speaking, chewing and swallowing, and breathing also are affected. Eventually respiratory muscles fail.
- The person is kept active and independent to the extent possible.

Head Injuries

- Traumatic brain injury (TBI) occurs from violent injury to the brain. Common causes include falls, traffic accidents, violence, sports, explosive blasts, and combat injuries. Review Box 49.3 (p. 744), Traumatic Brain Injury—Signs and Symptoms, in the Textbook.
- Disabilities from TBI include cognitive problems, sensory problems, communications problems, and emotional problems.

Spinal Cord Injury

- Spinal cord injuries can permanently damage the nervous system. Common causes are motor vehicle crashes, falls, violence, sports injuries, alcohol use, and cancer and other diseases.
- The higher the level of injury, the more functions lost.
  - Lumbar injuries—sensory and muscle functions in the legs are lost. The person has **paraplegia**—paralysis and loss of sensory function in the legs and lower trunk.
  - Thoracic injuries—sensory and muscle function below the chest is lost. The person has paraplegia.
  - Cervical injuries—sensory and muscle functions of the arms, legs, and trunk are lost. Paralysis in the arms, legs, and trunk is called **quadriplegia** or **tetraplegia**.
- Review Box 49.4 (p. 746), Paralysis—Care Measures, in the Textbook.

Musculoskeletal Disorders

Arthritis

- Arthritis means joint inflammation.
- *Osteoarthritis (degenerative joint disease).* The fingers, spine (neck and lower back), and weight-bearing joints (hips, knees, and feet) are often affected.
- *Rheumatoid arthritis.* Rheumatoid arthritis (RA) causes joint pain, swelling, stiffness, and loss of function. Fatigue and fever may occur.
- Treatments for osteoarthritis and RA are similar.
    - o Pain control
    - o Heat and cold
    - o Exercise
    - o Rest and joint care
    - o Assistive (adaptive) devices
    - o Weight control
    - o Healthy lifestyle
    - o Safety
    - o Joint replacement surgery

Fractures

- A fracture is a broken bone. Falls, accidents, sports injuries, bone tumors, and osteoporosis are some causes.
- Signs and symptoms of a fracture include:
    - o Severe pain
    - o Swelling and tenderness
    - o Problems moving the part
    - o Deformity (the part looks out of place)
    - o Bruising and skin color changes at the fracture site
    - o Bleeding (internal or external)
    - o Numbness and tingling
- Review Box 49.7 (p. 751), Cast Care, Box 49.8 (p. 752), Traction Care, Box 49.9 (p. 754), Hip Fracture Care, in the Textbook.

CHAPTER 49 REVIEW QUESTIONS

Circle the BEST answer

1. Which action would the nursing assistant perform for a person who had a stroke?
    a. Keep the side rails up at all times
    b. Reposition the person every 2 hours
    c. Assist the person to a supine position
    d. Place personal items on the affected side
2. Which finding would the nursing assistant expect when caring for a person with hemiplegia?
    a. Paralyzed on one side of the body
    b. Paralyzed in both arms
    c. Paralysis in both legs
    d. Paralysis in all extremities
3. What is a leading cause of disability in the United States?
    a. Head injuries
    b. Arthritis
    c. Stroke
    d. Spinal cord injuries
4. Which term describes paralysis in the legs and lower trunk?
    a. Quadriplegia
    b. Paraplegia
    c. Hemiplegia
    d. Tetraplegia
5. What should the nursing assistant do on noticing that a person who has a cast on the left wrist is wearing a wedding ring?
    a. Advise to remove the ring and store it in a safe place
    b. Check to see if there is swelling or discoloration near the ring
    c. Do nothing; people have a right to wear personal jewelry
    d. Inform the nurse about the observation

Answers to these questions are on p. 578.

CHAPTER 50 CARDIOVASCULAR, RESPIRATORY, AND LYMPHATIC DISORDERS

Cardiovascular Disorders

- *Hypertension.* Hypertension (high blood pressure) occurs when the systolic pressure is 140 mm Hg or higher or the diastolic pressure is 90 mm Hg or higher. Narrowed blood vessels are a common cause. Review Box 50.1 (p. 760), Cardiovascular Disorders—Risk Factors, in the Textbook.
- *Coronary artery disease (CAD).* In CAD, the coronary arteries become hardened and narrow and the heart muscle gets less blood and oxygen. The most common cause is atherosclerosis, or plaque buildup on artery walls. Complications of CAD are angina, heart attack, heart failure, irregular heartbeats, and sudden death. CAD complications may require cardiac rehabilitation, which consists of exercise training and education, counseling, and training for lifestyle changes.
- *Angina.* Angina is chest pain. It is caused by reduced blood flow to part of the heart muscle. Chest pain is described as tightness, pressure, squeezing, or burning in the chest. Pain can occur in the shoulders, arms, neck, jaw, or back. The person may be pale, feel faint, and perspire. Dyspnea, nausea, fatigue, and weakness may occur. Some persons complain of "gas" or indigestion. Chest pain lasting longer than a few minutes and not relieved by rest and nitroglycerin may signal heart attack. The person needs emergency care.
- *Myocardial infarction (MI).* MI is also called *heart attack, acute myocardial infarction (AMI),* and *acute coronary syndrome (ACS).* Blood flow to the heart muscle is suddenly blocked. Part of the heart muscle dies. MI is an emergency. Sudden cardiac death *(sudden cardiac arrest)* can occur. Review Box 50.2 (p. 762), Myocardial Infarction—Signs and Symptoms, in the Textbook.
- *Heart failure.* Heart failure or congestive heart failure occurs when the heart is weakened and cannot pump normally. Blood backs up. Tissue congestion occurs. Drugs are given to strengthen the heart. They also reduce the amount of fluid in the body. A sodium-controlled diet is ordered. Oxygen is given. Semi-Fowler's position is preferred for breathing. Intake and output (I&O), daily weight, elastic stockings, and ROM exercises are part of the care plan.
- *Dysrhythmias.* Dysrhythmias are abnormal heart rhythms. Rhythms may be too fast, too slow, or irregular. Dysrhythmias are caused by changes in the

heart's electrical system. Some abnormal rhythms are treated with a pacemaker.

Respiratory Disorders

Chronic Obstructive Pulmonary Disease

- Chronic bronchitis and emphysema are two types of *chronic obstructive pulmonary disease (COPD)*. These disorders obstruct airflow. Lung function is gradually lost.
- *Chronic bronchitis*. Bronchitis means inflammation of the bronchi. Chronic bronchitis occurs after repeated episodes of bronchitis. Smoking is the major cause. Smoker's cough is the main symptom of chronic bronchitis. Over time, the cough becomes more frequent. The person has difficulty breathing and tires easily. The person must stop smoking. Oxygen therapy and breathing exercises are often ordered. If a respiratory tract infection occurs, the person needs prompt treatment.
- *Emphysema*. In emphysema, the alveoli enlarge and become less elastic. They do not expand and shrink normally when breathing in and out. Air becomes trapped when exhaling. Smoking is the most common cause. The person has shortness of breath and a cough. Fatigue is common. The person works hard to breathe in and out. Breathing is easier when the person sits upright and slightly forward. The person must stop smoking. Respiratory therapy, breathing exercises, oxygen, and drug therapy are ordered.

Asthma

- In asthma, the airway becomes inflamed and narrow. Extra mucus is produced. Dyspnea results. Wheezing, coughing, pain, and tightening in the chest are common. Asthma usually is triggered by allergies. Other triggers include air pollutants and irritants, smoking and secondhand smoke, respiratory tract infections, and exertion. Asthma is treated with drugs. Severe attacks may require emergency care.

Sleep Apnea

- Pauses in breathing last a few seconds to over a minute and can occur many times during sleep.
- The most common cause is blockage of the airway.
- During sleep, the person may use: continuous positive airway pressure (CPAP) or Bilevel positive airway pressure (BiPAP).
- In these therapies, a mask is attached to a pump. Air pressure is forced through the mask. The air keeps the airway open.

Pneumonia

- Pneumonia is an inflammation and infection of lung tissue. Bacteria, viruses, and other microbes are causes.
- High fever, chills, painful cough, chest pain on breathing, and rapid pulse occur. Shortness of breath and rapid breathing also occur. Cyanosis may be present.
- Drugs are ordered for infection and pain. Fluid intake is increased. Intravenous (IV) therapy and oxygen may be needed. The semi-Fowler's position eases breathing. Rest is important. Standard Precautions are followed. Isolation precautions are used depending on the cause.

Tuberculosis

- Tuberculosis (TB) is a bacterial infection in the lungs. TB is spread by airborne droplets with coughing, sneezing, speaking, singing, or laughing. Those who have close, frequent contact with an infected person are at risk. TB is more likely to occur in close, crowded areas. Age (very young or very old), poor nutrition, and human immunodeficiency virus (HIV) infection are other risk factors.
- Signs and symptoms are tiredness, loss of appetite, weight loss, fever, and night sweats. Cough and sputum production increase over time. Sputum may contain blood. Chest pain occurs.
- Drugs for TB are given. Standard Precautions and airborne precautions are needed. The person must cover the mouth and nose with tissues when sneezing, coughing, or producing sputum. Tissues are discarded in a no-touch waste container. Handwashing after contact with sputum is essential.

Lymphatic Disorders

Lymphedema

- Lymphedema usually occurs in an arm or a leg because of a blockage or damage to the lymph system. Treatment may include careful exercise, good skin care, massage therapy, and pressure garments (compression sleeves, lymphedema sleeves, or stockings). It is important to avoid putting pressure on the affected limb (e.g., no blood pressure cuff). See Box 50.5 (p. 769), Lymphedema—Care Measures, in the Textbook.

CHAPTER 50 REVIEW QUESTIONS

Circle the BEST answer

1. What is the most important information to remember when caring for a person who has angina?
   a. You should know the person's typical pain and symptom pattern and how drugs and rest usually affect the symptoms.
   b. The person should stop all activities, rest, and have nitroglycerin tablets available before angina occurs.
   c. Systolic pressure that is 140 mm Hg or higher or diastolic pressure that is 90 mm Hg or higher should be immediately reported.
   d. Pain that is severe, lasts longer than a few minutes, or is not relieved by rest or drugs may signal a heart attack.
2. Which task would the nursing assistant perform for a person who has heart failure?
   a. Measure intake and output
   b. Measure weight every week
   c. Promote a diet that is high in salt
   d. Encourage fluids for hydration
3. Which position is usually best for the person with pneumonia?
   a. Semi-Fowler's
   b. Prone
   c. Supine
   d. Trendelenburg's

4. In which situation would the nursing assistant expect to use airborne precautions?
   a. Person is being treated for an acute asthma attack.
   b. Person has chronic bronchitis and continues to smoke.
   c. Person has signs and symptoms of tuberculosis.
   d. Person has emphysema and is coughing up sputum.

Answers to these questions are on p. 578.

CHAPTER 51 DIGESTIVE AND ENDOCRINE DISORDERS

Digestive Disorders

Gastroesophageal Reflux Disease

- Gastroesophageal reflux disease (GERD) occurs when stomach contents flow back up into the esophagus. Drugs to prevent stomach acid production or to promote stomach emptying may be ordered. Lifestyle changes include limiting smoking and alcohol, losing weight, eating small meals, wearing loose belts and clothing, sitting upright for 3 hours after meals, and raising the head of the bed 6 to 9 inches so that head and shoulders are higher than the stomach.

Vomiting

- These measures are needed.
  - o Follow Standard Precautions and the Bloodborne Pathogen Standard.
  - o Turn the person's head well to the side. This prevents aspiration.
  - o Place a kidney basin under the person's chin.
  - o Move vomitus away from the person.
  - o Provide oral hygiene.
  - o Observe vomitus for color, odor, and undigested food. If it looks like coffee grounds, it contains undigested blood. This signals bleeding. Report your observations.
  - o Measure, report, and record the amount of vomitus. Also record the amount on the intake and output (I&O) record.
  - o Save a specimen for laboratory study.
  - o Dispose of vomitus after the nurse observes it.
  - o Eliminate odors.
  - o Provide for comfort.

Hepatitis

- Hepatitis is an inflammation of the liver. It can be mild or cause death. Signs and symptoms are listed in Box 51.1 (p. 777), Hepatitis, in the Textbook. Some people do not have symptoms.
- Protect yourself and others. Follow Standard Precautions and the Bloodborne Pathogen Standard. Isolation precautions are ordered as necessary. Assist the person with hygiene and handwashing as needed.

Endocrine Disorders

Diabetes

- In this disorder, the body cannot produce or use insulin properly. Insulin is needed for glucose to move from the blood into the cells. Sugar builds up in the blood. Cells do not have enough sugar for energy and cannot function.
- Diabetes must be controlled to prevent complications. Complications include eye problems, renal failure, nerve damage, stroke, heart attack, and slow healing. Foot and leg wounds can lead to infection and amputation.
- Blood glucose is monitored for:
  - o *Hypoglycemia*—low sugar in the blood.
  - o *Hyperglycemia*—high sugar in the blood.
- Review Table 51.1 (p. 780), Hypoglycemia and Hyperglycemia, in the Textbook. Either condition can lead to death if not corrected. You must call for the nurse at once.

CHAPTER 51 REVIEW QUESTIONS

Circle the BEST answer

1. What should the nursing assistant do first on observing that the person is in a supine position and vomiting?
   a. Obtain a kidney basin
   b. Notify the nurse immediately
   c. Turn the person's head to one side
   d. Observe emesis for blood, color, and odor
2. Which task is part of the nursing assistant's responsibility in helping a person with GERD successfully achieve the lifestyle modifications for this disorder?
   a. Remind the person to eat three large meals per day
   b. Remind that taking a nap is recommended after eating
   c. Assist the person to select and don a loose-fitting belt and loose clothes
   d. Place the person in the supine position to rest after dinner
3. Which symptom is the person most likely to report during a "gallbladder attack"?
   a. Pain in the right upper abdomen
   b. Constipation and pain with straining
   c. Rectal bleeding and bloody stools
   d. Severe itching and hot dry skin
4. What is the most important measure for infection control when caring for a person who has hepatitis A?
   a. Follow isolation precautions
   b. Good hand hygiene
   c. Take antiviral medications
   d. Cough etiquette
5. Which nursing measure would the nursing assistant use when a person who has diabetes is trembling, sweating, and feels hungry and faint?
   a. Get the person a cool cloth and a fan
   b. Get the person a glass of water
   c. Place him in a supine position with feet up
   d. Tell the nurse immediately

Answers to these questions are on p. 578.

CHAPTER 52 URINARY AND REPRODUCTIVE DISORDERS

Urinary System Disorders

Urinary Tract Infections

- Urinary tract infections (UTIs) are common. Urologic exams, intercourse, poor perineal hygiene, immobility, and poor fluid intake are common causes. Urinary catheters create a high risk; UTIs is a common health care–associated infection.

Prostate Enlargement

- The prostate grows larger as a man grows older. This is called benign prostatic hyperplasia (BPH). The enlarged prostate presses against the urethra. This obstructs urine flow through the urethra.

Urinary Diversion

- A urinary diversion is a surgically created pathway for urine to leave the body.
- Often an ostomy is involved. Good skin care is needed to prevent skin breakdown. Observe and report skin changes around the stoma. See "The Person With an Ostomy" in Chapter 29 (p. 461).

Kidney Stones

- Kidney stones (calculi) can cause severe pain and changes in urination: pain, frequency, urgency, hematuria (blood in urine), and cloudy foul-smelling urine.
- Urine is strained for stones. Fluids help to flush the stone; 2000 to 3000 mL/day is encouraged.

Kidney Failure

- In kidney failure (renal failure), the kidneys do not function or are severely impaired. Waste products are not removed from the blood. Fluid is retained.
- With chronic kidney failure, the kidneys cannot meet the body's needs. Hypertension and diabetes are common causes. Review Box 52.2 (p. 787), Chronic Kidney Disease—Signs and Symptoms, and Box 52.2 (p. 787), Chronic Kidney Disease—Care Measures, in the Textbook.

Reproductive Disorders

Sexually Transmitted Diseases

- A sexually transmitted disease, also known as sexually transmitted infection, is spread by oral, vaginal, or anal sex. Some people do not have signs and symptoms or are not aware of an infection. Standard Precautions and the Bloodborne Pathogen Standard are followed. Review Box 52.3 (p. 789), Sexually Transmitted Diseases/Sexually Transmitted Infections, in the Textbook.

CHAPTER 52 REVIEW QUESTIONS

Circle the BEST answer

1. Which symptom is an older man who has benign prostatic hyperplasia (BPH) most likely to report?
   a. Hiccups
   b. Fever and chills
   c. Flank pain
   d. Dribbling after voiding
2. What important role does the nursing assistant have when caring for a person with chronic renal failure that helps the doctor and the nurse to monitor the kidney function?
   a. Performing perineal care
   b. Measuring intake and output
   c. Adhering to Standard Precautions
   d. Straining the urine
3. Which action would the nursing assistant take before reporting to the nurse on noticing a sore on the shaft of an elderly person's penis?
   a. Gently cleanse the sore with mild soap and apply an antiseptic cream
   b. Initiate contact and wound precautions with gloving and gowning
   c. Use Standard Precautions and the Bloodborne Pathogen Standard
   d. Ask the person how long the sore has been there and if it is painful

Answers to these questions are on p. 578.

CHAPTER 53 MENTAL HEALTH DISORDERS

- **Mental health** involves a person's emotional, psychological, and social well-being.
- **Mental health disorders** are serious illnesses that can affect a person's thinking, mood, behavior, function, and ability to relate to others. Review Box 53.1 (p. 793), Mental Health Disorders, in the Textbook for warning signs and risk factors.
- **Stress** is the response or change in the body caused by any emotional, psychological, physical, social, or economic factor.

Anxiety Disorders

- **Anxiety** is feeling of worry, nervousness, or fear about an event or situation. Anxiety is a normal reaction to stress and helps a person to stay alert and focused and to cope.
- Coping and defense mechanisms are used to relieve anxiety. Review Box 53.3 (p. 794), Defense Mechanisms, in the Textbook.
- Some common anxiety disorders are generalized anxiety disorder, panic disorder, obsessive-compulsive disorder (OCD), phobias, and posttraumatic stress disorder (PTSD).
- *Generalized anxiety disorder.* **Generalized anxiety disorder** is characterized by extreme anxiety, fear, or worry that occurs most days for at least 6 months. The person has worry and concern about many things.
- *Panic disorder.* **Panic** is an intense and sudden feeling of fear, anxiety, or dread. Onset is sudden with no obvious reason. The person cannot function. Review Box 53.2 (p. 793), Anxiety—Signs and Symptoms, in the Textbook.
- *OCD.* An **obsession** is frequent, upsetting and unwanted thoughts, ideas, or images. **Compulsion** is an overwhelming urge to repeat certain rituals, acts, or behaviors.
- *Phobias.* **Phobia** means an intense fear. The person has an intense fear of an object, situation, or activity that has little or no actual danger. The person avoids what is feared. When faced with the fear, the person has high anxiety and cannot function.

- *PTSD.* PTSD occurs in some people after a terrifying, traumatic, scary or dangerous event that involved physical harm or threat of physical harm. Review Box 53.4 (p. 795), Posttraumatic Stress Disorder: Signs and Symptoms, in the Textbook. Flashbacks are common. A **flashback** is reliving the trauma in thoughts during the day and in nightmares during sleep. The traumatic event can seem like it is happening all over again. Some people recover within 6 months, for others the condition is chronic.

Psychotic Disorders

- **Schizophrenia** is a serious brain illness affecting how a person thinks feels and behaves. Symptoms include:
  - *Psychosis*—a condition that affects the mind and causes a loss of contact with reality
  - *Hallucinations*—seeing, hearing, smelling, or feeling something that is not real.
  - *Delusion*—a false belief.
  - *Delusion of grandeur*—an exaggerated belief about one's importance, wealth, power, or talents.
  - *Delusion of persecution*—the false belief that one is being mistreated, abused, or harassed.
  - *Emotional and behavioral problems*—normal functions are impaired or absent, including losing motivation or interest in daily activities, being unable to plan, lacking emotions, neglecting personal hygiene, and withdrawing socially.
  - *Cognitive problems*—trouble paying attention, understanding, or remembering information.
- The person with schizophrenia has problems relating to others. The person may be paranoid. The person may have difficulty organizing thoughts. Responses are inappropriate. Communication is disturbed. The person may withdraw. Some people regress to an earlier time or condition. Some persons with schizophrenia attempt suicide.

Mood Disorders

Bipolar Disorder

- The person with bipolar disorder has severe extremes in mood, energy, and ability to function. There are emotional lows (depression) and emotional highs (mania). This disorder must be managed throughout life. Review Table 53.1 (p. 796), Bipolar Disorder—Signs and Symptoms, in the Textbook. Bipolar disorder can damage relationships and affect school or work performance. Some people are suicidal.

Depression

- Depression causes distressing symptoms that affect feeling, thinking, and daily activities. Review Table 53.1 (p. 796), Bipolar Disorder—Signs and Symptoms; Depressive Episode in the Textbook.
- Depression is common in older persons. There are many losses—death of family and friends, loss of health, loss of body functions, and loss of independence. Loneliness and the side effects of some drugs also are causes. Review Box 53.6 (p. 797), Depression in Older Persons—Signs and Symptoms, in the Textbook. Depression in older persons is often overlooked or a wrong diagnosis is made.

Substance Abuse Disorder

- Addiction is a chronic disease involving substance seeking behaviors and use that is compulsive and hard to control despite the harmful effects. The person must have the substance. Persons addicted to drugs or alcohol cannot stop taking the substance without treatment.
- ***Alcoholism***—alcohol dependence involves:
  - *Craving*—a strong need to drink
  - *Loss of control*—not being able to stop drinking once started
  - *Physical dependence*—withdrawal symptoms
  - *Tolerance*—the need for more alcohol for the same effect
- **Withdrawal syndrome** is the physical and mental response after stopping or severely reducing use of a substance that was used regularly. The body responds with anxiety, restlessness, insomnia, irritability, poor attention, and physical illness.

Suicide

- **Suicide** means to end one's life on purpose.
- Suicide is most often linked to depression, alcohol or substance abuse, or stressful events. Review Box 53.10 (p. 800), Suicide, in the Textbook.
- If a person mentions or talks about suicide, take the person seriously. Call for the nurse at once. Do not leave the person alone.

Care and Treatment

- Treatment of mental health disorders involves having the person explore their thoughts and feelings. Often drugs are ordered.
- The care plan reflects the person's needs. The physical, safety and security, and emotional needs of the person must be met.
- Communication is important. Be alert to nonverbal communication.
- Protect yourself. Call for help. Do not try to handle the situation on your own.
- Keep a safe distance between you and the person.
- Be aware of your setting. Do not let the person block your exit.

CHAPTER 53 REVIEW QUESTIONS

Circle the BEST answer

1. Which action would be included in the care plan for a person with mysophobia?
   a. Carefully clean the over-the-bed table before bringing the meal tray
   b. Make sure that the room always has light; at night turn on a nightlight
   c. Reassure the person that the activity is conducted in a small private room
   d. Allow the person to choose a shower, tub bath, or a small basin of water

2. Which condition could have similar physical symptoms as a panic attack?
   a. A seizure
   b. A heart attack
   c. An opioid overdose
   d. A urinary tract infection
3. Which behavior is characteristic of bulimia nervosa and needs to be reported to the nurse?
   a. Eats only a small amount of certain foods
   b. Goes to the bathroom and induces vomiting
   c. Eats a large amount of food and asks for more
   d. Plays with food by pushing it around the plate
4. What would the nursing assistant do when a person says, "Everyone would be better off without me."?
   a. Convince the person of individual value
   b. Give the person privacy to consider thoughts
   c. Help the person focus on the reality of life
   d. Take the person seriously; notify the nurse
5. Which person has the greatest risk for suicide contagion?
   a. Grandmother whose grandson has suicidal thoughts
   b. Teenager whose best friend committed suicide
   c. Nursing assistant knows a patient who committed suicide
   d. Nursing instructor who teaches students about suicide prevention
6. What would the nursing assistant do first when entering a room to care for a person in the manic phase of bipolar disorder, and the person throws a shoe and shouts profanities?
   a. Tell her to quiet down and stop throwing things
   b. Quickly close the door and immediately get the nurse
   c. Stand in the open doorway and calmly call for assistance
   d. Cautiously approach her and use a friendly caring tone of voice

Answers to these questions are on p. 578.

CHAPTER 54 CONFUSION AND DEMENTIA

- Changes in the brain and nervous system occur with certain diseases and aging. Review Box 54.1 (p. 804), Nervous System Changes from Aging, in the Textbook.
- **Cognitive function** involves memory, thinking, reasoning, ability to understand, judgment, and behavior.

Confusion

- Confusion is a state of being disoriented to person, time, place, situation, or identity. Diseases, brain injury, infections, fever, alcohol or drug use, and drug side effects are some of the causes.
- The care of the confused person includes treatment that is aimed at the cause. Some measures help to improve function and basic needs must be met. Review Box 54.2 (p. 805), Confusion—Care Measures, in the Textbook.

Delirium

- **Delirium** is a state of sudden, severe confusion and rapid changes in brain function. Usually temporary and reversible, it occurs with physical or mental illness. Delirium is an emergency. Be alert for signs and symptoms and notify the nurse. Review Box 54.3 (p. 805), Delirium—Signs and Symptoms, in the Textbook.

Dementia

- **Dementia** is the loss of cognitive function that interferes with routine personal, social, and occupational activities.
- Dementia is not a normal part of aging; however, risk does increase with age.
- Some early warning signs include problems with language, dressing, cooking, personality changes, poor or decreased judgment, and driving, as well as getting lost in familiar places and misplacing items.
- Alzheimer disease (AD) is the most common type of permanent dementia.

Alzheimer Disease

- AD is a brain disease. Memory, thinking, reasoning, judgment, language, behavior, mood, and personality are affected. Onset is gradual.

Signs of AD

- Warning signs include:
  - Gradual loss of short-term memory.
  - Asking the same questions over and over again.
  - Repeating the same story—word for word, again and again.
  - Forgetting activities that were once done regularly with ease.
  - Losing the ability to pay bills or balance a checkbook.
  - Getting lost in familiar places. Or misplacing household objects.
  - Neglecting to bathe or wearing the same clothes over and over again. Meanwhile, the person insists that a bath was taken or that clothes were changed.
  - Relying on someone else to make decisions or answer questions that the person would have handled.
- Review Box 54.5 (p. 807), Signs of Alzheimer Disease—Early Signs and Symptoms, in the Textbook for other signs of AD.

Behaviors

- The following behaviors are common with AD.
  - *Wandering*. Persons with AD are not oriented to person, place, and time. They may wander away from home and not find their way back. The person cannot tell what is safe or dangerous.
  - *Sundowning*. With sundowning, signs, symptoms, and behaviors of AD increase during hours of darkness. As daylight ends, confusion, restlessness, anxiety, agitation, and other symptoms increase.

- *Hallucinations*. The person with AD may see, hear, or feel things that are not real.
- *Delusions*. People with AD may think that they are some other person. A person may believe that the caregiver is someone else.
- *Paranoia*. The person has false beliefs and suspicion about a person or situation.
- *Catastrophic reactions*. The person reacts as if there is a disaster or tragedy.
- *Agitation and aggression*. The person may pace, hit, or yell.
- *Communication changes*. The person has trouble expressing thoughts and emotions.
- *Screaming*. Persons with AD may scream to communicate.
- *Repetitive behaviors*. Persons with AD repeat the same motions over and over again.
- *Rummaging and hiding things*. The person may search for things by moving things around, turning things over, or looking through something such as a drawer or closet. The person may hide things, throw things away, or lose something.
- *Changes in intimacy and sexuality*. The person with AD may depend on and cling to their partner or may not remember life with or feelings for their partner. Sexual behaviors may involve the wrong person, the wrong time, and the wrong place. Persons with AD cannot control behavior.

Care of Persons With AD and Other Dementias

- People with AD do not choose to be forgetful, incontinent, agitated, or rude. Nor do they choose to have other behaviors, signs, and symptoms of the disease. The disease causes the behaviors.
- Safety, hygiene, nutrition and fluids, elimination, comfort, sleep, and activity needs must be met. Review Box 54.9 (p. 813), Dementia Care: Behavior and Changes, in the Textbook.
- The person can have other health problems and injuries. However, the person may not recognize pain, fever, constipation, incontinence, or other signs and symptoms. Carefully observe the person. Report any change in the person's usual behavior to the nurse.
- Infection is a risk. Provide good skin care, oral hygiene, and perineal care after bowel and bladder elimination.
- Supervised activities meet the person's needs and cognitive abilities.
- Impaired communication is a common problem. Avoid giving orders, expecting the truth, or correcting the person's errors.
- Always look for dangers in the person's room and in the hallways, lounges, dining areas, and other areas on the nursing unit. Remove the danger if you can.
- Every staff member must be alert to persons who wander. Such persons are allowed to wander in safe areas.

The Family

- The family may have physical, emotional, social, and financial stresses. The family often feels hopeless. No matter what is done, the person only gets worse. Anger and resentment may result. Guilt feelings are common.
- The family is an important part of the health team. They may help plan the person's care. For many persons, family members provide comfort. The family also needs support and understanding from the health team.

CHAPTER 54 REVIEW QUESTIONS

Circle the BEST answer

1. Which method would be the best way to accomplish morning care for a person who has AD?
   a. Rotate nursing assistants to increase the person's socialization
   b. Follow the same routine every morning; assign same staff member
   c. Check the person every morning and adapt care as needed
   d. Complete care, whenever the person seems willing to participate
2. Which clothing item would be the best choice for a confused person?
   a. Wrap-around skirt that ties on the side
   b. Jeans that button in front
   c. Pullover sweatshirt
   d. Shoes with Velcro fasteners
3. What is the major risk when a person with AD wanders?
   a. Potential for life-threatening accidents
   b. Disruption of routine activities of daily living
   c. Liability for the staff and facility
   d. Insufficient rest and sleep
4. Which item on the bedside table should be removed and given to the nurse for a person who has AD?
   a. Plastic bottle of water
   b. Cigarette lighter
   c. Picture of deceased spouse
   d. Alarm clock

Answers to these questions are on p. 578.

CHAPTER 58 EMERGENCY CARE

Emergency Care

- Rules for emergency care include:
  - Call for help.
  - Wait for help if the scene is not safe enough to approach.
  - Know your limits. Do not do more than you are able.
  - Stay calm.
  - Know where to find emergency supplies.
  - Follow Standard Precautions and the Bloodborne Pathogen Standard to the extent possible.
  - Check for life-threatening problems. Check for breathing, a pulse, and bleeding.
  - Keep the person lying down or as you found them.
  - Move the person only if the setting is unsafe.
  - Perform necessary emergency measures.
  - Do not remove clothes unless necessary.

- o Keep the person warm. Cover the person with a blanket, coat, or sweater.
- o Reassure the person. Explain what is happening and that help was called.
- o Do not give the person food or fluids.
- o Keep onlookers away. They invade privacy.

- Review Box 58.1 (p. 863), Emergency Care Rules, in the Textbook for more information.

Cardiopulmonary Resuscitation

- Cardiopulmonary resuscitation (CPR) supports breathing and circulation. It provides blood and oxygen to the heart, brain, and other organs until advanced emergency care is given. See Fig. 58.9 (p. 867) in the Textbook for additional information.
- CPR involves:
  - o *Chest compressions*—person must be on a hard, flat surface. Compressions are given at a rate of 100 to 120 per minute.
  - o *Opening the airway and giving breaths*—airway is opened using the head tilt-chin lift method. For an adult, two breaths are delivered after 30 compressions.
  - o *Defibrillation*—ventricular fibrillation (VF, V-fib) is an abnormal heart rhythm. Rather than beating in a regular rhythm, the heart shakes and quivers. The heart, brain, and other organs do not receive blood and oxygen. A *defibrillator* is used to deliver a shock to the heart and reestablish a regular rhythm. Defibrillation as soon as possible after the onset of VF (V-fib) increases the person's chance of survival.
  - o *Child and Infant CPR*—CPR for children and infants is different from adults and varies by age range. Review Table 58.1 (p. 871), CPR—Differences by Age Group.

Respiratory Arrest

- Breathing stops but the heart action continues for several minutes; if breathing is not restored cardiac arrest occurs.
- Open the airway.
- Give one breath every 6 seconds for adults.
- Give one breath every 2 to 3 seconds for infants and children.

Heart Attack

- Heart attack (myocardial infarction) occurs when part of the heart muscle dies from the sudden blockage of blood flow in a coronary artery. If you suspect a heart attack, activate Emergency Medical Services (EMS).
- Signs and symptoms include:
  - o Chest pain (not relieved by rest)
  - o Pain or discomfort in one or both arms, the back, neck, jaw, or stomach
  - o Shortness of breath
  - o Perspiration and cold, clammy skin
  - o Feeling light-headed
  - o Nausea and vomiting

Hemorrhage

- Hemorrhage is the excessive loss of blood in a short time. It can be internal or external. Follow the Emergency Care Rules in Box 58.1 (p. 863), in the Textbook; this includes activating the EMS system.
- Internal bleeding can cause pain, shock, vomiting of blood, coughing up blood, cold and moist skin, and loss of consciousness. Keep the person warm, flat, and quiet until help arrives. Do not give fluids.
- To control external bleeding:
  - o Do not remove any objects that have pierced or stabbed the person.
  - o Place a sterile dressing directly over the wound. Or use any clean material.
  - o Apply firm pressure directly over the bleeding site. Do not release pressure or remove the dressing.

Fainting

- **Fainting** is the sudden loss of consciousness from an inadequate blood supply to the brain.
- Warning signals are dizziness and perspiration, pale skin, and weak pulse. Have the person sit or lie down before fainting occurs.

Shock

- **Shock** results when tissues and organs do not get enough blood. Blood loss, poisoning, heart attack (myocardial infarction), burns, and severe infection are causes. Allergic reactions can cause anaphylaxis. Anaphylactic shock is an emergency.

Stroke

- **Stroke** occurs when the brain is suddenly deprived of its blood supply.
- Major signs include:
  - o Sudden numbness or weakness of the face, arm, or leg, especially on one side of the body
  - o Sudden confusion or trouble speaking or understanding speech
  - o Sudden trouble seeing in one or both eyes
  - o Sudden trouble walking, dizziness, or loss of balance or coordination
  - o Sudden, severe headache with no known cause
- If stroke is suspected, immediately activate the EMS system. The most effective stroke treatments must be given within 3 hours of symptom onset.

Seizures

- You cannot stop a seizure. However, you can protect the person from injury.
  - o Lower the person to the floor.
  - o Turn the person onto their side. Make sure the head is turned to the side. Do not put any object or your fingers between the person's teeth. Follow the Emergency Care Rules in Box 58.1 (p. 863), in the Textbook. Know when to call EMS for seizures.

Concussion

- Head injuries can be minor or serious and life threatening. Symptoms include difficulty thinking and concentrating, headaches, fuzzy or blurred vision, nausea and vomiting, feelings of tiredness or low energy, irritability and sadness, mood swings, and more or less sleep than usual. Some of the danger signs that signal the need for emergency care include: headache that gets worse or does not go away, weakness, numbness, or decreased coordination, nausea or vomiting more than once, slurred speech, and confusion.

Cold- and Heat-Related Illness

- **Hypothermia** is an abnormally low body temperature. Prolonged exposure to cold temperatures is the most common cause. Other causes include being cold and wet or being under cold water for too long.
- **Frostbite** is an injury to the body caused by freezing of the skin and underlying tissues. The nose, ears, cheeks, chin, fingers, and toes are the most common sites for frostbite. Damage can be permanent. Severe cases may require amputation
- **Heat-related illness** is caused by staying out in the heat too long. Exercising and working outside during hot, humid weather are other causes. Persons at risk for heat-related illness include infants, young children, and older persons. Other risk factors include obesity, fever, dehydration, heart disease, mental health disorders, poor circulation, prescription drug use, and alcohol use. Review Table 58.2 (p. 878), Heat-Related Illness, in the Textbook.
- **Burns** typically occur in the home. Infants, children, and older persons are at risk.
- First aid measures include:
  - Remove the person from the fire or burn source but do not touch the person if they are in contact with an electrical source.
  - Stop the burning process.
  - Apply cold or cool water for 10 to 15 minutes.
  - Remove hot clothing and jewelry that is not sticking to the skin.
  - Cover burns with sterile, dry dressings. Or use a sheet or any other clean cloth.
  - Keep blisters intact. Do not break blisters.
  - Elevate the burned area above heart level if possible.

CHAPTER 58 REVIEW QUESTIONS

Circle the BEST answer

1. Who determines when to activate the EMS system when a resident in a long-term care center shows signs and symptoms of sudden cardiac arrest?
   a. The doctor on call
   b. The charge nurse
   c. The facility administrator
   d. The staff member who witnessed the symptoms
2. Which action should the nursing assistant take on finding a person lying on the floor?
   a. Keep the person lying down
   b. Help the person back to the bed
   c. Elevate the person's head
   d. Obtain a wheelchair
3. Where would the nursing assistant place the hands when preparing to give chest compressions?
   a. On the sternum between the nipples
   b. On the upper half of the sternum
   c. On the left side of the sternum
   d. Slightly below the end of the sternum
4. Which nursing measure would the nursing assistant use if a person reports dizziness or feeling faint?
   a. Hold the person up to prevent falls
   b. Let the person walk to increase circulation
   c. Assist the person to sit or lie down
   d. Fan the person and encourage cool fluids
5. Which observation indicates that rescue breathing is being performed correctly?
   a. The chest muscles expand and contract
   b. Air is heard passing in and out of the mouth
   c. The chest rises with each breath
   d. The abdomen inflates with each breath

Answers to these questions are on p. 578.

CHAPTER 59 END-OF-LIFE CARE

Attitudes About Death

- Attitudes about death often change as a person grows older and with changing circumstances.

Culture and Spiritual Needs

- Practices and attitudes about death differ among cultures.
- Many religions practice rites and rituals during the dying process and at the time of death.

Age

- For children, their understanding and interpretation of death is based on their developmental age.
- Adults fear pain and suffering, dying alone, and the invasion of privacy. They also fear loneliness and separation from loved ones. Adults often resent death because it affects plans, hopes, dreams, and ambitions.
- Older persons usually have fewer fears than younger adults. Some welcome death as freedom from pain, suffering, and disability. Like younger adults, they often fear dying alone.

The Stages of Dying

- Dr. Kübler-Ross described five stages of dying. They are:
  - *Stage 1: Denial*. The person refuses to believe they are going to die.
  - *Stage 2: Anger*. There is anger and rage, often at family, friends, and the health team.
  - *Stage 3: Bargaining*. Often the person bargains with God or a higher power for more time.
  - *Stage 4: Depression*. The person is sad and mourns things that were lost.
  - *Stage 5: Acceptance*. The person is calm and at peace. The person accepts death.
- Dying persons do not always pass through all five stages. A person may never get beyond a certain stage. Some move back and forth between stages.

Comfort Needs

- Comfort is a basic part of end-of-life care. It involves physical, mental and emotional, and spiritual needs. Comfort goals are to:
  - o Prevent or relieve suffering to the extent possible.
  - o Respect and follow end-of-life wishes.
- Dying persons may want to talk about their fears, worries, and anxieties. You need to listen and use touch.
  - o *Listening*. Let the person express feelings and emotions in their own way. Do not worry about saying the wrong thing or finding the right words. You do not need to say anything.
  - o *Touch*. Touch shows caring and concern. Sometimes the person does not want to talk but needs you nearby. Silence, along with touch, is a meaningful way to communicate.
- Some people may want to see a spiritual leader. Or they may want to take part in religious practices.

Physical Needs

- As the person weakens, basic needs are met. The person may depend on others for basic needs and activities of daily living (ADLs). Every effort is made to promote physical and psychological comfort. The person is allowed to die in peace and with dignity.

Pain

- Some dying persons do not have pain. Others may have severe pain. Always report signs and symptoms of pain at once. Pain management is important. The nurse can give pain-relief drugs. Preventing and controlling pain is easier than relieving pain.

Breathing Problems

- Shortness of breath and difficulty breathing (dyspnea) are common end-of-life problems. The semi-Fowler's position and oxygen are helpful.
- Noisy breathing (death rattle) is common as death nears. This is due to mucus collecting in the airway. The side-lying position, suctioning by the nurse, and drugs to reduce the amount of mucus may help

Vision, Hearing, and Speech

- Vision blurs and gradually fails. Explain what you are doing during care measures or for environmental comfort. Provide good eye care.
- Hearing is one of the last functions lost. Always assume that the person can hear.
- Speech becomes difficult. Anticipate the person's needs. Do not ask questions that need long answers.

Mouth, Nose, and Skin

- Frequent oral hygiene is given as death nears.
- Crusting and irritation of the nostrils can occur. Carefully clean the nose.
- Skin care, bathing, and preventing pressure injuries are necessary. Change linens and gowns whenever needed.

Nutrition

- Nausea, vomiting, and loss of appetite are common at the end of life. Drugs for nausea and vomiting are given.
- Some persons are too tired or too weak to eat. You may need to feed them.
- As death nears, loss of appetite is common. The person may choose not to eat or drink. Do not force the person to eat or drink. Report refusal to eat or drink to the nurse.

Elimination

- Urinary and fecal incontinence may occur. Give perineal care as needed.

The Person's Room

- The person's room should be comfortable and pleasant. It should be well lit and well ventilated. Remove unnecessary equipment.
- Mementos, pictures, cards, flowers, and treasured items provide comfort. The person and family arrange the room as they wish.

The Family

- This is a hard time for family. The family goes through stages like the dying person. Be available, courteous, and considerate.
- The person and family need time together. However, you cannot neglect care because the family is present. Most agencies let family members help give care.

Legal Issues

- *Advance directives*. Advance directives give persons rights to accept or refuse treatment. The advance directive is a document stating a person's wishes about health care when that person cannot make their own decisions.
- *Living wills*. A living will is a document about measures that support or maintain life when death is likely.
- *Durable power of attorney for health care*. This gives the power to make health-care decisions to another person. When a person cannot make health-care decisions, the person with durable power of attorney can do so.
- *"Do Not Resuscitate" (DNR) order*. This means the person will not be resuscitated. The person is allowed to die with peace and dignity. The orders are written after consulting with the person and family.
- You may not agree with care and resuscitation decisions. However, you must follow the person's or family's wishes and the doctor's orders. These may be against your personal, religious, and cultural values. If so, discuss the matter with the nurse. An assignment change may be needed.

Signs of Death

- There are signs that death is near.
  - o Movement, muscle tone, and sensation are lost.

  - o Abdominal distention, fecal incontinence, nausea, and vomiting are common.
  - o Body temperature changes. The person feels cool, looks pale, and perspires heavily.
  - o The pulse is fast or slow, weak, and irregular. Blood pressure starts to fall.
  - o Slow or rapid and shallow respirations are observed. Mucus collects in the airway. You may hear the death rattle.
  - o Pain decreases as the person loses consciousness. Some people are conscious until the moment of death.
- The signs of death include no pulse, no respirations, and no blood pressure. The pupils are dilated and fixed.

Care of the Body After Death

- Postmortem care is done to maintain a good appearance of the body.
- Moving the body when giving postmortem care can cause remaining air in the lungs, stomach, and intestines to be expelled. When air is expelled, sounds are produced.
- When giving postmortem care, follow Standard Precautions and the Bloodborne Pathogen Standard.

CHAPTER 59 REVIEW QUESTIONS

Circle the BEST answer

1. Which action will the nursing assistant use when caring for a person who is dying and having trouble speaking?
   a. Smile frequently, but do not talk
   b. Speak slowly and clearly
   c. Ask the family to anticipate needs
   d. Ask yes or no questions, as needed
2. What behavior characterizes the denial stage of dying?
   a. Person is angry
   b. Person bargains with God
   c. Person refuses to believe that they are dying
   d. Person is calm and at peace
3. What is the focus of care measures when a person who has advanced Alzheimer disease is dying?
   a. Comfort is provided by using the senses
   b. Confusion is reduced by maintaining a routine
   c. Happiness is offered by retrieving long-term memories
   d. Support is given by relying on the person's family
4. Which action would the nursing assistant take on hearing the *death rattle* while caring for a dying person?
   a. Obtain the bag-valve mask with oxygen
   b. Turn the person to a side-lying position
   c. Take the person's hand: death is near
   d. Elevate the head of the bed
5. Which action would the nursing assistant use when assisting with postmortem care and the person's mouth will not stay closed?
   a. Place the neck in hyperextension
   b. Use a small strip of tape across the lips
   c. Place a rolled towel under the chin
   d. Roll an ace wrap around the chin and head
6. Which legal document states a person's wishes about health care when that person cannot make their own decisions?
   a. A living will
   b. An advance directive
   c. A durable power of attorney for health care
   d. A "Do Not Resuscitate" order

Answers to these questions are on p. 578.

Practice Examination 1

This test contains 80 questions. For each question, circle the BEST answer.

1. Which response would the nursing assistant give when a nurse says to give a person his medication when he is done in the bathroom?
   A. "I will give the drug, but I don't know what to do if something goes wrong, or if he refuses it."
   B. "I will ask the other nursing assistant to give the drug. She has more experience and she knows what to do."
   C. "I am sorry but I cannot give that drug. I will let you know when he is out of the bathroom."
   D. "I refuse to give that drug. It's not part of my job responsibilities and we could both get fired."
2. Which member of the health-care team is demonstrating ethical behavior?
   A. Nurse remarks, "That IV was so hard to start; drug users ruin their own veins. "
   B. Physical therapist says, "I prefer people who have religious and moral values."
   C. Doctor states, "That man is refusing all life-saving treatments; I just can't stand it."
   D. Nursing assistant says, "I saw that nurse hit a patient; I have to report what I saw."
3. Which action would the nursing assistant take on smelling alcohol on the breath of a coworker?
   A. Ignore the situation
   B. Tell the coworker to get counseling
   C. Give the coworker a breath mint
   D. Tell the nurse at once
4. Which circumstance is grounds for negligence?
   A. Call light goes unanswered; resident gets out of bed, falls, and breaks a leg.
   B. Nursing assistant tells a resident that her family refuses to come and visit her.
   C. Resident repeatedly removes incontinence pants; no one wants to help for her.
   D. Resident is restrained for being rude and impolite to a staff member.
5. How would the nursing assistant respond when a close relative asks about a patient?
   A. "She is walking better now that she is receiving physical therapy."
   B. "I must respect the patient's privacy and confidentiality."
   C. "Don't tell anyone I told you but she is getting worse."
   D. "She has been very sad recently and needs visitors."
6. Which response would the nursing assistant use at the end of the shift when the oncoming nursing assistant is available and a call light goes on?
   A. "I'm ready to go. I will let you answer that light."
   B. "I've been here all day so I am not answering that light."
   C. "Everyone usually answers the lights when they come on duty."
   D. "I will answer the light; you can organize your workload."
7. Which nursing assistant has correctly used the computer to record patient information?
   A. Nursing assistant A saves data and logs off after charting.
   B. Nursing assistant B gives care after lunch, but charts 0800.
   C. Nursing assistant C gets permission to use the nurse's password.
   D. Nursing assistant D does the recording for a coworker to help out.
8. Which action would the nursing assistant take when assigned to answer the phone?
   A. Wait to answer the phone, until full attention can be given to the caller
   B. Give a courteous greeting, identify the unit, and give your name and title
   C. Ask the caller to call back, because the nurse is not available
   D. Give patient information to family members or close family friends
9. What is the best action when a person who was recently admitted to the nursing center does not feel safe?
   A. Tell the person that nothing in the routine care is harmful
   B. Reassure the person that the place will soon feel like home
   C. Show the person around the nursing center
   D. Quickly give care to decrease the person's anxiety
10. Which care measure would the nursing assistant use when a person is angry and shouting very loudly?
    A. Inform the person that shouting is unacceptable
    B. Stay calm and try to understand the person
    C. Remove the person away from others
    D. Call the family and explain the situation
11. Which nursing assistant is using a good communication technique?
    A. Nursing assistant A says, "Oral hygiene prevents halitosis."
    B. Nursing assistant B softly mumbles, "Good morning, sir."
    C. Nursing assistant C says, "Do you want to bath, eat, rest, or talk?"
    D. Nursing assistant D clearly says, "Please straighten your arm."
12. Which person has a condition that would prompt the nursing assistant to check with the nurse and the care plan before using a gait belt?
    A. Person A has weakness in his right arm.
    B. Person B has urinary incontinence.
    C. Person C had recent abdominal surgery.
    D. Person D had a stroke several years ago.

13. Which response would the nursing assistant use when listening to a person?
    A. Say, "I only have a few minutes, what do you need?"
    B. Stand in the doorway and nod your head
    C. Say, "mmm" while you are performing tasks
    D. Face the person and make eye contact
14. Which nursing assistant displays the best interaction with a comatose person?
    A. Nursing assistant A makes jokes that she thinks the person would like.
    B. Nursing assistant B skillfully cares for the person without talking.
    C. Nursing assistant C assumes that the person can hear and explains actions.
    D. Nursing assistant D talks to another nursing assistant while giving care.
15. Which action would the nursing assistant take when trying to give hygienic care to an elderly female when a visitor is present?
    A. Politely show the visitor where to wait until the care is complete
    B. Do care in the presence of any visitor who is also a female
    C. Tell the visitor that the nurse's permission to stay is required
    D. Tell the visitor that hygienic care is not allowed if anyone is present
16. Which care measure would the nursing assistant use when a person asks to talk with a minister?
    A. Ask the person to share concerns and listen carefully
    B. Tell the person that the nurse will be notified right away
    C. Ask why the person wants to talk with the minister
    D. Advise that the minister only comes on Sunday
17. Which care measure would be included in the care plan for a person who has a restraint?
    A. Observe the person every 15 minutes or as often as directed by the nurse
    B. Release the restraints and reposition the person every 4 to 6 hours
    C. Check to see if the restrained person is okay at the end of the shift
    D. Apply the restraint and cover the person with a warm blanket
18. Which care measure will be included in the care plan for an elderly person who has frequent nighttime urination?
    A. Put an extra diaper on the person
    B. Wake the person during the night to void
    C. Withhold fluids throughout the day
    D. Give fluids before 1700 hours
19. Which action would the nursing assistant take if a person who lives in an assisted living facility and has medication reminders says, "This pill looks different"?
    A. Call the person's family and ask about any changes to prescriptions
    B. Reassure that pills can look different but are chemically the same
    C. Tell the person that the nurse will be contacted right away
    D. Use the computer to locate a picture of the pill for comparison
20. Which action would the nursing assistant use when pushing a person in a wheelchair up a ramp?
    A. Pull the chair backward
    B. Ask the person to help by using his feet
    C. Push the chair forward
    D. Ask the person to push on the wheel rims
21. Which action would the nursing assistant take if unable to read the person's name on the identification (ID) bracelet?
    A. Tell the nurse so a new bracelet can be made
    B. Ignore the bracelet, because the person is familiar
    C. Ask another nursing assistant to identify the person
    D. Ask the family to verify the person's identity
22. What is the universal sign of choking?
    A. Holding the breath
    B. Clutching at the throat
    C. Waving the hands
    D. Coughing up mucus
23. Which action would be on the care plan for a person who is on a diabetic diet?
    A. Serve meals early, so the person has plenty of time to eat
    B. Give the person snacks whenever they are hungry
    C. Make the person finish any food that is left on the tray
    D. Tell the nurse about changes in the person's eating habits
24. What is anticipated when a person has a mild airway obstruction?
    A. The person is usually unconscious.
    B. The person cannot speak.
    C. Finger sweep should be attempted.
    D. Forceful coughing may clear airway.
25. Which action would the nursing assistant use to relieve a severe airway obstruction in a conscious adult?
    A. Abdominal thrusts
    B. Back thrusts
    C. Chest compressions
    D. Finger sweeps
26. Which action would the nursing assistant take on finding faulty electrical equipment?
    A. Use if it is functional
    B. Report item to the nurse
    C. Replace it as soon as possible
    D. Use only with alert persons

27. Which action would the nursing assistant take when a warning label has been removed from a hazardous substance container?
    A. Use the substance if the contents of the container are known
    B. Open the container to determine the properties of the substance
    C. Take the container to the nurse and explain the problem
    D. Discard the container and contents immediately in the trash
28. What should the nursing assistant do when assigned to care for a person whose beliefs and values are different?
    A. Refuse to care for the person
    B. Delegate care to another nursing assistant
    C. Tell the nurse about concerns
    D. Explain personal beliefs to the person
29. What should the nursing assistant do on finding a person smoking in the nursing center?
    A. Ignore the smoking if no one is using oxygen
    B. Tell the person to leave the nursing center
    C. Call security to report the smoking violation
    D. Remind the person about designated smoking areas
30. What is the first action that the nursing assistant would take during a fire?
    A. Rescue persons in immediate danger
    B. Sound the nearest fire alarm
    C. Close doors and windows to confine the fire
    D. Extinguish the fire
31. Which nursing measure would be include in the care plan for a person with Alzheimer disease who has increased restlessness and confusion toward the end of the day?
    A. Try to reason with the person
    B. Ask the person to explain what is needed
    C. Provide a calm, quiet setting late in the day
    D. Complete treatments and activities late in the day
32. During which nursing task, would the nursing assistant increase vigilance to prevent suffocation?
    A. Helping an elderly person to the toilet
    B. Supervising a person during smoking
    C. Assisting an older person during mealtime
    D. Helping a person with morning hygiene
33. Which action would the nursing assistant take when using a wheelchair?
    A. Lock both wheels before transferring a person to and from the wheelchair
    B. Lock one wheel to prevent the person from moving the wheelchair
    C. Let the person move feet along the floor while being pushed in the chair
    D. Ask the person to step over the footplates before pivoting to sit
34. What should the nursing assistant do first when an obese elderly person falls to the floor, but appears uninjured and wants help to get up?
    A. Apply a gait belt and assist the person to stand up slowly
    B. Tell the person to lie still; the nurse is coming to check
    C. Inform the person that assistance and the manual lift are coming
    D. Have the person sit up first, ask if anything hurts, then help him to stand
35. Which serious complication is prevented when the nursing assistant reports to the nurse that someone has put the person's vest restraint on backward?
    A. Contracture
    B. Strangulation
    C. Humiliation
    D. Incontinence
36. Which nursing measure would the nursing assistant perform before feeding a person?
    A. Ask the nurse if the person has a health-care-associated infection
    B. Wash hands with alcohol-based hand sanitizer
    C. Wash hands with soap and water
    D. Put on personal protective equipment
37. Which action does the nursing assistant perform when wearing gloves?
    A. Wears them until they become visibly soiled or contaminated
    B. Wears the same gloves if remaining in the same room
    C. Uses sterile gloves to give care if the person has risk for infection
    D. Changes gloves when they become contaminated with urine
38. Which action does the nursing assistant use when washing the hands?
    A. Use hot water and a disinfectant to create a rich lather
    B. Dry hands and then use that towel to turn off the faucet
    C. Shake the excessive water from the hands before drying
    D. Keep the hands and forearms lower than the elbows
39. Which action does the nursing assistant use when moving a box from the floor to the counter in the utility room?
    A. Bend from the waist to pick up the box
    B. Hold the box away from the body as it is picked it up
    C. Bend the knees and squat to lift the box
    D. Stand with feet close together as box is picked up
40. What would the nursing assistant do when putting a person in Fowler's position?
    A. Put the bed flat
    B. Raise the head of the bed 15 degrees
    C. Raise the head of the bed between 45 and 60 degrees
    D. Raise the head of the bed between 80 and 90 degrees

41. What does the nursing assistant do when the baby needs to go to sleep?
    A. Dress the baby in a sleepwear that covers the head
    B. Place pillows around the baby for comfort and security
    C. Place the baby on the stomach with head turned to the side
    D. Lay the baby on the back on a firm, flat mattress
42. How does the nursing assistant position a person in a chair to achieve good body alignment?
    A. Have the person's back and buttocks against the back of the chair
    B. Leave the person's feet unsupported for freedom of movement
    C. Have the backs of the person's knees touch the edge of the chair
    D. Have the person sit on the edge of the chair and hold arm rests
43. Which action does the nursing assistant use when transferring a person with a weak left leg from the bed to the wheelchair?
    A. Get the person out of bed on the left side
    B. Get the person out of bed on the right side
    C. Get help and manually lift the person out of bed
    D. Ask the person which they prefer to move first
44. Which nursing measure would the nursing assistant use first when a person tries to scratch and kick?
    A. Protect self from harm
    B. Restrain the person
    C. Tell the nurse about the behavior
    D. Ignore the behavior and continue care
45. Which circumstance is most likely to cause shearing?
    A. Person is logrolled so that soiled underpad can be removed.
    B. Person slips down in bed when head of the bed is raised.
    C. Person reports feeling dizzy when first sitting up to dangle.
    D. Person is sleeping in a supine position with pillow under the head.
46. Which environmental adjustment would provide comfort for most older persons?
    A. Rooms that are cool with circulating ceiling fans
    B. Restrooms that resemble a home bathroom
    C. Cheerful talking and laughing at the nurses' station
    D. Lighting that meets their needs
47. Which location is the best for call lights?
    A. Placed on the person's strong side
    B. Positioned near the bathroom door
    C. Stored in a bedside drawer
    D. Placed near the dominant hand
48. What would the nursing assistant do when a nurse asks that a person's closet be inspected?
    A. Ask the nurse for permission to handle the person's property
    B. Inspect the closet when the person is in the dining room
    C. Ask the person for permission to check contents of the closet
    D. Tell the nurse that inspecting the closet is not an assistant task
49. Which action would the nursing assistant use when changing bed linens?
    A. Take the linen cart from room to room
    B. Shake the linens to remove dust and debris
    C. Take only needed linens into the person's room
    D. Put dirty or used linens on the floor
50. In which circumstance would the nursing assistant attempt to fight the fire by using a fire extinguisher?
    A. There is a fire in the resident's trash can.
    B. A grease fire in the kitchen is spreading.
    C. Cigarette ash ignites the blankets and mattress.
    D. A resident is trapped behind a wall of flames.
51. Which nursing measure for mouth care would be included in the care plan for an unconscious person?
    A. Wipe the mouth and teeth with a damp cloth
    B. Give mouth care at least every 2 hours
    C. Place the person in a supine position
    D. Open the mouth with fingers of dominant hand
52. How would the nursing assistant respond to a person who is angry because morning care was delayed due to staff shortage?
    A. "It's not my fault. A co-worker called off today and we are short-staffed."
    B. "I'm sorry the care has been late this morning. I will try to plan better."
    C. "I am doing the best I can. We had some unexpected problems today."
    D. "I have been very busy and you know that I usually get morning care done."
53. Which action would the nursing assistant use when asked to clean a person's dentures?
    A. Use hot water and scrub away food particles and mucous
    B. Hold the dentures firmly and line the sink with a towel
    C. Wrap the dentures in tissues after cleaning
    D. Store the denture cup with the person's room number on it
54. Which action would the nursing assistant take when bathing a person and noticing a rash that was not there before?
    A. Apply a thin layer of lotion to soothe the rash
    B. Ask if the water temperature is causing the rash
    C. Tell the nurse and record it in the medical record
    D. Ask the person if the rash itches or is contagious
55. Which nursing measure would the nursing assistant use when washing a person's eyes?
    A. Use sterile irrigating eye drops
    B. Clean the right eye first, then the left eye
    C. Wipe from the inner to the outer aspect of the eye
    D. Wipe beneath the eye but avoid the upper lid

56. Which nursing assistant is using a correct step when giving a back massage?
    A. Nursing assistant A uses cool lotion to soothe the skin.
    B. Nursing assistant B uses light feathery strokes.
    C. Nursing assistant C gently massages red bony areas.
    D. Nursing assistant D looks for bruises and breaks in the skin.
57. Which nursing measure would the nursing assistant use when giving perineal care to a female?
    A. Separate the labia and clean downward from front to back
    B. Cleanse entire genital area with gentle upward strokes
    C. Wear gloves only if there is drainage or secretions
    D. Use plain tap water and rub the tissue with a soft cloth
58. What would the nursing assistant do when giving a person a tub bath or shower?
    A. Stand beside the person until they are finished
    B. Turn the hot water on first, then the cold water
    C. Stay within hearing distance if the person can be left alone
    D. Direct the person to adjust the water temperature
59. Which nursing measure for grooming facial hair would be included in the care plan for a person who takes an anticoagulant medication?
    A. Use a safety razor
    B. Use an electric razor
    C. Use a straight razor
    D. Use a pair of scissors
60. What would the nursing assistant do when a person with a weak left arm wants to take off a sweater?
    A. Encourage the person to independently take off the sweater
    B. Help the person remove the sweater from the right arm first
    C. Help the person remove the sweater from the left arm first
    D. Suggest that the person keep the sweater on
61. Which nursing assistant is demonstrating a communication barrier?
    A. Nursing assistant A calls residents by preferred name and title.
    B. Nursing assistant B says, "Don't worry, everything will be alright."
    C. Nursing assistant C is quiet and calm when the person seems tearful.
    D. Nursing assistant D says, "Could you say that again, please?"
62. Which care measure would be included in the care plan for a person who has an indwelling catheter?
    A. Instruct the person on how to position the tubing
    B. Disconnect the catheter from the drainage tubing every 8 hours
    C. Secure the catheter to the lower leg
    D. Measure and record the amount of urine in the drainage bag
63. Which nutritional benefits are provided by eating a diet that contains carbohydrates?
    A. Boosts tissue repair and growth
    B. Provides energy and fiber for bowel elimination
    C. Adds flavor to food and helps the body use certain vitamins
    D. Facilitates nerve and muscle function
64. What would the nursing assistant do when taking a rectal temperature with an electronic thermometer?
    A. Insert the thermometer, provide privacy, and return in 2 minutes
    B. Place the person in a prone position
    C. Insert the thermometer 1 inch into the rectum
    D. Insert the thermometer ½ inch into the rectum
65. Which action would the nursing assistant take when a patient has a blood pressure (BP) of 86/58 mm Hg?
    A. Report the BP to the nurse at once
    B. Record the BP and tell the nurse at the end of the shift
    C. Report the BP along with vital signs from other patients
    D. Retake the BP in 30 minutes and then tell the nurse
66. For which person would the nursing assistant take an oral temperature?
    A. An unconscious person
    B. A person receiving oxygen
    C. A child who breathes through the mouth
    D. A cooperative adult
67. Which action would the nursing assistant use when caring for a person who is blind or visually impaired?
    A. Offer arm and the person walks a half step behind
    B. Do as much for the person as possible
    C. Talk very loudly to get the person's attention
    D. Touch the person before indicating the presence
68. Which nursing measure would be included in the care plan for a resident with dementia?
    A. Encourage resident to select seasonal appropriate clothes
    B. Show the resident the calendar for social activities
    C. Ask the resident which belongings should sent home
    D. Give the resident step-by-step instructions for dressing
69. Which information would the nursing assistant need to get from the nurse and the care plan for a person who needs amputee rehabilitation?
    A. Type of dietary restrictions
    B. Type of communication device
    C. Type of prosthetic device
    D. Type of incontinence training
70. Which nursing measure would the nursing assistant use while bathing a person?
    A. Keep the windows open for good ventilation
    B. Wash the dirtiest areas first; then change gloves
    C. Encourage the person to help as much as possible
    D. Rub the skin dry with several dry paper towels

71. Which assumption does the health-care team make in the care of a person who is dying?
    A. Hearing is retained.
    B. Swallowing is impossible.
    C. Vision is retained.
    D. Movement causes discomfort.
72. What action does the nursing assistant perform when a patient is on intake and output?
    A. Measure only liquids such as water and juice
    B. Measure ice cream and gelatin as part of intake
    C. Measure intravenous (IV) fluids
    D. Measure tube feedings
73. What is the priority action when a person who has been on bed rest needs to get up and start walk around again?
    A. Help the person to get up and encourage walking
    B. Have the person dangle before getting out of bed
    C. Have the person sit in a chair for at least 10 minutes
    D. Help the person to do range-of-motion exercises
74. Which aspect of the nursing assistant's personal grooming and attire can help to prevent skin tears when working with elderly patients?
    A. Wearing soft clothing and long sleeves
    B. Keeping fingernails short and smooth
    C. Wearing arm and leg protectors
    D. Keeping skin well moisturized
75. Which circumstance is an example of maintaining a resident's privacy?
    A. Giving information to staff who are directly involved in the care of the resident
    B. Discussing the resident's care with another nursing assistant in the lunch room
    C. Opening the resident's mail because she will not remember to open it herself
    D. Keeping the door open while assisting a resident with toileting to reduce odors
76. How often should the nursing assistant check on the person who is on a bedpan?
    A. Every 5 minutes
    B. Every 10 minutes
    C. After 30 minutes
    D. Wait until person calls
77. Which activity is included in the care plan for a person who is on bed rest?
    A. May be allowed to perform some activities of daily living (ADLs)
    B. Can use the bedside commode for elimination needs
    C. Will remain in bed and needs help with all ADLs
    D. Can use the bathroom for elimination needs
78. What would the nursing assistant do to identify person who is being admitted?
    A. Ask the person to state full name
    B. Check the admission form and identification bracelet
    C. Call the admitting office and ask about the identity of the person
    D. Ask the charge nurse to identify the person
79. Which body system brings oxygen (O_2) into the lungs and removes carbon dioxide (CO_2)?
    A. Renal system
    B. Circulatory system
    C. Nervous system
    D. Respiratory system
80. Which behavior is associated with sudden onset of a "gallbladder attack"?
    A. Smoking a cigarette
    B. Lifting heavy objects at work
    C. Eating a heavy evening meal
    D. Straining during bowel movements

Practice Examination 2

This test contains 77 questions. For each question, circle the BEST answer.

1. In which circumstance would the nursing assistant refuse to do a delegated task?
   A. Too busy with other tasks
   B. Not familiar with the task
   C. Task is not in job description
   D. It is the end of the shift
2. Which nursing measure would the nursing assistant use when Mr. Smith does not want lifesaving measures?
   A. Explain to Mr. Smith why he should have lifesaving measures
   B. Respect his decision and support his right to self-determination
   C. Ask the family to speak with him and change his mind
   D. Tell the spiritual advisor about Mr. Smith's decision
3. What is occurring when the nursing assistant hears a nurse shouting at a resident?
   A. Battery
   B. Malpractice
   C. Verbal abuse
   D. Neglect
4. Which nursing measure would the nursing assistant use when caring for a patient who speaks a different language?
   A. Speak loudly and clearly to the patient
   B. Change patient assignments
   C. Use words the patient seems to understand
   D. Speak quickly and pantomime actions
5. What would the home health nursing assistant do on observing that the elderly patient is living with a daughter who is a hoarder?
   A. Help the daughter clear pathways to exit the house
   B. Check the environment for unsafe sources of heat
   C. Report situation to the nurse and follow nurse's instructions
   D. Suggest that the daughter take the elderly patient to a safer place
6. Which action would the nursing assistant take to prevent equipment accidents?
   A. Use two-pronged plugs on all electrical devices
   B. Follow the manufacturer's instructions
   C. Place a barrier around spills and wipe up later
   D. Use old equipment if new equipment is unfamiliar
7. Which action is part of the safety check that the nursing assistant would perform after visitors leave?
   A. Make sure that the call light is within reach
   B. Straighten the bed linens and empty the trash cans
   C. Show interest in how the visit went
   D. Check to see if visitors had any problems
8. When does the nursing assistant need to wash the hands?
   A. After documenting a procedure
   B. After removing gloves
   C. After talking with a person
   D. After taking a lunch break
9. Which action would the nursing assistant use to move a person weighing 250 lbs. (113.4 kg) in bed?
   A. Do the procedure alone and ask the person to help
   B. Keep the door open in case help is needed
   C. Roll the person back and forth while shifting weight
   D. Ask for assistance from at least two other staff members
10. Which action would the nursing assistant use when transferring a person from a bed to a wheelchair?
    A. Lock the wheels on the bed and wheelchair before transfer
    B. Pull on the front of the transfer belt as the person stands up
    C. Have the person put their arms around your neck
    D. Have the person sit and dangle while getting the wheelchair
11. Which action would the nursing assistant use when making a bed?
    A. Keep the bed in the low position
    B. Wear gloves when removing linens
    C. Raise the head of the bed
    D. Raise the foot of the bed
12. Which nursing measure would the nursing assistant use to give perineal care to a male?
    A. Use a circular motion and work toward the meatus
    B. Use a circular motion and start at the meatus and work outward
    C. Clean the shaft first using long firm upward strokes
    D. Clean the scrotum first using a circular motion
13. Which information would the nursing assistant get from the nurse before changing the gown of a person with an intravenous (IV) infusion?
    A. If the person has an IV pump
    B. Can the tubing be disconnected
    C. What type of IV solution is infusing
    D. If IV infusion can be turned off for gown change
14. What would the nursing assistant do with the drainage bag when a person has an indwelling catheter?
    A. Place the drainage bag on the floor
    B. Hang the drainage bag on the bedside stand
    C. Hang the drainage bag on a bed rail
    D. Hang the drainage bag from the bed frame

15. Which nutritional benefit comes from including protein in the a diet?
    A. Increases tissue repair and growth
    B. Provides energy and fiber
    C. Adds flavor to food
    D. Allows nerve conduction
16. What is an expected behavior for older persons related to their fluid needs?
    A. Have an increased sense of thirst
    B. Need less water than younger persons
    C. May not feel thirsty
    D. Usually ask for water if they need it
17. What would the nursing assistant do when a person is nil per os (NPO)?
    A. Post a sign in the bathroom
    B. Keep the water pitcher filled at the bedside
    C. Remove the water pitcher and glass from the room
    D. Provide oral hygiene once a day
18. How much intake would the nursing assistant record when a person drank 3 oz of milk at lunch?
    A. 30 mL
    B. 60 mL
    C. 90 mL
    D. 120 mL
19. What would the nursing assistant do when feeding a person?
    A. Offer fluids at the end of the meal
    B. Use a fork and a knife
    C. Sit silently while the person talks
    D. Allow time to chew and swallow
20. In planning care, which person is likely to require the most assistance with range-of-motion (ROM) exercises?
    A. Person A is in a coma and needs passive ROM
    B. Person B is self-care, but needs reminders to do active ROM
    C. Person C has some weakness in the arm and needs active-assistive ROM
    D. Person D needs active ROM for legs and active-assistive ROM for the left arm
21. Which instruction about assistive devices would the nursing assistant give to a person who has a weak left leg?
    A. Hold the cane in the left hand
    B. Hold the cane in the right hand
    C. Use two canes; one in each hand
    D. Use a walker
22. Which nursing measure would the nursing assistant use to promote comfort and relieve pain?
    A. Help the person get out of bed when changing the linens
    B. Place pillows to support the body in good alignment
    C. Talk, make jokes, and distract the person from the pain
    D. Wait 10 minutes after pain medication is given before giving care
23. What would the nursing assistant do when a person is receiving oxygen through a nasal cannula?
    A. Turn the oxygen higher when the person is short of breath
    B. Fill the humidifier when it is not bubbling
    C. Check behind the ears and under the nose for signs of irritation
    D. Remove the cannula when the person goes to the dining room
24. What would the nursing assistant do when a glass thermometer accidentally breaks?
    A. Tell the nurse at once
    B. Get a broom and sweep it up
    C. Put the glass in the sharps container
    D. Call the infection control nurse
25. What would the nursing assistant do when taking a person's pulse?
    A. Locate the brachial pulse
    B. Take the pulse for 30 seconds if it is irregular
    C. Tell the nurse if the pulse is less than 60
    D. Place the thumb on the pulse
26. What would the nursing assistant do when counting respirations on a person?
    A. Make friendly conversation with the person to show interest
    B. Count for 1 minute if an abnormal breathing pattern is noted
    C. Report a rate of 16 to the nurse at once
    D. Check breaths with a stethoscope if an abnormal pattern is noted
27. Which action would the nursing assistant take when an older patient has a blood pressure (BP) of 158/96 mm Hg?
    A. Report the BP to the nurse at once
    B. Finish taking BP on all assigned patients
    C. Tell the patient to relax and recheck the BP in 20 minutes
    D. Look at the record to see if the BP is normal for that patient
28. For which patient would the nursing assistant take a rectal temperature?
    A. Patient A has diarrhea.
    B. Patient B is confused.
    C. Patient C is an infant.
    D. Patient D is agitated.
29. Which nursing measure would the nursing assistant use when a person is being admitted to the nursing center?
    A. Check belongings for dangerous items
    B. Defer all questions to the nurse
    C. Speak respectfully in a calm welcoming voice
    D. Leave the person alone, for privacy
30. What would the nursing assistant do when taking a person's height and weight?
    A. Have the person completely undress
    B. Have the person void before being weighed
    C. Weigh the person after a bath or shower
    D. Balance the scale after every usage

31. Which nursing measure to prevent pressure injuries would be included in the care plan for a person who is bedfast?
   A. Reposition the person at least every 3 hours
   B. Gently massage reddened areas and bony prominences
   C. Perform range-of-motion on legs every 2 hours
   D. Keep the skin free of moisture from urine, stools, or perspiration
32. Which communication method would the nursing assistant use for a person who has a hearing problem?
   A. Invite the person to large social gatherings
   B. Chat about own personal interests
   C. Face the person when speaking
   D. Speak very loudly and give details
33. Which nursing measure would the nursing assistant use when caring for a person who is blind or visually impaired?
   A. Position equipment for the staff's convenience
   B. Keep the lights off; the person cannot see
   C. Explain the location of food and beverages
   D. Rearrange furniture to minimize clutter
34. Which nursing assistant is safeguarding right to privacy in caring for a person with dementia?
   A. Nursing assistant A reads the person's mail for him
   B. Nursing assistant B tells the family about the person's condition
   C. Nursing assistant C protects the person's confidential information
   D. Nursing assistant D exposes the person's body to expedite care
35. Which nursing assistant is using an appropriate care measure for a person who is confused?
   A. Nursing assistant A uses terms of endearment to increase trust
   B. Nursing assistant B explains actions only if the person shows interest
   C. Nursing assistant C gives simple, clear directions and answers to questions
   D. Nursing assistant D removes clocks and calendars to decrease distractions
36. Which safety measure would be included in the care plan for a person with Alzheimer disorder who likes to wander?
   A. Keep the person in their own room
   B. Restrain the person in a chair
   C. Follow the person around the facility
   D. Allow person to wander in a safe space
37. What is the general goal of restorative nursing programs?
   A. Return the person to independent life at home
   B. Promote independence in performing self-care measures
   C. Assist the physician to repair the person's disability
   D. Help the person admit to limitations and restrictions
38. Which nursing measure would the nursing assistant use when caring for a person with a disability?
   A. Sympathize with limitations and show kindness by taking over care
   B. Tell the person that progress is faster, when cooperating
   C. Remind about progress made in the rehabilitation program
   D. Support denial of the disability if it helps the person to cope
39. Which action violates the person's rights after death?
   A. Draping and screening the body during postmortem care
   B. Collecting, bagging, and labeling personal possessions
   C. Discussing the family's reactions with other staff members
   D. Allowing the family to view the body in a private area
40. Which action would the nursing assistant perform first on entering a person's room and finding a fire in the wastebasket?
   A. Remove the person from the room
   B. Close the door and open the window
   C. Call for help and put out the fire
   D. Activate the fire alarm and evacuate
41. What has occurred when a person is left lying in urine and a pressure injury develops?
   A. Fraud
   B. Neglect
   C. Assault
   D. Battery
42. Which action would the nursing assistant take when a nurse says to assess a small foot wound, clean it, place a topical medication and a sterile dressing on the wound?
   A. Agree to do the task if the nurse will show how to do it
   B. Ask another nursing assistant to help with the task
   C. Politely say that the task is not included in the nursing assistant's training
   D. Do the task, but afterward, report the nurse to the director of nursing
43. What is the nursing assistant's first action on observing that a person's urine is foul-smelling and dark amber?
   A. Measure the urine
   B. Ask the person about fluid intake
   C. Tell the nurse
   D. Record the observation
44. How would the nursing assistant respond when a daughter asks for some water for her mother?
   A. "I am not caring for your mom. I will get her nursing assistant for you."
   B. "I do not have time right now, but if you can wait 30 minutes, I'll get it."
   C. "She might be on a special diet or fluid restrictions that I don't know about."
   D. "Of course but first let me make sure she is not on fluid restrictions."

45. Which restraint alternative would be a good choice for a person with dementia who has wandering behavior?
    A. Take vital signs and give reassurance every 15 minutes
    B. Lock the person in his bedroom and turn on the television
    C. Alert staff and others about person's wandering behavior
    D. Tell the person to use the call bell whenever he begins to wander
46. Which action would the nursing assistant use to place a person in the supine position?
    A. Elevate the head of the bed 45 degrees
    B. Elevate the foot of the bed 15 degrees
    C. Place the person on the back with the bed flat
    D. Place the person on the abdomen
47. What is the most important action to prevent or avoid spreading infection?
    A. Washing the hands
    B. Covering nose when coughing
    C. Using disposable gloves
    D. Wearing a mask
48. Which action would the nursing assistant take when a coworker begins to gossip about a person?
    A. Join the conversation and talk about the person
    B. Remove self from the group
    C. Try to say something nice about the person
    D. Change the subject or talk about someone else
49. What would the nursing assistant do to move a person up in bed?
    A. Raise the head of the bed
    B. Ask the person to remain still
    C. Apply a transfer belt
    D. Ask a coworker for help
50. What is expected when a person is on a sodium-controlled diet?
    A. Canned vegetables are omitted from the diet
    B. Small amounts of salt are added to food at the table
    C. Expensive salt products are less harmful
    D. Small servings of ham, sausage, or bacon are served
51. Which nursing assistant is performing a correct nursing measure for a patient who needs elastic stockings?
    A. Nursing assistant A helps patient to put on the stocking after breakfast
    B. Nursing assistant B ensures that the stockings are smooth and wrinkle free
    C. Nursing assistant C tells the patient that the stockings prevent pneumonia
    D. Nursing assistant D helps patient to put on the stockings before bedtime
52. Which action would the nursing assistant take when the person begins to fall while ambulating in the hallway?
    A. Call for help and ask for a wheelchair
    B. Grab the gait belt; hold on to prevent a fall
    C. Bring person close to self; ease to the floor
    D. Quickly move items that could cause injury
53. Which care measure would the nursing assistant use before assisting a person to bathe?
    A. Help person to go to the toilet
    B. Partially undress the person
    C. Raise the head of the bed
    D. Instruct person to brush the teeth
54. What is the correct depth of insertion when taking a rectal temperature on an adult with an electronic thermometer?
    A. ½ inch
    B. 1½ inches
    C. 2 inches
    D. 2½ inches
55. Which care measure would be included in the care plan for a child who has spina bifida; type myelomeningocele?
    A. Frequently check child for bowel or bladder incontinence
    B. Feed the child small spoonfuls of food and give extra time for swallowing
    C. Repeat instructions several times using the same phrasing
    D. Same caregiver should be assigned to give care as much as possible
56. Which nursing assistant is appropriately sharing information about a person's care and condition?
    A. Nursing assistant A reports to other staff who are caring for the person
    B. Nursing assistant B gives information to the person's only daughter
    C. Nursing assistant C shares some information with a close friend
    D. Nursing assistant D tells other nursing assistants about care issues
57. Which action would the nursing assistant take when a person has pain on urination?
    A. Tell the nurse
    B. Ask the person to describe the pain
    C. Ask the person how often it happens
    D. Obtain a midstream urine specimen
58. Which action should the nursing assistant take when caring for the newborn and the cord stump still attached?
    A. Very gently pull the stump off
    B. Apply the diaper below the umbilicus
    C. Give the baby a tub bath to soak the stump
    D. Cover the cord with a dry sterile dressing
59. Which nursing assistant is performing a correct action to maintain a sterile field?
    A. Nursing assistant A talks without donning a mask
    B. Nursing assistant B keeps the sterile field within sight
    C. Nursing assistant C places saline bottle on sterile field
    D. Nursing assistant D reaches across sterile field to assist the doctor

60. What would the nursing assistant do when an older person who is normally alert seems disoriented and confused?
   A. Try to stimulate the person with activities
   B. Ignore the confusion; this condition is common
   C. Check to see if the person is confused later in the day
   D. Report specific behavioral changes to the nurse
61. Which action would the nursing assistant take first when a person says he feels faint during his morning walk?
   A. Help the person to sit down
   B. Call for the nurse
   C. Obtain a wheelchair
   D. Encourage slow deep breaths
62. Which nursing measure would be included in the care plan to encourage fluids for a person?
   A. Offer fluids frequently
   B. Measure fluid before offering
   C. Withhold food and have the person drink fluids first
   D. Give coffee, soda, beer, or whatever the person wants
63. Which nursing assistant is failing to effectively communicate?
   A. Nursing assistant A uses words the other person understands.
   B. Nursing assistant B always talks about herself and her own issues.
   C. Nursing assistant C lets others express their feelings and concerns.
   D. Nursing assistant D listens while a person talks about an uncomfortable topic.
64. What is the pulse deficit when the apical rate is 90 beats per minute and the radial rate is 86 beats per minute?
   A. Pulse deficit is 0
   B. Pulse deficit is 4
   C. Pulse deficit is 86
   D. Pulse deficit is 90
65. Which child's behavior should be reported to the supervising nurse because of possible developmental delay?
   A. A 6-month old rolls from front to back and reaches for toys
   B. A 9-month old is afraid of strangers and clings to familiar adults
   C. An 18-month old stands up alone, but is not taking steps
   D. A 3-year old can string large beads and joins other children to play
66. Which nursing assistant needs a reminder about measuring blood pressure?
   A. Nursing assistant A applies the cuff to a bare upper arm
   B. Nursing assistant B encourages 20 minutes of rest before the procedure
   C. Nursing assistant C locates the brachial artery
   D. Nursing assistant D uses the arm with an IV infusion
67. Which nursing assistant has performed the correct action on finding clean linens on the floor in a person's room?
   A. Nursing assistant A uses the linens to make the bed
   B. Nursing assistant B return the linens to the linen cart
   C. Nursing assistant C put the linens in the laundry
   D. Nursing assistant D reports the incident to the nurse
68. Which care measure would the nursing assistant use when doing mouth care on an unconscious person?
   A. Use a large amount of fluid to rinse secretions
   B. Position the person on the side
   C. Entertain the person by talking about current events
   D. Insert the dentures when done
69. Which action would the nursing assistant use when brushing or combing a person's hair?
   A. Cut matted or tangled hair
   B. Encourage self-care as much as possible
   C. Style the hair so it looks nice
   D. Perform the task weekly
70. Which nursing measure would the nursing assistant use when providing nail and foot care?
   A. Cut fingernails with scissors
   B. Trim toenails for all assigned persons
   C. Carefully clip ingrown toenails
   D. Check between the toes for cracks and sores
71. What would the nursing assistant do when an indwelling catheter becomes disconnected from the drainage system?
   A. Quickly reconnect the tubing to the catheter
   B. Tell the nurse at once
   C. Get a new drainage system
   D. Flush the catheter with antiseptic solution
72. Which action would the nursing assistant perform at the end of the shift to complete duties related to a urinary drainage bag?
   A. Discard the bag
   B. Wash and store the bag
   C. Clean and rinse the bag and reattach
   D. Empty and measure urine in the bag
73. Which action would the nursing assistant use when a person needs a condom catheter applied?
   A. Use a soft rubber band to secure the catheter
   B. Apply adhesive tape to secure the catheter
   C. Wrap elastic tape to secure the catheter
   D. Apply catheter adhesive cream to secure the catheter
74. What would the nursing assistant do to increase comfort and to facilitate the urge to have a bowel movement?
   A. Have the person use the commode for privacy
   B. Talk to and distract the visitors while the person is on the toilet
   C. Keep the door slightly ajar and partially draw the privacy curtain
   D. Leave the person alone if possible

75. Where would the nursing assistant place the wheelchair when transferring a person with a weak left side from the wheelchair to the bed?
   A. On the left side of the bed with the person facing the foot of the bed
   B. On the right side of the bed with the person facing the head of the bed
   C. At the bottom of the bed with the person facing the head of the bed
   D. At the top of the bed with the person facing the foot of the bed
76. Which position would be the best an elderly person to assume if the doctor wants to perform a rectal examination?
   A. Knee-chest position
   B. Lithotomy position
   C. Side-lying position
   D. Horizontal recumbent position
77. Which patient comment would the nursing assistant immediately report to the nurse as a symptom of myocardial infarction?
   A. Heaviness in the left side of the chest
   B. Cough that is productive of mucus
   C. Swelling in the feet, ankles, and legs
   D. Painless swelling in the lymph nodes in the neck

Skills Evaluation Review

Each state has its own policies and procedures for the skills test. The following information is an overview of what to expect.

- To pass the skills evaluation, you typically will need to perform five of all the skills available.
- To pass the skills evaluation, you must perform skills correctly. Some states require all five to be performed correctly; others require four of five.
- Be prepared to perform at least one measurement skill, such as blood pressure, radial pulse, respirations, urine output or weight; performance includes recording and documentation.
- A nurse aide evaluator evaluates your performance of certain skills. Having someone watch as you work is not a new experience. Your instructor evaluated your performance during your training program. While you are working, your supervisor evaluates your skills.
- Mannequins and people are used as "patients" or "residents," depending on the skills you are performing. Speak to the person as you would a patient or resident.
- If you make a mistake, tell the evaluator what you did wrong. Then perform the skill correctly. Do not panic.
- Take whatever equipment you normally take to or use at work. Wear a watch with a second hand. You may need it to measure vital signs and check how much time you have left.

Before and During the Procedure

- Handwashing is evaluated at the beginning of the skills test. You are expected to know when to wash your hands. Therefore you may not be told to do so. Follow the rules for hand hygiene during the test.
- Before entering a person's room, knock on the door. Greet the person by name and introduce yourself before beginning a procedure. Check the identification (ID) or the photo ID to make certain you are giving care to the right person.
- Explain what you are going to do before beginning the procedure and as needed throughout the procedure.
- Always follow the rules of medical asepsis. For example, remove gloves and dispose of them properly. Keep clean linens separated from used linens.
- Always protect the person's rights throughout the skills test.
- Communicate with the person as you give care. Focus on the person's needs and interests. Always treat the person with respect. Do not talk about yourself or your personal problems.
- Provide privacy. This involves pulling the privacy curtain around the bed, closing doors, and asking visitors to leave the room.
- Promote safety for the person. For example, lock the wheelchair when you transfer a person to and from it. Place the bed in the lowest horizontal position when the person must get out of bed or when you are done giving care.
- Make sure the call light is within the person's reach. Attaching it to the bed or bed rail does not mean the person can reach it.
- Use good body mechanics. Raise the bed and over-bed table to a good working height.
- Provide for comfort.
  - o Make sure the person and linens are clean and dry. The person may have become incontinent during the procedure.
  - o Change or straighten bed linens as needed.
  - o Position the person for comfort and in good alignment.
  - o Provide pillows as directed by the nurse and the care plan.
  - o Raise the head of the bed as the person prefers and allowed by the nurse and the care plan.
  - o Provide for warmth. The person may need an extra blanket, a lap blanket, a sweater, socks, and so on.
  - o Adjust lighting to meet the person's needs.
  - o Make sure eyeglasses, hearing aids, and other devices are in place as needed.
  - o Ask the person if they are comfortable.
  - o Ask the person if there is anything else you can do.
  - o Make sure the person is covered for warmth and privacy.

Skills

Ask your instructor to tell you which of the following skills are tested in your state. Place a checkmark in the box in front of each tested skill so it will be easy for you to reference. The skills marked with an asterisk (*) are used with permission from the National Council of State Boards of Nursing. These skills are offered as a study guide to you. The word "client" refers to the resident or person receiving care. You are responsible for following the most current standards, practices, and guidelines in your state.

The steps in boldface type are critical element steps. Critical element steps must be done correctly to pass the skill. If you miss a critical element step, you will not pass the skills evaluation. For example, you are to transfer a client from the bed to a wheelchair. You will fail if you do not lock the wheels on the wheelchair before transferring the person. An automatic failure is one that could potentially cause harm to a person. Your state may mark critical element steps in another way—underline or italics. If your state has one, review the candidate's handbook.

*Reproduced and used with permission from the *Nurse Assistant Candidate Handbook* from the National Council of State Boards of Nursing (NCSBN), Chicago, Illinois, © 2019.

❑**Hand Hygiene (Handwashing) (see Chapter 17)*

1. Addresses client by name and introduces self to client by name
2. Turns on water at sink
3. Wets hands and wrists thoroughly
4. Applies soap to hands
5. **Lathers all surfaces of wrists, hands, and fingers, producing friction for at least 20 seconds keeping hands lower than the elbows and the fingertips down**
6. Cleans fingernails by rubbing fingertips against palms of the opposite hand
7. **Rinses all surfaces of wrists, hands, and fingers, keeping hands lower than the elbows and the fingertips down**
8. Uses clean, dry paper towel/towels to dry all surfaces of fingers, hands, wrists, starting at the fingertips, and then disposes of paper towel/towels into waste container
9. Uses clean, dry paper towel/towels to turn off faucet and then disposes of paper towel/towels into waste container or uses knee/foot control to turn off faucet
10. Does not touch inside of sink at any time

❑**Applies One Knee-High Elastic Stocking (see Chapter 40)*

1. Explains procedure, speaking clearly, slowly, and directly, maintaining face-to-face contact whenever possible
2. Privacy is provided with a curtain, screen, or door
3. Client is in the supine position (lying down in bed) while stocking is applied
4. Turns stocking inside-out, at least to heel
5. Places foot of stocking over toes, foot, and heel
6. Pulls top of stocking over foot, heel, and leg
7. Moves foot and leg gently and naturally, avoiding force and overextension of limb and joints
8. **Finishes procedure with no twists or wrinkles and heel of stocking, if present, is over heel and opening in toe area (if present) is either under or over toe area; if using mannequin, candidate may state stocking needs to be wrinkle-free**
9. Signaling device is within reach, and bed is in low position
10. After completing skill, washes hands

❑**Assists to Ambulate Using a Transfer Belt (see Chapter 15 and 35)*

1. Explains procedure, speaking clearly, slowly, and directly, maintaining face-to-face contact whenever possible
2. Privacy is provided with a curtain, screen, or door
3. **Before assisting to stand, client is wearing nonskid shoes/footwear**
4. Before assisting to stand, bed is at a safe level
5. Before assisting to stand, checks and/or locks bed wheels
6. **Before assisting to stand, client is assisted to sitting position with feet flat on the floor**
7. Before assisting to stand, applies transfer belt securely at the waist over clothing/gown
8. Before assisting to stand, provides instructions to enable client to assist in standing including prearranged signal to alert client to begin standing
9. Stands facing client positioning self to ensure safety of candidate and client during transfer. Counts to three (or says other prearranged signal) to alert client to begin standing
10. On signal, gradually assists client to stand by grasping transfer belt on both sides with an upward grasp (candidate's hands are in upward position), and maintaining stability of client's legs by standing knee to knee, or toe to toe with client
11. Walks slightly behind and to one side of client for a distance of 10 feet, while holding onto the belt
12. Assists client to bed and removes transfer belt
13. Signaling device is within reach, and bed is in low position
14. After completing skill, washes hands

❑**Assists With Use of Bedpan (see Chapter 27)*

1. Explains procedure speaking clearly, slowly, and directly, maintaining face-to-face contact whenever possible
2. Privacy is provided with a curtain, screen, or door
3. Before placing bedpan, lowers head of bed
4. Puts on clean gloves before placing bedpan under client
5. Places bedpan correctly under client's buttocks
6. Removes and disposes of gloves (without contaminating self) into waste container and washes hands
7. After positioning client on bedpan and removing gloves, raises head of bed
8. Toilet tissue is within reach
9. Hand wipe is within reach, and client is instructed to clean hands with hand wipe when finished
10. Signaling device within reach and client is asked to signal when finished
11. Puts on clean gloves before removing bedpan
12. Head of bed is lowered before bedpan is removed
13. Ensures client is covered except when placing and removing bedpan
14. Empties and rinses bedpan and pours rinse into toilet

15. Places bedpan in designated dirty supply area
16. Removes and disposes of gloves (without contaminating self) into waste container and washes hands
17. Signaling device is within reach, and bed is in low position

❑*Cleans Upper or Lower Denture (see Chapter 23)

1. Puts on clean gloves before handling dentures
2. Bottom of sink is lined and/or sink is partially filled with water before denture is held over sink
3. Rinses denture in moderate temperature running water before brushing them
4. Applies denture toothpaste to toothbrush
5. Brushes all surfaces of denture
6. Rinses all surfaces of denture under moderate temperature running water
7. Rinses denture cup and lid
8. Places denture in denture cup with moderate temperature water solution and places lid on cup
9. Rinses toothbrush and places in designated toothbrush basin/container
10. Maintains clean technique with placement of toothbrush and denture
11. Sink liner is removed and disposed of appropriately and/or sink is drained
12. Removes and disposes of gloves (without contaminating self) into waste container and washes hands

❑*Counts and Records Radial Pulse (see Chapter 34)**

1. Explains procedure, speaking clearly, slowly, and directly, maintaining face-to-face contact whenever possible
2. Places fingertips on thumb side of client's wrist to locate radial pulse
3. Counts beats for 1 full minute
4. Signaling device is within reach
5. Before recording, washes hands
6. **Records pulse rate within plus or minus 4 beats of evaluator's reading**

❑*Counts and Records Respirations (see Chapter 34)†

1. Explains procedure (for testing purposes), speaking clearly, slowly, and directly, maintaining face-to-face contact whenever possible
2. Counts respirations for 1 full minute
3. Signaling device is within reach
4. Washes hands
5. **Records respiration rate within plus or minus 2 breaths of evaluator's reading**

❑*Dresses Client With Affected (Weak) Right Arm (see Chapter 26)

1. Explains procedure, speaking clearly, slowly, and directly, maintaining face-to-face contact whenever possible
2. Privacy is provided with a curtain, screen, or door
3. Asks which shirt the client would like to wear and dresses in shirt of choice
4. Avoids overexposure of client by ensuring client's chest is covered
5. Removes gown from the left (unaffected) side first and then removes gown from the right (affected/weak) side
6. Before dressing client, disposes of gown into soiled linen container
7. **Assists to put the right (affected/weak) arm through the right sleeve of the shirt before placing garment on the left (unaffected) arm**
8. While putting on shirt, moves body gently and naturally, avoiding force and overextension of limbs and joints
9. Finishes with clothing in place
10. Signaling device is within reach, and bed is in low position
11. After completing skill, washes hands

❑*Feeds Client Who Cannot Feed Self (see Chapter 31)

1. Explains procedure to client, speaking clearly, slowly, and directly, maintaining face-to-face contact whenever possible
2. Before feeding, looks at name card on tray and asks client to state name
3. **Before feeding client, client is in an upright sitting position (75–90 degrees)**
4. Places tray where the food can be easily seen by client
5. Cleans client's hands before beginning feeding
6. Sits facing client during feeding
7. Tells client what foods and beverages are on tray
8. Asks client what they would like to eat first
9. Using spoon, offers client one bite of each type of food on tray, telling client the content of each spoonful

**Count for 1 full minute.

†Count for 1 full minute. For testing purposes, you may explain to the client that you will be counting the respirations.

10. Offers beverage at least once during meal
11. Asks client if they are ready for next bite of food or sip of beverage
12. At end of meal, cleans client's mouth and hands
13. Removes food tray
14. Leaves client in the upright sitting position (75–90 degrees) with signaling device within client's reach
15. After completing skill, washes hands

❑**Gives Modified Bed Bath (Face and One Arm, Hand, and Underarm) (see Chapter 24)*

1. Explains procedure, speaking clearly, slowly, and directly, maintaining face-to-face contact whenever possible
2. Privacy is provided with a curtain, screen, or door
3. Removes gown and places directly in soiled linen container while ensuring client's chest and lower body are covered
4. Before washing, checks water temperature for safety and comfort and asks client to verify comfort of water
5. Puts on clean gloves before washing client
6. **Beginning with eyes, washes eyes with wet washcloth (no soap), using a different area of the washcloth for each stroke, washing inner aspect to outer aspect, then proceeds to wash face**
7. Dries face with dry cloth towel/washcloth
8. Exposes one arm and places cloth towel underneath arm
9. Applies soap to wet washcloth
10. Washes fingers (including fingernails), hand, arm, and underarm keeping rest of body covered
11. Rinses and dries fingers, hand, arm, and underarm
12. Moves body gently and naturally, avoiding force and overextension of limbs and joints
13. Puts clean gown on client
14. Empties, rinses, and dries basin
15. Places basin in designated dirty supply area
16. Disposes of linen into soiled linen container
17. Avoids contact between own clothing and used linens
18. Removes and disposes of gloves (without contaminating self) into waste container and washes hands
19. Signaling device is within reach, and bed is in low position

Makes an Occupied Bed (Client Does Not Need Assistance to Turn) (see Chapter 22)

1. Explains procedure, speaking clearly, slowly, and directly, maintaining face-to-face contact whenever possible
2. Privacy is provided with a curtain, screen, or door
3. Lowers head of bed before moving client
4. Client is covered while linens are changed
5. Loosens top linen from the end of the bed
6. Raises side rail on side to which client will move and client moves toward raised side rail
7. Loosens bottom used linen on working side and fanfolds bottom used linen toward center of bed
8. Fanfolds and places clean bottom linen or fitted bottom sheet on working side and tucks linen folds under client
9. Before going to other side, client rolls back onto clean bottom linen
10. Raises side rail then goes to other side of bed
11. Removes used bottom linen
12. Pulls and tucks in clean bottom linen, finishing with bottom sheet free of wrinkles
13. Client is covered with clean top sheet and bath blanket/used top sheet has been removed
14. Changes pillowcase
15. Linen is centered and tucked at foot of bed
16. Avoids contact between own clothing and used linens
17. Disposes of used linens into soiled linen container and avoids putting linens on floor
18. Signaling device is within reach, and bed is in low position
19. Washes hands

❑**Measures and Records Blood Pressure (see Chapter 34)*

1. Explains procedure, speaking clearly, slowly, and directly, maintaining face-to-face contact whenever possible
2. Before using stethoscope, wipes bell/diaphragm and earpieces of stethoscope with alcohol
3. Client's arm is positioned with palm up, and upper arm is exposed
4. Feels for brachial artery on inner aspect of arm, at bend of elbow
5. Places blood pressure cuff snugly on client's upper arm with sensor/arrow over brachial artery site
6. Earpieces of stethoscope are in ears, and bell/diaphragm is over brachial artery site
7. Inflates cuff between 160 and 180 mm Hg. If beat heard immediately upon cuff deflation, completely deflate cuff. Reinflate cuff to no more than 200 mm Hg.
8. Deflates cuff slowly and notes the first sound (systolic reading), and last sound (diastolic reading) (If rounding needed, measurements are rounded UP to the nearest 2 mm Hg)
9. Removes cuff

10. Signaling device is within reach
11. Before recording, washes hands
12. **After obtaining reading using BP cuff and stethoscope, records both systolic and diastolic pressures each within plus or minus 8 mm Hg of evaluator's reading**

❑**Measures and Records Urinary Output (see Chapter 32)*

1. Puts on clean gloves before handling bedpan
2. Pours the contents of the bedpan into measuring container without spilling or splashing urine outside of container
3. Rinses bedpan and pours rinse into toilet
4. Measures the amount of urine at eye level with container on flat surface (if between measurement lines, round up to nearest 25 mL/cc)
5. After measuring urine, empties contents of measuring container into toilet
6. Rinses measuring container and pours rinse water into toilet
7. Before recording output, removes and disposes of gloves (without contaminating self) into waste container and washes hands
8. **Records contents of container within plus or minus 25 mL/cc of evaluator's reading**

❑**Measures and Records Weight of Ambulatory Client (see Chapter 37)*

1. Explains procedure, speaking clearly, slowly, and directly, maintaining face-to-face contact whenever possible
2. Client has nonskid shoes/footwear on before walking to scale
3. Before client steps on scale, sets scale to zero
4. Ask client to step on center of scale and obtains client's weight
5. Asks client to step off scale
6. Before recording, washes hands
7. **Records weight based on indicator on scale. Weight is within plus or minus 2 lb of evaluator's reading. (If weight recorded in kg, weight is within plus or minus 0.9 kg of evaluator's reading.)**

❑**Positions on Side (see Chapter 20)*

1. Explains procedure, speaking clearly, slowly, and directly, maintaining face-to-face contact whenever possible
2. Privacy is provided with a curtain, screen, or door
3. Before turning, lowers head of bed
4. Raises side rail on side to which body will be turned
5. Assists client to slowly roll onto side toward raised side rail
6. Places or adjusts pillow under head for support
7. Repositions arm and shoulder so that client is not lying on arm
8. Supports top arm with supportive device
9. Places supportive device behind client's back
10. Places supportive device between legs with top knee flexed; knee and ankle supported
11. Makes sure the client's face, nose, and mouth are not obstructed (blocked) by a pillow or other device
12. Signaling device is within reach, and bed is in low position
13. After completing skill, washes hands

❑**Provides Catheter Care for Female (see Chapter 28)*

1. Explains procedure, speaking clearly, slowly, and directly, maintaining face-to-face contact whenever possible
2. Privacy is provided with a curtain, screen, or door
3. Before washing checks water temperature for safety and comfort and asks client to verify comfort of water
4. Puts on clean gloves before washing
5. Places linen protector under perineal area including buttocks before washing
6. Exposes area surrounding catheter (only exposing client between hip and knee)
7. Applies soap to wet washcloth
8. **While holding catheter at meatus without tugging, cleans at least 4 inches of catheter from meatus, moving in only one direction, away from meatus, using a clean area of the cloth for each stroke**
9. **While holding catheter at meatus without tugging, using a clean washcloth, rinses at least 4 inches of catheter from meatus, moving only in one direction, away from meatus, using a clean area of the washcloth for each stroke**
10. While holding catheter at meatus without tugging, dries at least 4 inches of catheter moving away from meatus using a dry cloth towel/washcloth
11. Empties, rinses, and dries basin
12. Places basin in designated dirty supply area
13. Disposes of used linen into soiled linen container and disposes of linen protector appropriately
14. Avoids contact between own clothing and used linen
15. Removes and disposes of gloves (without contaminating self) into waste container and washes hands
16. Signaling device is within reach, and bed is in low position

Provides Fingernail Care on One Hand (see Chapter 25)

1. Explains procedure, speaking clearly, slowly, and directly, maintaining face-to-face contact whenever possible
2. Before immersing fingernails, checks water temperature for safety and comfort and asks client to verify comfort of water
3. Basin is in a comfortable position for client
4. Puts on clean gloves before cleaning fingernails
5. Fingernails are immersed in basin of water
6. Cleans under each fingernail with orangewood stick
7. Wipes orangewood stick on towel after each nail
8. Dries fingernail area
9. Feels each nail and files as needed
10. Disposes of orangewood stick and emery board into waste container (for testing purposes)
11. Empties, rinses, and dries basin
12. After rinsing basin, places basin in designated used supply area
13. Disposes of used linens into used linens container
14. Removes and disposes of gloves (without contaminating self) into waste container and washes hands
15. Signaling device is within reach

❑**Provides Foot Care on One Foot (see Chapter 25)*

1. Explains procedure, speaking clearly, slowly, and directly, maintaining face-to-face contact whenever possible
2. Privacy is provided with a curtain, screen, or door
3. Before washing, checks water temperature for safety and comfort and asks client to verify comfort of water
4. Basin is in a comfortable position for client and on protective barrier
5. Puts on clean gloves before washing foot
6. Client's bare foot is placed into the water
7. Applies soap to wet washcloth
8. Lifts foot from water and washes foot (including between the toes)
9. Foot is rinsed (including between the toes)
10. Dries foot (including between the toes) with dry cloth towel/washcloth
11. Applies lotion to top and bottom of foot (excluding between the toes) removing excess with a towel/washcloth
12. Supports foot and ankle during procedure
13. Empties, rinses, and dries basin
14. Places basin in designated dirty supply area
15. Disposes of used linen into soiled linen container
16. Removes and disposes of gloves (without contaminating self) into waste container and washes hands
17. Signaling device is within reach

❑**Provides Mouth Care (see Chapter 23)*

1. Explains procedure, speaking clearly, slowly, and directly, maintaining face-to-face contact whenever possible
2. Privacy is provided with a curtain, screen, or door
3. Before providing mouth care, client is in the upright sitting position (75–90 degrees)
4. Puts on clean gloves before cleaning mouth
5. Places cloth towel across chest before providing mouth care
6. Secures cup of water and moistens toothbrush
7. Before cleaning mouth applies toothpaste to moistened toothbrush
8. **Cleans mouth (including tongue and all surfaces of teeth) using gentle motions**
9. Maintains clean technique with placement of toothbrush
10. Holds emesis basin to chin while client rinses mouth
11. Wipes mouth and removes clothing protector
12. Disposes of used linen into soiled linen container
13. Rinses toothbrush and empties, rinses, and dries basin
14. Removes and disposes of gloves (without contaminating self) into waste container and washes hands
15. Signaling device is within reach, and bed is in low position

❑**Provides Perineal Care (Peri-Care) for Female (see Chapter 24)*

1. Explains procedure, speaking clearly, slowly, and directly, maintaining face-to-face contact whenever possible
2. Privacy is provided with a curtain, screen, or door
3. Before washing checks water temperature for safety and comfort and asks client to verify comfort of water
4. Puts on clean gloves before washing perineal area
5. Places pad/linen protector under perineal area, including buttocks, before washing
6. Exposes perineal area (only exposing between hips and knees)
7. Applies soap to wet washcloth
8. **Washes genital area, moving from front to back, while using a clean area of the washcloth for each stroke**

9. **Using clean washcloth, rinses soap from genital area, moving from front to back, while using a clean area of the washcloth for each stroke**
10. Dries genital area moving from front to back with dry cloth towel/washcloth
11. After washing genital area, turns to side, then washes rectal area moving from front to back using a clean area of washcloth for each stroke.
12. Using clean washcloth, rinses soap from rectal area, moving from front to back, while using a clean area of washcloth for each stroke
13. Dries rectal area moving from front to back with dry cloth towel/washcloth
14. Repositions client
15. Empties, rinses, and dries basin
16. Places basin in designated dirty supply area
17. Disposes of used linen into soiled linen container and disposes of linen protector appropriately
18. Avoids contact between own clothing and used linen
19. Removes and disposes of gloves (without contaminating self) into waste container and washes hands
20. Signaling device is within reach, and bed is in low position

❑**Transfers From Bed to Wheelchair Using Transfer Belt (see Chapter 21)*

1. Explains procedure, speaking clearly, slowly, and directly, maintaining face-to-face contact whenever possible
2. Privacy is provided with a curtain, screen, or door
3. Before assisting to stand, wheelchair is positioned along the side of bed, at head of bed, facing the foot, or foot of bed facing head
4. Before assisting to stand, footrests are folded up or removed
5. **Before assisting to stand, locks wheels on wheelchair**
6. Before assisting to stand, bed is at a safe level
7. Before assisting to stand, checks and/or locks bed wheels
8. **Before assisting to stand, client is assisted to a sitting position with feet flat on the floor**
9. Before assisting to stand, client is wearing shoes
10. Before assisting to stand, applies transfer belt securely at the waist over clothing/gown
11. Before assisting to stand, provides instructions to enable client to assist in transfer including prearranged signal to alert when to begin standing
12. Stands facing client, positioning self to ensure safety of self and client during transfer. Counts to three (or says other prearranged signal) to alert client to begin standing
13. On signal, gradually assists client to stand by grasping transfer belt on both sides with an upward grasp (hands are in upward position) and maintaining stability of client's legs by standing knee to knee, or toe to toe with the client
14. Assists client to turn to stand in front of wheelchair with back of client's legs against wheelchair
15. Lowers client into wheelchair
16. Positions client with hips touching back of wheelchair, and transfer belt is removed
17. Positions feet on footrests
18. Signaling device is within reach
19. After completing skill, washes hands

❑**Performs Modified Passive Range of Motion (PROM) for One Knee and One Ankle (see Chapter 35)*

1. Explains procedure, speaking clearly, slowly, and directly, maintaining face-to-face contact whenever possible
2. Privacy is provided with a curtain, screen, or door
3. Ensures that client is supine in bed and instructs client to report if pain is experienced during exercise
4. **While supporting the leg at knee and ankle, bends the knee then returns leg to client's normal position (extension/flexion) (AT LEAST 3 TIMES unless pain is verbalized). Moves joints gently, slowly, and smoothly through the range of motion, discontinuing exercise if client verbalizes pain**
5. **While supporting the foot and ankle close to the bed, pushes/pulls foot toward head (dorsiflexion), and pushes/pulls foot down, toes point down (plantar flexion) (AT LEAST 3 TIMES unless pain is verbalized). Moves joints gently, slowly, and smoothly through the range of motion, discontinuing exercise if client verbalizes pain**
6. Signaling device is within reach, and bed is in low position
7. After completing skill, washes hands

❑**Performs Modified Passive Range of Motion (PROM) for One Shoulder (see Chapter 35)*

1. Explains procedure, speaking clearly, slowly, and directly, maintaining face-to-face contact whenever possible
2. Privacy is provided with a curtain, screen, or door
3. Instructs client to report if pain is experienced during exercise
4. **While supporting arm at the elbow and at the wrist, raises client's straightened arm from side position upward toward head to ear level and returns arm down to side of body (flexion/extension) (AT LEAST 3 TIMES unless pain is verbalized). Moves joint**

gently, slowly, and smoothly through the range of motion, discontinuing exercise if client verbalizes pain

5. **While supporting arm at the elbow and at the wrist, moves client's straightened arm away from the side of body to shoulder level and returns to side of body (abduction/adduction) (AT LEAST 3 TIMES unless pain is verbalized). Moves joint gently, slowly, and smoothly through the range of motion, discontinuing exercise if client verbalizes pain**
6. Signaling device is within reach, and bed is in low position
7. After completing skill, washes hands

❑*Performs Passive Range of Motion of Lower Extremity (Hip, Knee, Ankle) (see Chapter 35)*

1. Washes hands before contact with client
2. Identifies self to client by name and addresses client by name
3. Explains procedure to client, speaking clearly, slowly, and directly, maintaining face-to-face contact whenever possible
4. Provides for client's privacy during procedure with curtain, screen, or door
5. Positions client in supine and in good body alignment
6. Supports client's leg by placing one hand under knee and other hand under heel
7. Moves entire leg away from body (performs AT LEAST 3 TIMES unless pain occurs)
8. Moves entire leg toward body (performs AT LEAST 3 TIMES unless pain occurs)
9. Bends client's knee and hip toward client's trunk (performs AT LEAST 3 TIMES unless pain occurs)
10. Straightens knee and hip (performs AT LEAST 3 TIMES unless pain occurs)
11. Flexes and extends ankle through range-of-motion exercises (performs AT LEAST 3 TIMES unless pain occurs)
12. Rotates ankle through range-of-motion exercises (performs AT LEAST 3 TIMES unless pain occurs)
13. **While supporting limb, moves joints gently, slowly, and smoothly through range of motion to point of resistance, discontinuing exercise if pain occurs**
14. Provides for comfort
15. Before leaving client, places signaling device within client's reach
16. Washes hands

❑*Performs Passive Range of Motion of Upper Extremity (Shoulder, Elbow, Wrist, Finger) (see Chapter 35)*

1. Washes hands before contact with client
2. Identifies self to client by name and addresses client by name
3. Explains procedure to client, speaking clearly, slowly, and directly, maintaining face-to-face contact whenever possible
4. Provides for client's privacy during procedure with curtain, screen, or door
5. Supports client's extremity above and below joints while performing range of motion
6. Raises client's straightened arm toward ceiling and back toward head of bed and returns to flat position (flexion/extension) (performs AT LEAST 3 TIMES unless pain occurs)
7. Moves client's straightened arm away from client's side of body toward head of bed, and returns client's straightened arm to midline of client's body (abduction/adduction) (performs AT LEAST 3 TIMES unless pain occurs)
8. Moves client's shoulder through rotation range-of-motion exercises (performs AT LEAST 3 TIMES unless pain occurs)
9. Flexes and extends elbow through range-of-motion exercises (performs AT LEAST 3 TIMES unless pain occurs)
10. Provides range-of-motion exercises to wrist (performs AT LEAST 3 TIMES unless pain occurs)
11. Moves finger and thumb joints through range-of-motion exercises (performs AT LEAST 3 TIMES unless pain occurs)
12. **While supporting body part, moves joint gently, slowly, and smoothly through range of motion to point of resistance, discontinuing exercise if pain occurs**
13. Before leaving client, places signaling device within client's reach
14. Washes hands

❑*Makes an Unoccupied (Closed) Bed (see Chapter 22)*

1. Washes hands
2. Collects clean linens
3. Places clean linens on a clean surface
4. Raises the bed for good body mechanics
5. Puts on gloves
6. Removes linens without contaminating uniform. Rolls each piece away from self
7. Discards linens into laundry bag
8. Moves the mattress to the head of the bed
9. Applies mattress pad
10. Applies bottom sheet, keeping it smooth and free of wrinkles
11. Places the top sheet and bedspread on the bed, keeping them smooth and free of wrinkles
12. Tucks in top linens at the foot of the bed. Makes mitered corners

13. Applies clean pillowcase with zippers and/or tags to inside of pillowcase
14. Lowers the bed to its lowest position. Locks the bed wheels
15. Washes hands

❑**Donning and Removing Personal Protective Equipment (Gown and Gloves) (see Chapter 18)*

1. Picks up gown and unfolds
2. Facing the back opening of gown, places arms through each sleeve
3. Fastens the neck opening
4. Secures gown at waist making sure that back of clothing is covered by gown (as much as possible)
5. Puts on gloves
6. Cuffs of gloves overlap cuffs of gown
7. **Before removing gown, with one gloved hand, grasps the other glove at the palm, removes glove**
8. **Slips fingers from ungloved hand underneath cuff of remaining glove at wrist, and removes glove turning it inside-out as it is removed**
9. Disposes of gloves into designated waste container without contaminating self
10. After removing gloves, unfastens gown at neck and at waist
11. After removing gloves, removes gown without touching outside of gown
12. While removing gown, holds gown away from body, without touching the floor, turns gown inward and keeps it inside-out
13. Disposes of gown in designated container without contaminating self
14. After completing skill, washes hands

❑*Performs Abdominal Thrusts (see Chapter 14)*

1. Asks client if they are choking
2. Stands behind the client
3. Wraps arms around client's waist
4. Makes a fist with one hand
5. Places thumb side of fist against the client's abdomen
6. Positions fist in middle above navel and well below sternum (breastbone)
7. Grasps your fist with your other hand
8. Presses fist and other hand into abdomen with a quick upward thrust
9. Repeats thrusts until object is expelled or client becomes unresponsive

❑*Ambulation With Cane or Walker (see Chapter 35)*

1. Explains procedure to client, speaking clearly, slowly, and directly, maintaining face-to-face contact whenever possible
2. **Locks bed wheels or wheelchair brakes**
3. Assists client to a sitting position
4. **Before ambulating, puts on and properly fastens slip-resistant footwear**
5. Applies transfer (gait) belt (if directed by nurse or care plan)
6. Positions cane or walker correctly. Cane is on the client's strong side
7. Assists client to stand, using correct body mechanics
8. Stabilizes cane or walker and ensures that client stabilizes cane or walker
9. Stands behind and slightly to the side of client on the person's weak side; grasps transfer (gait) belt (if used)
10. Ambulates client at least 10 steps
11. Assists client to pivot and sit, using correct body mechanics
12. Before leaving client, remove transfer belt (if used); places signaling device within client's reach
13. Washes hands

❑*Fluid Intake (see Chapter 32)*

1. Observes dinner tray
2. Determines, in milliliters, the amount of fluid consumed from each container
3. Determines total fluid consumed in milliliters
4. Records total fluid consumed on intake and output (I&O) sheet
5. Calculated total is within required range of evaluator's reading

❑*Brushes or Combs Client's Hair (see Chapter 25)*

1. Explains procedure to client, speaking clearly, slowly, and directly, maintaining face-to-face contact whenever possible
2. Collects brush or comb and bath towel
3. Places towel across client's back and shoulders or across the pillow
4. Asks client how they wants the hair styled
5. Combs/brushes hair gently and completely
6. Leaves hair neatly brushed, combed, and/or styled
7. Removes towel
8. Removes hair from comb or brush
9. Before leaving client, places signaling device within client's reach
10. Washes hands

❑*Transfers a Client Using a Mechanical Lift (see Chapter 21)*

1. Assembles required equipment; performs safety check of slings, straps, hooks, and chains
2. Checks client's weight to ensure that it does not exceed the lift's capacity
3. Asks a coworker to help
4. Explains procedure to client, speaking clearly, slowly, and directly, maintaining face-to-face contact whenever possible
5. Provides for privacy during procedure with curtain, screen, or door
6. Locks the bed wheels
7. Raises the bed for proper body mechanics
8. Lowers the head of the bed to a level appropriate for the client
9. Stands on one side of the bed; coworker stands on the other side
10. Lowers the bed rails if up
11. Centers the sling under the client following the manufacturer's instructions
12. Ensures that the sling is smooth
13. Positions the client in semi-Fowler's position
14. Positions a chair to lower the client into it
15. Lowers the bed to its lowest position
16. Raises the lift to position it over the client
17. Positions the lift over the client
18. Attaches the sling to the sling hooks and checks fasteners for security
19. Crosses the client's arms over the chest
20. Raises the lift high enough until the client and sling are free of the bed
21. Instructs coworker to support the client's legs as candidate moves the lift and the client away from the bed
22. Positions the lift so the client's back is toward the chair
23. Slowly lowers the client into the chair
24. Places client in comfortable position, in correct body alignment
25. Lowers the sling hooks and unhooks the sling
26. Removes the sling from under the client unless otherwise indicated. Moves lift away from client
27. Puts footwear on the client
28. Covers the client's lap and legs with a lap blanket
29. Positions the chair as the client prefers
30. Places signaling device within client's reach
31. Washes hands

❑*Provides Mouth Care for an Unconscious Client (see Chapter 23)*

1. Explains procedure to client, speaking clearly, slowly, and directly, maintaining face-to-face contact whenever possible
2. Provides for privacy during procedure with curtain, screen, or door
3. Washes hands
4. Positions client on side with head turned well to one side
5. Puts on gloves
6. Places the towel under the client's face
7. Places the kidney basin under the chin
8. Uses swabs or toothbrush and toothpaste or other cleaning solution
9. Uses a bite block or plastic tongue depressor (if needed) to hold the person's mouth open
10. Cleans inside of mouth including the gums, tongue, and teeth
11. Cleans and dries face
12. Removes the towel and kidney basin
13. Applies lubricant to the lips
14. Positions client for comfort and safety
15. Removes and discards the gloves
16. Places signaling device within the client's reach
17. Washes hands

❑*Provides Drinking Water (see Chapter 32)*

1. Washes hands
2. Assembles equipment—ice, scoop, pitcher, cup, straw
3. Explains procedure to client, speaking clearly, slowly, and directly, maintaining face-to-face contact whenever possible
4. Uses the scoop to fill the pitcher with ice; does not let the scoop touch the rim or inside of the pitcher
5. Places scoop in appropriate receptacle after each use
6. Adds water to pitcher
7. Places the pitcher, disposable cup, and straw (if used) on the over-bed table, within the person's reach
8. Before leaving, places signaling device within client's reach
9. Washes hands

❑*Provides Perineal Care for Uncircumcised Male (see Chapter 24)*

1. Explains procedure to client, speaking clearly, slowly, and directly, maintaining face-to-face contact whenever possible
2. Provides for privacy during procedure with curtain, screen, or door

3. Washes hands
4. Fills basin with comfortably warm water
5. Puts on gloves
6. Elevates bed to working height
7. Places waterproof pad under buttocks
8. Gently grasps penis
9. Retracts the foreskin
10. Using a circular motion, cleans the tip by starting at the meatus of the urethra and working outward
11. Rinses the area with another washcloth
12. Returns the foreskin to its natural position
13. Cleans the shaft of the penis with firm, downward strokes and rinses the area
14. Cleans the scrotum
15. Pats dry the penis and the scrotum
16. Cleans the rectal area
17. Removes the waterproof pad
18. Lowers the bed
19. Removes and discards the gloves
20. Washes hands
21. Before leaving, places signaling device within client's reach

❑*Empties and Records Content of Urinary Drainage Bag (see Chapter 28)*

1. Explains procedure to client, speaking clearly, slowly, and directly, maintaining face-to-face contact whenever possible
2. Washes hands
3. Puts on gloves
4. Places a paper towel (or disposable waterproof pad) on the floor
5. Places the graduate on the paper towel (or disposable waterproof pad)
6. Places the graduate under the collection bag
7. Ensures that the bag is below the bladder, and the drainage tube is not kinked
8. Opens the clamp on the drain
9. Lets all urine drain into the graduate—does not let the drain touch the graduate
10. Closes clamp and positions drain in holder
11. Measures urine
12. Removes and discards the paper towel (or disposable waterproof pad).
13. Empties the contents of the graduate into the toilet and flushes
14. Rinses and dries the graduate with clean, dry paper towels
15. Returns the graduate to its proper place
16. Removes the gloves
17. Washes hands
18. Records the time and amount on the intake and output (I&O) record
19. Provides for client comfort
20. Places the signaling device within reach of client

❑*Applies a Vest Restraint (see Chapter 16)*

1. Obtains the correct type and size of restraint
2. Checks straps for tears or frays
3. Washes hands
4. Explains procedure to client, speaking clearly, slowly, and directly, maintaining face-to-face contact whenever possible
5. Provides for privacy during procedure with curtain, screen, or door
6. Makes sure the client is comfortable and in good alignment
7. Assists the client to a sitting position; as far back in wheelchair as possible with buttocks against chair back.
8. Applies the restraint following the manufacturer's instructions—the "V" part of the vest crosses in front
9. Makes sure the vest is free of wrinkles in the front and back
10. Brings the straps through the slots if vest crisscrosses.
11. Makes sure the client is comfortable and in good alignment
12. Secures the straps to the chair or to the movable part of the bed frame
13. Uses buckle or a quick release tie
14. Makes sure the vest is snug—slide an open hand between the restraint and the client
15. Places the signaling device within the client's reach
16. Washes hands

❑*Performs a Back Rub (Massage) (see Chapter 36)*

1. Washes hands
2. Explains procedure to client, speaking clearly, slowly, and directly, maintaining face-to-face contact whenever possible
3. Provides for privacy during procedure with curtain, screen, or door
4. Raises the bed for good body mechanics
5. Lowers the bed rail near self, if up
6. Positions the client in the prone or side-lying position
7. Exposes the back, shoulders, upper arms, and buttocks
8. Warms the lotion

9. Rubs entire back in upward, outward motion for approximately 2 to 3 minutes; does not massage reddened bony areas
10. Straightens and secures clothing or sleepwear
11. Returns client to comfortable and safe position
12. Places the signaling device within reach
13. Lowers the bed to its lowest position
14. Washes hands

❑*Positions a Foley (Indwelling) Catheter (see Chapter 28)*

1. Explains procedure to client, speaking clearly, slowly, and directly, maintaining face-to-face contact whenever possible
2. Washes hands
3. Puts on gloves
4. Secures catheter and drainage tubing according to facility procedure
5. Places tubing over leg
6. Positions drainage tubing so urine flows freely into drainage bag and has no kinks
7. Attaches bag to bed frame, below level of bladder
8. Washes hands

❑*Applies a Cold Pack or Warm Compress (see Chapter 43)*

1. Washes hands
2. Collects needed equipment
3. Explains procedure to client, speaking clearly, slowly, and directly, maintaining face-to-face contact whenever possible
4. Provides for privacy during procedure with curtain, screen, or door
5. Positions the client for the procedure
6. Covers cold pack or warm compress with towel or other protective cover
7. Properly places cold pack or warm compress on site
8. Checks the client for complications every 5 minutes
9. Checks the cold pack or warm compress every 5 minutes
10. Removes the application at the specified time—usually after 15 to 20 minutes
11. Provides for comfort
12. Places the signaling device within reach
13. Washes hands

❑*Positions for an Enema (see Chapter 29)*

1. Washes hands
2. Explains procedure to client, speaking clearly, slowly, and directly, maintaining face-to-face contact whenever possible
3. Provides for privacy
4. Positions the client in a left side-lying position
5. Covers client with a bath blanket
6. Provides for comfort
7. Places the signaling device within reach
8. Washes hands

❑*Positions Client for Meals (see Chapter 31)*

1. Washes hands
2. Explains procedure to client, speaking clearly, slowly, and directly, maintaining face-to-face contact whenever possible
3. If the person will eat in bed:
   a. Raises the head of the bed to a comfortable position—usually Fowler's or high-Fowler's position is preferred
   b. Removes items from the over-bed table and cleans the over-bed table
   c. Adjusts the over-bed table in front of the client
   d. Places the client in proper body alignment
4. If the client will sit in a chair:
   a. Positions the client in a chair or wheelchair
   b. Provides support for the client's feet
   c. Removes items from the over-bed table and cleans the table
   d. Adjusts the over-bed table in front of the client
   e. Places the client in proper body alignment
5. Places the signaling device within reach
6. Washes hands

❑*Takes and Records Axillary Temperature, Pulse, and Respirations (see Chapter 34)*

1. Washes hands before contact with client
2. Identifies self to client by name and addresses client by name
3. Explains procedure to client, speaking clearly, slowly, and directly, maintaining face-to-face contact whenever possible
4. Provides for client's privacy during procedure with curtain, screen, or door
5. Turns on digital oral thermometer
6. Dries axilla and places thermometer in the center of the axilla
7. Holds thermometer in place for appropriate length of time
8. Removes and reads thermometer
9. Records temperature on pad of paper
10. **Report abnormal temperature at once**
11. Discards sheath from thermometer
12. Places fingertips on thumb side of client's wrist to locate radial pulse
13. Counts beats for 1 full minute

14. Records pulse rate on pad of paper
15. **Report abnormal pulse at once**
16. Counts respirations for 1 full minute
17. Records respirations on pad of paper
18. **Report abnormal respirations at once**
19. Before leaving client, places signaling device within client's reach
20. Washes hands

❑*Transfers Client From Wheelchair to Bed (see Chapter 21)*

1. Washes hands before contact with client
2. Identifies self to client by name and addresses client by name
3. Explains procedure to client, speaking clearly, slowly, and directly, maintaining face-to-face contact whenever possible
4. Provides for client's privacy during procedure with curtain, screen, or door
5. Positions wheelchair close to bed with arm of wheelchair almost touching bed
6. Before transferring client, ensures that client is wearing nonskid footwear
7. Before transferring client, folds up footplates
8. Before transferring client, places bed at safe and appropriate level for client
9. **Before transferring client, locks wheels on wheelchair and locks bed brakes**
   a. *With transfer (gait) belt*: Stands in front of client, positioning self to ensure safety of self and client during transfer (e.g., knees bent, feet apart, back straight), places belt around client's waist, and grasps belt. Tightens belt so that fingers can be slipped between transfer/gait belt and client
   b. *Without transfer belt*: Stands in front of client, positioning self to ensure safety of self and client during transfer (e.g., knees bent, feet apart, back straight, arms around client's torso under arms)
10. Provides instructions to enable client to assist in transfer, including prearranged signal to alert client to begin standing
11. Braces client's lower extremities to prevent slipping
12. Counts to three (or says other prearranged signal) to alert client to begin transfer
13. On signal, gradually assists client to stand
14. Assists client to pivot and sit on bed in manner that ensures safety
15. Removes transfer belt, if used
16. Assists client to remove nonskid footwear
17. Assists client to move to the center of bed
18. Provides for comfort and good body alignment
19. Before leaving client, places signaling device within client's reach
20. Washes hands

❑*Applies an Incontinence Brief (see Chapter 27)*

1. Washes hands before contact with client
2. Identifies self to client by name and addresses client by name
3. Explains procedure to client, speaking clearly, slowly, and directly, maintaining face-to-face contact whenever possible
4. Chooses correct brief and size per facility instructions
5. Provides privacy for the client
6. Elevates bed to comfortable working height
7. Puts on gloves
8. Places waterproof underpad under client, asking client to raise buttocks or turning the client to the side
9. Loosens tabs on each side of the product
10. Turns the client away from you
11. Removes the product from front to back, observes for urine amount (small, moderate, large) color, or blood; rolls the product up and places the product into trash bag
12. Opens the new brief, folding it in half, lengthwise along the center, and inserts it between the client's legs from front to back; unfolds and spreads the back panel
13. Turns the client onto their back, with the product under buttocks with top of absorbent pad aligned just above the buttocks crease
14. Grasps and stretches the leg portion of front panel to extend elastic for groin placement
15. Rolls ruffles away from groin
16. Snuggly places bottom tabs angled toward abdomen on both sides
17. Places top tabs on each side angled toward bottom tabs
18. Removes gloves
19. Washes hands
20. Covers client appropriately and provides for comfort
21. Places signaling device within reach

After the Procedure

After you demonstrate a skill, complete a safety check of the room.

- The person is wearing eyeglasses, hearing aids, and other devices as needed.
- The call light is plugged in and within reach.
- Bed rails are up or down according to the care plan.
- The bed is in the lowest horizontal position.
- The bed position is locked if needed.
- Manual bed cranks are in the down position.

- Bed wheels are locked.
- Assistive devices are within reach. Walker, cane, and wheelchair are examples.
- The over-bed table, filled water pitcher and cup, tissues, phone, TV controls, and other needed items are within reach.
- Unneeded equipment is unplugged or turned off.
- Harmful substances are stored properly. Lotion, mouthwash, shampoo, aftershave, and other personal care products are examples.

After the Test

- Celebrate—you have completed the competency evaluation! The length of time for you to get your test results varies with each state. In the meantime, try to relax. Continue your daily routine and be the best nursing assistant you can be.

Answers to Review Questions in Textbook Chapters Review

Chapter 1
1. a
2. b
3. c

Chapter 2
1. d
2. a
3. b
4. d

Chapter 3
1. d
2. a
3. b
4. a

Chapter 4
1. b
2. a
3. d

Chapter 5
1. c
2. a
3. b
4. a
5. a
6. a
7. a
8. b

Chapter 6
1. b
2. c
3. a
4. d
5. a
6. b

Chapter 7
1. b
2. d
3. d
4. d
5. b
6. a
7. a
8. c
9. c
10. d
11. c
12. c
13. b
14. b

Chapter 8
1. a
2. d
3. c
4. c
5. a

Chapter 9
1. b
2. c
3. b

Chapter 11
1. d
2. b
3. b

Chapter 12
1. a
2. d
3. a
4. c
5. d
6. c

Chapter 13
1. c
2. b
3. a
4. a
5. d
6. c
7. d

Chapter 14
1. b
2. d
3. c
4. b
5. c
6. c
7. b
8. a
9. a
10. b

Chapter 15
1. b
2. b
3. c
4. a
5. a
6. d

Chapter 16
1. d
2. c
3. b
4. a
5. b
6. c

Chapter 17
1. b
2. b
3. a
4. b
5. c

Chapter 18
1. c
2. d
3. a
4. c
5. b

Chapter 19
1. c
2. b
3. a
4. d

Chapter 20
1. d
2. a
3. b

Chapter 21
1. d
2. c
3. d

Chapter 22
1. b
2. d
3. a
4. b
5. c

Chapter 23
1. b
2. a
3. b
4. a

Chapter 24
1. a
2. b
3. d
4. d
5. b
6. c

Chapter 25
1. d
2. c
3. d
4. b
5. d
6. d
7. a
8. b
9. a
10. b

Chapter 26
1. d
2. a
3. c
4. d
5. c

Chapter 27
1. d
2. a
3. c
4. a
5. c

Chapter 28
1. d
2. a
3. c
4. a

Chapter 29
1. b
2. d
3. b
4. a

Chapter 30
1. a
2. d
3. d
4. a

Chapter 31
1. a
2. d
3. b

Chapter 32
1. b
2. a
3. c
4. c
5. b

Chapter 34
1. c
2. a
3. b
4. b

Chapter 35
1. c
2. a
3. c
4. a

Chapter 36
1. a
2. c
3. d
4. a
5. c

Chapter 37
1. c
2. a
3. a
4. b

Chapter 39
1. b
2. c
3. d
4. b

Chapter 40
1. b
2. d
3. d

Chapter 41
1. a
2. b
3. a

Chapter 42
1. b
2. c
3. b
4. c

Chapter 43
1. c
2. a

Chapter 44
1. b
2. b
3. a
4. b
5. a

Chapter 46
1. a
2. c
3. d
4. c
5. b

Chapter 47
1. d
2. c
3. b
4. c

Chapter 48
1. d
2. a
3. a
4. c

Chapter 49
1. b
2. a
3. c
4. b
5. d

Chapter 50
1. d
2. a
3. a
4. c

Chapter 51
1. c
2. c
3. a
4. b
5. d

Chapter 52
1. d
2. b
3. c

Chapter 53
1. a
2. b
3. b
4. d
5. b
6. c

Chapter 54
1. b
2. d
3. a
4. b

Chapter 58
1. b
2. a
3. a
4. c
5. c

Chapter 59
1. d
2. c
3. a
4. b
5. c
6. b

Answers to Practice Examination 1

1. **C** Nursing assistants do not give drugs, without additional medication assistant training and certification. Politely refusing to do a task that is outside the scope of nursing assistant practice is acceptable. The nurse must be informed that the request is being declined, not ignored. Page 26, Chapter 3.
2. **D** An ethical person does not judge others or cause harm to another person; harm must be immediately reported. Ethical behavior excludes personal prejudices or biases. Ethical behavior also includes giving care to persons whose standards and values are different. Page 41, Chapter 5.
3. **D** An ethical person is knowledgeable of what is right conduct and wrong conduct. Health-care workers do not drink alcohol before coming to work and do not drink alcohol while working. Page 41, Chapter 5.
4. **A** Negligence is an unintentional wrong and a failure to act in a reasonable and prudent manner that results in harm. Page 43, Chapter 5.
5. **B** The person's information is confidential. Information about the patient or resident is shared only among health team members involved in the care. Page 44, Chapter 5.
6. **D** End-of-shift is a time for good teamwork. Continue to do the job. Attitude is important. Page 96, Chapter 8.
7. **A** If data are not saved if can be lost. Logging off prevents someone else from using the computer under a secure personal password. The time should accurately reflect when the care was given. Using someone else's password or charting for a coworker are incorrect actions. Page 97, Chapter 8.
8. **B** Give a courteous greeting and identify location and self. Answer calls promptly ideally on the first ring. Take a message if someone is not available to come to the phone. Confidential information about a patient or employee is not given to any caller. Page 99, Chapter 8.
9. **C** Showing the person the nursing center is the best action. Health-care agencies are strange places with strange routines and equipment. People feel safer if they know what to expect. Reassuring and making vague statements or rushing care will not reduce the person's anxiety. Page 70, Chapter 7.
10. **B** When a person is angry or hostile, stay calm and professional. The person is usually not angry with the individual staff member. The person may be angry with the situation. Page 80, Chapter 7.
11. **D** Use words that are familiar to the person. Speak clearly, slowly, and distinctly. Also, ask one question at a time and wait for an answer. Page 75, Chapter 7.
12. **C** Conditions that involve the chest or abdomen should be discussed with the nurse before using the gait belt. Weakness of the arm, urinary problems, and history of stroke are not contraindications for use of a gait belt; however, always check with the nurse, as needed. Page 214, Chapter 15.
13. **D** Listening requires care and interest in the other person. Have good eye contact with the person. Focus on what the person is saying. Page 78, Chapter 7.
14. **C** Assume that a comatose person hears and understands. Talk to the person and explain actions and care measures. Page 74, Chapter 7.
15. **A** Protect a person's right to privacy when giving care. Politely ask visitors to leave the room. Do not expose the person's body in front of them. Show visitors where to wait. Page 81, Chapter 7.
16. **B** If a person wants to talk with a minister or spiritual leader, tell the nurse. It is not the nursing assistant's responsibility to act as a spiritual counselor. Page 71, Chapter 7.
17. **A** Observe the person with a restraint at least every 15 minutes (or as often as directed by the nurse or care plan). Remove the restraint and reposition the person every 2 hours. Checking the person at the end of the shift is not incorrect, but checks should be performed every 15 minutes throughout the shift. Restraints and the restrained body part should be in plain view. Page 223, Chapter 16.
18. **D** For persons who experience frequent nighttime urination, most fluids are given before 1700. Diapering, withholding fluid, and waking the person at night are incorrect measures. Consult the nurse and the care plan as needed. Page 150, Chapter 12.
19. **C** The nurse should be contacted as soon as possible to investigate the medication for possible error. People who are prescribed medications for chronic conditions are often familiar with the appearance and dosage of each pill. Page 859, Chapter 57.
20. **C** Push the chair forward when transporting the person. Do not pull the chair backward unless going through a doorway. If the person tries to help, hands or feet could be injured. Page 305, Chapter 21.
21. **A** Tell the nurse at once. It is important to do the correct procedure on the right person. The nursing assistant must be able to read the person's name on the ID bracelet or use the photo ID to identify the person. Page 178, Chapter 14.
22. **B** Clutching at the throat is the "universal sign of choking." Page 186, Chapter 14.
23. **D** When a person is on a diabetic diet, tell the nurse about changes in the person's eating habits. The person's meals and snacks need to be served on time. If the person is snacking between meals, tell the nurse. The nursing assistant cannot make the person eat, but amounts consumed should be reported. Page 476, Chapter 30.

24. **D** With mild airway obstruction, the person is conscious and can speak. Often forceful coughing can remove the object. Page 186, Chapter 14.
25. **A** Abdominal thrusts are used to relieve severe airway obstruction. Page 186, Chapter 14.
26. **B** Do not use faulty electrical equipment in nursing centers. Take the item to the nurse. Page 191, Chapter 14.
27. **C** If a warning label is removed or damaged, do not use the substance. Take the container to the nurse and explain the problem. Page 193, Chapter 14.
28. **C** An ethical person realizes that other people's values and standards may differ from one's own. Sharing concerns with the nurse is a good first step; the nurse can assist with values clarification. Page 41, Chapter 5.
29. **D** Politely remind the person to smoke in designated smoking areas. Page 197, Chapter 14.
30. **A** During a fire, remember the word *RACE* (rescue, alarm, confine, extinguish). Page 197, Chapter 14.
31. **C** If a person with Alzheimer disease has sundowning (increased restlessness and confusion as daylight ends), provide a calm, quiet setting late in the day. Do not try to reason with the person or ask the person to explain. Reason and communication are impaired, and these attempts may increase agitation. Complete treatments and activities early in the day. Page 813, Chapter 54.
32. **C** Mealtime provides opportunities for choking. Remember to cut food into small pieces and make sure that the person can chew and swallow the food served. Report loose teeth or dentures to the nurse. Page 204, Chapter 14.
33. **A** Lock both wheels before transferring a person to and from the wheelchair. Locking wheels can be considered a form of restraint; follow agency's policy. The person's feet are on the footplates before moving the chair. The footplates should be raised before transfer. Page 307, Chapter 21.
34. **B** The nurse needs to check him for injuries before he gets up; then the nurse will determine which method should be used to move the person. Page 218, Chapter 15.
35. **B** Death from strangulation is the most serious risk factor if the vest restraint has been put on backward. The other complications can be associated with restraint use, but are less directly related to the improper application of a vest restraint. Page 225, Chapter 16.
36. **C** Wash hands with soap and water before eating or helping others to eat. Page 241, Chapter 17.
37. **D** Gloves need to be changed when they become contaminated (contamination is not always visible) with blood, body fluids, secretions, and excretions. Page 252, Chapter 17.
38. **D** When washing hands, keep hands and forearms lower than elbows. Use warm water (not hot) and a mild soap (not a disinfectant) to protect the integrity of the skin. Use a clean dry paper towel to turn off the faucet. Do not shake or wave hands during the procedure. Page 243, Chapter 17.
39. **C** Bend knees and squat to lift a heavy object. Hold items close to the body when lifting a heavy object. For a wider base of support and more balance, stand with feet apart. Do not bend from the waist when lifting objects. Page 276, Chapter 19.
40. **C** The head of the bed is raised between 45 and 60 degrees for Fowler's position. Page 279, Chapter 19.
41. **D** Lay babies on their backs for sleep. Do not lay babies on their stomachs for sleep. This can interfere with chest expansion and breathing. The baby can suffocate. Page 831, Chapter 56.
42. **A** Have the person's back and buttocks against the back of the chair. Feet are flat on the floor or on the wheelchair footplates. The backs of the person's knees and calves are slightly away from the edge of the seat. Page 281, Chapter 19.
43. **B** Help the person out of bed on the strong side. In transferring, the strong side moves first. It pulls the weaker side along. Page 307, Chapter 21.
44. **A** When a person tries to bite, scratch, pinch, or kick, protect the person, others, and self from harm. Telling the nurse is the next action; the nurse may contact the doctor if restraints are needed. The nurse may recommend ignoring the behavior, but this would be used in conjunction with other behavioral management techniques. Page 80, Chapter 7.
45. **B** When the head of the bed is raised, skin on the buttocks stays in place and internal structures move forward as the person slides down in bed. This creates a shearing force. Page 286, Chapter 20.
46. **D** For comfort, adjust lighting to meet the person's changing needs. Nursing centers maintain a temperature range of 71°F to 81°F (21.6°C–27.2°C). Home bathrooms do not always have the safety features or assistive devices that older people need. Many older persons are sensitive to noise. Page 161, Chapter 13.
47. **A** Call lights are placed on the person's strong side and kept within the person's reach. The person's dominant side is usually stronger, but disease or injury can result in weakness. All call lights are answered promptly, but calls from the bathroom should be answered first if several lights are activated at the same time. Page 173, Chapter 13.
48. **C** The nursing assistant must have the person's permission to open or search closets or drawers. Page 173, Chapter 13.
49. **C** When handling linens, do not take unneeded linens to a person's room. Once in the room, extra linens are considered contaminated. The linen cart is kept in a central location so that all staff have access to it. To prevent the spread of microbes, never shake linens. Never put clean or used linens on the floor. Page 329, Chapter 22.
50. **A** Handheld fire extinguishers are used to fight small fires that have not spread. For personal safety and the safety of others, notify the fire department for large or spreading fires. Page 197, Chapter 14.

51. **B** Mouth care is given at least every 2 hours for an unconscious person. Wiping the teeth is insufficient. To prevent aspiration, position the person on the side with the head turned well to the side. Use a plastic tongue depressor to keep the person's mouth open. Wear gloves. Page 349, Chapter 23.
52. **B** A good attitude is needed at work. Be pleasant and respectful. Avoid making excuses or being defensive. Page 60, Chapter 6.
53. **B** During cleaning, firmly hold dentures over a sink half-filled with water and lined with a towel. This prevents them from falling onto a hard surface and breaking. Clean and store dentures in cool water. Hot water causes dentures to lose their shape. To prevent losing dentures, label the denture cup with the person's name. Page 351, Chapter 23.
54. **C** Report and record the location and description of the rash. Page 360, Chapter 24.
55. **C** Gently wipe the eye from the inner aspect to the outer aspect of the eye. Clean the far eye first. The eyelids (upper and lower) are cleansed with a clean damp washcloth. Page 363, Chapter 24.
56. **D** When giving a back massage, observe for and report bruises or skin damage. If skin is damaged, ask the nurse for instructions before starting the massage. Wear gloves if the person's skin has open areas. Warm the lotion before applying it to the person. Use firm strokes. Do not massage reddened bony areas. This can lead to more tissue damage. Page 569, Chapter 36.
57. **A** Separate the labia and clean downward from front to back. Wear gloves and use soap. Page 374, Chapter 24.
58. **C** Stay within hearing distance if the person can be left alone. Standing close to the person is sometimes necessary to maintain safety, but privacy is respected whenever possible. Cold water is turned on first, then hot water. Some people are able to adjust the water temperature, but it is safer if the cold water is turned on first and then adjusted by adding hot water. Page 369, Chapter 24.
59. **B** Electric razors are used when a person is on an anticoagulant. An anticoagulant prevents or slows down blood clotting. Bleeding occurs easily. A nick or cut from a safety razor can cause bleeding. Page 388, Chapter 25.
60. **B** Remove clothing from the strong (unaffected) side first. Page 398, Chapter 26.
61. **B** Pat answers ("Don't worry") are barriers to communication. Using preferred name and title is a sign of respect. Remaining silent when a person is upset and asking for clarification are good communication techniques. Page 79, Chapter 7.
62. **D** Measure and record the amount of urine in the drainage bag. The catheter is secured to the person's thigh or abdomen. Do not disconnect the catheter from the drainage tubing. The nurse may teach the person about positioning the tubing. Page 433, Chapter 28.
63. **B** Carbohydrates provide energy and fiber for bowel elimination. Page 470, Chapter 30.
64. **D** When taking a rectal temperature with an electronic thermometer, the thermometer is inserted ½ inch into the rectum. Privacy is provided by drawing the curtain, but the thermometer must be held in place. Side-lying position is preferred. Page 524, Chapter 34.
65. **A** It is the nursing assistant's responsibility to immediately report any systolic pressure below 90 mm Hg and any diastolic pressure below 60 mm Hg. Page 537, Chapter 34.
66. **D** Oral temperatures are not taken on unconscious persons, persons receiving oxygen, or persons who breathe through their mouth. Page 519, Chapter 34.
67. **A** To assist with walking, offer the person an arm and have the person walk a half step behind. When caring for a person who is blind or visually impaired, let the person do as much for self as possible. Use a normal voice tone. Do not shout at the person. Identify self when entering the room. Do not use touch until the person is aware that someone else is in the room. Page 721, Chapter 47.
68. **D** Step-by-step instructions help the resident to perform actions that are complex. A resident with confusion and dementia has the right to personal choice, but choices should be limited. Dementia is likely to cause difficulty with interpreting or remembering calendar events. The resident also has the right to keep and use personal items, but decision-making should be simplified. Page 812, Chapter 54.
69. **C** Persons requiring amputation rehabilitation will often (not always) need to learn how to use and adapt to a prosthetic (artificial) arm or leg. Special diets are used for many conditions, for example, those who have trouble swallowing may require a dysphagia diet. Communication devices, such as picture boards, are used to assist persons with speech disorders. Bowel and bladder programs are used for persons with various urinary disorders or spinal cord injuries. Page 704, Chapter 46.
70. **C** Encourage the person to help as much as possible. Doors and windows are closed to reduce drafts. Wash from the cleanest areas to the dirtiest areas. Pat the skin dry with a soft towel to avoid irritating or breaking the skin. Page 359, Chapter 24.
71. **A** When a person is dying, always assume that the person can hear. Reposition the person every 2 hours to promote comfort. Ability to swallow and see will vary. Skin care, personal hygiene, back massages, oral hygiene, and good body alignment promote comfort. Page 884, Chapter 59.
72. **B** Foods that melt at room temperature (ice cream, sherbet, custard, pudding, gelatin, and ice pops) are measured and recorded as intake. The nurse measures and records IV fluids and tube feedings. Page 495, Chapter 32.
73. **B** After bed rest, activity increases slowly and in steps. First the person dangles. Sitting in a chair follows.

Next the person walks in the room and then in the hallway. Page 297, Chapter 20.

74. **B** For personal grooming and attire, keep nails trimmed and smooth; this decreases the chances of tearing a person's fragile skin. The other options could be used to protect the nursing assistant's skin. Page 637, Chapter 41.

75. **A** Treat the resident with respect and ensure privacy. The resident has a right not to have private affairs exposed or made public without giving consent. Only staff involved in the resident's care should see, handle, or examine the resident's body. Page 15, Chapter 2.

76. **B** Check on the person every 5 minutes. Page 414, Chapter 27.

77. **A** When a person is on bed rest, they are allowed to do some ADLs, such as self-feeding, oral hygiene, bathing, shaving, and hair care. For strict or complete bed rest, everything is done for the person who must remain in bed. For bed rest with commode privileges, the commode is at the bedside. For bed rest with bathroom privileges, the bathroom is used for elimination. Page 547, Chapter 35.

78. **B** Identification is always done by using two identifiers. On admission, use the admission form and the ID bracelet. Asking the person to state full name is polite and correct, but some people are not able. If name is correctly stated a second identifier is still needed. Calling the admission office is incorrect. The nurse should be consulted if two identifiers are not available. Page 580, Chapter 37.

79. **D** The respiratory system brings oxygen (O_2) into the lungs and removes carbon dioxide (CO_2). The renal system removes waste products and maintains water, electrolyte, and acid-base balance. The circulatory system pumps blood to the body. The nervous system controls, directs, and coordinates body functions. Page 764, Chapter 50.

80. **A** "Gallbladder attack" or "gallstone attack" usually occurs in the evening or at night after having a heavy meal. Signs and symptoms include nausea, vomiting, and pain in the upper right abdomen, back, or right shoulder. Page 776, Chapter 51

Answers to Practice Examination 2

1. **C** You may politely refuse to do a task that is not in your job description. If you are not familiar with the task, you should ask for instruction and supervision. Page 37, Chapter 4.
2. **B** You may not agree with advance directives or resuscitation decisions. However, you must respect the person's wishes. In addition, it is not the nursing assistant's responsibility to have this discussion with the person, his family, or others. Page 45, Chapter 5, and Page 884, Chapter 59.
3. **C** Verbal abuse is using oral or written words or statements that speak badly of, sneer at, criticize, or condemn. Page 48, Chapter 5.
4. **C** Speak in a normal tone. Use words the patient seems to understand and speak slowly and distinctly. Asking for translation help is reasonable; changing assignments is not always possible and could be viewed as unethical. Page 75, Chapter 7.
5. **C** Report the situation to the nurse and follow the nurse's instructions. It is the nurse's responsibility to assess for dangers and talk to the daughter about solutions. Page 202, Chapter 14.
6. **B** Follow the manufacturer's instructions for equipment. Use three-pronged plugs on all electrical devices. Wipe up spills right away. Ask for training if you are unfamiliar with something. Page 192, Chapter 14.
7. **A** After the visitors leave, the purpose of the safety check is too ensure that nothing was moved, removed, or left behind. Unintentional alterations to the person's environment could cause harm. Page 160, Chapter 13.
8. **B** Perform hand hygiene after removing gloves. Page 243, Chapter 17.
9. **D** Sometimes multiple people or a mechanical lift are needed for moving and turning persons in bed. If the person weighs more than 200 lbs (90.8 kg), at least three staff members should help with the move. Page 290, Chapter 20.
10. **A** The wheels of the bed and wheelchair should be locked before attempting the transfer. When using a transfer belt, grasp the belt from underneath and pull upward as the person stands up. A person must not put their arms around your neck. The person can pull you forward or cause you to lose your balance. Equipment should be obtained before starting a procedure. Person may become dizzy while dangling and should not be left alone. Page 299, Chapter 21.
11. **B** Wear gloves when removing linens. Linens may contain blood, body fluids, secretions, or excretions. Raise the bed for good body mechanics. Put the bed flat, then place the clean linens. Page 329, Chapter 22.
12. **B** Use a circular motion, start at the meatus, and work outward. The shaft is cleaned after the tip of the penis using long firm downward strokes. The scrotum is cleaned with a clean washcloth. Page 376, Chapter 24.
13. **A** Before changing a gown on a person with an IV, you need this information from the nurse and the care plan. Which arm has the IV, if the person has an IV pump, which gown to use—IV therapy gown, standard gown. Page 406, Chapter 26.
14. **D** The drainage bag hangs from the bed frame. It must not touch the floor. The bag is always kept lower than the person's bladder. The drainage bag does not hang on the bed rail, because when the rail is moved it could place tension on the catheter or drainage tubing. Page 433, Chapter 28.
15. **A** Protein is needed for tissue repair and growth. Page 470, Chapter 30.
16. **C** Older persons may not feel thirsty (decreased sense of thirst). Frequently offer water. Page 494, Chapter 32.
17. **C** The water pitcher and glass are removed from the room. Nil per os (NPO) means that the person should not take food or fluids by mouth. An NPO sign is posted above the bed. Oral hygiene is performed frequently. Page 494, Chapter 32.
18. **C** 1 oz equals 30 mL. 3 oz equals 90 mL. Page 495, Chapter 32.
19. **D** Allow time to chew and swallow. Fluids are offered during the meal. A teaspoon, rather than a fork and knife, is used for feeding. Engage in normal conversation during the meal. Page 486, Chapter 31.
20. **A** A person in a coma cannot move, turn, or transfer and needs frequent passive range of motion (ROM). All motions must be done for the person. In active ROM, the person does the exercise. In active assisted the person does the exercise, but some requires help. Page 548, Chapter 35.
21. **B** A cane is held on the strong side of the body. If the left leg is weak, the cane is held in the right hand. Page 556, Chapter 35.
22. **B** Position the person in good alignment. Getting out of bed is generally encouraged, but for some people movement can disrupt comfort and increase pain. Consult the nurse when in doubt. Talk softly and gently; jokes could irritate or offend someone who is uncomfortable. Thirty minutes is usually the amount of time required for most oral pain medications to have effect. Page 569, Chapter 36.
23. **C** Check behind the ears and under the nose for signs of irritation. Notify the nurse if the person is short of breath, needs the oxygen removed (for any reason), or if the oxygen system is not working properly. Page 684, Chapter 44.

24. **A** Tell the nurse at once. Glass thermometers may contain mercury, which is a hazardous substance. Follow special procedures for handling hazardous materials. Page 522, Chapter 34.
25. **C** Record and report at once a pulse rate less than 60 or more than 100 beats per minute. The radial pulse is used for routine vital signs. If the pulse is irregular, count it for 1 minute. Do not use your thumb to take a pulse. Page 529, Chapter 34.
26. **B** Count the respirations for 1 minute if an abnormal breathing pattern is noted. People change their breathing patterns if they are conversing. A healthy adult has 12 to 20 respirations per minute. Listening for breath sounds with a stethoscope is the nurse's responsibility. Page 536, Chapter 34.
27. **A** Immediately report any systolic pressure above 120 mm Hg and any diastolic pressure above 80 mm Hg. Record the BP and the time that the nurse was notified. Page 537, Chapter 34.
28. **C** Rectal temperatures are taken on infants and young children. Rectal temperatures are not taken if a patient has diarrhea, is confused, or is agitated. Page 519, Chapter 34.
29. **C** Use tone of voice to convey a warm welcome. Answer any questions that relate to your scope of practice. If you are not able to answer the question, tell the person that you will get the nurse. It is the nurse's responsibility to check for dangerous items. Before leaving, make sure that the person is safe and comfortable. Page 576, Chapter 37.
30. **B** Have the person void before being weighed. A full bladder adds weight. Person should be clothed for privacy and dignity. Weigh the person at the same time of day, usually before breakfast. Balance the scale before weighing the person. Page 582, Chapter 37.
31. **D** Keep the skin free of moisture from urine, stools, or perspiration. Re-position the person at least every 2 hours. Do not massage reddened areas or bony prominences. ROM to the legs is important, but this does not address pressure in other areas (e.g., back of head, sacrum, shoulders). Page 659, Chapter 42.
32. **C** Face the person when speaking. Large social gatherings create background noise that can be difficult for people with hearing problems. Chatting about your personal interests is generally not appropriate. Speak in a normal voice tone and do not include excessive details. Speak clearly, distinctly, and slowly. Page 714, Chapter 47.
33. **C** Explain the location of food and beverages. Furniture and equipment should be positioned according to the person's preferences, rather than the staff's convenience. Provide lighting as the person prefers. Do not rearrange furniture and equipment. Page 721, Chapter 47.
34. **C** The person with confusion and dementia has the right to privacy and confidentiality. Information about the person's care and condition is shared only with those involved in providing the care. Protect the person from exposure. Page 819, Chapter 54.
35. **C** Use simple, clear language. Explain what you are going to do and why. Call the person by name every time you have contact. Terms of endearment (honey, sweetie) can be demeaning for some people. Keep calendars and clocks in the person's room. Page 805, Chapter 54.
36. **D** Wandering in a safe place allows exercise, which can reduce wandering. Do not keep the person in their room. Involve the person in activities. Following the person is impractical; all staff members should be alert for the person's whereabouts. Page 809, Chapter 54.
37. **B** Restorative nursing programs promote self-care measures. They help maintain the person's highest level of function; this could be at home or in a nursing care facility. Repair of the disability is not a realistic goal; however, the person can regain health, strength, and independence. The focus is on abilities and progress, not restrictions or limitations. Page 701, Chapter 46.
38. **C** Remind the person of the progress in the rehabilitation program. Focus on the person's abilities and strengths. Progress may be slow, regardless of motivation or hard work. Denial is a coping mechanism but helping the person to deny the disability is not part of the nursing assistant role. Page 705, Chapter 46.
39. **C** The final moments of death are kept confidential. So are family reactions. Draping the body, treating personal possessions with respect, and allowing the family to have privacy for viewing are part of the dying person's rights. Page 889, Chapter 59.
40. **A** Remember the word *RACE*. Your first action is to Rescue the person in immediate danger. Then sound the Alarm, Confine the fire, and Extinguish the fire. Page 197, Chapter 14.
41. **B** Neglect is defined as failure to provide a person with the goods or services needed to avoid physical harm or mental anguish. Page 47, Chapter 5.
42. **C** Nursing assistants cannot perform assessment or give medications. Some facilities and state practice acts will allow nursing assistants to perform some wound care if properly trained. Do not perform tasks that are not in your job description. Page 26, Chapter 3.
43. **C** Ask the nurse to observe urine that looks or smells abnormal. Then record your observation. Page 433, Chapter 28.
44. **D** A good attitude is needed at work. You are expected to be pleasant, respectful and willing to help. Page 60, Chapter 6.
45. **C** Staff, other departments, and others (visitors, volunteers, etc.) should be alerted to watch out for people who wander. Doors that open to the outside may also have alarms. Taking frequent vital signs is not necessary; locking the person in the room would be a violation of rights, and a person with dementia who wanders is unlikely to be able to use the call bell for monitoring purposes. Page 223, Chapter 16.

46. **C** The supine position is the back-lying position. For good alignment, the bed is flat and the head and shoulders are supported on a pillow. Place arms and hands at the sides. Page 280, Chapter 19.
47. **A** Handwashing is the most important way to prevent or avoid spreading infection. Page 242, Chapter 17.
48. **B** To gossip means to spread rumors or talk about the private matters of others. Gossiping is unprofessional and hurtful. If others are gossiping, you need to remove yourself from the group. Do not make or repeat any comment that can hurt another person. Page 61, Chapter 6.
49. **D** Ask a coworker to help you. The head of the bed is lowered. The person flexes both knees. Assistive devices may be used, but a transfer belt is not the right device for this task. Page 275, Chapter 19.
50. **A** On a sodium-controlled diet, high-sodium foods such as ham and canned vegetables are omitted. Salt is not added to food at the table. The use of salt should be limited, regardless of the type or cost. Page 475, Chapter 30.
51. **B** Elastic stockings should not have wrinkles or creases after being applied. Wrinkles and creases can cause skin breakdown. Apply stockings before the person gets out of bed. Apply the correct size. Purpose is to decrease risk for thrombus and embolus. Page 629, Chapter 40.
52. **C** When a person begins to fall, pull the person close to your body and ease to the floor. Also protect the person's head. Page 216, Chapter 15.
53. **A** Before bathing, allow the person to use the bathroom, bedpan, or urinal. Page 361, Chapter 24.
54. **A** For an adult, insert an electronic thermometer ½ inch into the rectum. Page 524, Chapter 34.
55. **A** Children with severe forms of spina bifida are at risk for bladder, bowel, and mobility problems. Myelomeningocele is the most severe type. Page 826, Chapter 55.
56. **A** A person's information is confidential. The information is shared only among health team members involved in the person's care. Page 61, Chapter 6.
57. **A** Report to the nurses and record complaints of urgency, burning, dysuria, or other urinary problems. Page 423, Chapter 27.
58. **B**. Diaper is applied below the umbilicus if the cord stump has not healed. Stump should be kept dry and is never pulled off. Page 843, Chapter 56.
59. **B** Sterile field must always be within sight. Activities that cause air currents (e.g., talking, sneezing, drafts) and reaching over the sterile field are considered sources of contamination. Unsterile objects, such as saline bottles, should not be placed on the field. Page 253, Chapter 17.
60. **D** Report any changes from normal or changes in the person's condition to the nurse at once. Then record your observations. Page 89, Chapter 8.
61. **A** If a person is standing (or walking), have the person sit before fainting occurs. Page 874, Chapter 58.
62. **A** The person drinks an increased amount of fluid. You would measure the fluids, but this action does not encourage fluids. Withholding food is punitive and violates the rights of the person. Consult the nurse and the care plan before offering fluids, such as beer, coffee, or soda. These fluids might be harmful to some people because of medical conditions or medications. Page 494, Chapter 32.
63. **B** Communication fails when you talk too much and fail to listen. Page 79, Chapter 7.
64. **B 90 apical beats per minute – 86 radial beats per minute = 4**. For the pulse deficit, subtract the radial rate from the apical rate. (The radial rate is never greater than the apical rate.) Page 532, Chapter 34.
65. **C** At 18 months, children can usually stand, walk alone, walk up steps and may run. At 12 months, children are walking by holding on to furniture and will attempt several without holding on. Page 136, Chapter 11.
66. **D** Blood pressure is not taken on an arm with an IV infusion. When taking a blood pressure, apply the cuff to the bare upper arm. Ten to 20 minutes of rest prior to the procedure is correct technique. The diaphragm of the stethoscope is placed over the brachial artery. Page 539, Chapter 34.
67. **C** Never put clean or used linens on the floor. The floor is dirty. You cannot use the linens. Page 329, Chapter 22.
68. **B** To prevent aspiration, position the unconscious person on their side when you do mouth care. Use a small amount of fluid to clean the mouth. Tell the person what you are doing. Dentures are not worn when the person is unconscious. Page 349, Chapter 23.
69. **B** Encourage people to do their own hair care. Do not cut matted or tangled hair. The person chooses his or her hairstyle. Brushing and combing are done with morning care and whenever needed. Page 382, Chapter 25.
70. **D** Check between the toes for cracks and sores. If left untreated, a serious infection could occur. Fingernails are cut with nail clippers, not scissors. Nursing assistants do not trim or cut toenails if a person has diabetes, poor circulation, takes anticoagulant medications or has thickened nails, ingrown toenails, or nail fungus. Page 393, Chapter 25.
71. **B** If an indwelling catheter becomes disconnected from the drainage system, you tell the nurse at once. Page 436, Chapter 28.
72. **D** Urinary drainage bags are emptied, and the contents measured at the end of each shift. Drainage bags must not touch the floor. The bag is always kept lower than the person's bladder. Drainage bags are discarded, but not at the end of each shift. They are never stored. Cleaning and rinsing leg bags may be

done (in the home setting), but the larger drainage bags are usually discarded and replaced. Page 433, Chapter 28.

73. **C** Use elastic tape to secure a condom catheter. Elastic tape expands when the penis changes size. Adhesive tape and rubber bands do not. There is no adhesive cream that is used to secure catheters. Page 443, Chapter 28.

74. **D** For comfort during bowel elimination, leave the person alone if possible. Provide for privacy. Maintaining privacy is a little more difficult to ensure if the person is using the commode. Page 452, Chapter 29.

75. **A** Help the person from the wheelchair to the bed on their strong side. In transferring, the strong side moves first. It pulls the weaker side along. Placing the wheelchair at the head or bottom of the bed increases the transfer distance from wheelchair to bed. Page 310, Chapter 21.

76. **C** The side-lying position is the choice for elderly patients if the examiner needs to do a rectal examination. For adults or children, the knee-chest (genupectoral) position would be the first choice if they are able to assume that position. Page 593, Chapter 38.

77. **A** Heaviness or discomfort in the left chest or in the center of the chest should be immediately reported as possible symptom of myocardial infarction. A productive cough signals respiratory disorders, such as pneumonia or chronic obstructive pulmonary disease. Swelling in the lower extremities can occur with chronic heart failure. Swelling in the lymph nodes must be investigated for possible lymphoma. Page 762, Chapter 50.